Delirium: Acute Confusional States

Delirium: Acute Confusional States

Zbigniew J. Lipowski, M.D., F.R.C.P.(C)
Professor of Psychiatry
University of Toronto

New York Oxford
OXFORD UNIVERSITY PRESS *1990*

Oxford University Press

Oxford New York Toronto
Delhi Bombay Calcutta Madras Karachi
Petaling Jaya Singapore Hong Kong Tokyo
Nairobi Dar es Salaam Cape Town
Melbourne Auckland

and associated companies in
Berlin Ibadan

Published by Oxford University Press, Inc.,
200 Madison Avenue, New York, New York 10016

Library of Congress Cataloging-in-Publication Data
Lipowski, Z. J. (Zbigniew Jerzy)
Delirium : acute confusional states / by Zbigniew J. Lipowski.
p. cm. Subtitle of previous work: Acute brain failure in man.
Includes bibliographical references.
ISBN 0-19-506150-0
1. Delirium. 2. Delirium—Etiology. I. Title.
RC520.7.L56 1990 616.8′4—dc20 89-36826 CIP

This book is a revision of DELIRIUM: Acute Brain Failure in Man by Zbigniew J. Lipowski, published by Charles C Thomas, Springfield, Illinois, copyright © 1980 by Charles C Thomas, Publisher.

9 8 7 6 5 4 3 2 1

Printed in the United States of America
on acid-free paper

Preface

The first version of this book was published under the title *Delirium: Acute Brain Failure in Man* (1) in 1980. The present version has been completely rewritten and brought up-to-date. While no major advances in the understanding of delirium have occurred in the past decade and the syndrome has continued to be neglected by researchers, progress in the neurosciences and in many other areas relevant to it necessitated a thorough revision of the original text. The title was changed because the term "acute brain failure" has been cogently criticized for being misleading. The brain as a whole does not fail in delirium; instead, its highest integrative functions, those subserving reception, processing, and retrieval of information, become disorganized, rendering a delirious person more or less incapable of thinking and acting in a rational, goal-directed manner.

Delirium, or "phrenitis," was one of the first mental disorders to be recognized by Western medical writers 2,500 years ago. Excellent clinical descriptions of it can be found as early as the second century A.D. The English-language medical literature contains numerous references to it as far back as the sixteenth century, yet oddly enough, apart from a treatise by Frings (2) that appeared in 1746, not a single book devoted solely to this syndrome had been published before the first version of this book appeared. As far as I could ascertain, it remains the only monograph in English on this subject today. Hopefully, it will stimulate research on delirium and help clinicians recognize and treat it.

Delirium is likely to be more common today than ever before. It is most often encountered in later life, and the aging of the population together with the growing prevalence of dementia—two factors associated with a high incidence of the syndrome—make it highly probable that delirium will be encountered with increasing frequency. It can be found on any given day in the medical or surgical wards or the emergency department of a general hospital. While common, it is often unrecognized by the medical staff, which can have deplorable consequences for the patient. The formulation in 1980 (3) of explicit diagnostic criteria for delirium should facilitate its diagnosis, as well as research on it. It is a curious paradox that a syndrome so common in clinical practice and of such great theoretical interest has been almost totally bypassed by researchers. Delirium poses intriguing questions for everyone interested in brain–behavior relationships, cognition, consciousness, attention, the sleep-wake cycle, perceptual disturbances, and organization of the mind. It illustrates dramatically how the functioning of the mind can become disrupted by a wide range of cerebral and systemic diseases and toxic agents affecting the neurochemical processes in the brain. Delirium is an experiment of nature that may be observed daily on any medical or surgical ward.

One and a half centuries ago, an English surgeon, Gallway (4, p 46), noted that "the subject of delirium is generally looked upon by the practical physician as one of the most obscure in the chain of morbid phenomena he has to deal with; whilst the frequency of its occurrence under various diseased conditions of the system renders the affection not a little familiar to his eye. My object in approaching so acknowledged a terra incognita is not, I regret to say, that I have any fresh contribution towards its elucidation to bring into the field, but rather to awaken a more lively inquiry amongst the profession as to its real nature and causes." This quotation provides an apt motto for the present book. Its purpose is just that: "to awaken a more lively inquiry."

I acknowledge with gratitude the receipt of a grant-in-aid from the Commonwealth Fund of New York, which has been most helpful in compiling the material for this book. I also wish to thank Drs. D. F. Benson and H. Merskey for their helpful comments and my secretary, Ms. Debbie Virtue, for patiently typing and correcting the rather long manuscript.

References

1. Lipowski Z. J.: *Delirium: Acute Brain Failure in Man.* Springfield, Ill, Charles C Thomas, 1980.
2. Frings P.: *A Treatise on Phrensy.* London, Gardner, 1746.
3. *Diagnostic and Statistical Manual of Mental Disorders,* ed 3. Washington, DC, American Psychiatric Association, 1980.
4. Gallway M. D.: Nature and treatment of delirium. *Lond. Med. Gaz.* 1838;1:46–49.

Toronto
May 1989

Z.J.L.

Contents

Part I

Delirium: an Organic Mental Syndrome

1

History

Etymology of "delirium"

The term "delirium" stems from the Latin word *delirare,* which literally means to go out of the furrow (*lira,* Latin for furrow) but whose vernacular meaning is to be deranged, crazy, out of one's wits (1). From this root was derived the now obsolete English verb "delire," meaning to go wrong, to go astray from reason, to rave, to wander in mind, to be delirious or mad (1). "Delirium" has been used in English in two senses: first, to refer to a mental disorder due to disturbance of brain function and featuring incoherent speech, hallucinations, frenzied excitement, and restlessness; and second, to connote uncontrollable excitement or emotion, "frenzied rapture," or "wildly absurd thought or speech" (1). The word was first used in English in the late sixteenth century (1). The adjective "delirious" may refer to a person affected with delirium, particularly as a consequence or symptom of disease, or to one temporarily insane. It can also imply a characteristic feature of delirium, or refer to a person, thing, or action featuring wild excitement, or one that is frantic, crazy, or mad (1).

The word "delirium" was probably introduced into medical literature by Celsus (2) in the first century A.D., but its meaning remained ambiguous until at least the end of the eighteenth century. The ambiguity resulted from the fact that the term was used by medical writers in one of two ways: first, as a general designation for insanity; and second, more specifically, to refer to a transient, acute mental disorder associated mostly with febrile diseases. Despite this double meaning, however, the clinical descriptions of the syndrome have remained remarkably consistent since the second century A.D. This consistency is striking when one considers that a variety of terms have been applied over the centuries to the same set of symptoms of mental derangement. The following outline of the history of delirium bears this out.

History of delirium as a mental disorder

Delirium was one of the first mental disorders to be recognized by medical writers. The Hippocratic works contain numerous references to what we call delirium today, so that the history of the syndrome goes back some 2,500 years. To trace that history from the beginning proved an arduous but rewarding task that involved scanning several hundred books and articles, as no comprehensive outline of it has ever been published, to my knowledge. Books on the history of psychiatry have been of little help. I have not found a single book on delirium (other than on delirium tremens) in English, with the exception of a treatise on phrenitis by Frings (3), published in 1746. Apart from the *Index Medicus,* several works have been helpful in guiding me to the relevant original sources (4–7). Systematic scanning of the contents of old medical books and journals in several rare medical book collections proved invaluable, if time-consuming.

It would be both pedantic and pointless to record in detail all the confusing shifts in the terminology of delirium found in the medical literature over the ages. Far more interesting is the historical development of the concept of this disorder, which illustrates a remarkable continuity of Western medical thought in this area of psychopathology over many centuries. It shows that clinicians have excelled in observing and describing human behavior, even though they have shown disregard for the consistent use of terms with which to label what they have observed and recorded. Moreover, the history of delirium highlights the fact that the cluster of abnormalities of human mental function and behavior that this term has come to denote constitutes one of the basic forms of psychopathology to which we are prone. To trace this history is not merely an intellectual exercise. On the contrary, clinical observations recorded and explanatory hypotheses advanced by many medical writers over the centuries are still relevant today and provide a challenge for researchers who address them. Despite its long history, delirium remains a poorly understood mental disorder, yet one that raises fundamental questions about the nature of the brain–behavior relationship and its disturbances. Knowledge of its pathophysiology is still scanty and calls for more investigations. The high frequency of this syndrome in clinical practice today underscores the need to bring together the observations and speculations about it made by astute clinicians over the centuries. Their more salient contributions will be referred to in chronological order in the following sections of this chapter.

The ancients

Throughout Western ancient medical history, from the time of Hippocrates on, mental disorders were viewed in physiological terms and hence, like all other diseases, were considered to be essentially organic (8). The modern distinction between the organic and the so-called functional mental disorders was not yet made. As Drabkin (8) points out, however, a distinction was made between *essential* or idiopathic mental diseases, on the one hand, and *symptomatic* ones attendant on other diseases, especially febrile ones or those due to poisoning, on the other hand. Delirium, or phrenitis, was consistently included in the latter class. Greek and Roman medical writers whose works are extant recognized three main forms of mental disorders: *phrenitis, melancholia,* and *mania* (9). Phrenitis was described in ways that largely correspond to what we call delirium in this book. It was regarded as an acute disorder usually associated with fever, one featuring cognitive and behavioral disturbances as well as disruption of sleep. References to disordered sleep in this condition are found in practically all accounts of it from Hippocrates on. Phrenitis was typically described as marked by restless and excited behavior, and was contrasted with its opposite condition, namely, "lethargus" or "lethargy," a term derived from the Greek work *lethe,* meaning forgetfulness or oblivion. "Phrenitis" seemed to have a more complex origin, since the Greek words *phrên* or *phrenos* refer both to diaphragm and mind. This, however, is no coincidence, since the ancients believed that the mind had its seat in the diaphragm (8). Frings (3), writing in 1746, referred to those linguistic links explicitly to explain the derivation of the term "phrenitis" or "phrensy": "This Name squares exquisitely with the Diaphragma. Sebastian Bartholus . . . properly placed the Soul, or the Seat of Life, in the Diaphragma and nervous Center, which being any ways affected, the Mind and Senses are disordered through their Union with the Brain, by the Inflammation whereof, the Phrensy is caused" (p 3). Moreover, the Greek word "phreneticos" means frenzied, frantic, or mad.

Lethargus, or lethargy, was consistently described as the opposite of phrenitis, in that it featured listlessness, sleepiness, inertia, memory loss, and dulling of the senses. It also accompanied fever and was viewed as an ominous prognostic sign. Lethargus could change into phrenitis, and vice versa. A distinction between these two pathological conditions appears to have been made until the late eighteenth century, when the word "delirium" gradually came to replace both of the earlier terms. Moreover, two species of delirium were described: the low, which roughly corresponded to lethargus; and the raving, whose description resembled that of phrenitis of the ancients.

There are many references to delirium in the extant works of Hippocrates (460–366 B.C.). He did not speak of "delirium," a term of Latin and not of Greek origin, but used several Greek words to refer to it (10). Translators of his works into English, however, have usually employed the term "delirium" (10–12). Sprengell (12), for example, who translated into English and interpreted the aphorisms of Hippocrates in the early eighteenth century, uses the term "delirium" several times. Two of the aphorisms are worth quoting: "When a delirium or raving is appeased by sleep, it is a good sign" (p 21). Sprengell interpreted this statement as implying that lack of sleep can cause delirium, which, in turn, can be cured if sleep is restored. The other aphorism is: "Difficulty of breathing and delirium in continual fevers are mortal" (p 112). This remark suggests that Hippocrates was aware that delirium could be a feature of terminal illness.

A recent translation of the medical works of Hippocrates contains numerous references to delirium, especially in the *Books of Epidemics* (11). Many salient features of the syndrome are referred to, including its association with physical, especially febrile, diseases; unpredictable lucid intervals in the diurnal course of the disorder; nocturnal exacerbation of symptoms; insomnia; visual hallucinations; shifting moods; restlessness; and "wandering of the wits." Hippocrates observed that delirium occurring in a generally weakened patient was a bad prognostic sign. The disorder had its origin in the brain. Its manifestations could vary considerably, as illustrated by the case of a patient who became ill as a result of excessive drinking and was "delirious without excitement, being well-behaved and silent," yet a few days later "went mad," with "much tossing about" (p 80). When a delirious patient turned very quiet and "insensible," the prognosis was apt to be grave: "Cases of silent delirium, with restlessness, a changing gaze . . . are likely to prove fatal" (p 261).

As the above brief account clearly indicates, Hippocrates was a superb clinical observer, and even though he did not describe distinct psychiatric syndromes as such, he noted and recorded many of the essential features of delirium. The influence of his teaching, of his empirical approach to natural phenomena, and of the clinical observations he recorded was immense.

Celsus (25 B.C.–A.D. 50), a Roman aristocrat but not a physician, compiled the first great medical work since Hippocrates. His *De Medicina,* written about A.D. 30, consisted of eight books and offered the earliest extant effort at psychiatric nosology (2). He distinguished phrenitis, lethargy, hysteria, melancholia, and mania. He was the first medical writer known to use the term "delirium," even if he did so rather inconsistently. He included it among the signs of impending death and claimed that it was a particularly bad prognostic sign in disease of the "small intestine." Phrenitis, or "phrenesis" in his scheme, corresponded roughly to febrile insanity or delirium. It was an acute form of insanity, one that commonly accompanied fever and called for no treatment other than that for the latter. It could be followed at times by "dementia continua," a chronic insanity. This was probably the first time that the term "dementia" was used in the medical literature. Mettler (6) points out, however, that most terms with a psychiatric connotation used in Roman times had no clear-cut meaning and overlapped a great deal. Celsus considered lethargy as the opposite of phrenesis in that it featured somnolence and slow mentation, yet both of these conditions accompanied febrile diseases.

Three Roman medical writers active in the second century A.D. profoundly influenced Western medical thought for some 1,700 years: Aretaeus (A.D. 50–130), Soranus (A.D. 93–138), and Galen (A.D. 131–200). Of these three masters, Soranus of Ephesus, a Greco-Roman physician, has been called the first psychiatrist for having offered detailed descriptions and treatment of several mental disorders, including phrenitis or delirium (13).

Aretaeus of Cappadocia (14) divided diseases into *acute* and *chronic.* Among the former he included phrenitis and lethargy. Melancholia, mania, and senile dementia ("dotage") represented the chronic diseases. Phrenitis could be caused not only by fever but also by drunkenness and poisoning by mandragora and hyoscyamus. Aretaeus recommended putting a phrenitic patient in a dark place if he was disturbed by light and in the light if he was afraid of the dark. Moreover, the patient was to have rest and sleep, the latter best secured by poppies boiled in oil. We see in this advice the rudiments of modern management of a delirious patient and a remarkable concern for his well-being. Lethargy, another acute mental disorder and one featuring symptoms opposite to those of phrenitis, called for different treatment, namely, stimulation rather than sedation. Aretaeus was probably the first medical writer to distinguish senile dementia, or "dotage," which started in old age, accompanied the patient until death, and featured "a torpor of the senses, and a stupefaction of the gnostic and intellectual faculties" (14, p 103).

Soranus (13,15), whose work was compiled by his Latin interpreter, Caelius Aurelianus, in the fifth century A.D., offered a remarkably accurate description of phrenitis or delirium. He insisted that it could never occur without fever, yet he pointed out that mania, or insanity, also frequently started with it. He proposed that in phrenitis the whole body was affected and ought to be the object of treatment, but allowed that certain signs indicated that the head was affected more than other body parts. Soranus argued that phrenitis derived its name from the fact that it involved a disturbance of the mind *(deliratio)* and defined it as an "acute mental derangement accompanied by acute fever." His most important contribution to our subject, however, was a brilliant account of the clinical features of delirium, as well as of its treatment. He observed that a person about to develop phrenitis displayed "continual sleeplessness or troubled sleep with confused dreams." Once the disorder had fully developed, the patient showed "quiet or loud laughter, singing or a state of sadness, silence, murmuring, crying, or a barely audible muttering to one's self; or such a state of anger that the patient jumps in a rage and can scarcely be held back, is wrathful at everyone, shouts, beats himself or tears his own clothing and that of his neighbors, or seeks to hide in fear, or weeps, or fails to answer those who speak to him, while he speaks not only with those who are not present but with the dead, as if they were in his presence" (15, p 23). Moreover, in phrenitis the patient tended to pluck threads from the covers *(crocydismos)* and pick small pieces of straw from the walls *(carphologia)*. These symptoms helped to distinguish phrenitis from mania with fever. Speaking of treatment, Soranus stressed the need to ensure sleep. He taught that people whom the delirious person disliked should be kept out so as to avoid aggravating his condition but "permit people who are regarded by the patient with awe or veneration to enter, yet only at intervals, for familiarity breeds contempt" (15, p 43). In some cases, venesection might be required.

Galen, one of the most influential medical writers of all times, used the term "delirium" freely but rather ambiguously. His major contribution was to recognize that mental disorders could be primary or secondary, according to whether the basic disturbance was located in the brain or if the latter was secondarily implicated by "consensus" or "sympathetically" in diseases such as pneumonia (7,9). Phrenitis was an acute disease located in the brain or the meninges, characterized by fever and delirium. Fever delirium, by contrast, was also an acute mental disease but resulted from a primary disease elsewhere in the body (9). The cause of phrenitis was abnormal dryness and heat, qualities associated with yellow bile. In one type of phrenitis, the diaphragm was primarily affected. Treatment should generally aim at cooling and calming the patient.

As this brief account of the contribution to our subject by the most influential Greek and Roman writers illustrates, they described with remarkable accuracy and consistency the salient features of delirium. Despite inconsistencies in the use of terms to label it, they left us a clinical picture that closely resembles what we call delirium today. Phrenitis, or delirium, was one of the main mental disorders recognized in antiquity (8,10,16). It was believed to be due to a primary or secondary brain disorder and to represent an acute form of madness, one invariably associated with a somatic illness. This view of its etiology still prevails. In accordance with the then dominant humoral theory of disease, phrenitis was regarded as a consequence of an excess of yellow bile, whose chief properties were heat and dryness. In spite of the strictly organic view of its etiology and pathogenesis, the ancient writers recommended treatment that included both a physiological and a psychological approach. The needs of both the mind and the body of the patient had to be met. This two-pronged therapeutic approach still constitutes a model for the management of delirium, and may be regarded as one of the most important contributions of the ancient writers not only to the treatment of this syndrome, but also to psychiatry and medicine generally.

The medieval period

Medieval medical writers were largely influenced by the teachings of their Greek and Roman predecessors (16). They contributed relatively little that was original to the development of the concept of delirium.

Cassius Felix, active in the fifth century A.D., is credited by some authors with being the first medical writer to link drunkenness explicitly with delirium (17). The Talmud, compiled mostly in the fourth and fifth centuries A.D., contains the description of a disorder named *kordiakos,* a temporary mental derangement due to excessive drinking of wine and having a good prognosis (18). In modern translations of the Talmud, *Kordiakos* is usually rendered as "delirium" (18).

In late antiquity, the center of medieval thought and writing moved to Byzantium; hence the term "Byzantine medicine" (7,16). Oribasius of Pergamon (325–403), Alexander of Tralles (525–605), and Paulus of Aegina (625–90) were the main medical authorities of that period (16). They were mostly compilers and interpreters of the works of Hippocrates, Galen, and Soranus, and their writings were merely elaborations of the views of their illustrious predecessors. Paulus of Aegina viewed phrenitis as an inflammation of the brain or the meninges, while delirium he considered to be a subspecies of it brought about by the brain's "sympathizing" with the diaphragm (7).

From Byzantium the center of medieval learning and writing shifted to the Arabs, who dominated the field from about the seventh to the twelfth century (6,7). They added little of note to our subject. Two of the most outstanding Arab writers came from Persia: Rhazes (865–925) and Avicenna (980–1037). The former described a condition named *sirsen,* which corresponded to both lethargus and phrenitis and was due to fever or indulgence in wine (7). As such, it was a precursor of a unified concept of delirium. Avicenna's most famous work, *Canon of Medicine,* contained many references to mental disorders (7). He distinguished phrenitis, lethargus, delirium, amentia or fatuity, disorders of memory and imagination, mania, melancholia, and lycanthropy (7). He referred to delirium as either a symptom of phrenitis or a separate disorder, and considered it to be a manifestation of brain disease caused by black, yellow, or red bile, or by hot and burning blood reaching the brain, or as a disorder originating at times in that organ itself (7).

With the decline of Arabic medicine in the twelfth century, the interest in mental disorders waned. Bartholomeus Anglicus, active in the thirteenth century, provided a notable exception. His influential encyclopedia, *De Proprietatibus Rerum,* first published in 1470, offered authoritative teaching on mental disorders (6). Following the ancient writers, he recognized four forms of mental aberration: melancholia, mania, dementia, and "frenesie," or delirium. The last he believed to be due to disease of the brain and its membranes, and distinguished it from "perafrenesi," or delirium secondary to febrile and other systemic diseases. His description of frenesie featured anguish, frequent waking from sleep, restlessness, laughing, singing, weeping, and attempts to get out of bed (6). For treatment he recommended bleeding the patient and safeguarding sleep. The distinction between frenesie and perafrenesi, one that reflected Galen's etiological concepts, prevailed until the eighteenth century (3). Frenesie probably represented encephalitis and meningitis with delirium.

The sixteenth century

The medical writings of the sixteenth century reflect both the influence of and the growing challenge to Galenic medicine (16). Some interesting developments in the concept of delirium took place during this period. Antonio Guainerio, an Italian physician whose textbook *Practica* was published in 1517, emphasized the importance of a thorough medical study of a delirious patient because delirium could occur in a wide range of systemic diseases such as those of the lungs, heart, liver, kidneys, stomach, or uterus (19). He asserted that one could recognize a predelirious phase ("paraphrenitis"), which might or might not be followed by a full-blown delirium. The outcome of the latter depended on the patient's constitution, the nature of the underlying disease, and the method of treatment applied (19).

Girolamo Fracastoro (1483–1553), another Italian physician, gave a good description of delirium in the course of typhus (6). He noted disorientation and observed that some patients displayed vigilance, others torpor. These two contrasting states could occur in the same patient on a single day or a few days apart.

From the late 1560s on, a large number of dissertations on phrenitis and delirium were printed in Germany and Switzerland (19). Probably the earliest of them, by Cnobloch (20), appeared in 1569 and dealt with delirium, or paraphrenitis. Another one, by Haunoldt (21), consisted of 49 theses about delirium—its causes, pathophysiology, and treatment. It was a concise summary of the views of the earlier medical writers and contained nothing innovative. Other dissertations from that period emphasized the need to recognize the prodromal symptoms of phrenitis such as insomnia, headache, and disturbing dreams (19). The psychopathological features of the syndrome involved abnormalities of imagination (visual hallucinations), reason, and memory. Dissertations by the students of Felix Platter (1536–1614), a famous professor at the University of Basle, further clarified the symptomatology of delirium; this was their main contribution (19). Platter himself described its features and pathogenesis in his textbook but offered no new insights (19).

In England, the term "delirium" was probably first used by Cosin (4) in 1592. He defined it as "that weakenes of conceite and consideration, which we call dotage: when a man, through age or infirmitie, falleth to be a childe againe in discretion: albeit he understand what is said, and can happely speak somwhat pertinently unto sundry matters" (p 44). An interesting account of delirium ("frenesie") can be found in Philip Barrough's (22) textbook *The Method of Physick,* first published in 1583. He defined it as a "continuall madness and fury joyned with a sharp fever" (p 21). Frenetics displayed the derangement of the three main "internall senses": imagination, cogitation, and memory; some suffered from a disorder of imagination alone. They had a continuous fever and could not sleep. Some of them had "troublesome sleepes, so that they rise up and leap, and cry out furiously" (p 22). The prognosis of delirium was poor: it was "indeed incurable and deadly for the most part." Treatment had to involve attention to the patient's needs: if he was troubled by the light, he had to be placed in a dark room. Moreover, "Let his dearest friends come to him, and let them somtime speake gently and softly unto him, and sometime rebuke him sharply." His diet had to be light. The patient had to be left undisturbed, since "perturbations of the mind do hurt frenetick persons exceedingly" (p 23). If his strength allowed it, the patient had to be bled from the "uttermost veine of the arme called Cephalica." If bleeding was contraindicated, cupping had to be done and the patient's head sprinkled with the oil of roses to cool it. Sleep needed to be ensured by the use of appropriate medications such as opium or henbane, taking care not to oversedate the patient, as this could turn "frenesie into a lethargie, wherby you may cause him to sleepe so, that you can awake him no more" (p 24). Barrough defined lethargie as "nothing else but a dull oblivion" and "inexpugnable desire of sleeping." It was caused by overcooling of the brain by phlegm and was always associated with fever. It had to be treated by bleeding and stimulants. Lethargie might at times be followed by loss of memory, either alone or with concurrent impairment of reason.

One is struck by Barrough's excellent description of delirium, and especially by his careful and humane attention to its treatment. His account of it bore the stamp of the best teachings of the Greek and Roman writers, whom he quoted.

One other sixteenth-century contribution is worth mentioning. Ambroise Paré (1510–1590), a famous French surgeon, discussed delirium complicating surgical conditions and procedures. His works, translated into English in 1634 (23), referred to delirium as an affliction of fantasy, one marked by "raving, talking idly or doting." It was a transient disturbance that commonly followed fever and pain due to wounds, gangrene, and operations involving excessive bleeding of the patient.

The seventeenth century

Important developments took place in medicine during this century. Work on anatomy by Vesalius, on physiology by Harvey, and on the brain by Willis advanced knowledge of the structure and functions of the human body. Thomas Sydenham, the "English Hippocrates," became a true founder of modern medicine. He emphasized direct observation rather than theorizing as the best approach to establishing the etiology of a disease. His work on hysteria was a landmark in the development of that concept. Robert Burton's *The Anatomy of Melancholy,* first published in 1621, was another major addition to the literature on mental disorders.

An interesting, if not fundamental, contribution to the concept of delirium came from a great physician, neuroanatomist, and neurophysiologist, Thomas Willis (1621–1675). In his treatise on mental disorders, *De Anima Brutorum,* published in 1672 and translated into English in 1683 (24), he offered a good description of delirium and discussed its etiology and pathogenesis. He pointed out that it was not a disease but rather a *symptom.* Patients suffering from it "think, speak, or do absurd things" and experience "incongruous conceptions, and confused thoughts." Moreover, their visual perceptions were distorted, and they tended to display "incongruous speeches" and "absurd gestures of the body." Delirium was usually associated with a fever but might also result from drunkenness, poisoning with mandrake, hemorrhage, lack of sleep, "hysterical passions," or gangrene. The immediate cause of the "symptom" might be blood either swollen with too much heat or carrying "venomous particles." Its prognosis was generally favorable and this distinguished it from phrensie, which was "longer or continuall" but was also usually associated with fever and sometimes resulted from drunkenness or succeeded "violent passions" such as love or hate. Phrensie depended on the soul rather than on disordered humors or particles carried by the blood. The "burning" began in the brain, where the animal spirits were inflamed. Phrensie could sometimes pass into lethargy, or madness, or melancholy.

One should note that Willis departed from the traditional humoral theory of delirium and phrensie and explained its pathogenesis in terms reflecting the new chemical and corpuscular theories of disease (16). A similar explanation was offered by his contemporary, Richard Morton (1637–1698), who proposed that delirium was the consequence of increased velocity of blood caused by fever, which resulted in disordered secretion of the brain glands

(6). Moreover, Morton claimed the delirium represented a *waking dream,* a notion that took firm hold in the next century.

The eighteenth century

By the end of the seventeenth century, the essential features of delirium had been adequately described and only needed to be further refined. By contrast, the relevant terminology was still inconsistent and confusing. This confusion persisted throughout much of the eighteenth century: "delirium" implied madness or raving, while "phrenitis" or "phrensy" referred to delirium associated with febrile and sometimes other somatic diseases, and was usually divided into primary and secondary ("paraphrensy"). The views on the etiology and pathogenesis of mental disorders, including phrenitis, came to reflect the influence of the new chemical and corpuscular theories, as indicated in the preceding section. Another interesting trend was to equate delirium with waking dreams and to ascribe it to disordered sleep. Finally, an important event was the appearance, in 1746, of the first, and probably the only, treatise on phrenitis in English.

The meaning of the term "delirium" in the first half of the eighteenth century can be gleaned from two representative English medical dictionaries, those of Quincy (1719) and James (1745), respectively. Quincy (25) defined it as follows: "Delirium, is an Incapacity in the Organs of Sensation to perform their Function in due Manner, so that the Mind does not reflect upon and judge of external Objects as usual; as is the Case frequently in Fevers, from too impetuous a Hurry of the Blood, which alters so far the Secretion in the Brain, as to disorder the whole Nervous System" (p 103). Mania, or madness, is "a Delirium without Fever." Moreover, "A Delirium is therefore the Dreams of waking Persons, wherein Ideas are excited without Order or Coherence and the animal Spirits are drove into irregular Fluctuations" (p 243).

James (26) added further observations on the relationship between delirium and the disorder of the sleep-wake cycle: "a Delirium is always attended with Want of Sleep, and both proceed from the same Cause"; "Sleeps which are tumultuous and disturbed, as also those unsound Slumbers, during which the Patient is, as it were, half awake, or cries out, and starts up, are the Forerunners of a future Delirium."

George Cheyne (1671–1743) (27) also stressed the importance of sleep in delirium: "Sleep in Phrenzies and all Deliria is a main Intention Physicians aim at" (p 369). If delirious patients managed to sleep soundly, they became "perfectly restored to their Intellects." On the other hand, as long as the "Fury of the Spirits continues, Sleep is utterly banished" (p 369).

In 1746, the first, and to my knowledge the only, treatise on delirium (phrensy) in English, that by Frings (3), was published. In it he proceeded to refute the views of Galenists on the cause of that disorder and to "explode" their method of treating it. He defined delirium as "the Loss of Sense and Reason, which deviate from their natural Law and Order" (p 4). Not only reason, however, but also imagination and memory were disturbed: "When the Imagination is only affected, absurd and incoherent Objects present themselves, and absent Things seem to be in Sight" (p 6). Frings used the term "delirium" to refer to insanity generally and spoke of "deliriums" with or without or after a fever. Those without the latter included mania and melancholia. Phrensy was never without fever and was attended by constant delirium. It might be primary, that is, due to the brain and its membranes being affected, or secondary, that is, paraphrensy, resulting from overheating of the brain in consequence of an inflamed viscus, especially inflammation of the diaphragm. Delirium in fever could be of two types: ridiculous, when the patient was cheerful, and serious, when he talked at random and tended to be angry. The latter had a poorer prognosis. Frings' description of the prodromal and actual symptoms of phrensy followed the classical model and added nothing worth noting. Regarding its etiology, he derided the notion of the Galenists that it was due to "Choleric Blood" and put forth his own view: "The Cause of Phrensy is the Overheating the Spirits, and an Effervency first in the Heart, and next in the Brain; so that the whole Disorder lies in the Spirits, and that in various and different Ways, as the Spirits are diversly affected. The human Soul is immutable and unalterable, being always the same; neither can it be inflamed, or receive any Hurt from any internal or external Cause whatsoever" (pp 20–21). Frings went on to insist that it was the inflamed spirits that were to blame for all the mental aberrations observed in phrensy. Fever began with the excessive heat of the vital spirits in the heart or the brain. The spirits of the blood, becoming increasingly inflamed, affected the brain, causing mental derangement. The cause of their being overheated was excessive heat of the blood, and this, in turn, might be due to the "sulphurous, salt, and sharp Particles begotten in the human Body, out of its Nourishment"; or to too much exercise; or to anger and other "Passions of the Mind." Phrensy was usually fatal; however, the prognosis was hopeful if the patient could sleep. Frings criticized bitterly the treatment advocated by the Galenists, saying that they were the "most expert in the Art of Killing," since they held that bleeding was the best therapy for phrensy. He himself recommended a proper diet as the mainstay of treatment of this disorder and stressed the need for rest and sleep. Only an extremely agitated patient should be bled. Opium could be used to sedate patients but had to be administered cautiously to avoid transition to lethargy and death.

As the above summary of his book makes clear, Frings explicitly rejected the humoral theory of disease and the treatment of phrensy based on it. His account of the etiology and pathogenesis of that disorder combined the elements of both the chemical theory—he spoke of "fermentation" of the assorted "particles" in the blood—and the corpuscular one in his reference to the particles (16). The inflammation of the animal spirits was responsible for the mental derangement, but the soul remained unaffected. This notion appeared to reflect Descartes' dualistic conception of soul and body, and his physiological explanation of mental activity as mediated by the animal spirits of the nervous system (16).

Three years after the publication of Frings' treatise, there appeared a remarkable book by David Hartley (1705–1757) (28), an English physician and philosopher and a founder of associational psychology. It asserted that the insane differed from normal people only relatively, insofar as they displayed failures and abnormalities of memory, judgment, emotions, reasoning, consciousness, and actions. In his classification of mental disorders, Hartley included "The deliriums attending acute or other distempers." His description of delirium was quite accurate and included "disgustful" associations; distortion of reasoning; "a vivid train of visible images" forcing itself on the eyes; incoherent speech; and disorientation for place. A patient was most likely to be delirious on going to or waking from sleep or when placed in a dark room. When his room was lit, he tended to recover and talk rationally until the candle was withdrawn. Hartley asserted that, in the dark, internally derived images and associations overpowered "impressions from real objects."

In the second half of the eighteenth century, William Cullen (1710–1790) became a predominant medical authority. The brain and the nervous system, rather than the heart and the vascular system, were central elements in his physiology (16). His theory of disease was based on the notions of "excitement," that is, conditions ranging from normal wakefulness to mania, and "collapse," that is, states ranging from normal sleep to syncope and death (16). Speaking of delirium, Cullen stated that it was a frequent symptom of fever, one that depended on the "inequality in the excitement of the brain" and involved "diminution in the energy of the brain" (29, p 37). This is surely an intriguing idea if one considers that an influential current theory of the pathogenesis of delirium posits reduced cerebral metabolism.

Two major medical figures of the late eighteenth century, Erasmus Darwin (1731–1802) and John Hunter (1728–1793), made important contributions to the theory of delirium. Darwin (30), an English physician and the grandfather of Charles Darwin, classified delirium among the diseases of sensation, specifically as one with increased sensation and action of the sense organs. He distinguished several species of it, including the febrile ("paraphrosyne"), maniacal, and drunken, and asserted that dreams constituted "the most complete kind of delirium." A hallucination represented a partial delirium. Darwin differentiated febrile delirium from madness, in which "the patients well know the persons of their acquaintance, and the place where they are; and perform all the voluntary actions with steadiness and determination" (p 495). The ideas in delirium consisted of those "excited by the sensation of pleasure or pain." Maniacal delirium was caused by the increase of the pleasurable or painful sensation and belonged to a different class of insanities. Drunken delirium in no way differed from the febrile one, except that it was caused by alcohol or "other poisons." Darwin compared delirium to a dream and proposed that dreaming might protect one against developing it. In fevers dreaming was interfered with, and hence protection against the syndrome was lost. In both dreams and delirium, there was a "defect or paralysis of the voluntary power," while the capacity for attending to external objects is suspended.

Hunter (31), an eminent Scottish anatomist and surgeon, carried the above line of thought still further. He defined delirium as "a dream arising from disease, whether the dream is in the brain itself or in the body . . . a delirium is a diseased dream arising from what may be called diseased sleep" (p 333). Sleep was a "cessation of susceptibility of sensation," as a consequence of which there was a "cessation of consciousness in the animal of its own existence." It is not clear, however, if this whole process arose in the brain or in the nerves. Delirium and sleep differed from insanity in that a person might be roused from the former and perceive his situation properly, whereas an insane person could not distinguish truth from error. Delirium, in turn, differed from dreams: "In natural sleep the more the brain puts on that peculiar state the less we have of dreaming; but the more the other state is put on the greater the delirium" (p 334). Both in delirium and in dreams, "what the mind thinks about appears to be real."

Darwin and Hunter developed and refined the notion, referred to by many eighteenth-century writers, that delirium constituted a form of dreaming while the person was awake, and hence, that both dreams and the mental contents of a delirious individual had a close affinity. This provocative hypothesis waits to be addressed by researchers. Hunter also referred to "consciousness" in this context and clearly understood by this term the awareness of one's self, one's body, and one's environment. It was only in the next century that consciousness came to be regarded as a distinct mental state or function, one whose disturbance ("clouding") was believed to be a core abnormality in delirium.

In the last year of the eighteenth century, an interesting article on mental disorders was published by James Sims (32). He referred to delirium as a form of "alienation of mind," one very different from madness. It either succeeded or was followed be fever and was of one of two kinds: low or raving. The former resembled melancholia, while the latter could be mistaken for mania. In either case, however, the patient experienced hallucinations, his memory was blunted, his mind had no clear purpose, and his reason was deficient. In low delirium the patient was inattentive, muttered incoherently, tended to doze off, picked at his bed clothes, and was incontinent. By contrast, a patient suffering from a raving delirium was unable to sleep, was hyperalert, spoke with persons whom nobody else could see, and constantly tried to rise from bed. Thus, Sims clearly recognized two clinical variants of the syndrome distinguished by contrasting states of alertness and of psychomotor behavior. Moreover, he used the term "delirium" in its modern sense to denote a distinct mental disorder rather than to refer to insanity generally, as had been the custom. One may say that he offered a *unified concept* of delirium and avoided the terminological confusion of his predecessors and contemporaries.

The nineteenth century

Several important developments in the evolution of the concept and treatment of delirium took place in this century. The syndrome became increasingly recognized as a transient cognitive and behavioral disorder brought about by brain dysfunction resulting from a wide range of physical (organic) causes. The terminology lost some of its earlier confusion; the term "delirium" came to be applied, at least in the English medical literature, consistently to an acute mental disorder with distinct identifying features, and not to insanity or mental derangement in general. Old terms, such as "phrenitis," "phrensy," "lethargy," and "paraphrensy," were gradually dropped from the medical vocabulary. A remarkably sophisticated discussion of the psychopathology of delirium and its relationship to dreams was published by Greiner early in the century. Delirium tremens, thought to be due to alcohol or its withdrawal, was described at about the same time. The concepts of clouding of consciousness and confusion were formulated and applied to delirium. Finally, treatment of the syndrome advanced beyond bleeding and the use of herbal concoctions, without, however, losing sight of the delirious patient's psychological needs. These developments will be presented in a more or less chronological order.

Encyclopedias and dictionaries offer a fair idea of how a particular term was applied in a given historical period. A dictionary by Rees (33), published about 1818, reflected clarification in the use of the term "delirium" early in the nineteenth century. It defined delirium as an "alienation of mind connected with fever" and added the following comment: "This is the sense in which delirium is *commonly understood:* but by some writers, as Hoffman, Sauvages, etc., delirium is the term employed to denote the whole class of mental derangements, including the different forms of mania, melancholy, febrile delirium, and so forth" (italics added). Rees went on to say that febrile delirium's distinguishing feature was that it "originates from a certain physical condition of the brain." This statement reaffirmed the organic etiology of the syndrome. Delirium "first occurs between sleeping and waking, especially in the dark"—an accurate observation—and hence may be regarded as a "sort of waking dream." Two "species" of the disorder could be distinguished: violent and low. The former reflected an increased quantity and force of blood in the brain and called for treatment that would lessen both—by the application of leeches to the head, for example. By contrast, in low delirium, circulation of the blood in the brain was sluggish, and the patient was inattentive and close to a stupor. In such cases, wine might help the patient. In both types of delirium the patient experienced a "perpetual flow of ideas," he was disoriented for place and person, his powers of imagination and association were morbidly increased, and his judgment was faulty. An analogous situation prevailed when the person was asleep and dreaming.

The above description of delirium resembles that given by Benjamin Rush (1745–1813), the author of the first American textbook of psychiatry, published in 1812 (34). He argued that delirium and dreaming shared the incoherence of thought; hence "a dream may be considered as a transient paroxysm of delirium, and delirium as a permanent dream" (p 300).

A year later, Sutton (35) published his tract on "delirium tremens," a term he coined. This disorder had to be distinguished from phrenitis and was characterized by a marked tremor of the hands. Delirium tremens was either caused by excessive drinking or reflected the person's constitutional sensitivity to alcohol. Pearson (36) wrote *Observations on Brain Fever* in 1801 and published it in 1813. He offered an accurate description of delirium tremens, antedating that of Sutton, but did not call it so, even though he acknowledged that brain fever due to alcohol should be distinguished from that accompanying infections ("putrid fever"). Following Sutton's account, many writers in Britain and America published observations on delirium tremens. An important point, one already made by Sutton, was that it had to be treated by large, repeated doses of opium, not by bloodletting, which made it worse.

In 1817, there appeared a remarkably thoughtful and comprehensive account of the psychopathology of delirium written in German by F. C. Greiner (37). In the introduction, he observed that two somatopsychic phenomena, dreams and delirium or "febrile madness," were so common that one tended to pay little attention to them. These conditions deserved serious study, as they might offer deep insights into the innermost life of human beings. In both dreams and delirium the consciousness became clouded *(verdunkelt)*, the usual laws of thinking were suspended, and the normal distinction between internally derived images and the perceptions of external objects became blurred and confused. The affinity of delirium to dreams was suggested by the fact that the former arose as a true dream, yet one that, as the fever increased, continued during the waking state. The fever brought about a disturbance in the organ of consciousness in the brain, and a clouding of consciousness *(Verdunkelung des Bewusstseins)* resulted. Such a disturbance followed either excessive arterial function or an inflammation of the brain's or the nervous system's capillaries. As brain function and consciousness became disordered, the animal soul *(Tierseele)* came to the fore—it was normally suppressed—and imposed on the psyche impressions that did not correspond to reality. The animal soul also interfered with the capacity to distinguish between what was real and what was not. The consciousness being disturbed, the psyche became disordered too. The senses, the awareness of one's self and one's body, the emotions, and the memory, were all affected. Both distortions of perception and actual false perceptions resulted from the senses being afflicted. The clarity of awareness of one's self and one's personality became blurred. The experience of one's own body was also disturbed, so that it might be perceived as abnormally heavy or as falling, for example. Drives and instincts were also affected, as manifested by increased thirst or aversion to certain foods. Anxious feelings were readily aroused and, in turn, influenced body functions. The patient felt tired and restless. As his reason, judgment, and understanding were disturbed, he might come to misinterpret his abnormal bodily perceptions and to believe that his bones were broken or his limbs had been torn off. Such false beliefs tended to increase his restlessness, and he might try to get out of bed and leave the room. Memory was also affected. The distinction between the past and the present became blurred, and spontaneous recall of memories that the patient might not have been able to invoke at will while he was healthy tended to occur. He might believe that dead persons he knew in the past were alive and speak to them, yet fail to recognize those familiar to him and present at his bedside. While he readily forgot events that had taken place recently, he tended to remember clearly those that occurred long before. The fantasy of a delirious patient was unrestrained, and he tended to confuse its productions with his perceptions of the environment. He might live largely in the past and believe himself to be in school facing a teacher or to command a regiment in wartime, for example. Moreover, the patient tended to speak and act in accordance with his fantasies, perceptual distortions, and false beliefs.

The course and severity of delirium, as well as its clinical picture, were influenced by the patient's constitution and by the duration and degree of the fever. If the latter was not strong, the delirium tended to be quieter and barely noticeable. The patient might just wake up and continue to remain in his dream world for a while, or experience vivid fantasies only when he closed his eyes. As the fever fluctuated, so did the patient's clarity of consciousness; he might be quite lucid at times. The actual contents of a delirious patient's fantasies and other morbid productions depended on his habits, education, morals, and lifestyle. A soldier, a peasant, or a scholar experienced delirium differently, but the laws that caused its occurrence were the same. Moreover, as the strength of the fever increased, all resistance to the pressure of fantasies failed, regardless of how strong the personality and the will of the patient might be.

The onset of delirium in the patient had to be a matter of concern to the physician. He might draw some conclusions regarding the nature of the underlying illness from the symptoms exhibited by the patient. For example, if delirium came on in the early stage of the illness, one might suspect that inflammation of the brain was present. Those taking care of a delirious patient had an obligation to do everything possible to lessen his anxiety. They had to avoid speaking freely in his presence, since he might have lucid moments and grasp what was being said. The patient had to be treated with even greater respect than when he was healthy. Objects that might disturb him had to be removed so as not to frighten him. The same applied to persons whom he disliked and who increased his restlessness. A person whom he did like had to try to calm him by speaking to him gently and softly, by addressing him by his name to enhance his self-awareness, and by drawing his attention to objects and subjects in which he showed interest. Those in attendance had to put aside their prejudices and conventional attitudes, and see in the patient nothing but a suffering human being. His utterances and actions ought to be regarded as occurring without his intent or free will. Hence, he could not be held responsible for what he said or did. Moreover, it was not right to judge his moral standards from his delirious behavior or to regard his statements as an expression of his secrets. A testament made by a delirious patient could not be considered valid unless the attending physician deemed him capable of making it and witnessed it himself. Greiner ended his book with some noteworthy remarks about the bright points in the dark picture of the mind in delirium. Even though the psyche was disturbed, some of its capacities showed through the confusion and allowed hope for its full recovery. One had to respect the human dignity of one whose innermost life is broken up in delirium and to offer him protection. Every person who approaches the bed of a delirious patient should think: "I am also human, and no man's fate is foreign to my heart."

The above is but a short summary of a remarkable book of 264 pages. It contains the most insightful and compassionate account of the psychopathology and treatment of delirium of which this writer is aware. Moreover, Greiner was probably the first author to invoke the concept of clouding of consciousness, one that came to be generally regarded as a hallmark of delirium later in the century.

Two clinical articles on delirium published around the middle of the nineteenth century by Gallway and Salter are worth mentioning. Gallway (38) observed that "The subject of delirium is generally looked upon by the practical physician as one of the most obscure in the chain of morbid phenomena he has to deal with; whilst the frequency of its occurrence under various diseased conditions renders the affection not a little familiar to his eye" (p 46). He went on to argue that delirium was by no means confined to inflammation of the brain and meninges, but might occur in diseases in which the brain was found to be normal after the patient's death. He asserted that obstruction of the passage of blood through the lungs, due to either pulmonary or cardiac disease, might lead to its being "maloxygenated" and hence deleterious to the brain. This hypothesis is interesting in that Gallway added a new and important factor to account for the etiology and pathogenesis of some cases of delirium, namely, that of hypoxemia. He made the useful suggestion that one must not bleed a patient so afflicted, as this would further deprive the brain of the stimulation necessary for the discharge of its function.

Salter (39) argued that it was always essential to diagnose the disease causing delirium in order to treat it properly. He pointed out that insanity could sometimes be mistaken for delirium, or vice versa, but the two conditions of mental derangement could be distinguished by their clinical picture and by the fact that delirium was generally associated with "much well-marked bodily disease," and was usually acute, not chronic. Salter gave an excellent description of delirium tremens, noted that it could be due to either intoxication with or withdrawal from liquor, and pointed out the close clinical resemblance between the delirium of drunkards and that due to other causes such as heart disease. He observed that loss of sleep in the latter contributed to the occurrence of delirium and was due to irregular breathing, with periods of apnea (probably Cheyne-Stokes breathing) that kept the patient awake. Salter also referred to a close relationship between delirium and epilepsy: the former might usher in the latter, or vice versa.

The above two articles were written by practicing physicians and reflected their clinical experience. They added useful observations to the development of the concept of delirium and went beyond the traditional notion that the latter was invariably associated with either a febrile illness or intoxication.

Several other works published in the first half of the nineteenth century are worthy of note. Hallaran (40), an Irish physician, asserted that a distinction should be made between "mental" insanity and that due to primary or secondary disease of the brain. Such a distinction was necessary in order to choose appropriate treatment for the patient. Delirium was a condition marked by excitement, maniacal symptoms, and hallucinations; hence, it was not unlike mental insanity, but was associated with and readily traceable to a disease of the body. Fordyce (41), an authority on fevers, gave an excellent clinical description of delirium in the course of various febrile illnesses. Armstrong (42) not only described the features of the syndrome occurring in typhus but also offered an account of his personal experience of it. A patient suffering from this infectious disease showed a gradual progression of mental symptoms. At first he was distractible, restless, sleepless, and forgetful; then he became garrulous, like a drunken person. After a few days his "mental confusion" became obvious and, as the disease progressed, passed into delirium, with visual and auditory "deceptions," excitement, and ultimately collapse. Sir Henry Holland (43), an eminent English physician, distinguished between delirium and insanity: "Delirium and intoxication may be considered transient effects, from temporary causes, of that condition of sensorium which, more deeply fixed and longer continued, obtains the name and produces all the aspects of mental derangement" (p 135). Thus the main distinction lay in the reversibility or transience of delirium, in contrast to the permanence of insanity. In a fully developed delirium, "every function of the mind is disordered by the unreal images and false combinations which possess it, uncontrolled by impressions from without" (p 142). Both insanity and delirium were closely related to dreaming: insanity might be called "a waking and active dream." Dupuytren (44), a French surgeon, described "traumatic" delirium occurring after accidental or surgical trauma. Patients affected by it displayed "confusion of things, places, and persons," insomnia, restlessness, preoccupation with personally important matters, a flushed and animated face, and insensitivity to pain. Such delirium was transient and its prognosis was good, but at times it might end in death for no obvious reason. Surprisingly, fever and tachycardia were often absent. Laudanum enema was the best treatment for this condition.

All the above works were written by physicians and surgeons, not by psychiatrists. It was only in the early nineteenth century that the treatment of mental disorders gradually became monopolized by a group of physicians (alienists) and the specialty of psychiatry emerged. This development coincided with and was fostered by the establishment of asylums for the treatment of the insane. Concurrently, polemics were taking place about the causation of mental disorders. The somaticists viewed them as manifestations of brain dysfunction, and hence as organic, while the psychicists advocated "moral" theories of insanity and ascribed it to an affliction of the mind. By the middle of the century, the somatic theories of mental disorders had largely prevailed, both in Europe and America. Once more, the brain came to be viewed as the organ of the mind, and physiological psychology began to dominate the field of psychopathology (45). This development was clearly articulated in a British textbook of psychiatry by Bucknill and Tuke (46), first published in 1858, which remained the foremost statement on mental disorders in Britain for several decades. Insanity was defined as "a disease of the brain (idiopathic or sympathetic) affecting the integrity of the mind, whether marked by intellectual or emotional disorder; such affection not being the mere symptom or immediate result of fever or poison" (p 21). This last exclusion is of special interest to the student of delirium. Bucknill and Tuke explicitly excluded the latter from the classification of mental disorders. Even though all forms of insanity were viewed as connected with "a previous or present affection of some organ in the body," delirium, which fully met this criterion, was excluded, since it was but a fleeting disorder of the mind, one arising as a complication of other diseases that passed with the patient's bodily affliction; it was a "mere accident of such disease." The authors pointed out that this exclusion was not really scientific, but made only for practical purposes.

One may speculate that the exclusion of delirium from psychiatric classification and from an authoritative textbook of psychiatry reflected no more than the fact that the nineteenth century was the *age of the asylum* and of isolation of psychiatry from medicine. Consequently, a mental disorder that was acute and invariably occurred as a transient manifestation and complication of a physical illness was neither familiar nor of practical importance to the asylum psychiatrist, with his almost exclusive concern with *chronic* mental disorders. This may well account for the meager contribution of psychiatry to the development of the concept of delirium throughout much of the nineteenth century. By contrast, most seminal works on this subject were written by nonpsychiatric physicians.

CLOUDING OF CONSCIOUSNESS AND CONFUSION

An important theoretical development in the history of the concept of delirium in the second half of the nineteenth century was to view it as a disorder of consciousness (47). The word "consciousness" had already appeared in this context in the late eighteenth century in the writings of Hunter (31), but was used to denote awareness of the self and the environment rather than a distinct mental faculty. Greiner (37) used the term freely in his discussion of delirium and spoke of an "organ of consciousness" in the brain whose disorder resulted in the clouding of consciousness in that condition. He was, to my knowledge, the first writer to invoke that concept in the medical literature. It was only later in the nineteenth century that consciousness came to be regarded as a distinct mental function, one whose disturbances became a major form or aspect of psychopathology. The work of Hughlings Jackson (48), an eminent English neurologist, in the 1860s was particularly important in this regard.

Jackson viewed mental disorders as the most complex forms of diseases of the nervous system. They were the consequence of dysfunction of the highest nervous centers, those constituting the physical basis of the "mind" or "consciousness," terms used by Jackson synonymously. In accordance with the theory of evolution, he considered the functional organization of the central nervous system—or the "nervous centers"—to be arranged hiearchically in three layers or levels: highest, middle, and lowest. The highest centers were the most complex and voluntary, the least organized, and the most susceptible to disorganization. They represented the "climax of nervous evolution." The mind, or consciousness, was a concomitant of the activity of the highest nervous centers. In every mental and nervous disorder, one could distinguish two basic components: the negative and the positive, respectively. The negative component reflected *dissolution,* that is, the reverse of evolution, and resulted from local or uniform losses of function of the nervous centers. The positive component, or symptoms, reflected activity of the intact lower centers released from inhibition by the higher centers. In uniform dissolution, there was a reversal of the whole nervous system in the direction of more organized, automatic, and primitive functioning.

Delirium exemplified the application of this theory to mental disorders generally. The psychopathology of a delirious patient could be regarded as partly negative and partly positive. The negative aspect resulted from some loss of function of the topmost layer of the highest centers. Defective orientation, impairment of memory and thinking, and confusion constituted negative symptoms, or deficits of consciousness. By contrast, misidentification of people and places, illusions, hallucinations, delusions, abnormal emotions, and disturbed behavior reflected activity of the second, lower, layer of the highest centers, which had been released from the control of the topmost layer; they comprised the remaining consciousness. The latter was defective, since to be confused implied that one had a defect of consciousness. Clinically, one encountered all degrees of defective or reduced consciousness in delirium, ranging from the "slightest confusion of thought to deepest coma" (48, v 1, p 187). Jackson compared the three degrees of defective consciousness to sleep without dreams, deeper sleep with somnambulism, and deep sleep without dreams, respectively. Delirium corresponded to the first two of these levels of reduced consciousness. The less the dissolution of the topmost layer, the more elaborate the mental manifestations of a delirious patient were liable to be. The milder the dissolution or the less defective the person's consciousness, the more marked was the influence on his symptoms of the rate of dissolution, of his personality, of his bodily states, and of external circumstances. In other words, the more the positive symptoms prevailed due to a relatively mild degree of dissolution of consciousness, the more complex and rich in variety and content was the delirious patient's clinical picture.

Jackson's theoretical views provided a novel approach to the interpretation of the psychopathology of delirium. The latter represented an intermediate state of consciousness between its clear normal state, on the one hand, and stupor and coma, on the other. The more profound the loss of function of the highest nervous centers, the more impoverished the delirious patient's mental contents were or the more pronounced the negative symptoms. These concepts provided a plausible theoretical basis for a unified view of delirium as a manifestation of reduced consciousness and for an interpretation of the patient's clinical picture. One must remember, however, that Jackson considered his theory of dissolution to be applicable to *all* mental disorders not just to delirium, which he saw as a rather simple form of mental derangement. Moreover, he used the terms "consciousness," "mind," and "mentation" synonymously and thus diminished the explanatory power of the concept of disordered consciousness as applied specifically to the syndrome of delirium. It was one thing to equate consciousness with mind, as Jackson did, and another to regard the former as a function or faculty of the latter.

In 1870, Bastian (49) published a lengthy article on consciousness in which he criticized those authors who equated it with the mind and proposed that it should be regarded as a "*special function* of some part or parts of the brain—the principal organ of mind" (italics added) (p 522). Consciousness was a product of molecular change in brain tissue. It was closely related to, if not coterminous with, attention.

In the years to follow, the above concept took hold and a variety of mental disorders, including delirium, came to be regarded as forms of disordered consciousness, the newly adopted independent mental function. Krafft-Ebing (50), for example, devoted a chapter in his textbook of psychiatry to what he designated "the elementary disturbances of consciousness," including psychic twilight states, dream states of waking life (delirium was included under this heading), stupor, and ecstasy. The clarity of consciousness had different levels indicated by the degree of distinctness of perceptions. Moreover, this author spoke of the "sphere of unconscious psychic life," one that was more important than the self-conscious "I" and whose activity was manifested in deliria and hallucinations.

Müller (51) published a monograph on the psychopathology of consciousness in 1889, devoting a chapter to states of inanition and fever delirium. He stated clearly that "delirium" meant a morbid alteration of consciousness in which the grasp of the external world became obscured by hallucinations. Not only fever, but also loss of blood, deprivation of food and drink, and severe illnesses could lead to this state. Children and the elderly were particularly prone to develop it.

In the same year, there appeared a paper by a Russian psychiatrist, Orschansky (52), devoted to the disturbances of consciousness and their relation to madness and dementia. The author listed a number of mental disorders, including confusion *(Verwirrtheit)*, characterized by a profound *clouding of consciousness* and a related beclouded state of the whole psychic activity. The recognition of external reality and the boundary between the "I" and "not I" disappeared. The ability to recall memories and to orient oneself in time and space were abolished. The behavior of the patient was without a purpose, and his feelings, drives, and impulses were unclear and weak. Depending on the degree of clouding, the condition of the patient could vary a great deal. Lucid intervals might occur. When the clouding was severe, the patient was close to stupor and coma. Hallucinations, illusions, and delusions were common. The confusion was usually either a brief episode or a phase in the evolution of a complicated psychosis. It was usually seen in the course of such conditions as hysteria, epilepsy, and neurasthenia. Psychopathological states dependent on organic brain disorders were not particularly suitable for the study of disturbances of consciousness, since they featured organic deficits that complicate the clinical picture.

Orschansky described a state rather closely resembling delirium but considered it a functional disorder. Berrios (47) claimed that clouding of consciousness became recognized during the second half of the nineteenth century as the clinical criterion distinguishing delirium from the other insanities. As the works quoted here illustrate, however, this statement is incorrect. It is true that delirium was usually included among disorders featuring altered or clouded consciousness, but so were some functional mental disorders. Even the seventh edition of Kraepelin's (53) textbook spoke of clouding of consciousness occurring in transient hysterical states, delirious mania, melancholia of involution, and catatonic stupor and excitement. The same comment applied to the concept of confusion.

The concept of "confusion" was elaborated first in France *(confusion mentale)* and later in Germany *(Verwirrtheit)* in the second half of the nineteenth century, although forerunners of it may be found even earlier in the French psychiatric literature (47,54). Actually the words "confusion" and "confused" had been used informally by medical writers for centuries to refer to disturbed cognition, especially in delirium and allied states. Willis (24), for example spoke of "confused thoughts" in this context. A disturbance of cogitation (thinking), imagination (perception), and memory as a core abnormality in delirium can be found in descriptions of it since at least the sixteenth century. The very notion—one so persistently expressed by many writers since the seventeenth century—that this syndrome, if not insanity generally, represents a waking dream, implies an altered state of mentation that amounts to confusion. Delasiauve (55) is usually credited with formalizing this concept in 1851. Not surprisingly, he saw it as being analogous to sleep with dreams. Confusion was further elaborated by Chaslin (56), who viewed what he called *"La confusion mentale"* as a core psychological impairment, one that featured an inability to think coherently and logically, reduced perceptual discrimination, and defective memory. One notes here a close resemblance to the traditional descriptions of the psychopathology of delirium. Superimposed on these basic deficits are hallucinations and dream-like (oneiric) mentation, seen in many delirious patients and most typically in delirium tremens. The confusional-oneiric syndrome can be idiopathic, or secondary to a whole range of organic disorders, or psychogenic. An analogous concept appeared in the German psychiatric literature under the terms *Verwirrtheit, Amentia,* and *Dysnoia* (47,54,57).

These two new concepts, clouding of consciousness and confusion, are closely related to each other and to delirium. They may be seen as attempts by nineteenth century psychiatrists to define a basic psychological disturbance characteristic of a whole class of mental disorders, one including, but not confined to, delirium. Some of these disorders were considered organic, some psychogenic. Since the second century A.D. delirium had been distinguished from other forms of psychopathology not so much on the basis of its constituent symptoms but rather on two criteria: association with fever or intoxication and acuteness. By contrast, insanity, mostly melancholia and mania, had been traditionally defined as chronic and occurring in the absence of fever. The concepts of clouding of consciousness and confusion allowed a redefinition of delirium on the basis of its characteristic psychopathological features, namely cognitive impairment and dream-like mentation. This could be seen as a certain refinement in the development of the concept of delirium and hence as an advance. Matters became complicated, however, as those two features were also found in some mental disorders lacking clear organic etiology. What followed was a deplorable tendency to coin a host of new terms to designate those disorders. This created a terminological and nosological confusion that came to bedevil this area of psychiatry for decades (54). Terms such as acute delirium, delirium acutum, acute delirious mania, delirium of collapse, amentia, confusional states, acute confusional insanity, and so forth, came to be used to refer to assorted mental disorders which shared certain clinical features with delirium caused by infectious, toxic, and other organic diseases. That terminological and conceptual chaos undoubtedly delayed progress in the further clarification of the concept of delirium and in the exploration of its etiology, pathogenesis, and psychophysiology. Moreover, the terms like clouding of consciousness and confusion were quite vague and poorly defined. They reflected nineteenth-century trends in psychology, such as the preoccupation with the concept of consciousness, and the prevailing notions about the mind-body and mind-brain relations. On the positive side, the introduction of these new concepts helped to attract attention to an important, and to this day poorly investigated, area of psychopathology, and to collect a wealth of interesting clinical observations. With time, the terminological mess got partly cleaned up and many of the superfluous terms were discarded. To trace their fate here would be confusing and pointless. Interested readers are referred to historical sources (47,54).

By the end of the nineteenth century the concept of delirium had been well established, at least in the English-language literature. This is reflected in the excellent discussion of it in Tuke's *Dictionary of Psychological Medicine* (58), published in 1892. The main impairment in delirium concerns the area of intellectual or cognitive functions. To this basic psychopathological core are added secondary features, i.e. disturbances of attention and perception, restlessness, incoherent speech, and delusions. Delirium represents a transient complication of a wide range of bodily diseases. The *Dictionary* made no reference to either clouding of consciousness or confusion.

An American psychiatrist, Worcester (59), published a clear account of delirium in 1889. He lamented that the syndrome had been taken for granted by most medical writers, who made no effort to differentiate it on the basis of its essential symptoms, rather than of its putative etiology, from other forms of insanity. Consequently, he proceeded to separate its "essential" from its "accidental" features. The former encompassed sensory disturbances, i.e., illusions and hallucinations, and mental bewilderment or confusion, with "failure to identify surrounding persons and objects." Either one or both of these core abnormalities had to be present. The accidental symptoms included abnormal emotions, reduced or increased psychomotor activity, delusions, and so forth. The patient might display lucid intervals. His emotional state tended to be influenced by hallucinations and delusions, and varied from case to case. Some patients were anxious, some amused, some despairing. They might sustain, or inflict on others, injuries resulting from attempts to attack or escape imaginary foes. The patient had an incomplete, if any, memory of the delirious experience once it was over, but might occasionally remember its more vivid fragments and refuse to accept that they did not reflect true external events. Delirium could be compared to dreaming. It constituted a well-defined, constant cluster of symptoms that distinguished it from most other forms of insanity, such as mania, melancholia, dementia, and delusional states.

Worcester's delineation of the core features of delirium came close to its modern definition. A similar attempt to define clearly the boundaries of this syndrome was made in an article by Hirsch (60), published at the very end of the century. He defined delirium as a "psychical state characterized by an abolition of self-consciousness, by an incoherence in the chain of conceptions, and by the appearance of symptoms of sensory and motor irritation" (p 109). The description that follows resembles that given by the earlier writers. What deserves mention, however, is the author's laudable effort to discuss the differential diagnosis between delirium, a condition due to a wide range of organic diseases, on the one hand, and similar psychopathological states of "agitated confusion which arise from pathological passions and affections," and may be seen in "hysteria and in most of the psychoses," on the other hand. In all these cases, a marked "cloudiness of self-consciousness" could be observed, and the differential diagnosis from delirium presented difficulties but should be attempted. Hirsch complained that this task was rendered even more arduous by the misguided tendency of many writers to introduce new terms to label the same disorder, and hence to create a false impression that many different yet similar disorders existed.

The above two clinical papers provide a welcome counterpoint to the conceptual and terminological muddle that arose in the wake of the introduction of the terms "clouding of consciousness" and "confusion." They provide a fit closure to the nineteenth-century efforts to define the clinical concept of delirium along descriptive lines with reasonable clarity.

The twentieth century

As noted in the preceding section, by the turn of this century the syndrome of delirium had been clearly delineated and linked etiologically with cerebral dysfunction due to a wide range of somatic diseases. Despite this progress, however, much remained to be studied and clarified. In particular, little was still known about this syndrome's pathogenesis and pathophysiology, its incidence and prevalence in various patient populations and clinical settings, and its relation to similar disorders occurring in the absence of physical disease. Moreover, much more needed to be done to improve the methods of its treatment and prevention and to formulate criteria for its diagnosis. Some progress has been achieved in all these areas during the course of this century, even though delirium has been largely ignored by both medical and psychiatric investigators. What advances have been made in elucidating the above issues owe much to the development of general hospital psychiatry in this century and the opportunity it offered psychiatrists to become better acquainted with psychiatric complications of physical illness. Delirium is one of the most common such complication to be encountered in general hospital settings.

A major development in the area of psychopathology due to somatic diseases took place early in this century with the appearance of Bonhoeffer's work (61,62). This German psychiatrist proposed that acute mental concomitants of physical illness fell into a single class of what he called "acute exogenous reaction types," including *delirium, epileptiform excitement, twilight state, hallucinosis,* and *amentia.* "Exogenous" in this context implied origin of the disorder in the body outside the brain, a notion not unlike that advanced by Galen in the second century A.D. In other words, Bonhoeffer's reaction types could be the result only of *systemic* diseases and not of those originating in the brain. They differed symptomatically from the endogenous, or functional, mental disorders, and to diagnose one of them on clinical grounds offered presumptive evidence that a cerebral disorder, one secondary to a systemic illness, was indeed present. The particular exogenous syndrome so diagnosed was in no way indicative of the nature of the underlying physical illness, however. In other words, the exogenous reaction types were *nonspecific* mental manifestations of somatic diseases, and no such disease gave rise to a uniquely specific mental disorder. Bonhoeffer's formulation of such diagnostic nonspecificity of the disorders under discussion ran directly counter to the then prevailing tendency, most prominently represented by Kraepelin (53), to look for and describe an allegedly characteristic mental disorder in every infectious, toxic, and other organic disease, a tendency that proved to be misleading. The main psychopathological feature showed by most exogenous reaction types is a disorder, a *clouding,* of consciousness. Bonhoeffer's work, despite some flaws to be discussed, was a major step in the development of psychiatry of somatic diseases and helped to advance it beyond the futile search for disease-specific mental syndromes, as Kraepelin and others had done. His work was based on meticulous clinical observations rather than on theoretical preconceptions. As Hoch (63), an American psychiatrist and his contemporary, observed, he had "greatly advanced our knowledge of delirium tremens and of deliria in general." Hoch himself followed Bonhoeffer's lead and investigated delirium induced by various drugs. He concluded that both delirium tremens and the drug-induced delirium shared the same core abnormality: "a constant tendency to dip down to a lower level of consciousness" and a "condition of mental dissociation analogous to dreaming or to the hypnagogic state, in which hallucinations are also present" (p 86).

In the decades that followed the publication of Bonhoeffer's work, some of his conceptions were modified and his terminology was changed. It became clear that not only acute systemic diseases but also the primary cerebral ones, as well as intoxication by assorted drugs and poisons, could give rise to one of the exogenous reaction types. The list of the latter has been shortened by the elimination of amentia, epileptic excitement, and twilight states. Only the terms "delirium" and "hallucinosis" have survived. Moreover, the importance of clouding of consciousness as a core feature of psychiatric concomitants of somatic diseases has been deemphasized (the term has been dropped from the list of the criteria of delirium in the revised edition of the American classification of mental disorders, or *DSM-III-R*).

In the United States, Adolf Meyer (64), a contemporary of Bonhoeffer, developed his own classification of mental disorders, or "mental reaction types," which included the so-called *dysergastic reactions,* whose prototype was delirium, with hallucinosis as its variant. This class of reactions included mental disorders due to "impaired nutritive and circulatory support" of the brain. Meyer's dysergastic reaction was meant to replace such overlapping terms as "symptomatic psychoses," "acute delirious mania," "delirium due to fever and drugs," and "toxic-infectious psychoses." The terms "delirium" and "dysergastic reaction" were synonyms and aimed at overcoming the terminological muddle in this area of psychiatry. As it happened, however, despite Meyer's preeminence in American psychiatry in the first half of this century, his terminology and classification never took hold. The term "dysergastic" has seldom been used, and "delirium" has become established as the designation for the most common and most important acute organic mental syndrome. This development became finally enshrined in *DSM-III*.

The description of delirium was further refined as a result of a classic clinical study by Wolff and Curran (65), published in 1935. A fine example of meticulous observation, that study has been much quoted in the literature of the past half-century despite its serious flaws. Its main flaw is the fact that it was carried out on a skewed patient population. The patients studied were those admitted to psychiatric wards, presumably on account of their severely disturbed and disturbing behavior, which interfered with their management on medical and surgical wards. Nearly one-third of them had abused alcohol, a fact judged by the investigators to be causally related to the delirium. Consequently, this clinical population was strongly prone to display the more flamboyant and inconstant features of the syndrome, such as marked restlessness, excitement, and vivid hallucinations. These symptoms characterize delirium associated with alcohol and drug withdrawal but are often lacking in the delirium of patients, especially the elderly, suffering from metabolic, toxic, and other diseases. Wolff and Curran's description of those conspicuous symptoms has been extensively and uncritically quoted and misrepresented as characterizing delirium generally. As a result, quiet, delirious patients have often been overlooked and undiagnosed by medical staff. Despite its methodological flaws, however, this study stands out as a laudable effort at painstaking description of the symptoms of delirium and provides an example worth following by future clinical investigators.

While Wolff and Curran advanced knowledge of the *symptoms* of delirium, other clinicians went beyond description and focused on its *pathogenesis* and *pathophysiology*, i.e., its two crucially important yet sorely neglected aspects. Two articles published in the 1930s address that issue. Hart (66) discussed the pathogenesis of delirium and pointed out how little was known about it. He asserted that a syndrome of delirium could not be precisely marked off, as it shaded into clinically similar pathological states, usually referred to in the literature as "acute confusional insanity," which were associated with functional psychoses and hysteria, and might arise in conditions of excessive fatigue and emotional stress. Turning to its pathogenesis, Hart stated: "Of the precise processes by which delirium is mediated we know nothing." He concluded that, in the great majority of cases, "the *primary* causal factors are 'organic,' and consist in a modification of brain substance produced either by a toxin or a degenerative process" (p 749).

In the second article, Robinson (67) discussed the important subject of delirium (acute confusional states) in later life. He referred to the recent work on brain function and proposed that cerebral arteriosclerosis and general aging of the brain lowered its metabolism and rendered it more susceptible to a variety of endogenous and exogenous toxic agents, which reduced its metabolic rate even further. Robinson considered this pathophysiological process responsible for "senile delirium," as distinct from senile dementia. He recommended intravenous dextrose infusions as appropriate treatment, since dextrose was vital to the brain.

Robinson's paper was important for two reasons: first, he drew attention to the common occurrence of delirium in the elderly, a subject of growing current importance on account of the aging of the population; and second, he was, as far as I am aware, the first writer to acknoweldge the crucial role of *cerebral oxidative metabolism* in the pathogenesis of delirium, a hypothesis further developed and tested in the 1940s.

Between about 1940 and 1946, a group of American investigators, one led by Romano and Engel, carried out pioneering work on delirium, published in a series of papers and summarized in a much-quoted article by Engel and Romano (68) in 1959. The researchers attempted to correlate clinical, psychological, and encephalographic (EEG) data in patients with delirium due to a variety of systemic diseases. Their approach combined clinical and experimental research methodology on a scale never before applied to the study of the syndrome. Their findings, first summarized in 1944 (69), led them to the following main conclusions. Delirium was a disturbance in the level of consciousness, one established clinically by patients' responses to tests of cognition. The syndrome depended on the presence of a cerebral disorder indicated by the general slowing of the EEG background activity. A lowering of the rate of brain metabolism was a necessary condition for the EEG slowing and the concomitant cognitive impairment, both of which tended to vary simultaneously: the greater the slowing, the more profound the degree of impairment. Psychiatric symptomatology of delirium reflected fluctuations in the level of awareness (consciousness). Those psychological variables that correlated best with the slowing of the EEG background activity included attention, memory, and comprehension. Manifest behavior of a delirious patient might range from overactivity and hyperarousal to lethargy and stupor.

The above studies represent a turning point in the development of the concept of delirium. The investigators went beyond the traditional descriptive and speculative approach and embarked on a *scientific inquiry* into the pathophysiological mechanisms underlying delirium. They also offered a measurable objective indicator for its diagnosis in the form of the EEG recording. Moreover, Romano and Engel formulated, more clearly than anyone before them, a *unified concept* of the syndrome, one that transcended the superficial variability of its behavioral features, such as the level of psychomotor activity, and was based on its essential psychopathological features. This development made it possible at last to differentiate delirium from symptomatically similar mental disorders that had baffled earlier writers. Unfortunately, the investigators soon abandoned this field of research and found few successors who attempted to replicate and extend their important findings. No comparably extensive studies of the syndrome have been carried out to date and are overdue.

Application of the work of Romano and Engel to all clinical variants of delirium was challenged by the neurologists Adams and Victor (70), who considered delirium tremens as the prototype of delirium, one in which slowing of the EEG background activity was absent. These authors used a different terminology and discounted the validity of the unified concept of delirium proposed by Romano and Engel. This controversy is discussed in a later chapter.

In the last 40 years, research on delirium has been relatively uninspired and has produced no breakthroughs. The most important studies were those on *experimental* delirium, induced by various anticholinergic agents, carried out in the 1960s and summarized by Itil and Fink (71). Those investigations highlighted the role of the disturbed balance of cerebral *neurotransmitters,* notably acetylcholine and noradrenaline, in the pathogenesis of delirium, and hence created an important new approach to the scientific inquiry into this subject. Otherwise, most recent studies on delirium have focused on such relatively narrow topics as delirium tremens, intoxication with various drugs, and metabolic encephalopathies. No systematic research on delirium as such, regardless of its specific etiology, has been reported. Trends in psychiatric research and theory had largely bypassed organic mental disorders until very recently. With the growing interest in the psychiatry of later life over the past decade, however, much attention has lately been paid to these disorders, notably to dementia. Aging of the population, and the high prevalence and incidence of cognitive disorders in the elderly, have made this trend inevitable. One may expect that it will soon extend to delirium, a very common disorder in the elderly.

The need to advance the development of the concept of delirium and to stimulate research on its various aspects called for an attempt to summarize what knowledge about it had accrued over the centuries. Moreover, it was necessary to review critically the relevent terminology and to try to bring some order to it. The article by Engel and Romano (68) went a long way to accomplish these tasks. Their effort was followed by Lipowski's (72) review of the syndrome in 1967 and to the publication of his monograph on this subject, the first to appear in English in modern times, in 1980 (73). Two of his overviews of delirium in later life came out subsequently (74,75). Moreover, Lipowski (76) proposed a new classification of organic mental (brain) syndromes, one that was largely adopted in the third edition of the classification of mental disorders of the American Psychiatric Association, published in 1980 (77). The latter, followed by its revision in 1987 (78), has not only firmly established delirium as one of the organic mental syndromes, but has also offered for the first time explicit criteria for its diagnosis. These publications have prepared the ground for the much-needed research on the syndrome that is yet to begin. Recent advances in the neurosciences and in the methodology of psychiatric research should also facilitate such future investigations.

This historical account covers 2,500 years. It documents an unbroken continuity of the clinical descriptive concept of delirium over the centuries despite the confusing vagaries of relevant terminology. The history of this concept underscores the value of clinical observation as the empirical cornerstone of progress in both medicine and psychiatry. Moreover, it constitutes an important chapter not only in the history of those two fields, but also in the development of ideas about the nature of humanity, of mind, and of the mind–body relationship.

References

1. Murray J. A. H. (ed): *A New English Dictionary on Historical Principles.* Vol 3, Oxford, Clarendon Press, 1897, p 165.
2. Celsus: *De Medicina.* 3 vols. Trans. by W. G. Spencer. London, Heinemann, 1938.
3. Frings P.: *A Treatise on Phrensy.* London, Gardner, 1746.
4. Hunter R., Macalpine I.: *Three Hundred Years of Psychiatry, 1535–1860.* London, Oxford University Press, 1963.
5. Laehr H.: *Die Literatur der Psychiatrie, Neurologie and Psychologie von 1459 bis 1889.* Berlin, Reiner, 1900.
6. Mettler C. C.: *History of Medicine; A Correlative Text, Arranged According to Subjects.* Philadelphia, Blakiston, 1947.
7. Whitwell J. R.: *Historical Notes on Psychiatry.* Philadelphia, Blakiston, 1937.
8. Drabkin I. E.: Remarks on ancient psychopathology. Isis 1955;46:223–234.
9. Jackson S. W.: Galen—on mental disorders. *J. Hist. Behav. Sci.* 1969;5:365–384.
10. Simon B.: *Mind and Madness in Ancient Greece.* Ithaca, N.Y.: Cornell University Press, 1978.
11. *The Medical Works of Hippocrates.* Trans. by J. Chadwick and W. N. Mann. Oxford, Blackwell, 1950.
12. Sprengell C.: *The Aphorisms of Hippocrates, and the Sentences of Celsus,* ed 2. London, Wilkin, Bonwick, Birt, et al, 1735.
13. Veith I.: The infancy of psychiatry. *Bull. Menninger Clin.* 1964;28:186–197.
14. *The Extant Works of Aretaeus, the Cappadocian.* F. Adams (ed). London, Sydenham Society, 1861.
15. Aurelianus C.: *On Acute Diseases and on Chronic Diseases.* I. E. Drabkin (ed). Chicago, University of Chicago Press, 1950.
16. Jackson S. W.: *Melancholia and Depression.* New Haven, Conn, Yale University Press, 1986.

17. Liebowitz J. O.: Studies in the history of alcoholism. II. Acute alcoholism in ancient Greek and Roman medicine. *Br. J. Addict.* 1967;62:83–86.
18. Hankoff L. D.: Ancient descriptions of organic brain syndrome: the "Kordiakos" of the Talmud. *Am. J. Psychiatry* 1972;129:147–150.
19. Diethelm O.: *Medical Dissertations of Psychiatric Interest.* Basal, Karger, 1971.
20. Cnobloch J.: *De Paraphrosyne s. Delirio et Diferentii's Suis.* Halle, 1569.
21. Haunoldt A.: *Disputatio de Delirio.* Witebergae, Gronenbergii, 1593.
22. Barrough P.; *The Method of Physick,* ed 3. London, Field, 1596.
23. *The Works of That Famous Chirurgion Ambrose Parey.* Trans. by T. Johnson. London, Cotes and Young, 1634.
24. Willis T.: *Two Discourses Concerning the Soul of Brutes.* London, Bring, Harper and Leigh, 1683.
25. Quincy J.: *Lexicon Physico-Medicum.* London, Bell, Taylor, Osborn, 1719.
26. James R.: *A Medicinal Dictionary.* London, Osborne, 1745.
27. Cheyne G.: *An Essay on Health and Long Life.* London, Strahan, 1725.
28. Hartley D.: *Observations on Man, His Duty, and His Expectations.* London, Leake and Frederick, 1749.
29. Cullen W.: *First Lines of the Practice of Physic.* ed 3. Vol 1. Edinburgh, Creech, 1781.
30. Darwin E.: *Zoonomia; or the Laws of Organic Life.* ed 3. Vol III. London, Johnson, 1801.
31. The Works of John Hunter, F. R. S., J. F. Palmer (ed.) Vol 1. London, Longman, Rees, Orme, Brown, Green and Longman, 1835.
32. Sims J.: Pathological remarks upon various kinds of alienation of mind. *Memoirs of the Royal Society of London,* 1799;5:372–406.
33. Rees A.: *The Cyclopedia; or Universal Dictionary of Arts, Sciences, and Literature.* First American ed. Philadelphia, S. F. Bradford, 1818.
34. Rush B.: *Medical Inquiries and Observations upon the Diseases of the Mind.* Philadelphia, Kimber & Richardson, 1812.
35. Sutton T.: *Tracts on Delirium Tremens, on Peritonitis and on Some Other Inflammatory Affections.* London, Underwood, 1813.
36. Pearson S. B.: Observations on brain fever. *Edinburgh Med. Surg. J.* 1813;9:326–332.
37. Greiner F. C.: *Der Traum and das fieberhafte Irreseyn.* Altenburg, F. A. Brockhaus, 1817.
38. Gallway M. B.: Nature and treatment of delirium. *Lond. Med. Gaz.* 1838;1:46–49.
39. Salter T.: Practical observations on delirium. *Prov. M. S. J. Lond.* 1850;677–684.
40. Hallaran W. S.: *Practical Observations on the Causes and Cure of Insanity.* Cork, Hodges & McArthur, 1818.
41. Fordyce G.: *Five Dissertations on Fever.* 2nd American ed. Boston, Bedlington and Ewer, 1823.
42. Armstrong J.: *Practical Illustrations of Typhus Fever.* New York, Duckinck, Long, Collins & Co; Collins & Hannay, 1824.
43. Holland H.: *Medical Notes and Reflections.* Philadelphia, Haswell, Barrington, and Haswell, 1839.
44. Dupuytren B. G.: On nervous delirium (traumatic delirium)—successful employment of laudanum lavements. *Lancet* 1834;1:919–923.
45. Jacyna L. S.: Somatic theories of mind and the interests of medicine in Britain, 1850–1879. *Med. Hist.* 1982:26:233–258.

46. Bucknill J. C., Tuke D. H.: *A Manual of Psychological Medicine.* ed 4. London, J & A Churchill, 1879.
47. Berrios G. E.: Delirium and confusion in the 19th century: A conceptual history. *Br. J. Psychiatry* 1981;139:439–449.
48. Jackson J. H.: *Selected Writings.* 2 vols. J. Taylor (ed). London, Hodder and Stoughton, 1932.
49. Bastian H. C.: Consciousness. *J. Ment. Sci.* 1870;15:501–523.
50. Krafft-Ebing R. von: *Lehrbuch der Psychiatrie.* Stuttgart, Enke, 1879.
51. Müller F. C.: *Psychopathologie des Bewusstseins.* Leipzig, Abel, 1889.
52. Orschansky J.: *Ueber Bewasstseinsstörungen und deren Beziehungen zur Verrücktheit und Dementia. Arch. Psychiatr. Nervenkr.* 1889;20:309–353.
53. Diefendorf A. R.: *Clinical Psychiatry.* Abstracted and adapted from the seventh German edition of Kraepelin E.: *Lehrbuch der Psychiatrie.* New York, Macmillan, 1915.
54. Gomirato G., Gamna G.: *Die Verwirrtheitszustände.* Basel, Karger, 1957.
55. Delasiauve M.: Du diagnostic differentiel de le lypémanie. *Ann. Med.-Psychol.* 1851;3:370–442.
56. Chaslin P.: *La Confusion Mentale Primitive.* Paris, Asselin et Houzeau, 1895.
57. Wille L.: Die Lehre von der Verwirrtheit. *Arch. Psychiatr.* 1888;19:328–351.
58. Tuke H. (ed): *Dictionary of Psychological Medicine.* 2 vols. London, Churchill, 1892.
59. Worcester W. L.: Delirium. *Am. J. Insanity* 1889;46:22–27.
60. Hirsch W.: A study of delirium. N.Y. *Med. J.* 1899;70:109–115.
61. Bonhoeffer K.: *Die Geistesstörungen der Gewonheitstrinker.* Jena, Fischer, 1901.
62. Bonhoeffer K.: Die Psychosen im Gefolge von akuten Infektionen, Allgemeinerkrankungen und inneren Erkrankungen, in Aschaffenburg G. L. (ed): *Handbuch der Psychiatrie,* Spez Teil 3. Leipzig, Deuticke, 1912, pp 1–60.
63. Hoch A.: A study of some cases of delirium produced by drugs. *Stud. Psychiatry* 1912;1:75–93.
64. Meyer A.: The problems of mental reaction-types, mental causes and diseases. *Psychol. Bull.* 1908;5:245–257.
65. Wolff H. G., Curran D.: Nature of delirium and allied states. The dysergastic reaction *A.M.A. Arch. Neurol. Psychiatry* 1935;33:1175–1215.
66. Hart B.: Delirious states. *Br. Med. J.* 1936;2:745–749.
67. Robinson G. W.: Acute confusional states of old age. *South. Med. J.* 1939;32:81–88.
68. Engel G. L., Romano J.: Delirium, a syndrome of cerebral insufficiency. *J. Chronic Dis.* 1959;9:260–277.
69. Romano J., Engel G.L.: Physiologic and psychologic considerations of delirium. *Med. Clin. North Am.* 1944;28:629–638.
70. Adams R. D., Victor M.: *Principles of Neurology,* ed 2. New York, McGraw-Hill, 1981.
71. Itil T., Fink M.: Anticholinergic drug-induced delirium: experimental modification, quantitative EEG and behavioral correlations. *J. Nerv. Ment. Dis.* 1966;143:492–507.
72. Lipowski Z. J.: Delirium, clouding of consciousness and confusion. *J. Nerv. Ment. Dis.* 1967;145:227–255.
73. Lipowski Z. J. *Delirium: Acute Brain Failure in Man.* Springfield, Ill, Charles C. Thomas, 1980.

74. Lipowski Z. J.: Transient cognitive disorders (delirium, acute confusional states) in the elderly. *Am. J. Psychiatry* 1983;140:1426–1436.
75. Lipowski Z. J.: Acute confusional states (delirium) in the elderly, in Albert M. L. (ed): *Clinical Neurology of Old Age.* New York, Oxford University Press, 1984, pp 277–297.
76. Lipowski Z. J.: A new look at the organic brain syndromes. *Am. J. Psychiatry* 1980;137:674–678.
77. *Diagnostic and Statistical Manual of Mental Disorders,* ed 3. Washington D.C., American Psychiatric Association, 1980.
78. *Diagnostic and Statistical Manual of Mental Disroders,* ed 3 revised. Washington, D.C., American Psychiatric Association, 1987.

2

Definition of Terms

A semantic muddle

In Chapter 1, the evolution of the clinical concept of delirium was traced back to the earliest Western medical writings, documenting the fact that a distinct syndrome corresponding to what we call "delirium" has been consistently identified and described by clinicians from the beginning. Furthermore, this syndrome has always been linked with physical illness, and has been considered to represent mental and behavioral manifestations of acute brain dysfunction due to primary or secondary cerebral diseases or to intoxication with some exogenous poison. Thus, delirium has been regarded throughout medical history as an organic mental syndrome par excellence. This view has prevailed despite the repeated failure to find gross cerebral pathology in delirious patients who came to autopsy. Fordyce (1), for example, writing in the early nineteenth century, marveled at the commonly normal appearance of the brain in patients dying in febrile delirium and wondered if the syndrome might arise as an "affection of the mind only." Such a "psychogenic" interpretation never took hold, however.

By contrast to the consistency of the *clinical description,* the term "delirium" was often used ambiguously, as pointed out in Chapter 1. Some writers used it to refer to the syndrome under discussion, while others applied it to insanity generally. That double connotation of the term persisted until the end of the eighteenth century. To make matters worse, numerous other designations have been used for the syndrome, resulting in a deplorable semantic muddle and skewed communication. This problem has persisted to this day. Liston (2) has recently found 30 synonyms for delirium in the medical literature. Overlapping, inconsistently used, and poorly defined terms have bedeviled this area of psychiatry and likely retarded progress in it. Terms such as "acute brain syndrome," "encephalopathy," "acute confusional states," "clouded states," "toxic psychosis," "toxic delirium," "acute organic psychosyndrome," "exogenous psychosis," "acute brain failure," "acute confusion," and so forth, have been applied indiscriminately by various writers to what is called "delirium or acute confusional states" in this book.

Welcome efforts to introduce consistency and order into the prevailing nosological and terminological chaos in this area have been made in recent years. The new classification of mental disorders of the American Psychiatric Association, *DSM-III* (3), has played a pioneering and crucial role in this regard. Not only has it established the term "delerium" as the only official designation for the syndrome, it has provided a set of explicit diagnostic criteria, further modified in its revised version, i.e., *DSM-III-R* (4). It has included delirium among the organic mental syndromes, i.e., those due to manifest cerebral dysfunction. This approach is being followed in the tenth edition of the *International Classification of Diseases,* whose 1987 draft of Chapter V (5) defines delirium as an "etiologically nonspecific organic cerebral syndrome characterized by concurrent disturbances of consciousness and attention, perception, thinking, memory, psychomotor behaviour, emotion, and the sleep-wake cycle" (p 27). The word "delirium" is stated to replace such terms as "acute confusional state," "acute brain syndrome," and "acute psycho-organic syndrome."

The above recent developments in the nosology and terminology of mental disorders may be expected to improve communication and to facilitate research. In regard to delirium, its position in the nosological system has at last become unambiguously and firmly established. To further clarify its status as a recognized organic mental syndrome, the definition and classification of these syndromes in *DSM-III-R* (4) needs to be discussed.

Delirium—an organic mental syndrome

Since the nineteenth century, it has been customary to divide mental disorders into organic and functional; this division is still in force today. An organic mental disorder constitutes a manifestation of *brain dysfunction,* either transient, permanent, or both (4,6). Such dysfunction may be caused by focal or widespread primary cerebral disease, or by a systemic disease affecting the brain secondarily, or by intoxication with an exogenous chemical agent such as a drug or a poison. In all these cases, there must be involvement of the anatomical and physiological substrate of one or more psychological functions for a mental disorder to become manifest. These functions encompass cognition, attention, consciousness, psychomotor behavior, emotions, drives, motivation of behavior, and personality. One or more of them may be implicated, depending on the localization, degree of spread, rate of progression, and other features of the underlying brain pathology. The psychopathological symptoms so induced tend to cluster together to form more or less distinct so-called *organic mental syndromes* (4). Identification of one of them on clinical grounds constitutes presumptive evidence that cerebral dysfunction due to one or more organic etiologic factors is present. Consequently, the diagnosis of such a syndrome should direct the clinician's attention to the underlying brain disorder, one whose nature needs to be identified in order to apply cause-specific treatment, if this is currently available. Therein lies the practical value of distinguishing a separate class of organic mental disorders. Such differentiation by no means implies that nonorganic, i.e., functional, psychopathological states occur independently of brain activity (4,6). On the contrary, all psychological functions, states, and processes are assumed to depend on it. For practical purposes, however, in the current state of our knowledge it is helpful to distinguish between those mental disorders *directly* caused by cerebral disease and those that reflect the personal meaning for the individual of information impinging on him, or representing a deviant personality or learned behavior patterns, or whose specific etiological organic factor has not yet been discovered (4,6,7).

In general, psychopathological manifestations of cerebral dysfunction include the following (7): 1. impairment of cognitive functions, i.e., thinking, memory, and perception; 2. disorders of consciousness (awareness), wakefulness, and attention; 3. personality change; and 4. compensatory and protective strategies displayed by the patient suffering from cognitive impairment.

Turning to the current psychiatric classification, a distinction is made between an "organic mental syndrome" and an "organic mental disorder" (4). The former term designates a set of psychological or behavioral symptoms due to the brain dynfunction without reference to etiology, while the latter refers to a particular mental syndrome whose etiology has been conclusively or presumptively established (4). The *DSM-III-R* (4) includes the following organic mental syndromes:

1. Delirium
2. Dementia
3. Amnestic disorder
4. Organic delusional disorder

5. Organic hallucinosis
6. Organic mood disorder
7. Organic anxiety disorder
8. Organic personality disorder
9. Intoxication
10. Withdrawal
11. Organic mental disorder not otherwise specified (NOS)

Delirium, dementia, intoxication, and withdrawal are the most common organic mental syndromes (4). The first two are noteworthy not only because they are the most important on account of their frequent occurrence, but also because both of them involve *global impairment of cognitive functions* (6,7), a feature that sets them apart from the other syndromes.

Definition of delirium

Having reviewed the position of delirium in the current classification of mental disorders I can offer its definition:

Delirium is a transient organic mental syndrome of acute onset, characterized by global impairment of cognitive functions, a reduced level of consciousness, attentional abnormalities, increased or decreased psychomotor activity, and a disordered sleep-wake cycle (4,5–7).

The above definition includes several important components that call for a comment. First, it is a *syndrome,* i.e., a set of concurrent psychopathological symptoms that constitute its essential diagnostic features. Second, it is an *organic* syndrome, i.e., one that involves cerebral dysfunction due to a specific etiological organic factor (or factors) as a necessary condition. Third, it is *acute* and *transient,* i.e., of sudden onset and relatively brief duration. It seldom lasts for more than one month and is never chronic. Fourth, its constituent psychopathological symptoms involve a *wide range* of psychological or behavioral functions, not merely those usually referred to as "cognitive" or "intellectual." Fifth, it is regarded, in part, as a *disorder of consciousness,* or awareness, but the old concepts of clouding of consciousness and confusion are no longer included in its definition. And sixth, it comprises a disorder of the *sleep-wake cycle,* a feature emphasized by medical writers for centuries but often ignored in the more recent literature.

The clinical features of delirium will be discussed in more detail in subsequent chapters, and the criteria for its diagnosis will be provided. Meanwhile, it is appropriate to review briefly the other designation used in the title of this book, i.e., "acute confusional states," as well as several other common and more or less synonymous terms still encountered in the medical literature.

"Acute confusional states" and related terms

"Acute confusional states" is the most often used synonym for "delirium," and for this reason only appears in the title of this book. The historical derivation of this term was discussed in Chapter 1. It stems from the word "confusion," which is devoid of a generally agreed upon meaning and hence is ambiguous. Even a cursory search of the recent medical and psychiatric sources bears this out. A recently published medical dictionary (8) offers separate definitions of "confusion" and "mental confusion." The former is defined as "disorientation resulting from memory impairment, hallucinations, mistaken interpretation of events, and/or uncertainty about one's role or identity" (p 621). "Disorientation" is not defined in this context, and it is not clear what it means. "Mental confusion" is defined as "a state of disorientation, often occurring in association with memory disturbances as part of a delirium" (p 621). A standard psychiatric dictionary (9) offers a somewhat different definition of "confusion": "In psychiatry this generally means a state of disordered orientation. It represents a disturbance of consciousness in the sense that awareness of time, place, or person is unclear. Confusion may be occasioned by *organic or psychic causes*" (italics added) (p 149). The latest edition of a representative medical textbook (10) focuses on disordered thinking: confusion is "a general term denoting an incapacity of the patient to think with customary speed and clarity" (p 127).

The word "confusion" is frequently encountered in the geriatric literature, where its meaning is so vague as to prompt an exasperated geriatrician to complain that "elderly patients who are disoriented are often referred to as being 'confused.' This overworked term covers a wide range of eccentricities of speech and behaviour and should not be applied as if it were a diagnosis" (11). Various writers have defined "confusion" as disorientation; inability to think clearly and coherently; and tenuous contact with reality and reduced awareness of one's relation to the environment (12–15). Moreover, for some authors, "confusion" is synonymous with "clouding of consciousness," while others assert that it features some degree of, or is actually caused by, the latter. Clearly, this term has been inconsistently defined and is highly ambiguous. It exemplifies the semantic and conceptual muddle referred to earlier in this chapter. One cannot but agree with Lishman (16), who deplores the fact that a term as vague as "confusion" has been presented by some writers as a hallmark of acute organic mental disorders and even incorporated into designations for them, as in "acute confusional states" and "acute confusion."

Just how ambiguous the term "confusion" really is has been demonstrated by Simpson (17). He sent a questionnaire to 274 doctors and nurses attached to a large teaching hospital in Britain and offered them a list of symptoms and signs, with a request to indicate which of them suggested that a patient was "confused." The variation in the responses was so great that no consistent meaning of the word emerged. Simpson concluded that the term "confused" should be used only if it was clearly defined.

The derivative term "acute confusional states" is hardly more unambiguous than the word it is derived from. It appeared for the first time in French and German psychiatric writings in the second half of the nineteenth century. Gomirato and Gamna (18) traced its history and shifting meaning up to the 1950s. They found that some writers used it more or less as a synonym for "delirium," while others applied it to designate delirium-like idiopathic or explicitly nonorganic mental disorders. The boundary between the acute confusional states and other psychiatric syndromes had never been satisfactorily defined. Lishman (16) points out that as confusion may be encountered in both organic and nonorganic mental disorders, it is advisable to avoid the use of this term in nosology. Some authors (19,20) have actually applied the term "acute confusional state" to a psychiatric condition bearing some superficial resemblance to delirium but usually induced by a stressful life event or change and lacking evidence of an etiological organic factor. The official French classification of mental disorders (21) distinguishes between confusional states with and without an organic etiology; the latter are considered schizophrenic.

While the term "acute confusional states" has been expurgated from the current American classification of mental disorders, it continues to be widely used in the medical, neurological, and geriatric literatures. Moreover, some medical writers insist on making a distinction between delirium and acute confusional states, two admittedly allied conditions (10,22). The latest edition of a widely used medical textbook (10), for example, distinguishes delirium from acute confusional states, which are associated with reduced altertness and decreased psychomotor activity. Delirium is said to denote a variant of confusional state—a broader diagnostic category—characterized by gross disorientation, heightened alertness, illusions, vivid hallucinations, psychomotor overactivity, and increased autonomic nervous activity. It is classically represented in an alcoholic patient. Thus, delirium tremens is viewed as a prototype of delirium generally. A mild form of this syndrome, often encountered in febrile diseases, lacks motor and autonomic overactivity and is sometimes called a "quiet," or "hypokinetic," delirium. By contrast, acute confusional states typically feature marked reduction of alertness and attentiveness, as well as of psychomotor activity.

It is difficult to fathom the logic of the above classification. Frankly idiosyncratic, it can hardly be justified on either clinical or etiological grounds. The two proposed syndromes overlap to a large extent, and it seems pointless to set them apart and attach different labels to them. Lishman (16) rightly observes that this classification is both cumbersome and of questionable clinical usefulness. Nor is enough known about the pathophysiology of the two syndromes to base the distinction on it. In this writer's opinion, this classification is quite arbitrary and liable to confuse clinicians, and should not be used. One term, "delirium," must suffice, unless and until future research provides adequate justification to split the syndrome on pathophysiological and pathogenetic grounds. It should be noted that for nearly two centuries many writers have observed that delirium can present in two contrasting *clinical forms* in regard to the level of alertness and psychomotor activity displayed by the patient. In some conditions, such as alcohol and hypnotic-sedative withdrawal states, the hyperalert and hyperactive form is the rule, but it may also be observed in delirium due to many other causes. Despite these opposed clinical presentations, delirium has been traditionally regarded as comprising them both, and hence a *unitary* view of the syndrome has largely prevailed. This viewpoint has been explicitly stated by the writers who carried out the most extensive research on delirium due to various causes reported to date, namely, Engel and Romano (23). Neither they nor the present writer (24–26) see a valid reason to split the syndrome asunder on the basis of its nonessential clinical manifestations. A transient global disorder of cognition, consciousness, and attention is a core feature of delirium, regardless of the level of consciousness (awareness) or psychomotor activity that a given patient exhibits, and which may often change from one extreme to another in the course of a single day. The same viewpoint has been adopted in *DSM-III-R* (4) and is expected to be incorporated in the forthcoming tenth edition of the *International Classification of Diseases* (5).

In conclusion, the terms "confusion" and "acute confusional states" are vague and ambiguous, and have been inconsistently used since their introduction into psychiatric nomenclature a century ago. The term "acute confusional states" should be considered a *synonym* for "delirium," albeit a clumsy and cumbersome one. Once the newly adopted psychiatric nomenclature becomes generally known and accepted, this term may be relegated to the annals of history.

Several other terms, more or less synonymous with "delirium," need to be mentioned. "Acute brain syndrome" was a term widely used in the psychiatric literature to denote a reversible organic mental disorder; since 1980 it has been replaced by "delirium" (3) and is now obsolete. "Toxic psychosis" refers to a severe organic mental syndrome caused by a drug or poison. It does not refer to any specific syndrome and has no place in the currently adopted psychiatric nomenclature, and its use is discouraged. "Infective-exhaustive psychosis" is an obsolete designation for a severe organic mental syndrome associated with an infectious disease. "Encephalopathy," a term used mostly by neurologists, refers to clinical, including psychopathological, manifestations of widespread failure of cerebral metabolism due to metabolic, toxic, or infectious diseases. Those manifestations typically involve a disorder of consciousness or awareness, such as delirium, stupor, or coma, as well as a variety of focal neurological signs and sometimes seizures. "Exogenous" or "symptomatic" psychoses are terms used mostly in the German psychiatric literature to refer to acute organic mental syndromes associated with systemic diseases.

In summary, the term "delirium" denotes a transient organic mental syndrome of acute onset and featuring concurrent disturbance of consciousness, a global cognitive and attentional disorder, reduced or increased psychomotor activity, and a disrupted sleep-wake cycle. This definition is in accordance with the currently adopted psychiatric nomenclature, and the term "delirium" replaces all related designations for the sake of clear communication. "Acute confusional states" is a synonym for "delirium," one still widely used in the nonpsychiatric medical literature.

References

1. Fordyce G.: *Five Dissertations on Fever.* 2nd American ed. Boston, Bedlington and Ewes, 1823.
2. Liston E. H.: Delirium in the aged. *Psychiatry Clin. North Am.* 1982;5:49–66.
3. *Diagnostic and Statistical Manual of Mental Disorders,* ed 3. Washington, DC, American Psychiatric Association, 1980.
4. *Diagnostic and Statistical Manual of Mental Disoders,* ed 3 revised. Washington, DC, American Psychiatric Association, 1987.
5. Draft of Chapter V, Mental, behavioural and developmental disorders in *International Classification of Diseases,* ed 10. Geneva, World Health Organization, June 1987.
6. Lipowski Z. J.: Organic mental disorders: Introduction and review of syndromes, in Kaplan H. I., Freedman A. M., Sadock B. J. (eds): *Comprehensive Textbook of Psychiatry,* ed 3. Baltimore, Williams & Wilkins, 1980, pp. 1359–1392.
7. Lipowski Z. J.: *Psychosomatic Medicine and Liaison Psychiatry. Selected Papers.* New York, Plenum, 1985.
8. Landau S. I. (ed.): *International Dictionary of Medicine and Biology.* Vol I. New York, Wiley, 1986.
9. Hinsie L. E., Campbell R. J.: *Psychiatric Dictionary,* ed 3. New York, Oxford University Press, 1960.
10. Braunwald E., Isselbacher K. J., Petersdorf R. G., et al (eds): *Harrison's Principles of Internal Medicine,* ed 11. New York, McGraw-Hill, 1987.
11. Adams G.: *Essentials of Geriatric Medicine.* Oxford, Oxford University Press, 1977.
12. Bedford P. D.: General medical aspects of confusional states in elderly people. *Br. Med. J.* 1959;2:185–188.
13. Isaacs B.: *An Introduction to Geriatrics.* London, Bailliere, Tindall and Cassell, 1965.
14. Roth M.: The psychiatric disorders of later life. *Psychiatr. Ann.* 1976;6:417–445.
15. Stengel E.: The organic confusional state and the organic dementias. *Br. J. Clin. Pract.* 1969;2:719–724.

16. Lishman W. A.: *Organic Psychiatry.* Oxford, Blackwell Scientific Publications, 1979.
17. Simpson C. J.: Doctors and nurses use of the word confused. *Br. J. Psychiatry* 1984; 441–443.
18. Gomirato G., Gamna G.: *Die Verwirrtheitszustände.* Basel, Karger, 1957.
19. Carlson H. B.: Identity-confusion (acute confusional state): Research design for identification of the syndrome and analysis of preliminary results. *Int. J. Neuropsychiatry* 1965;1:452–465.
20. Skoog G.: The course of acute confusional states. *Acta Psychiatr. Scand. Suppl.* 1968;203:29–32.
21. *Classification Française des Troubles Mentaux.* Bulletin de L'Institut National de la Santé et de la Recherche Médicale, Suppl. 2, 1969.
22. Adams R. D., Victor M.: *Principles of Neurology,* ed 2. New York, McGraw-Hill, 1981.
23. Engel G. L., Romano J.: Delirium: A syndrome of cerebral insufficiency. *J. Chronic Dis.* 1959;9:260–277.
24. Lipowski Z. J.: Delirium, clouding of consciousness and confusion. *J. Nerv. Ment. Dis.* 1967;145:227–255.
25. Lipowski Z. J.: Delirum (acute confusional state), in Frederiks J. A. M. (ed.): *Handbook of Clinical Neurology.* Vol 2 (No. 46): *Neurobehavioural Disorders.* Amsterdam, Elsevier, 1985, pp. 523–559.
26. Lipowski Z. J.: Delirum (acute confusional states). *J.A.M.A.* 1987;248:1789–1792.

3

Incidence and Prevalence

Few epidemiological studies of delirium have been reported to date. There is general agreement that the syndrome is common among general hospital patients, especially the elderly, but hard data are difficult to find. There are several likely reasons for this state of affairs. First, delirium is, by definition, a transient disorder of relatively brief duration, and as such may be considered by researchers to be both unimportant and difficult to study. Second, the syndrome occurs in the physically ill, and while physicians tend to see it mainly as a temporary nuisance, psychiatrists have limited access to patients suffering from it. As a result, neither group has enough motivation to study it. Third, lack of a generally accepted definition, terminology, and diagnostic criteria until lately may have deterred potential investigators. And fourth, no reliable and specific diagnostic test or scale for delirium has yet been developed, which hinders the search for cases.

Noting a variation in the reported incidence and prevalence data on delirium, Liston (1) cautions that they should be taken with a grain of salt. Such data may be divided into several categories, depending on the patient population studied and the clinical setting in which the study was carried out. For example, some investigators have focused exclusively on elderly patients admitted to general medical or psychiatric wards or specialized geriatric facilities. Clearly, the reported incidence and prevalence of delirium are liable to reflect the selective nature of this patient population. Other workers have screened all adult inpatients on one or more general medical wards, or those hospitalized in an intensive care unit, or those who had undergone some form of surgery. Lastly, a number of reports are confined to patients referred for psychiatric consultation from medical and surgical wards of a general hospital—hardly a representative sample. For clarity's sake, these studies will be reviewed under separate headings.

General medical inpatients

Engel (2) estimates that 10 to 15% of patients on acute medical and surgical wards are likely to exhibit delirium of varying severity. Swiss investigators (3) offer a lower estimate: 5 to 10%. These two estimates were made in the 1960s and may no longer hold, since the composition (mainly the age) of general hospital patients has changed in the past 20 years. Recent data show about 40% of all acute hospital beds are currently occupied by those aged 65 years and older (4). It is such elderly patients who are most likely to suffer from delirium.

In two large Swiss studies of psychiatric morbidity among medical and surgical patients, Modestin (5) found that 16.6% and 18.9%, respectively, suffered from an "acute exogenous reaction type," a term roughly equivalent to "delirium." Knights and Folstein (6) detected cognitive impairment in 33% of 57 medical inpatients but made no distinction between delirium and dementia. Considering, however, that the mean age of those patients was only 55, it is unlikely that many of them were demented. Cavanaugh (7) administered the Mini Mental Status Examination to 335 randomly selected hospitalized medical patients, 28% of whom showed evidence of cognitive dysfunction. In this study the mean age was 57, and it is likely that a large proportion of the subjects were delirious. The co-occurrence of delirium and dementia has been demonstrated in a Finnish study of 2,000 patients aged 55 years and older admitted to a department of medicine (8). The combined prevalence of the two syndromes was 20.4%. On admission, 15.1% were delirious and nearly 25% were subsequently found to be also demented; delirium was diagnosed in 41.4% of the latter group.

The above studies are hardly conclusive, given the differences in research methodology. One may tentatively accept Engel's (2) estimate that *10% to 15%* of medical and surgical inpatients are delirious at any point in time.

Hospitalized elderly patients

The elderly are particularly prone to develop delirium even in the course of a mild physical illness or as a side effect of medical drugs (9,10). Its incidence in later life has been claimed to be four times higher than that in younger adults and to be highest among patients older than 70 years (9,10). These claims are to some extent supported by the published data.

A geriatric multicenter British study (11) found that 35% of patients aged 65 years and older had delirium on admission or developed it during index hospitalization. Of 534 patients aged 60 or older admitted to psychiatric wards of the San Francisco General Hospital in 1959, 55% were diagnosed as having an acute brain syndrome (delirium), which in about 80% of the cases was associated with chronic brain disease (12). An even higher incidence (80%) was found among 5,000 patients 65 years and older admitted to the Oxford Geriatric Unit (13).

The above three studies were carried out in specialized, i.e., geriatric or psychiatric, clinical settings and may not be representative of general hospital medical inpatients. Two studies of such patients admitted to general medical wards reported an identical incidence of delirium on admission, i.e., 16% (14,15). Two more recent investigations of patients aged 70 years or older admitted to general medical wards found that 30% and 50%, respectively, showed delirium at some point during the index admission (16,17). By contrast, other investigators (18) reported a much lower incidence and prevalence of delirium in a comparable medical patient population, i.e., 10% and 17%, respectively. The researchers point out that their lower figures likely reflect different criteria for case finding. There is an obvious need for a carefully designed study of elderly medical patients from the time of hospital admission to discharge. Only such a study can resolve the discrepancies in the published incidence and prevalence data. Meanwhile, one may tentatively and conservatively estimate that *15% to 20%* of elderly medical inpatients are delirious at some point during the index admission.

Turning to elderly *surgical* patients, three studies report that 10% to 14% of those who underwent *general surgery* developed delirium postoperatively (19–21). The figures are much higher, i.e, 44% to 50%, following surgery for *hip fracture* (22,23). Cognitive impairment after such fracture prior to surgery was reported in 40% of the subjects (24,25). The high prevalence of dementia in female patients with hip fracture undoubtedly predisposes them to postoperative delirium. Overall, almost 50% of elderly patients with this injury develop delirium during their hospitalization (26). *Cataract surgery* has been reported to be followed by delirium in 0.3% to 15.9% of cases (27), but its current incidence is probably about 3% (28). *Myocardial revascularization* in elderly patients may induce transient delirium in about 10% of cases (29). However, in one series studied, only 2 out of 50 such patients who had undergone *open-heart surgery* became delirious postoperatively (30).

Specialized units

Delirium has been reported in 2% to 30% of patients hospitalized in *coronary and medical intensive care units* (31–34) and in 2% to 30% of those in *surgical intensive care units* (35–37). Anesthetists have reported *postoperative* "emergence" delirium in 5% to 6% of a large series of surgical patients (38). In a random sample of 200 *surgical* patients, delirium was found in 7.8% (39). Finally, the incidence of the syndrome following *burns* has been variously reported to range from 5% to 57% (40–44).

Medical and surgical inpatients referred for psychiatric consultation

Patterns of referral for psychiatric consultation of medical and surgical inpatients have been the subject of many published studies (45–49). In most of these reports, however, no distinction is made between delirium and dementia, the most commonly encountered organic mental syndromes in general hospital patients. Investigators usually refer to the "organic brain syndrome" or "organic mental disorder," without further specifying the type of syndrome so diagnosed. In general, there has been a marked increase in recent years in the number of *elderly* medical and surgical inpatients referred for psychiatric consultation, a trend reflecting the aging of the population. Currently, patients aged 60 years and older account for 20% to 30% of the referrals (45–48). As these patients are the ones who most often display symptoms of delirium or dementia, or both, it is not surprising that these syndromes constitute about 27% of all psychiatric diagnoses assigned by the consultants (45,49). Delirium accounts for about one-half of these diagnoses, i.e., about 10% to 15% of all patients referred for psychiatric consultation from medical and surgical wards (49–52). In *surgical* inpatients, the syndrome is reported reported to account for a much higher proportion of the diagnoses assigned to referred patients, i.e., 26% (53).

In summary, little is known about the epidemiology of delirium. Published data about its incidence and prevalence are few, discrepant, and of questionable reliability. It is generally accepted that it is most common in children and the elderly; however, no information can be found in the literature about its incidence in pediatric settings. The available data tend to support the contention that delirium is most often encountered in hospitalized, medically ill, elderly patients. Because the proportion of such patients in the population at large and in the general hospitals is steadily growing, one may expect that the incidence and prevalence of the syndrome will rise in the years to come. Meanwhile, one may tentatively estimate that between 10% and 15% of medical and surgical general hospital inpatients are delirious at any given time. This percentage is likely to be higher if one considers only the patients aged 60 years and older. The higher the average age of a given patient population, the greater the incidence and prevalence of delirium are likely to be.

References

1. Liston E. H.: Delirium in the aged. *Psychiatr. Clin. North. Am.* 1982;5:49–66.
2. Engel G. L.: Delirium, in Freedman A. M., Kaplan H. S. (eds.): *Comprehensive Textbook of Psychiatry.* Baltimore, Williams & Wilkins, 1967, pp 711–716.
3. Bleuler M., Willi J., Buhler H. R.: *Akute psychische Begleiterscheinungen Körperlicher Krankheiten.* Stuttgart, Thieme, 1966.
4. *Utilization of Short-Stay Hospitals: Annual Summary for the United States, 1980.* Series 13, No. 64. Washington, D. C., U. S. Dept of Health and Human Services, National Center for Health Statistics, 1982.
5. Modestin J.: Psychiatrische Morbidität bei intern-medizinisch hospitalisierten Patienten. *Schweiz. Med. Wochenschr.* 1977:107:1354–1361.
6. Knights E. B., Folstein M. F.: Unsuspected emotional and cognitive disturbance in medical patients. *Ann. Intern. Med.* 1977;87:723–724.
7. Cavanaugh S.: The prevalence of emotional and cognitive dysfunction in a general medical population: Using the MMSE, GHQ and BDI. *Gen. Hosp. Psychiatry* 1983;5:15–24.
8. Erkinjuntti T., Wikström J., Palo J., et al: Dementia among medical inpatients. *Arch. Intern. Med.* 1986;146:1923–1926.
9. Lipowski Z. J.: Transient cognitive disorders (delirium, acute confusional states) in the elderly. *Am. J. Psychiatry* 1983;140:1426–1436.
10. Lipowski Z. J.: Acute confusional states (delirium in the elderly, in Albert M. L. (ed): *Clinical Neurology of Old Age.* New York, Oxford Universtiy Press, 1984, pp 277–297.
11. Hodkinson H. M.: Mental impairment in the elderly. *J. R. Coll. Physicians Lond.* 1973;7:305–317.
12. Simon A., Cahan R. B.: The acute brain syndrome in geriatric patients. *Psychiatric Res. Rep.* 1963;16:8–21.
13. Bedford P. D.: General medical aspects of confusional states in elderly people. *Br. Med. J.* 1959;2:185–188.
14. Bergmann K., Eastham E. J.: Psychogeriatric ascertainment and assessment for treatment in an acute medical ward setting. *Age Ageing* 1974;2:174–188.
15. Seymour D. G., Henschke P. J., Cape R. D. T., et al: Acute confusional states and dementia in the elderly: The role of dehydration/volume depletion, physical illness and age. *Age Ageing,* 1980;9:137–146.
16. Gillick M. R., Serrell N. A., Gillick L. S.: Adverse consequences of hospitalization in the elderly. *Soc. Sci. Med.* 1982;16:1033–1038.
17. Warshaw G. A., Moore J. T., Friedman S. W., et al: Functional disability in the hospitalized elderly. *J.A.M.A.* 1982;248:847–850.
18. Johnson J., Sullivan E., Gottlieb G., et al: Delirium in elderly patients on internal medicine services. *J. Am. Geriatr. Soc.* 1987;35:972.
19. Seymour D. G., Pringle R.: Post-operative complications in the elderly surgical patient. *Gerontology* 1983;29:262–270.
20. Millar H. R.: Psychiatric morbidity in elderly surgical patients. *Br. J. Psychiatry* 1981;138:17–20.
21. Chung F., Meier R., Lautenschlager E., et al: General or spinal anesthesia: Which is better for the elderly? *Anesthesiology* 1987;67:422–427.
22. Berggren D., Gustafson Y., Eriksson B., et al: Postoperative confusion after anesthesia in elderly patients with femoral neck fractures. *Anesth. Analg.* 1987; 66:497–504.

23. Williams M. A., Campbell E. B., Raynor W. J., et al: Predictors of acute confusional states in hospitalized elderly patients. *Res. Nurs. Health* 1985;8:31–40.
24. Billig N., Ahmed S. W., Kenmore P., et al: Assessment of depression and cognitive impairment after hip fracture. *J. Am. Geriatr. Soc.* 1986;34:499–503.
25. Haljamae H., Stefansson T., Wickstrom I.: Preanesthetic evaluation of the female geriatric patient with hip fracture. *Acta Anaesth. Scand.* 1982;26:393–402.
26. Campion E. W., Jette A. M., Cleary P. D., et al: Hip fracture: A prospective study of hospital course, complications, and costs. *J. Gen. Intern. Med.* 1987;2:78–82.
27. Summers W. K., Reich T. C.: Delirium after cataract surgery: A review and two cases. *Am. J. Psychiatry* 1979;136:385–391.
28. Karhunen U., Orko R.: Psychiatric reactions complicating cataract surgery: A prospective study. *Ophthalmic Surg.* 1982;13:1008–1012.
29. Calabrese J. R., Skwerer R. G., Gulledge A. D., et al: Incidence of postoperative delirium following myocardial revascularization. *Cleve. Clin. J. Med.* 1987;54:29–32.
30. Pelletier L. C., Castonguay Y. R., Chaitman B. R.: Open-heart surgery in elderly patients. *Can. Med. Assoc. J.* 1983;128:409–412.
31. Holland J., Sgroi S. M., Marwit S. J., et al: The ICU syndrome: Fact or fancy? *Psychiatry Med.* 1973;4:241–249.
32. Cay E. L., Vetter N., Philip A. E., et al: Psychological reactions to a coronary care unit. *J. Psychosom. Res.* 1972;16:437–447.
33. Parker D. L., Hodge J. R.: Delirium in a coronary care unit. *J.A.M.A.* 1967;201:702–703.
34. Hackett T. P., Cassem N. H., Wishnie H. A.: The coronary-care unit. An appraisal of its psychologic hazards. *N. Engl. J. Med.* 1968;279:1365–1370.
35. Hale M., Koss N., Kerstein M., et al: Psychiatric complications in a surgical ICU. *Crit. Care Med.* 1977;5:199–203.
36. Katz N. M., Agle D. P., De Palma R. G., et al: Delirium in surgical patients under intensive care. *Arch. Surg.* 1972;104:310–314.
37. Wilson L. M.: Intensive care delirium. *Arch. Intern. Med.* 1972;130:225–226.
38. Coppolino G. A.: Incidence of post-anesthetic delirium in a community hospital: A statistical study. *Milit. Med.* 1963;128:238–241.
39. Titchener J. L., Zwerling L., Gottschalk L., et al: Psychosis in surgical patients. *Surg. Gynecol. Obstet.* 1956;102:59–65.
40. Andreasen N. J. C., Noyes R., Hartford C. E., et al: Management of emotional reactions in seriously burned adults. *N. Engl. J. Med.* 1972; 286:65–69.
41. Antoon A. Y., Volpe J. J., Crawford J. D.: Burn encephalopathy in children. *Pediatrics* 1972;50:609–616.
42. Steiner H., Clark W. R.: Psychiatric complications of burned adults: A classification. *J. Trauma* 1977;17:134–143.
43. May S. R., Ehleben C. M., De Clement F.: Delirium in burn patients isolated in a plenum laminar air flow ventilation unit. *Burns* 1984;10:331–338.
44. Mohnot D., Snead O. C., Benton J. W.: Burn encephalopathy in children. *Ann. Neurol.* 1981;12:42–47.
45. Mainprize E., Rodin G.: Geriatric referrals to a psychiatric consultation-liaison service. *Can. J. Psychiatry* 1987;32:5–9.
46. Popkin M. K., MacKenzie T. B., Callies A. L.: Psychiatric consultation to geriatric medically ill inpatients in a university hospital. *Arch. Gen. Psychiatry* 1984;41:703–707.

47. Rabins P., Lucas J., Teitelbaum M., et al: Utilization of psychiatric consultation for elderly patients. *J. Am. Geriatr. Soc.* 1983; 31:581–585.
48. Wallen J., Pincus H. A., Goldman H. H., et al: Psychiatric consultations in short-term hospitals. *Arch. Gen. Psychiatry* 1987;44:163–168.
49. McKegney F. P., McMahon T., King J.: The use of *DSM-III* in a general hospital consultation-liaison service. *Gen. Hosp. Psychiatry* 1983;5:115–121.
50. Lee M. B.: Organic brain syndromes seen in psychiatric consultation in a general hospital. *J. Formosan Med. Assoc.* 1981;80:119–128.
51. Montero I., Sanjuan J., Frades B.: A Spanish experience of *DSM-III* in a consultation-liaison psychiatric service. *Acta Psychiatr. Scand.* 1986;74:536–541.
52. Trzepacz P. T., Teague G. B., Lipowski Z. J.: Delirium and other organic mental disorders in a general hospital. *Gen. Hosp. Psychiatry* 1985;7:101–106.
53. Golinger R. C.: Delirium in surgical patients seen at psychiatric consultation. *Surg. Gynecol. Obstet.* 1986;163:104–106.

4

Clinical Features, Course, and Outcome

Chapter 1 traced the historical development of the concept of delirium as a clinical syndrome whose essential features have been consistently described since the second century A.D. This consistency is remarkable in view of the fact that the syndrome's clinical presentation may be quite variable, as pointed out by Fothergill (1) more than 100 years ago: "each differs somewhat from every other case, and there are peculiarities in each and every one. In order, then to meet such cases with a fair attention to their needs, the first thing requisite is a pretty clear comprehension of delirium as a whole" (p 400). This chapter tries to achieve that purpose by elucidating both the essential and the associated features of delirium, paying proper attention to its clinical variants. This task was facilitated in the 1980s by the publication of the new psychiatric classification, *DSM-III* (2), and its revised version, *DSM-III-R* (3), which provide both a standard description of the syndrome and explicit criteria for its diagnosis. The clinical features, course, and outcome of delirium will now be presented. Its psychopathology will be discussed in considerable detail in Chapter 5.

Essential characteristics

The following features of delirium are considered essential for its identification in clinical practice and for research (3–5):

1. Impaired awareness of self and surroundings (also referred to as "reduced level of consciousness").
2. Impairment of directed thinking.
3. Disorder of attention, with hypo- or hyperalertness.
4. Impairment of memory.
5. Diminished perceptual discrimination, with a tendency toward misperceptions, i.e., illusions and hallucinations.
6. Impairment of spatiotemporal orientation (may be absent in a mild case).
7. Disturbance of psychomotor behavior, with hyper- or hypoactivity, both verbal and nonverbal.
8. Disordered sleep-wake cycle, usually marked by drowsiness and naps during the day, insomnia at night, or both.
9. Unpredictable fluctuations in alertness and in severity of cognitive impairment during the day and overall exacerbation of symptoms at night and upon awakening.
10. Acute onset and relatively brief duration (hours to several weeks).
11. Laboratory evidence of widespread cerebral dysfunction, especially diffuse changes (slowing or fast activity) of background activity on the EEG.

The above list of essential features comprises the basic psychopathology of delirium and links it causally to cerebral dysfunction. The most constant features include global impairment of cognitive processes (thinking, remembering, and perceiving), as well as attentional abnormalities and a reduced level of awareness of the self and the environment. The patient displays *defective ability to extract, process, and retain information,* and to relate ongoing stimuli from the environment and his or her body to previously acquired knowledge. Consequently, the grasp of the situation is faulty, and the patient displays a diminished capacity to act in the customary purposeful, sustained, and goal-directed manner. Behavior tends to be erratic and unduly influenced by cognitive distortions and poorly controlled impulses.

In addition to the essential features just discussed, a delirious patient may display a gamut of inconstant and highly variable *associated symptoms* (3). These include emotional and mood disturbances ranging from apathy to rage and fear; increased autonomic nervous activity manifested by tachycardia, sweating, dilated pupils, flushed face, and elevated blood pressure; involuntary movements such as asterixis; dysnomia and dysgraphia; confabulation; and perseveration.

DSM-III-R (3, p 103) offers the following diagnostic criteria for delirium that include its essential features:

A. Reduced ability to maintain attention to external stimuli (e.g., questions must be repeated because attention wanders) and to appropriately shift attention to new external stimuli (e.g., perseverates answer to previous question).
B. Disorganized thinking, as indicated by rambling, irrelevant, or incoherent speech.
C. At least two of the following:
   (1) reduced level of consciousness, e.g., difficulty keeping awake during examination
   (2) perceptual disturbances: misinterpretations, illusions, or hallucinations
   (3) disturbance of sleep-wake cycle with insomnia or daytime sleepiness
   (4) increased or decreased psychomotor activity
   (5) disorientation to time, place, or person
   (6) memory impairment, e.g., inability to learn new material, such as the names of several unrelated objects after five minutes, or to remember past events, such as history of current episode of illness
D. Clinical features develop over a short period of time (usually hours to days) and tend to fluctuate over the course of a day.
E. Either (1) or (2):
   (1) evidence from the history, physical examination, or laboratory tests of a specific organic factor (or factors) judged to be etiologically related to the disturbance
   (2) in the absence of such evidence, an etiologic organic factor can be presumed if the disturbance cannot be accounted for by any nonorganic mental disorder, e.g., Manic Episode accounting for agitation and sleep disturbance

The above diagnostic criteria should be regarded as no more than the currently suggested *guidelines* for diagnosis; they are neither flawless nor immutable. Examined more closely, they imply that only two psychopathological features must be present in all cases: attentional disorder and disorganized thinking. Any of the remaining symptoms may be absent in a given case. It follows that neither a reduced level of consciousness nor global cognitive impairment need be present. This implication is erroneous and misleading. It contradicts clinical observations consistently reported for centuries. Moreover, the criteria include evidence not of cerebral dysfunction but rather of an "organic factor," and permit diagnosis of delirium even in the absence of such a factor, and hence by exclusion. Clinicians and researchers would be ill-advised to accept the above criteria literally and uncritically, as they are flawed and do not reflect clinical reality. The current draft of the tenth revision of the *International Classification of Diseases* (6) offers much more satisfactory guidelines for the diagnosis of the syndrome (pp 27–28):

1. Impairment of consciousness and attention;
2. Global disturbance of cognition;
3. Psychomotor disturbance;
4. Disturbance of the sleep-wake cycle; and
5. Emotional disturbances.

The following descriptive account of the symptoms of delirium and its course is intended to flesh out the rather abstract and schematic diagnostic criteria just discussed. It is based on personal clinical observation of delirious patients seen in general hospital settings.

Mode of onset

The onset of delirium is typically rapid, usually developing within a few hours or days. It often occurs *at night.* The mode of onset depends to some extent on the cause. Delirium resulting from concussion or following major surgery tends to come on immediately after the event, while that occurring in the course of an infection or with metabolic encephalopathy may have a more gradual onset. In the latter case, one may often distinguish a *prodromal stage* during which the patient tends to have some difficulty in concentrating and thinking clearly; feels restless and anxious; and may complain of irritability, fatigue, malaise, hypersensitivity to lights and sounds, drowsiness, insomnia, vivid dreams or nightmares, and even transient illusions and hallucinations. Many of us have experienced some of these symptoms in the course of a febrile illness and can attest to their unpleasantness. Every mental effort is unwelcome, and one tends to drift from reverie to sleep and back. At night one is apt to wake up startled, sometimes remembering a vivid, and likely an unpleasant dream, and to wonder for a moment where one is.

Symptoms and course

The patient may never progress beyond the prodromal stage. Or the symptoms may increase in intensity and the patient grows more restless or drowsy, experiences difficulty in thinking coherently, and becomes unsure of the time. Attention to the surroundings waxes and wanes, and illusions and hallucinations, mostly in the visual sphere, may now appear. A full-blown delirium often occurs at night. The patient wakes up and finds it difficult to tell if he or she is still dreaming. The dreams may now continue as hallucinations, and the patient tends to accept them as real happenings and to respond to them according to their content. If they are frightening, as they often are, he or she responds with fear and is likely to try to get out of bed and run away. This is most likely to happen if the patient is in an unfamiliar place, such as a hospital, and is not sure where he or she is and why. As Fothergill (1) put it so well, "Every sick person craves ardently to be at home amidst relatives and friends; and in delirium the craving commonly takes the direction of an attempt to get away home by immediate escape from the room occupied at the time" (p 404). If such behavior occurs on a hospital ward, the night nurse becomes alarmed, notes in the chart that the patient is confused, and asks the doctor on call to intervene. If the patient tries to resist attempts to be returned to bed, a wild struggle and an injection of a potent tranquilizer are liable to follow. The patient may then wake up the next morning relatively lucid and cooperative, and the nocturnal episode is apt to be ignored unless it recurs the next night or the patient shows evidence of being disturbed, disoriented, and agitated on awakening.

A mildly delirious patient may be aware of and alarmed by the increasing difficulty in marshaling and directing thoughts at will, by the misperceptions, and by difficulty recalling events of the preceding few days. He or she is liable to react to the awareness of these difficulties with anxiety, embarrassment, and attempts to appear normal. When spoken to, the patient may try to conceal the experienced confusion by answering questions briefly and avoiding topics that might expose his or her faulty memory, grasp, and orientaton. Some patients may explicitly deny being confused or try to cover up their cognitive deficits by voicing physical complaints or by asking politely how the doctor is feeling. When an examiner tries to assess such a patient's mental state by asking questions about orientation or memory, for example, the patient often evades the issue by attempts to change the subject or return the questions, by jokes or sarcastic remarks, by embarking on some irrelevant story, and at times by an outburst of anger or tears. Other patients make an earnest effort to answer questions, but do so slowly and hesitantly, and may actually complain of being forgetful and confused. Patients tend to vary markedly in their manner of coping with subjective awareness of being cognitively impaired. Such individual differences in response, both emotional and behavioral, reflect the patient's personality and contribute to the striking variability in the clinical manifestations of delirium that no diagnostic criteria can encompass (7).

If, for whatever reason, delirium progresses in severity, the initial symptoms become more conspicuous and the patient's subjective sense and objective signs of confusion intensify. The word "confusion" is commonly used in this context by both staff and patients. It is an imprecise term that usually implies a combination of incoherent thinking, difficulty in grasping the meaning of verbal and nonverbal stimuli, forgetfulness, bewilderment, and spatiotemporal disorientation. The patient usually exhibits some degree of defective orientation at least for time, but, in more severe delirium, also for place and person, becoming unable to identify correctly his or her whereabouts and familiar people. At first, the patient cannot give the correct day of the week and the date; this can progress to an inability to state correctly the month, the season, and the year. Yet some ability to orient oneself in time may still be present. For example, the writer once interviewed a delirious Vermont farmer hospitalized in New Hampshire. The patient was totally disoriented for time and place, but when asked to look through the window, he said: "This looks like apple-picking time." He was correct and demonstrated some intact ability to use relevant cues and to respond in keeping with his habitual experience. Orientation for place is liable to be impaired once that for time is seriously defective. The patient tends to mistake the hospital for home, a hotel, or a hospital with which he or she is most familiar. As the severity of delirium increases, the patient misidentifies not only the surroundings but also familiar persons. Nurses and doctors are mistaken for relatives or friends, or the patient views them as strangers engaged in other than their actual occupations: a doctor may be thought to be a chef because of his white coat, and nurses are often misidentified as waitresses. Some patients give truly delusional misidentifications presumably reflecting their cognitive distortions of the situation. For example, doctors may be referred to as butchers or undertakers and nurses as prostitutes. Such errors may offend some staff members, even though they are not likely to express the patient's desire to insult them. In the most severe delirium, patients may be unable to recognize their next of kin, but they hardly ever lose the sense of their own identity. On the whole, a delirious patient tends to mistake unfamiliar places and persons for familiar ones until even the latter can no longer be recognized.

Pari passu with progressive confusion and as the severity of delirium grows, the patient becomes increasingly distractible and either drowsy and lethargic or, at the other extreme, hyperalert and agitated. In either case, however, there is mounting difficulty in deploying, fixing, and directing attention at will. This is apparent to the examiner, who finds that the patient cannot maintain contact and communicate coherently for more than a brief period, if at all. Uncontrolled, often dream-like, thoughts lacking direction appear to dominate the patient's awareness; hallucinations may intrude; the question or the beginning of the sentence is forgotten; and the patient may doze off or seem to be preoccupied with hallucinatory images and sounds. Concurrently, thinking becomes increasingly labored and slow or rapid but incoherent. This disorganization of thought processes is evidenced by spontaneous utterances and responses to questions. Perceptual discrimination is likewise affected, and the patient's capacity to discriminate what is perceived and to interpret it correctly wanes. Misperceptions, i.e., illusions and hallucinations, most often visual but in some cases accompanied by auditory ones, are apt to be present at this stage, and the patient has difficulty in distinguishing them from true perceptions. Not all delirious patients hallucinate, however, and some may only do so at night. Typically, the patient accepts the hallucinations as real happenings and reacts to them accordingly. He or she may speak to, shout at, or curse the hallucinated images, follow them with the eyes, reach out to or recoil from them, or try to escape or attack them. Fear, anger, or amusement may all be experienced and expressed by the patient verbally in response to the hallucinations, and these emotions are usually reflected in his or her facial expression, gestures, and actions.

To an observer the patient may display a whole range of behavior, one of which may predominate yet shift unpredictably to a different one. He or she may look inert, sleepy, and withdrawn or, by contrast, restless, fidgety, and vigilant. A drowsy or an alert but quiet patient tends to respond to questions slowly, with a bewildered or indifferent facial expression, and with long pauses between words. Such a patient may ask to be left alone or otherwise indicate a wish not to be disturbed. This may be expressed in a moaning, pleading, or irritated voice. The examiner must make persistent effort to engage such a patient in a verbal exchange long enough to allow assessment of the mental status.

Other patients may scan the surroundings with their eyes and then suddenly exclaim as if in fear, cringe, speak excitedly to an invisible person or animal, or make a striking motion as if in self-defense or attack. The patient may seem to look for something on or under the bed, pick at bedclothes, mutter, laugh, sing, call for help, wail, or curse. Such noisy behavior is liable to alert and alarm the staff and to result in an urgent call for a psychiatric consultation. Attempts to get out of bed are commonly seen in restless and frightened patients, and injuries may readily result. When approached, a hyperactive and excitable patient looks bewildered, fearful, or annoyed. He or she may start to answer a question and then suddenly look away, point to a corner of the room, and shout that "they" must be thrown out. Noisy and fearful or angry vocalizations may be made repeatedly, and are particularly common and disturbing at night. Pleas to be allowed to go home, for example, can go on for hours, interrupted by bursts of low muttering, moaning, or screams for help. One delirious patient kept the whole ward awake by screaming "murder!" again and again throughout the night.

At any time, unpredictably, an agitated, restless, and obviously hallucinating patient may calm down, ask about his or her whereabouts, inquire about the time or a meal, ask to see a doctor or family member, and answer questions relatively coherently and precisely. Such "lucid intervals" constitute irregular breaks from the confusion during which the patient is transiently more attentive, coherent, and rational. These periods are quite characteristic of delirium. The waxing and waning of the patient's alertness, cognitive impairment, and psychomotor activity over the course of a day are usually referred to as "fluctuations" in the level of awareness. If present, as they often are, they strongly suggest the diagnosis of delirium. The lucid intervals can last for minutes or hours, and can start and end without warning. While lucid, the patient is in better contact and may be examined more easily, but is still liable to exhibit some memory impairment and disorientation. As a rule, the longest and most frequent lucid intervals tend to occur during the day. At night and in the dark, the patient is usually consistently disturbed and confused.

The behavior of a delirious patient may be at odds with his or her habitual conduct. Personality traits, as manifested in observable verbal and nonverbal behavior, may be either accentuated or altered. In the former case, the patient speaks and acts in a manner reflecting enhanced suspiciousness, timidity, pugnacity, or withdrawal. Rather than accentuation of habitual traits, however, unaccustomed tendencies may be displayed. Thus, a normally shy, retiring person may become loud and combative, or a placid individual may exhibit a frankly paranoid attitude and act in a belligerent and accusatory manner. The latter attitude may take the form of persecutory delusions, which are typically unsystematized and changeable in content in response to environmental stimuli. Such symptoms may occur in the presence of relatively mild cognitive impairment and may create a false diagnostic impression of a functional (e.g., schizophrenic) psychosis (8–10).

Uterrances reflecting the patient's experience during an episode of delirium may appear bland and impoverished, or fearful, or depressed, or dream-like and bizarre. It is the latter patients, those verbalizing hallucinatory experiences and delusional ideas, who are most likely to be misdiagnosed. Moreover, as Hughlings Jackson (11) so well observed over a century ago, the smaller the reduction in consciousness, the more room there is for florid psychotic phenomena. For the patient, such experiences are intensely real in the same way that a dream is usually experienced as real while it is occurring. A terminally ill, delirious patient, for example, woke up and, looking at his son, said: "I recognize you from my dreams." Unaccustomed and dream-like thoughts, images, and fantasies, which in many cases intermingle with actual dreams, illusions, and hallucinations, result in an experience not unlike that of a waking dream or nightmare. Conscious or unconscious wishes, impulses, conflicts, and guilt feelings may preoccupy a delirious patient and be reflected in speech (12–14). Intense fear, anger, shame, depression, or pleasure may accompany those inner experiences and may be expressed by the patient both verbally and nonverbally. External stimuli are readily incorporated into the experience, and the normally automatic distinctions that a person makes between dreams and imagery on the one hand, and external reality on the other, become blurred or even abolished.

A woman delirious in the course of uremia provided a good example of this blurring of the boundary between imagery and hallucinations on the one hand, and veridical perceptions on the other. She reported to the writer that she had awakened after a nightmare whose contents she could not recall, and saw a young man with a red moustache who started to massage her breasts until they became flat and then tried to push a thermometer into one of them but stopped after she yelled for help. The woman recounted this experience as a fact and would not accept the writer's suggestion that it was partly a hallucination and partly the result of a nurse's taking her temperature. In another case, an older physician who abused alcohol was hospitalized after a head injury. When visited by the writer one morning, he said excitedly that a strange event had taken place during the night. Several men came into his room, dragged him into a car, drove him to the country, and were about to shoot him, but for some reason returned him to the hospital instead. He had no doubt that this had actually happened.

Merging of dream contents, waking hallucinations and images, and true perceptions is a common feature of a delirious patient's experience, and gives it a weird and usually unpleasant subjective quality. Darkness, shadows, unexpected noises, monotonous sounds of monitoring apparatus in an intensive care unit, voices beaming from an intercom system—all these stimuli tend to enhance a delirious patient's dream-like experience, confusion, and perceptual-cognitive misinterpretations.

Delirium may begin to subside at any stage, and its maximum intensity will vary depending on its cause, the patient's age and physical condition, and timely treatment. Its worsening may take the form of gradual or sudden reduction in alertness and wakefulness, and a transition to sleep, stupor, and coma. In some cases, the patient shows increasing agitation and restlessness ending in collapse. A severely delirious patient may just mutter, oblivious of the surroundings and unresponsive to verbal stimuli. Involuntary movements, such as a course tremor, flapping motions of the hands and arms, groping, jerking, or persistent tossing about (jactitation), are displayed by some patients. Incontinence of urine and feces is usual in severe cases. Speech may vary from mutism to an almost constant flow of disjointed and apparently unrelated words and phrases. Signs of the autonomic nervous system's hyperarousal, with flushing or pallor of the face, sweating, tachycardia, dry mouth, and dilated pupils, may be observed in some patients. Others appear pale, dehydrated, and listless. Gradually the patient's cognitive processes become increasingly fragmented, labored, and impoverished in content. As the level of consciousness drops, contact with the patient becomes difficult, if not impossible. From this point on, there is progression either toward coma and possibly death, or to sleep from which the patient may awaken considerably more alert and on the road to recovery. Episodes of delirium may recur, especially and sometimes only at night for several weeks, and occasionally longer if the underlying physical illness or intoxication persists. On the average, however, the majority of patients, especially the younger ones, recover within a week or so.

The above composite description of the clinical picture of delirium is based on the literature, as well as on the writer's 25-year experience as a psychiatric consultant in medicine and surgery in several general hospitals and the Montreal Neurological Institute. He has personally examined more than 1,000 delirious patients and followed them during their hospitalization. A systematic account of the psychopathology of the syndrome is presented in the next chapter. Meanwhile, the most prominent variants of delirium, as well as its outcome, will be discussed next.

Clinical variants

The remarkable *variability* of the clinical picture of delirium has already been mentioned. Its manifestations may change not only among patients but also in the same patient even in the course of one day, as superbly described by Soranus of Ephesus in the second century A.D. (see Chapter 1 for the relevant quotation). Since the end of the eighteenth century, various writers on the subject have gone further and have distinguished two species or variants of the syndrome, variously referred to as "delirium ferox," or wild (acute, raving, active), and "delirium mite" or low (quiet) (15–18). In the former variant, the patient is "raving, noisy, and violent, requiring restraint" (17); in the latter, he or she is quiet, inattentive, and approaching stupor. Rees (16) argued that delirium was of "two species, and connected with two opposite conditions of the sensorium"; hence, its treatment should take prevailing conditions into account.

Thus, for two centuries, medical writers have clearly recognized these contrasting variants of the syndrome, distinguished by opposed levels of alertness and psychomotor activity. This division is still valid and based on clinical observation. Moreover, some patients may display features of both variants in the course of a single episode of delirium. We shall consequently distinguish three variants of the syndrome: the *hyperactive-hyperalert,* the *hypoactive-hypoalert,* and the *mixed.*

The hyperactive-hyperalert variant

This clinical variant features *psychomotor overactivity,* both verbal and nonverbal, as well as *hyperalertness,* i.e., abnormally increased responsivity to stimuli. The patient is visibly restless, excitable, and vigilant. He or she moves a great deal, gesticulates, and speaks loudly and under pressure. Behavior, posture, and facial expression reflect a hyperaroused state. The patient responds to stimuli promptly, excessively, and indiscriminately. If allowed to get out of bed, such a patient moves constantly, seems to search for something, shouts, and may be combative. More often than not, he or she tries to leave the bed and the ward without permission and is liable to resist attempts at restraint. Such patients can readily create an emergency situation on the ward and may sometimes injure others. Coupled with the above features are signs of increased autonomic, especially sympathetic, nervous system activity, involuntary movements, and extreme distractibility. Moreover, a hyperactive patient is also likely to experience vivid and often frightening hallucinations and to display intense fear or rage. If the hyperactive behavior is allowed to persist, the patient may eventually collapse. This type of behavior can be mistaken for a case of mania.

Delirium tremens (alcohol withdrawal delirium) offers a classic example of the hyperactive-hyperalert variant. It shows all of the characteristics described above to a high degree. This fact has prompted some writers, quoted in Chapter 2, to view it as a prototype of delirium as a whole. In this book, however, it is considered to be no more than a typical example of the variant under discussion.

The Hypoactive-Hypoalert Variant

This variant provides a striking contrast to the preceding one. It features a *reduced level* of psychomotor activity and alertness. The patient is generally quiet and listless, speaks little and is occasionally mute, tends to drift off into sleep even in the course of an examination, responds slowly to stimuli, and displays diminished psychomotor activity. This appearance may be misleading, since some of these patients may experience lively, if confused, mental activity and vivid hallucinations and imagery. Some patients are catatonic and may be mistakenly diagnosed as schizophrenic. Others lie with open eyes but appear indifferent, oblivious to what goes on around them, and absorbed in some inner, dream-like, world. They may mutter to themselves more or less incoherently and sometimes gesture incongruously. Such patients are often thought to be depressed and can actually be so, but many are merely apathetic. They are likely to be overlooked by the ward staff (19).

This variant of delirium corresponds to what the ancients called "lethargus" and some contemporary writers refer to as "acute confusional state," which is distinct from delirium (see Chapter 2). It is usually viewed by medical writers as a primary manifestation of the state of reduced (clouded) consciousness, somewhere between full alertness (or awareness, or consciousness) on the one hand, and stupor and coma on the other. The psychopathology of both this and the preceding variants will be discussed in Chapter 5. They are clearly distinct and presumably reflect different pathophysiological processes in the brain. Both of them, however, display the essential features of delirium defined as a psychopathological syndrome.

The mixed variant

This clinical picture is characterized by features of both of the foregoing variants. The patient's psychomotor activity and alertness *alternate irregularly* between a state of lethargy, inertia, and hypoalertness, on the one hand, and its opposite on the other. Such striking shifts in behavior and attention may occur unpredictably in the course of a delirious episode and even during a single day. As these changes tend to be relatively sudden and unexpected, they are likely to create crises and management problems for the clinical staff. It is easy to either oversedate or insufficiently sedate a patient of this type.

Because relevant statistics are unavailable, the frequency of the respective variants in clinical practice is unknown. The only study that addressed this issue found that 55% of a small series of delirious patients had an "active" delirium (20). There is some anecdotal evidence that elderly patients, as well as those suffering from a metabolic encephalopathy, tend to be hypoactive and hypoalert, while those who are delirious as a result of withdrawal from alcohol or sedative-hypnotics, or both, typically display features of the opposite variant. These impressions need to be validated by systematic clinical research.

Outcome

Delirium is, by definition, a *transient* organic mental syndrome, but this does not by any means imply that it is always followed by full recovery, even though this is the most common outcome. Transience in this context refers to the clinical syndrome as such, but not to the patient's overall psychological functioning and well-being or even survival. "Delirium" designates a cluster of psychopathological symptoms indicative of temporary cerebral dysfunction. It is the underlying cause (or causes) of the latter condition that determines whether the patient will survive the illness, return to the premorbid state, or display some form and degree of permanent psychological impairment or abnormality absent prior to the onset of the delirium. If it occurs in the course of a dementia, for example, the metabolic derangement causing the delirium may result in more brain damage and hence in an increase or acceleration of the dementing process. Thus, the nature of the patient's physical illness is of prognostic importance. The patient's age and overall physical condition are also relevant in this regard, as are the appropriateness, effectiveness, and timeliness of the treatment of the underlying disease and the management of the delirium itself.

The outcome of delirium includes the following possibilities:

1. Full recovery, usually within a week or so, but sometimes, especially in an elderly patient, after several weeks.
2. Progression to stupor and coma, or sudden cardiovascular collapse and death.
3. A transitional cognitive, affective, behavioral, or mixed abnormality and gradual full recovery.

4. Progression to an irreversible mental syndrome, with either global or relatively circumscribed cognitive deficits, or to an organic personality disorder.
5. A functional psychosis or postraumatic stress syndrome.

The most common outcome of delirium is *full recovery*. Sometimes the patient may experience recurrent episodes of it over a period of months or even years. This is most likely to happen in someone suffering from a progressive brain disease, such as a space-occupying lesion, or from a metabolic disease punctuated by recurrent exacerbations and concomitant cerebral dysfunction. Chronic renal, hepatic, cardiovascular, and pulmonary diseases offer relevant examples.

Death as an outcome of the syndrome has been observed by medical writers since Hippocrates. As an eighteenth-century medical dictionary put it, "to be in any manner delirious, or to be deprived, in whole or in part, of the use of his Reason, is a bad Prognostic, and, in acute Diseases, often portends Death" (21). Lately, the mortality from delirium has attracted some attention. In an early study, Curran (22) observed that of 106 patients with delirium, "some died," and that "physical prostration consequent upon restlessness and excitement may induce a fatal issue which otherwise would not have taken place" (p 874). Seven of his patients attempted suicide while delirious. A study of 117 patients with "organic syndrome" referred for psychiatric consultation from medical and surgical wards found that 17% died during the index admission, while the mortality of all admitted patients during the study period was only 3.7% (23). In a subsequent report on 262 patients from the same hospital suffering from "organic brain syndrome," the authors related that the index cases had twice the mortality of control subjects (24). The investigators concluded that the presence of an organic brain syndrome is associated with a markedly increased mortality during index admission. More recent studies have further documented high mortality from delirium (25–27), higher than that of medically ill demented, cognitively intact, and depressed patients (25). Those with delirium tended to be older and to suffer from multiple medical problems (26).

Several studies have focused on the mortality of delirious elderly patients (28–32). The reported mortality rates have ranged from 18% to 37%. The development of delirium in later life must be regarded as a grave prognostic sign (33). The syndrome is often a terminal event in diseases such as cancer (34,35).

Some patients pass through a *transitional or subacute* organic mental syndrome before recovering, one that may take the form of a reversible dementia, amnestic syndrome, organic hallucinosis, or an organic mood, anxiety, or personality disorder. There are no published data on the frequency of this development. Such patients not only display global or circumscribed cognitive deficits, but also often complain of mental fatigue, lack of initiative, poor concentration, impaired ability for sustained mental effort, irritability, and insomnia or hypersomnia. An amnestic syndrome most often follows cardiac arrest, Wernicke's encephalopathy, head injury, subarachnoid hemorrhage, encephalitis, and tuberculous meningitis (5).

An unknown percentage of delirious patients progress to a *chronic* organic mental syndrome, usually dementia, amnestic syndrome, or organic personality disorder. A patient who sustains severe head trauma, for example, will be comatose at first, then delirious, and finally may suffer from some form and degree of cognitive impairment, or an organic personality disorder (e.g., frontal lobe syndrome), or both (5). An irreversible amnestic syndrome may follow Wernicke's encephalopathy (36).

Delirium of any etiology may be followed by a *functional psychosis,* either schizophrenic, affective, or paranoid (14). The frequency of this occurrence is not known but appears to be very low (14). Delirium may occur at a time of high psychological stress for the patient occasioned by a severe physical illness and the threat of death or other traumatic events. During the syndrome, previously repressed and thus unconscious conflicts and disavowed impulses may become manifest in the form of uncontrolled thoughts, imagery, hallucinations, and delusions. The patient may also become uncharacteristically violent and abusive. Subsequent memory of these experiences may suffice to result in a breakdown of psychological defenses and a psychosis. It is remarkable that these events seem to be so uncommon. Some schizophrenic (14) and depressed (37) patients may actually show a remission of their mental illness after delirium. Finally, the very experience of the syndrome constitutes a stressful life event and may be followed by a *depression* or a *posttraumatic stress disorder* (38,39).

Complications

The course of delirium may be complicated by events related to the patient's behavior, the therapeutic intervention to control it, or both (40–42). Self-injury is an ever-present risk in an agitated, fearful patient. He or she may tear open sutures, pull out intravenous lines, attempt suicide, or sustain a fall and a fracture or concussion. A patient with delirium tremens, for example, left the ward on a winter day without being noticed, ran out of the hospital, slipped, fell, and sustained a fatal head injury. Another got into a laundry chute during the night, fell several stories, and suffered multiple fractures. Such mishaps can result in litigation. A hyperactive patient may suffer a fatal cardiac arrhythmia, while in a lethargic one atelectasis may occur (40). Moreover, an agitated, delirious patient may develop hypotension from an injection of a psychotropic drug, or may have to be physically restrained, with the consequent risk of deep vein thrombosis and pulmonary embolism (41). Such iatrogenic complications are avoidable.

Delirium in Childhood

There is a striking lack of studies of delirium in children and its outcome. Kanner (43) speaks of the "great frequency" of this syndrome among them and comments on how little attention has been paid to it in the literature. He claims that delirium may be recognized in an infant as young as 16 months of age. Prugh et al. (44) published the only study of delirium in children and adolescents to appear in recent years. They noted persistence of defective perceptual-motor performance, as well as of EEG abnormalities, in their subjects. Another writer (45) claimed that if the picture of delirium in a child is complicated by signs of oneirism that outlasts the febrile period, the prognosis is less favorable. About 3% of adult schizophrenics are said to have suffered one or more delirious episodes in childhood (45). Bender (46) asserts that terrifying hallucinations and panic experienced by a delirious child may be followed by a schizophrenic illness. In the course of one of the common nonneurotropic viral infections in childhood accompanied by delirium, the EEG is abnormal and the child may subsequently suffer from learning and behavior problems (47). There is an obvious need for more research on this important subject.

In summary, delirium usually ends in full recovery but may be followed by death or by a transitional or chronic mental disorder, either organic or functional. Its mortality appears to be highest in later life and in the presence of multiple medical problems. It often accompanies a terminal illness. Long-term sequelae of delirium remain to be studied to establish their frequency. Little is known about its possible effects on the subsequent development of psychiatric morbidity in children. On the whole, recent reports indicate that the appearance of delirium in a patient, especially an elderly one, must be taken seriously and viewed as a potentially grave prognostic sign. Medicolegal complications may result from self-injury or improper treatment of the syndrome.

References

1. Fothergill J. M.: The management of delirium. *The Practitioner* 1874;13:400–408.
2. *Diagnostic and Statistical Manual of Mental Disorders,* ed 3. Washington, DC, American Psychiatric Association, 1980.
3. *Diagnostic and Statistical Manual of Mental Disorders,* ed 3 revised. Washington, DC, American Psychiatric Association, 1987.

4. Lipowski Z. J.: Delirium (acute confusional state), in Frederiks J. A. M. (ed): *Handbook of Clinical Neurology*. Vol 2 (No. 46): *Neurobehavioral Disorders*. Amsterdam, Elsevier, 1985, pp 523–559.
5. Lipowski Z. J.: Organic mental disorders: Introduction and review of syndromes, in Kaplan H. I., Freedman A. M., Sadock B. J. (eds): *Comprehensive Textbook of Psychiatry*, ed 3. Baltimore, Williams & Wilkins, 1980, pp 1359–1392.
6. Draft of Chapter V, Mental, behavioural and developmental disorders in *International Classification of Diseases*, ed 10. Geneva, World Health Organization, June 1987.
7. Wolff H. G., Curran D.: Nature of delirium and allied states. The dysergastic reaction. *A.M.A. Arch Neurol Psychiatry* 1935;33:1175–1215.
8. Daniel D. G., Rabin P. L.: Disguises of delirium. *South. Med. J.* 1985;78:666–672.
9. Dubin W. R., Weiss K. J., Zeccardi J. A.: Organic brain syndrome. The psychiatric imposter. *J.A.M.A.* 1983;249:60–62.
10. Sullivan N., Fogel B. S.: Could this be delirium? *Am. J. Nurs.* 1986;1359–1363.
11. Jackson J. H.: *Selected Writings*. 2 vols. Ed. J. Taylor. London, Hadder and Soughton, 1932.
12. Blank K., Perry S.: Relationship of psychological processes during delirium to outcome. *Am J. Psychiatry* 1984;141:843–847.
13. Lipowski Z. J.: Delirium, clouding of consciousness and confusion. *J. Nerv. Ment. Dis.* 1967;145:227–255.
14. Willi J.: Delir, Dämmerzustand und Verwirrtheit bei körperlich Kranken, in Bleuler M., Willi J., Bühler H. R. (eds): *Akute psychische Begleiterscheinungen körperlicher Krankheiten*. Stuttgart, Georg Thieme, 1966, pp 27–158.
15. Sims J.: Pathological remarks upon various kinds of alienation of mind. *Memoirs R. Soc. Lond.* 1799;5:372–406.
16. Rees A.: *The Cyclopedia; or Universal Dictionary of Arts, Sciences, and Literature*. First American ed. Philadelphia, S. F. Bradford, 1818.
17. Verco: Delirium. *St. Bartholomews Hosp. Rep., Lond.* 1877;13:332–342.
18. Gowers W. R.: *A Manual of Diseases of the Nervous System*. Philadelphia, Blakiston, 1888.
19. Engel G. L., Romano J.: Delirium, a syndrome of cerebral insufficiency. *J. Chronic Dis.* 1959;9:260–277.
20. Ross C. A., Shapiro I., Tune L., et al. Phenomenological subtypes of delirium. Unpublished paper, 1987.
21. James R.: *A Medicinal Dictionary*. Vol 2. London, T. Osborne, 1945.
22. Curran D.: Prognosis in delirious states. *Lancet* 1937;2:873–875.
23. Guze S. B., Cantwell D. P.: The prognosis in "organic brain" syndromes. *Am. J. Psychiatry* 1964;120:878–881.
24. Guze S. B., Daengsurisri S.: Organic brain syndrome. *Arch. Gen. Psychiatry* 1967;17:365–366.
25. Rabins P. V., Folstein M. F.: Delirium and dementia: Diagnostic criteria and fatality rates. *Br. J. Psychiatry* 1982;140:149–153.
26. Trzepacz P. T., Teague G. B., Lipowski Z. J.: Delirium and other organic mental disorders in a general hospital. *Gen. Hosp. Psychiatry* 1985;7:101–106.
27. Weddington W. W.: The mortality of delirium: An unappreciated problem? *Psychosomatics* 1982;23:1232–1235.
28. Bedford P. D.: General medical aspects of confusional states in elderly people. *Br. Med. J.* 1959:2:185–188.

29. Bergmann K., Eastham E. J.: Psychogeriatric ascertainment and assessment for treatment in an acute medical ward setting. *Age Ageing* 1974;3:174–188.
30. Hodkinson H. M.: Mental impairment in the elderly. *J. R. Coll. Physicians Lond.* 1973;7:305–317.
31. Seymour D. G., Henschke P. J., Cape R. D. T., et al: Acute confusional states and dementia in the elderly: The role of dehydration/volume depletion, physical illness and age. *Age Ageing* 1980;9:137–146.
32. Simon A., Cahan R. B.: The acute brain syndrome in geriatric patients. *Psychiatric Res. Rep.* 1963;16:8–21.
33. Lipowski Z. J.: Transient cognitive disorders (delirium, acute confusional states) in the elderly. Am. J. Psychiatry *1983;140:1426–1436.*
34. Adams F.: Neuropsychiatric evaluation and treatment of delirium in the critically ill cancer patient. *Cancer Bull.* 1984; 36:156–160.
35. Massie M. J., Holland J. C., Glass E.: Delirium in terminally ill cancer patients. *Am. J. Psychiatry* 1983;140:1048–1050.
36. Victor M., Adams R. D., Collins G. H.: *The Wernicke-Korsakoff Syndrome.* Philadelphia, F. A. Davis, 1971.
37. Borchardt C. M., Popkin M. K.: Delirium and the resolution of depression. *J. Clin. Psychiatry* 1987;48:373–375.
38. Blank K., Perry S.: Relationship of psychological processes during delirium to outcome. *Am. J. Psychiatry* 1984;141:843–847.
39. MacKenzie T. B., Popkin M. K.: Stress response syndrome occurring after delirium. *Am J. Psychiatry* 1980;137:1433–1435.
40. Aita G. A.: Everyman's psychosis—the delirium. *Nebr. Med. J.* 1968;10:424–427.
41. Gillick M. R., Serrell N. A., Gillick L. S.: Adverse consequences of hospitalization in the elderly. *Soc. Sci. Med.* 1982;16:1033–1038.
42. Warshaw G. A., Moore J. T., Friedman S. W., et al: Functional disability in the hospitalized elderly. J.A.M.A. 1982;248:847–850.
43. Kanner L.: *Child Psychiatry,* ed 4. Springfield, Ill., Charles C Thomas, 1972.
44. Prugh D. G., Wagonfeld S., Metcalf D., et al: A clinical study of delirium in children and adolescents. *Psychosom. Med.* (Suppl) 1980;42:177–195.
45. Bollea G.: Acute organic psychoses in childhood, in Howells J. G. (ed): *Modern Perspectives in International Child Psychiatry.* New York, Brunner & Mazel, 1971, pp 706–732.
46. Bender L.: The maturation process and hallucinations in children, in Keup W. (ed): *Origin and Mechanisms of Hallucinations. New York, Plenum Press, 1970.*
47. Weinman H. M.: EEG changes in acute viral disease in infancy and childhood. *Electroencephalogr. Clin. Neurophysiol.* 1967;22:93.

5

Psychopathology

In Chapter 4 the clinical features of delirium, both essential and associated, were described to help clinicians diagnose it. In this chapter, the psychopathology of the syndrome will be discussed in a more formal and systematic manner. While many excellent clinical descriptions of delirium can be found in the literature, there is a dearth of reports of rigorous research on its assorted psychopathological features. The purpose of this chapter is to review these abnormalities, to point out the gaps in our knowledge of them, and to suggest areas for future research.

Delirium has been referred to by the various writers on the subject as a disorder of "consciousness," "attention," "cognition," or "wakefulness." While keeping in mind that all these terms have been inconsistently defined and are thus hardly unambiguous, one may propose that the syndrome involves abnormalities in *all* the areas of human function to which those concepts have been applied. To single out any of them as *the* basic abnormality seems unwarranted. The discussion to follow will, one hopes, bear out this contention.

Delirium as a disorder of consciousness

Since the late nineteenth century, it has been customary for psychiatric writers to refer to delirium as a disorder of "consciousness" (1–3). Ey (3) asserts that this term has traditionally been used to imply a disturbance of *wakeful-*

ness characterized by the *clouding of consciousness.* The historical roots of the link between delirium and the concept of consciousness and its so-called clouding were traced in Chapter 1. As that concept became embraced by the neurologists, such as Hughlings Jackson, and by psychologists, it filtered to psychiatry, where it was applied to explain the features of a wide range of psychopathological states, both organic and psychogenic. Delirium and allied states came to be regarded as classic examples of disordered consciousness. Hirsch (4) was probably the first American psychiatrist to propose this notion when he wrote that the syndrome was a "psychical state characterized by an abolition of self-consciousness," manifested by disorientation for place, disturbances of perception, and disorders of memory and thinking. He used the term "cloudiness of self-consciousness" to refer to the basic abnormality in delirium. Hoch (5) likewise asserted that the most specific and cardinal feature of delirium was a "constant tendency to dip down to a lower level of consciousness." He used the term "clouding of consciousness" in this context and claimed that this state was analogous to sleep, marked by a "general dissociation" of thought processes from external reality not unlike that of the act of dreaming. Disorientation, hallucinations, memory impairment, and attention disorder were all to be viewed as consequences and manifestations of the clouding of consciousness. In both of these early papers, the latter is seen as manifested essentially by a *disorder of cognition,* i.e., thinking, perceiving, and remembering, and Hoch adds *attention* to the cognitive abnormalities.

Thus, for about a century, the concept of delirium and a disorder (clouding) of consciousness have been inextricably linked, reflecting a contemporary fascination with the latter concept. The situation has become somewhat muddled, however, as some authors present the syndrome as a manifestation of the clouding, while for others that disorder constitutes a cardinal feature of delirium. More important, however, is to discern what all this really means. This question calls for a discussion of the concepts of "consciousness" and "clouding of consciousness" as they are currently conceived. We will see that both of them are cloudy indeed.

There is no generally accepted definition of "consciousness," and the connotations of this term are growing in number over time. A recent upsurge of interest in this concept on the part of psychologists, philosophers, and neuroscientists has resulted in a sizable literature but little consensus. As one author observed, "there are as many definitions of awareness or consciousness as there are writers (and readers)" (6, p 132). Natsoulas (7), in one of his papers on this topic, also points out that "conceptual confusions and difficulties in mutual comprehension" pervade scientific discourse on the subject of consciousness despite its central position in contemporary psychology. He himself discusses six distinct referents of this concept in an attempt to clarify its meaning. Frederiks (8), a neurologist, complains that uncertainty about the connotation of the term "consciousness" has led to the introduction of other equally inconsistently defined terms such as "vigilance," "alertness," "wakefulness," and "awareness." They can all be found in the literature on delirium, and they compound the semantic muddle. Yet, ambiguous as it is, the concept of consciousness is very much with us, as shown by a spate of recent books, articles, and symposia devoted to it (6–15). Moreover, the latest edition of the American classification of mental disorders (16) includes "reduced level of consciousness" among the essential features of delirium and its diagnostic criteria. Some medical writers (15) have concluded that even though "consciousness" is "bereft of scientific respectability," variations in it, or in the level of arousal, are too important for the practice of anesthesia and psychiatric medicine, for example, to be ignored. It is for this reason that this subject is being discussed here.

A comprehensive review of the concept of "consciousness" is beyond the scope of this book, and readers are referred to the relevant sources (6–15). Some discussion of it is needed, however, given the continued tendency to link it with delirium in the current literature. In particular, "clouding of consciousness," a concept still often encountered, needs to be critically appraised and explicated (1).

A recently published dictionary of psychology (17) states that "consciousness" is a term that "very loosely" refers to five overlapping states, the first and fourth of which are relevant to our subject. They are, first, the capacity of being aware or conscious of objects in the environment; and second, the capacity of human beings to have an organized mental life. The dictionary also defines disorders of consciousness as those of the awareness of the self and the external environment. They are said to include three main types: lowering of consciousness, narrowing of consciousness, and dream-like disorders. Lowering of consciousness is equivalent to its clouding and implies a reduced state of awareness on a continuum from slight diminution to stupor and coma. Narrowing implies awareness of only part of the environment, as in psychogenic twilight states. Finally, dream-like disorders involve severe impairment of consciousness, with spatiotemporal disorientation, misperceptions, and motor abnormalities; delirium is a typical example of this category. Thus, in contrast to the psychiatric literature, the dictionary distinguishes between clouding of consciousness and delirium. It is obvious that semantic and conceptual confusion pervades this area.

A notably lucid discussion of consciousness is offered by Hebb (18), who regards it as a state of being normally awake and responsive, and capable of engaging in complex thought processes to guide behavior. Insight, purpose, and immediate memory are the key features of consciousness so defined. Hebb's conception is thus applicable to delirium in that the syndrome involves deficits in all the aspects of functioning included by him. One must note, however, that wakefulness and consciousness are not synonymous: a person asleep but dreaming displays a mode of conscious experience (19).

Psychiatrists, neurologists, and other physicians have traditionally viewed consciousness in Jacksonian terms as a continuum of *levels* of awareness or arousal, i.e., of being aware of one's self and one's environment, and of being able to respond to external stimuli. In this usage, consciousness has a *quantitative* connotation: one may be more or less conscious. One can also talk of the contents of consciousness, which may be altered by drugs or hypnosis, or in delirium or reverie or dreaming, for example. This constitutes a *qualitative* aspect of conscious experience. In delirium, both of these aspects are disturbed. We actually have three pairs of polarities and continua to consider here: consciousness versus unconsciousness, wakefulness versus sleep, and normal versus altered consciousness.

"Clouding of consciousness," as the term has traditionally been used, cuts across all three of the above polarities and implies the presence of the following behavioral features:

1. The person is awake but may be drowsy.
2. Awareness of the self and the environment is reduced.
3. Both immediate and recent memory are impaired.
4. Thinking is disorganized and may be dream-like.
5. Perception is faulty, and misperceptions may occur.
6. The ability to learn new material is reduced.
7. The person is unable to overcome this state by deliberate effort.

The foregoing characteristics have been extracted from the descriptions of clouding of consciousness in the psychiatric literature (2). They represent no more than a catalogue of most of the essential features of delirium and add nothing new. This is noteworthy, since "clouding of consciousness" has often been used as an explanatory concept referring to some basic psychopathological phenomenon that could be independently ascertained and assessed. This has proved to be an illusory and misleading implication, since this concept is merely descriptive, not explanatory. In the writer's opinion, it is completely *redundant* and has actually been dropped from *DSM-III-R* (16). Getting rid of it may help open the way to a fresh and unbiased look at the clinical phenomena of delirium that it has served to label and obscure. A similar conclusion has been reached by Gloor (11) in regard to epileptic seizures. He argues, from the basis of clinical experience, that if we continue to describe various behavioral deficits encountered in epilepsy as "loss" or "impairment" of consciousness, we will never be able to advance our understanding of the pathophysiological mechanisms involved. Gloor recommends accumulating careful clinical observations of the patient's behavior during a seizure. He concludes that even though consciousness is a biological phenomenon dependent on brain function, it is neither definable nor analyzable in currently available scientific terms, and hence is not a useful concept for advancing knowledge of behavioral neurobiology. This writer fully agrees with this contention in regard to delirium.

In conclusion, to say that delirium is a disorder of consciousness, one characterized by its clouding, adds nothing to our understanding of the syndrome's psychopathology and pathophysiology. "Clouding of consciousness" is no more than a metaphor referring to a set of cognitive and attentional deficits and abnormalities that constitute the core of the syndrome of delirium. As these abnormalities *vary in degree,* depending on the patient's level of wakefulness and alertness, one may still speak of "levels" of consciousness or awareness to imply how readily he or she responds to stimuli, maintains the waking state, is able to process and store information, and is capable of acting purposefully.

Delirium as a disorder of wakefulness

Delirium may be viewed, in part, as a disorder of wakefulness (20). In a classic review published in 1846, Purkinje (21), the famous Czech physiologist, argued that the state of being awake *(Wachen)* was characterized by consciousness, its essential attribute, while sleep took place in its absence. A dream represented an intermediate state *(Schlafwachen).* Purkinje stressed, however, that consciousness and wakefulness were not identical, a point restated more recently by Kleitman (19), who defined the latter simply as a state of not being asleep and argued that sleep and wakefulness were states that could be objectively observed and measured. By contrast, in consciousness there is only one variable, whose criteria are, first, critical reactivity, involving an analysis of the incoming information in the light of one's individual experience and hence *thinking;* and second, the subsequent ability to recall events, i.e., *memory.* In consciousness the sleep-wakefulness dichotomy is absent, according to Kleitman, since dreaming represents a mode of conscious experience of the sleeper. In both sleep and wakefulness, certain cyclic or rhythmic events have been described that in the latter state appear to be related to gradation of alertness (19).

Thus, "wakefulness" and "consciousness" refer to distinct yet overlapping states. In the previous section, we discussed the notion that delirium is a disorder of consciousness and pointed out problems resulting from the lack of an agreed-upon definition of the latter term. The concept of disorders of wakefulness is less widely known, yet has been referred to by some writers. Luria (22), for example, asserts that "a study of the varied symptoms of disorders of wakefulness became a most important clinical task" (p 74). Broughton (9) observes that some of the so-called altered states of consciousness involve, primarily or exclusively, dysfunction of the sleep-wake mechanisms. In particular, in delirium one finds a breakdown of the normal boundaries between and the normal succession of sleep and wakefulness, with a resulting mixture of these two states during the day. Heinroth (23) expressed a similar idea about 150 years earlier, when he wrote that delirium was an intermediate state between sleep and wakefulness *(status medius est inter somnum atque vigiliam).* A concept closely related to wakefulness and consciousness is that of *vigilance.* Koella (24) defines it as the level of readiness of the organism to respond with a functionally successful behavioral act to a given set of external or internal stimuli, or both. Consequently, some writers have used the term "disorders of vigilance" (25). Finally, Feinberg (26) hypothesizes that in delirium, intrusion of rapid eye movement (REM) processes into the waking state may occur.

Delirium has been frequently linked with the concepts of vigilance, arousal, activation, alertness, and attention, all of which refer to various aspects of wakefulness, although some of them may pertain to sleep as well. Abnormalities of all of these aspects of the waking state are among the constant features of the syndrome. It is plausible to view them as intervening variables between acute cerebral dysfunction and the impairment of cognitive functions. A close association between a disordered sleep-wake cycle and delirium has been observed by many medical writers since Hippocrates, as was documented in Chapter 1. Frequent statements, from the seventeenth century on, that the syndrome represented a waking dream were more than mere analogies or metaphors. They were derived from clinical observations that need to be carefully examined in the light of present knowledge and subjected to research.

The relations between the sleep-wake cycle, dreaming, and delirium will be further discussed in Chapters 6 and 7. They are brought up at this point only to underscore their relevance to the notion that the syndrome is partly a disorder of wakefulness. Recent studies of the latter have shown that it is not a homogeneous state, but rather one with both tonic and phasic aspects modulated by brain neurotransmitters (27). Ultradian vigilance rhythms with a period of 60 to 110 minutes are detectable during the daytime (28). Recurrent REM periods occur not only during sleep but also during wakefulness. They do not, however, correlate with the periods of the most intense daydreaming, which occur at a rate of about 16 cycles per day and seem to coincide with a dream-like, hypnagogic state (29). Under conditions of reduced sensory input, such daydreaming, fantasies, and vivid imagery are readily experienced. There are some differences, however, between REM mentation and waking thought (30).

It is not yet clear what, if any, relevance the above findings may have for the psychopathology of delirium, but it is conceivable that in the course of this syndrome, the imagery that normally fluctuates during wakefulness, yet is recognized by the person as such, may become abnormally accentuated and uncontrolled and come to dominate awareness. Ey et al. (31) have shown that in confusional states the EEG tracings obtained during the day displayed fluctuations and transitions among wakefulness, somnolence, light sleep, and "microsleeps." Night recordings on the confused patients documented not only shortening of the total sleep time, but also relative loss of modulation and orderly progression of the stages of sleep. Discrimination between "rapid" and slow-wave sleep was more difficult than in normal control subjects because of the marked increase in intermediate (not REM-associated) phases of rapid sleep. The investigators concluded that in confusional states disorganization of the normal structure of sleep and its various constituents or, more to the point, of the total sleep-wake cycle, takes place. This study highlights the need for more investigations of this type in order to elucidate the relations between the disorganized sleep-wake cycle, abnormal wakefulness, dreaming, and delirium. Such explorations have only begun, and more of them are needed.

In conclusion, to hypothesize that delirium is partly a disorder of wakefulness is likely to prove more heuristically useful than to view it as a disorder of consciousness. To do so may help clarify the relation of the syndrome to the ubiquitous sleep-wake disturbance in it and to the dysfunction of specific neural systems and biochemical regulatory mechanisms subserving sleep and wakefulness.

Delirium as a disorder of attention

Confusional states are regarded by some writers as global disorders of attention (32). Attentional deficits and abnormalities had been relatively neglected in accounts of delirium until recently (2,20). They were usually referred to in passing as a feature of disordered consciousness (33). In the current American classification of mental disorders (16), however, they have gained a central position in the definition of delirium.

Attention has been defined in more than one way (18,34–45). Hebb (18), for example, defines it as a "state or activity of the brain predisposing the subject to respond to some part or aspect of the environment rather than other parts" (p 294). For Luria (37), attention implies *directivity* and *selectivity* of mental processes. Some authors recognize additional aspects of attention, such as *vigilance* or alertness and *distribution* (35). Other writers (39) distinguish three components of attention: *alertness,* i.e., the ability to develop and maintain optimal sensitivity to external stimulation; *selectivity,* i.e., the ability to select information from one source or of one kind rather than another; and *processing capacity,* i.e., the concept of a limited ability to process information inputs. A core problem in the study of attention is to "understand how the unity of conscious experience is related to the many levels of selectivity involved in processing external events" (40, p 107). While "consciousness" is said to refer to states that have content, "attention" pertains to those processes that organize the content into a conscious state (43). Attention influences the way information is processed and hence plays a crucial role in cognition. Hernandez-Peon (44) regards it as the primary process underlying perception, memory, and thinking, one related to the vigilance system, i.e., arousing neurons in the brain stem, which can be activated both by the specific sensory pathways and by descending projections from the cortex. Thus, some degree of attention is necessary for organized waking mental activity (37).

The neural substrate of attention will be discussed in Chapter 6. At this point, we must focus on attentional disturbances in delirium. They are believed to constitute one of its essential features. Luria (37) asserts that the principal characteristic of what he calls "oneiroid states" is the "loss of the selectivity of mental processes affecting all spheres of mental activity" (p 63). Both significant and insignificant stimuli tend to elicit the same type of response, since the train of thought becomes disorganized and incidental associations are evoked by common words. The normal waking state in humans is characterized by the capacity to mobilize, direct, focus, sustain, and shift attention not only in response to significant internal or external stimuli, but also voluntarily or intentionally. In delirium this capacity is impaired in all its aspects, and hence the processing of information as well as short-term memory are defective (20).

The following attentional deficits may be observed in delirium (20):

1. Impaired ability to mobilize attention.
2. Impaired ability to select information inputs.
3. Impaired ability to sustain attention, i.e., distractibility.
4. Impaired ability to shift attention.
5. Spontaneous fluctuations of alertness.
6. Abnormally reduced or increased alertness.

All of these disturbances of attention may be seen in delirious patients, especially of its directivity and selectivity. They occur in varying degrees and patterns, depending on the severity and type of delirium. In the predominantly hypoactive-hypoalert variant, the levels of arousal and alertness are reduced to some extent, and the patient displays difficulty in mobilizing, maintaining, and shifting attention both intentionally and in response to external stimuli. By contrast, in the hyperactive-hyperalert variant, exemplified by delirium tremens and other substance withdrawal deliria, the patient is highly distractible and shifts attention with excessive readiness, but the ability to deploy it selectively and in a sustained manner is impaired. In some delirious patients, one may observe spontaneous (i.e., independent of external stimuli) fluctuations of alertness during the day. These fluctuations appear to be brought about by changes in the activity of the ascending reticular system due to the metabolic derangement affecting it.

The foregoing account of attentional abnormalities in delirium is based on clinical impressions and not on systematic studies using standardized tests of attention, as such research has not been carried out and is badly needed. This is an obvious drawback, but clinical observations and speculations derived from them constitute the bulk of our knowledge of delirium today and are presented here in order to point to directions for future research.

In conclusion, several attentional deficits and abnormalities may be observed in delirious patients, notably reduced directivity and selectivity of attention. These disturbances are an integral part of the syndrome and need to be systematically studied. However, to state that they constitute the *basic* psychopathological feature of delirium, and that the latter is essentially a global disorder of attention (32), appears to be an arbitrary and reductionist assumption, one devoid of practical value for the diagnosis and treatment of delirious patients.

Delirium as a disorder of cognition

Disorganization and global impairment of cognitive processes is one of the core and diagnostic features of delirium. This statement has several implications. First, under normal waking conditions, cognitive processes are organized rather than chaotic. Second, a delirious patient displays impairment of *all* the major aspects of cognition; hence the use of the word "global." Third, the observed impairment represents a decrement in the patient's premorbid level of cognitive functioning.

The term "cognition" is used here to connote all the processes involving symbolic operations, namely, perceiving, remembering, thinking, and imagining. Cognition has been defined as "those mental processes that transform the sensory input in various ways, code it, store it in memory, and retrieve it for later use" (45, p 6). Such crucial mental operations as problem solving, decision making, reasoning, and action planning refer to the more complex cognitive processes. Cognition is currently conceptualized in terms of information processing, and the human mind is viewed as an information-processing system (35,45,46).

In delirium, one finds defective functioning of the above system in all of its key aspects: acquisition, processing, retention, retrieval, and utilization of information. All of these aspects are disordered to a greater or lesser extent. As a result, the affected individual is less able than normally to acquire and apply knowledge, to respond and to act purposefully, and to make sense of the incoming information inputs. Consequently, responses and behavior tend to be erratic and unpredictable, and the patient is helpless and may even be at risk of injury, being unable to guide actions in the interest of self-preservation.

A disorder of cognition has been regarded as a cardinal feature of delirium from the earliest accounts of it, as documented in Chapter 1. Barrough (47), for example, spoke of disordered imagination, cogitation, and reason in this context. That view of delirium as a cognitive disorder reflects accurate clinical observation and remains valid. In the sections to follow, the abnormalities of the main aspects of cognition in this syndrome are discussed in some detail.

Disorders of thinking

As noted above, disturbances of thinking processes have always been viewed as an integral feature of delirium. Terms such as "confusion" and "clouding of consciousness" that have been so often used to describe the core psychopathology of delirium connote a disturbance of normal thought processes (48). Thinking involves the ability to represent or imagine those events, situations, or things that are not physically present (45). Concept formation is a prerequisite for higher thought processes such as reasoning, judgment, planning, problem solving, and decision making. Moreover, human thought includes both verbal and visual representations and is continuous, as expressed in the notion of the "waking stream of consciousness" (49,50). It includes not only such relatively formal operations as logical reasoning, but also self-generated imagery or daydreaming or reverie, planning, anticipation, and fantasy (50).

One of the striking features of delirium is the disorganization and impairment of directed thinking coupled with a relative preponderance of free-floating, dream-like imagery. It is this feature that has fostered comparisons between delirium and dreaming and has given rise to such terms as "oneirism" and "oneiric state." They refer to the dream-like mode of mentation often encountered in delirious patients. Levin (51) maintains that disorientation, disturbances of association, illogical thinking, inability to grasp new and complex information, and unawareness of faulty and inconsistent reasoning constitute the most common forms of thought pathology in delirium.

Systematic studies of thinking in delirium remain to be carried out. As with all the other aspects of the psychopathology of this syndrome one is forced to rely on clinical impressions and anecdotal accounts—an unsatisfactory state of affairs from a scientific viewpoint. This discussion of thought disorders in delirium is a tentative attempt to present them in an organized manner. They will be considered under the following headings (20):

1. Organization, i.e., selective ordering of thoughts for the purpose of problem solving, decision making, action planning, and effective communication.
1. Dynamics, i.e., the evolution and state of progression of thoughts over time sequences.
3. Concept formation.
4. Thought content.

Clinical observation allows one to postulate that all of the above aspects of thinking are disturbed in delirium. *Organization* of thoughts is disrupted to a varying degree in that thinking is more or less incoherent, fragmented, illogical, and undirected. Logical contradictions are readily unappreciated by the patient. For example, the patient may address a physician as "Doctor" and yet, on direct questioning, deny the knowledge of his or her occupation (51). A sustained, selective, and intentionally directed train of thought is difficult for the patient to support and is liable to be disrupted by both internal and external factors. Internally, the patient tends to experience more or less unbidden and disjointed images, fantasies, and thoughts that interfere with, and may actually make impossible, goal-directed thought processes. Externally, he or she tends to respond indiscriminately to stimuli, which readily elicit irrelevant associations. The capacity to select thoughts and maintain their organized sequence for the purpose of solving problems, planning, and grasping the meaning of information inputs is generally reduced. As a result of this disorganization of the flow of thought, the patient is less able than normally to match the stimuli with long-term memories, and thus to interpret them according to past experience and accumulated knowledge. Consequently, judgment is also liable to be impaired.

The flow of a delirious patient's thoughts may be either abnormally slowed or accelerated, as reflected in speech that may be slow and hesitant or pressured but incoherent. This disturbed *dynamic* aspect of thinking seems to enhance its overall ineffectiveness.

Concept formation is impaired, with a tendency toward concrete thinking and a reduced ability to form and comprehend abstract concepts. This deficit can be elicited at the bedside by asking the patient to define words and offer their synonyms, list words belonging to a particular category, interpret proverbs, state similarities and differences between words, and so forth (52). Responses to such tasks must, of course, be assessed in the light of the patient's level of education and, if known, his or her cognitive functioning prior to the onset of the delirious episode.

Content of thought of a delirious patient may be simply impoverished, few thoughts being available. In some cases, however, such content may be rich in imagery, memories, and fantasies. They may dominate the patient's awareness largely to the exclusion of external stimuli, or the latter may give rise to and be woven into his or her stream of thought. This thinking activity tends to reflect the patient's particular concerns, conflicts, wishes, fears, and memories. As stated before, there is often a dream-like or oneiric quality to such thought content. In some cases, the patient may relive in imagery some recent or remote traumatic event (53). He or she may find it difficult to separate fact from fantasy, dream from waking imagery. This is hardly surprising, since recent studies have shown a continuity between dream content and waking mentation in normal subjects (54). A delirious patient, however, tends to blur the boundary between these two modes of thought. For example, a woman suffering from delirium and being interviewed by the writer asked repeatedly: "Are you there or am I dreaming?" Much thought content tends to focus on the delirious patient's current concerns, such as the likely impact of the illness on personal life and future prospects (55). Much of the imagery expresses, in a symbolic form, a preoccupation with and fear of disability, mutilation, or death. Thus, the thinking of at least some delirious patients is not totally disorganized and incoherent; rather, it is narrowly focused and relatively unaffected by environmental stimuli.

Pathology of thought content in delirium includes *delusions,* i.e., false beliefs incongruous with the patient's cultural and educational background. They are commonly but by no means invariably present and are not diagnostic of the syndrome. Typically, they are unsystematized, fleeting, and readily elicited and modified by internal and external stimuli. Thoughts expressing suspicion and mistrust are common but may not amount to frank delusions. The latter are usually persecutory. Patients may believe that they are about to be killed by the nurses or doctors, for example, or even that they are already dead. Delusions may also focus on the fate of people important to the patient, who may become convinced that his or her spouse has been murdered or is sick and hospitalized. One of the writer's patients developed the belief that his daughter was being raped outside his room. Such delusions may persist for a while, only to be replaced by new ones, for example, that the patient would be tortured, imprisoned, or abducted. Some patients insist that they have been robbed or have committed a crime.

Delusions merge imperceptibly with illusions and hallucinations in delirium, and to try and separate them in clinical practice may be both difficult and pointless. In fact, probably the most common is the delusion that what the patient hallucinates is real.

Delusions in delirium have been reported in 40% to 100% of cases (56–58). This discrepancy no doubt reflects the patient population studied and the investigator's definitions of delirium and delusion. The distinction between delusions and hallucinations or confabulations, for example, is often arbitrary. A patient may insist, for instance, that a dead relative has just paid a visit. Some patients explicitly deny being ill and may confabulate to the effect that they came to the hospital to visit someone or that they just returned from a walk. A delirious woman had an eye examination and afterward told the writer that a doctor had looked into her eyes and stated that he saw gold in them, which he would remove surgically. Is this a delusion or a confabulation? Does it really matter which label one atatches to this example of thought pathology? The latter may be viewed as a manifestation of the patient's impaired capacity for information processing. In general, delusions in delirium are an inconstant feature and usually accompany hallucinations. Their transient, shifting, and poorly organized character stands in sharp contrast to the typically systematized and relatively consistently held and elaborated delusions of a patient suffering from a functional psychosis—a fact of considerable importance for the differential diagnosis.

In summary, thinking is invariably disorganized to some extent in delirium. The capacity for directed and abstract thought, concept formation, and problem solving is always impaired to some degree. The ability to evaluate incoming information by relating it to past experience is defective, as is that for reasoning, judging, and drawing correct inferences from what one perceives. The patient's stream of thought may be dominated by free-floating imagery and by normally unconscious fantasies. As a result, the ability to act purposefully and communicte effectively is liable to be affected. Poorly systematized delusions are often but not invariably encountered.

Disorders of perception

"Perception" refers to the active process of extracting information from the environment and one's body, interpreting it, and integrating it in a meaningful way. It is closely linked with attention, memory, thinking, and learning. Attention, in particular, plays a crucial role in determining which sensory stimuli, or information, is selected and hence perceived. It appears that the ubiquitous attentional disorders in delirium interfere with perceptual processes, even though the patient's sense organs may be intact. As a result, perceptual functions are liable to be affected in that the patient's ability to interpret, integrate, and discriminate percepts is reduced. Deficient or excessive cerebral cortical arousal may adversely affect perceptual processes. Drowsiness and reduced alertness are often observed in delirious patients, especially in the hypoactive-hypoalert variant of the syndrome. A patient displaying it tends to show absence of expectancy and of perceptual searching (59). By contrast, hyperactive-hyperalert patients exhibit increased responsivity to stimuli, but their ability to select, discriminate, and integrate what they perceive is liable to be impaired. These defects in perceptual functions seem to facilitate distortions and misinterpretations of the sensory input. The distinction between figure and ground, images and percepts, and fantasy and reality is generally blurred.

Perceptual disorders in delirium may affect all sensory modalities: exteroceptive, proprioceptive, and interoceptive. The patient's perception of the passage of time (time sense), spatial relationships, and verbal communications is likely to be impaired. Disturbances of the body image, i.e., alteration in the perception of the actual size, shape, position, weight, and texture of one's body and its parts, as well as reduplication of the body, limbs, and head, may all occur (60). Perceptual distortions in the visual sphere involving perceived or hallucinated objects are not uncommon. They may include polyopsia (multiplication of a single perceived object); metamorphopsia (alteration of the size of objects—micropsia, macropsia); alteration of position in space, such as tilting; waviness of linear components; fragmentation of lines and gaps in the contours of objects; apparent movement of stationary objects or acceleration or slowing of moving ones; dysmorphopsia (alteration or distortion of shape); and autoscopy [visual hallucination of the self (60–63)].

Perceptual abnormalities in delirium include not only the distortions listed above, but also misperceptions, i.e., illusions and hallucinations. They are common but *not* invariably present. Impairment of attention and of information processing seems to facilitate their occurrence.

Illusions

Illusions have been defined as premature or improper labeling of aspects of the perceptual field (59). They are common in delirium, especially in the visual sphere. Misinterpretations of visual, auditory, tactile, kinesthetic, and somesthetic sensory stimuli may occur. They range from relatively simple to elaborate and symbolic misidentifications of the sensory input. The patient may mistake spots on a wall for crawling insects, folds in the bedcovers for snakes, or the sound of a falling object for a pistol shot. More complex illusions can be regarded as projections of personally meaningful thought content onto external or internal stimuli. For example, a female barbiturate addict, delirious as a result of withdrawal from the drug she had abused, misidentified her hospital room for a prison cell from which she would be taken to be executed for some unstated crime. She mistook a window for a door and was caught in the act of opening it in order to escape from the "prison." The staff person who prevented her from escaping thought that she was trying to jump out of the window to commit suicide. The psychiatric consultant found, however, that the patient simply wanted to run away from what she misperceived as a jail. She felt guilty over her addiction and feared punishment for it, but was not suicidal. Her illusions were closely bound with persecutory delusions, and both reflected her guilt feelings and conflicts. Such misinterpretations of the sensory input may result in behavior leading to injury or even death of the patient. Darkness, shadows, sounds of the hospital intercom system, and general unfamiliarity of the setting for the patient foster the occurrence of illusions.

Hallucinations

The word "hallucination" denotes an experience of perceptual vividness that occurs in the absence of a relevant sensory stimulus (64). Hallucinations in any sensory modality may occur in delirium, but the *visual* ones are the most common. In only one reported study did auditory hallucinations predominate. Farber (57) studied 122 patients with delirium of various etiologies and found that 54% of them experienced hallucinations: 21% auditory, 14% visual, and 16% both types. One notes, however, that 13% of his patients had a history of alcohol addiction, and some of them had previously been hospitalized for delirium tremens or acute alcoholic hallucinosis. These factors may have resulted in the high incidence of auditory hallucinations in this patient sample. Wolff and Curran (56) found visual hallucinations to be the most common: they occurred in 66% of 106 delirious patients studied, while auditory hallucinations were observed in 41%. A Swiss study of 300 patients with "exogenous psychosis," a term roughly equivalent to "delirium," revealed the following incidence: visual hallucinations in 75%, auditory in 23%, and both types combined in 17% (55).

The overall incidence of hallucinations in delirium varies in the published reports from about 40% to 75% (55–58). Some authors include hallucinations in their operational definition of delirium and thus imply that 100% of the cases display them. The reported incidence of hallucinations in the syndrome is liable to be influenced by the characteristics of the patient sample studied, as well as by the investigator's definition of delirium and hallucination. On the whole, patients with a hyperactive-hyperalert delirium are more likely to hallucinate than those with a hypoactive-hypoalert variant. Moreover, patients aged 60 years and older are reported to have a lower incidence of hallucinations—about 40%—than younger ones (58). Those delirious as a result of withdrawal from alcohol or sedative-hypnotics appear to hallucinate more often than sufferers from one of the metabolic encephalopathies. About 40% of patients who hallucinate tend to do so only at night (65).

Delirious patients may hallucinate in more than one sensory modality at the same time. The common combination is that of *visual and auditory* hallucinations (55–57,65). Some patients experience several types of misperceptions, not only exteroceptive but also proprioceptive and interoceptive. Tactile hallucinations are fairly common (65) and usually take the form of crawling, creeping, burning, and other sensations that are difficult to distinguish from paresthesias. Delusions of infestation, parasitosis, or sexual interference may accompany such tactile misperceptions. Vivid kinesthetic hallucinations of floating in the air, flying, or falling from heights have been described in typhus (66) and poliomyelitis (67), for example. Olfactory hallucinations, nearly always in the form of unpleasant odors, occur in about 10% of delirious patients (56,65), while gustatory ones are very uncommon (56,65).

Hallucinations may be viewed from two related perspectives: *formal features* and *content.* The formal aspects of visual hallucinations include their duration and frequency; the size, intensity, distinctness, color, shape, and motion of the hallucinated objects; the reality or true-to-life quality of the visions; projection into and placement in space; and the degree to which the patient believes in their veridical nature (65).

In terms of their *formal features,* visual hallucinations in delirium are usually projected to the nearby space and are experienced as bright-colored, clear, three-dimensional pictures whose elements frequently change in shape, size, or number and move about in the visual field (65). Lilliputian hallucinations may occasionally occur and usually consist of brightly colored little people (68). On the whole, the delirious patient's visual hallucinations tend to be relatively brief and often nocturnal, and commonly involve objects in motion (65). Moreover, they may be intermittent and fleeting or may take the form of a movie film-like experience. In the latter case, the pictures are likely to vary in the degree to which they are thematically connected, i.e., display a discernible theme. Some patients hallucinate only with their eyes closed, especially when they try to fall asleep. These hallucinations are probably hypnagogic and may make the patient afraid of falling asleep (69).

The *contents* of visual hallucinations in delirium are highly variable. The degree of their organization, complexity, and symbolic elaboration varies greatly. Three aspects of hallucinatory contents have been distinguished (70): noun, i.e., the predominant thing hallucinated; verb, i.e., the action within the hallucination in regard to the patient; and reaction, i.e., the patient's attitude to such action. Visual hallucinations in delirium comprise a wide variety of objects, ranging in complexity from relatively simple and unformed ones, such as colored spots, stars, balls, specks, flakes of light, geometric figures, and whorls at one end of the spectrum, to inanimate objects, animals, human figures, mythological or ghost-like apparitions, monsters, and complex panoramic scenes, at the other end. Wolff and Curran (56) reported that their delirious patients hallucinated figures in motion; all kinds of animals, from cockroaches to elephants; vividly colored objects, some of which seemed to have symbolic significance, such as hearses and coffins; and ghost-like figures. Patients suffering from pulmonary and cardiac diseases have been found to experience visions of white, black, or gray stationary figures (71). Hallucinations in delirium tremens typically teem with small animals, such as mice, rats, insects, or snakes, in vivid color and constant motion. Young children, aged 3 to 6 years, may hallucinate about being attacked by snakes or other animals and react with panic (72).

Actions of the assorted hallucinated objects with regard to the patient vary. They may appear to be indifferent or, by contrast, attacking, pursuing, or engulfing, for example. The patient's reactions are accordingly diverse. They may range from amused detachment to panic, and from a tendency to approach the visions to frantic attempts to escape them. In one series, 67% of the delirious patients responded to their visual hallucinations by taking some action, such as hitting at or trying to run away from the visions (65). One of my patients urged his wife to bring his revolver to the hospital so that he could shoot some black men entering his room through a nonexistent hatch in the ceiling and making threatening gestures. Fear is a typical response to hallucinations in delirium tremens. In general, unpleasant emotions of fear, anger, and despair appear to be more common in response to delirious hallucinations than amusement or other positive emotions. Most people become delirious in the course of an illness, often a life-threatening one, and their hallucinations and reactions to them tend to reflect their existential plight. Delirium itself is usually a highly disturbing experience that augments the sufferer's distress. The hallucinations and associated delusions tend to reflect this situation and call for empathic understanding on the part of those in attendance. The patient's unconscious conflicts, as well as guilt feelings over actual or imaginary misdeeds, may also influence the content of the hallucinations and the emotional and behavioral response to them.

Auditory hallucinations, alone or combined with visual ones, occur in about 30% to 50% of cases (55–57,67). They display as much variability as visual misperceptions. They can be relatively simple, such as sounds of shooting, or involve hearing whole conversations, music, singing, screams, and so forth. The patient may try to engage in a dialogue with the hallucinated voices, shout at them, or laugh at them.

There are several questions regarding hallucinatory experiences in delirium. First, why do delirious patients tend to hallucinate? Second, why do some of them hallucinate while others do not? Third, why do visual hallucinations predominate? And fourth, what determines the form and contents of hallucinations in delirium? These questions touch upon important theoretical issues concerned with the organization of human information processing and the consequences of its disruption. No satisfactory answers can be offered at this stage of our knowledge; we can only try to formulate hypotheses based on diverse indirect lines of evidence. I hope that the following discussion will stimulate badly needed research in this area. Considering that delirium is a very common condition and, as it were, an experiment of nature in which hallucinations often occur, its neglect by students of perceptual abnormalities is hard to understand.

Research on hallucinations carried out in recent years has gone beyond their phenomenology and generated explanatory hypotheses formulated from several vantage points: biochemical, neurophysiological, psychological, and sociocultural (64,69,73–78). Methodological approaches to the study of hallucinations have included the use of hallucinogenic drugs, direct electrical stimulation of the brain, sensory and sleep deprivation, hypnosis, and observations of patients with cerebral diseases. All of this research is relevant to the problem of hallucinations in delirium, but its review is outside the scope of this book. Hallucinations also need to be compared to other perceptual phenomena, such as imagery, daydreams, and dreams. Klüver (79) has rightly pointed out that all these subjective phenomena show similarities of content and form, and that transitions from one of them to another may occur. Such transitions seem to take place in delirious patients, who are relatively unable to control vivid daydreaming and to distinguish internally derived imagery from veridical perceptions. Thus, continuity is postulated to exist among the various perceptual phenomena, both normal and abnormal. In delirium, an accentuation of the imagery, both waking and hypnagogic, may contribute to the occurrence of hallucinations.

To try to answer the first question posed above: why do delirious patients hallucinate? The occurrence of hallucinations in delirium appears to be codetermined by the following factors: 1. disruption of the normal sleep-wake cycle; 2. reduced or excessive cerebral cortical activation and arousal; 3. fluctuating levels of attention and awareness; 4. stimulation or disinhibition of the activity of the temporal cortex and the limbic system structures; and 5. disorganization of thought processes and consequent impairment of reality testing.

Some authors (78) have proposed a *perceptual release* theory of hallucinations, which may be applied to account for their occurrence in delirium. Optimal sensory input is needed to keep currently irrelevant memory traces derived from past percepts out of awareness. Thus, during normal wakefulness, the steady information input to the brain enables the person to maintain scanning and screening activity. When that input is reduced or impaired for any reason, and simultaneously when adequate cerebral cortical arousal is maintained, perceptual or memory traces may be released and reexperienced with varying degrees of vividness. The higher the level of arousal, the greater the vividness of the released memories will be. They may be experienced by the person as fantasies, images, dreams, or hallucinations.

In delirium, the above conditions are present. The information input is either reduced or impaired, or both, as a result of the patient's lower receptivity to it in a state of abnormally lowered or heightened alertness, or due to fluctuations of attention. Moreover, the ability to process information is diminished. The normal sleep-wake cycle is disrupted, and mental contents that are usually associated with sleep, drowsiness, and daydreaming tend to dominate the patient's awareness. Alertness fluctuates, and hence the screening and inhibition of percepts, memories, and images become difficult to sustain. Cortical arousal is generally sufficient for wakeful awareness and may be abnormally increased. At the same time, either the stimulation or the release from inhibition of the temporal lobe structures allows uncontrolled intrusion of stored memories into awareness. Concurrent disorganization of thought processes impairs reality testing and discrimination between percepts derived from actual sensory stimuli, on the one hand, and released long-term memories, on the other. Reduced, ambiguous, discordant, novel, or excessive sensory input tends to impair perceptual discrimination even more, and to facilitate the appearance of hallucinations.

One may hypothesize that a combination of the above factors accounts for the frequent occurrence of hallucinations in delirium. They are most pronounced in the hyperactive-hyperalert variant of it, exemplified by delirium tremens and other substance withdrawal deliria, as well as in states of intoxication with anticholinergic agents, for example. By contrast, in the hypoactive-hypoalert variant, the cerebral cortical arousal, or activity of the temporal lobe structures, or both, appears to be reduced, and hence hallucinations are less common. This admittedly speculative account represents a testable hypothesis.

A different methodological approach to the study of hallucinations, one relevant to their occurrence in delirium, has focused on their postulated relationship to *dreams* (54,64,74,76). It has been hypothesized that hallucinations represent *waking dreams* (74). Jacobs (76) asserts that functional inactivation of the brain's serotonin system is a necessary, but not a sufficient, condition for the emergence of both dreams and drug-induced hallucinations. He allows, however, that the similarities of these two types of mental phenomena do not imply that they are identical. Some investigators argue that information during REM sleep is processed through increased activation of the right hemisphere; hence, the dreams reflect the functional mode of that hemisphere (80). That mode or style is observed to be predominantly visual rather than verbal, as well as metaphoric, synthetic, and holistic (80). Dreams are also postulated to reflect underlying biological states (81). Both of these hypotheses appear to be applicable to hallucinations in delirium. The latter are predominantly visual in character, and their contents often suggest the patient's sense that his or her life is in danger, i.e., awareness of an altered biological state. Moreover, the patient is particularly likely to hallucinate during the night.

The above hypotheses are provocative and deserve to be taken seriously. They propose a suggestive similarity, not to be mistaken as identity, between dreams and hallucinations. They are particularly intriguing in view of the long history, documented in Chapter 1, of the idea that delirium represents a waking dream arising from disordered sleep. That notion may not be literally correct, but recent research on both dreams and hallucinations indicates a link between them that is worth pursuing by studies on delirium.

The remaining questions concerning delirious hallucinations allow only brief speculative comments for lack of relevant information. Why do only some delirious patients hallucinate? One may postulate that individual differences exist in susceptibility to both delirium and hallucinations. Different neurochemical and neurophysiological changes in delirium due to various causative factors are likely to occur. Some etiological factors may have a greater potential for eliciting hallucinations than others. Why do visual misperceptions predominate? Several possible reasons may be given. First, studies of waking mentation show that about 70% of imagery during relaxed wakefulness is visual (82). It is striking how closely this percentage corresponds to the reported proportion of visual hallucinations in delirium (55,56). Second, about 80% of REM dream reports involves visual imagery (82). And third, visual imagery tends to predominate in hypnagogic states, i.e., those interposed between sleep and wakefulness (69). This statement also applies to the hypnagogic hallucinations and sleep mentation of narcoleptics (83,84). Thus, waking, dream, and hypnagogic imagery is predominantly visual. In delirium, all that imagery appears to be enhanced and occurs in a mostly waking state. Moreover, if one considers that the syndrome is, at least in part, a disorder of wakefulness, then the type of information processing that normally characterizes REM sleep mentation may be postulated to extend to the waking state (85). Given the reduced capacity for rational thought and judgment in the delirious patient, some of this intensified visual imagery that dominates the stream of consciousness may be projected onto the environment and misperceived as being externally derived and real. In other words, it may be experienced as what we refer to as "hallucinations."

Finally, what determines the form and content of delirious hallucinations? The determinants of the form are unknown, but clinical observations seem to throw some light on the factors that influence the content. Some writers have proposed that the delirious patient's misperceptions tend to reflect his or her remote and recent life events stored as episodic memory, as well as unconscious conflicts, impulses, guilt feelings, and defenses (64,86). These psychodynamic hypotheses are plausible and call for systematic studies of delirious subjects to validate them. Clinical impressions suggest that some hallucinations in these patients do indeed reflect highly meaningful mental contents and their symbolic representation (2,55,56). At the same time, however, many of the reported misperceptions appear to be relatively simple and devoid of personal meaning.

In summary, hallucinations are reported to occur in between 40% and 75% of cases. They are neither invariably present in nor diagnostic of delirium. Younger patients appear to hallucinate more often than the older ones, i.e., those aged 60 years and older. Visual and combined visual-auditory misperceptions predominate. A relationship between hallucinations, dreams, and waking and hypnagogic imagery has been postulated. All of them are hypothesized to reflect increased activity and the information-processing mode of the right cerebral hemisphere. Relevant pathophysiological and neurochemical mechanisms are discussed in Chapters 6 and 7.

Disorders of memory

Memory is the third major cognitive function to be impaired in delirium. Neuropsychologists distinguish two memory systems: *short-term* and *long-term* (46,87). Clinicians tend to recognize three kinds of memory rather than two. Some speak of *registration, immediate memory,* and *long-term memory* (52), while others distinguish *immediate, recent,* and *remote memory.* Immediate memory lasts for seconds, short-term memory for minutes, and long-term memory for days or years (87). The clinical terminology reflects not so much the underlying mechanisms as those aspects of memory assessment in a mental status examination (87).

In terms of clinical classification, all three kinds or stages of memory appear to be impaired in delirium to some extent (88). The level of alertness influences what and how much is remembered and learned (87). As that level is either abnormally increased or decreased in this syndrome, the amount of information that enters memory storage is liable to be reduced. Registration is affected, with a decreased amount of information being transferred to short-term memory storage. Immediate memory, regarded by some writers as the first phase of short-term memory (52), is impaired and the retention span is shortened, resulting in reduced acquisition of new information. Long-term memory also appears to be impaired to some extent. As systematic research on memory disorders in delirium has not been reported to date, their precise nature is unclear. The patient exhibits *anterograde amnesia,* i.e., inability or impaired ability to remember life events from the onset of delirium. There is also evidence of some degree of *retrograde amnesia,* i.e., loss of memory for events preceding the onset of delirium. The extent of this memory loss has not been systematically investigated in delirious patients, but it appears to extend for days or weeks rather than months or years. In such cases, clinicians usually state that the patient's recent memory is impaired but that remote memory is intact. Of course, if delirium develops in a demented patient, the extent of retrograde amnesia is liable to be much greater due to the underlying brain disease. In some conditions, such as tuberculous meningitis, herpes simplex encephalitis, and Wernicke's encephalopathy, the retrograde amnesia is also liable to be disproportionately severe while the patient is delirious (89). In such cases, one should probably speak of delirium superimposed on an amnestic syndrome.

Confabulation was observed in about 15% of delirious patients in one series (56). It refers to a tendency to fill gaps in memory with invented imaginary happenings that are elaborated to varying degrees (90). Delirious patients who do confabulate tend to give relatively simple, unembellished, and shifting confabulatory answers; such answers are difficult to tell apart from delusions, as noted in an earlier section of this chapter. In one study (56), the most frequent confabulations concerned familiar everyday activities such as imaginary visits from relatives. Another common type of confabulation found in that study was the patient's insistence that he or she had to keep an important appointment and therefore should be allowed to leave the hospital. Confabulations may be voiced by a patient spontaneously or in response to questions about recent activities, for example. The tendency to confabulate may be elicited by asking the patient to repeat a story read to him or her.

In summary, disorders of memory are an integral feature of delirium and form part of the global cognitive impairment. It appears that abnormally reduced or increased as well as fluctuating level of alertness and distractibility interfere with the patient's ability to register and retain information. Both anterograde and, to some extent, retrograde amnesia are present. Confabulation occurs in a minority of patients.

Disorders of orientation

As used in psychiatry, the term "orientation" refers to correct knowledge of one's spatial, temporal, and personal relationships (91–98). To orient oneself correctly in those respects requires reliable integration of attention, perception, and memory (52)."Orientation for time" indicates the ability to state correctly the day of the week, the date, and the time of day. "Orientation for place" refers to correct knowledge of the identity of the place one is in, as well as the ability to follow some normally familiar route and to appreciate the topographical arrangements of one's familiar surroundings. "Orientation for person" usually means the ability to identify correctly, by name and occupation, familiar people within one's field of vision. Sometimes it also connotes awareness of one's personal identity; to avoid ambiguity, this usage of the term is discouraged.

Orientation is discussed separately not because it represents a distinct cognitive function but because of its clinical importance in the diagnosis of delirium. As indicated earlier, orientation is not a basic cognitive function. On the contrary, it may be regarded as a product of integrated cognitive processes. Its abnormalities are traditionally subsumed under the global term "disorientation."

Some writers view disorientation as an essential feature of delirium (51), and it is so listed in *DSM-III-R* (16), which states, however, that it is "common." Some writers assert that in cases of relatively mild disturbance of awareness, the delirious patient is usually correctly oriented (88). In this writer's opinion, some degree of temporal disorientation at some period during the day is necessary for the diagnosis of the syndrome.

Disorientation for *time* varies in severity from case to case and often in the course of a single day. It is the first disorder of orientation to appear in delirium and the last to disappear. In its mildest form, it involves an inability to state correctly the date and the day of the week. Some investigators have proposed that temporal disorientation should be suspected if a patient with some college education misstates the day of the month by more than *1* day (96). A similar conclusion may be reached, according to those authors, if a patient with only a high school education misses the day of the month by more than *3* days. However, to state the exact degree of error that should be considered abnormal is to some extent arbitrary. Mistakes in giving the day and the week are not uncommon among healthy people. For example, a study of presumably normal passers-by at a university showed that about 12% of them made an error in response to the question "What day of the week is today?" (92). The mistakes involved mostly one day in the middle of the week and were readily corrected by the subjects—an important point. It is proposed that an error of *three* days in giving the date or the day of the week should be considered significant. Moreover, mistaking a weekday for the weekend should also be so regarded. Errors in giving the month, season, and year are clearly abnormal. Mistakes in stating the time of the day may be considered significant if they involve four or more hours. A more objective way of assessing temporal orientation involves scoring the answers to a set of five questions concerning the day of the week, day of the month, year, and time of day (95). Mistakes result in deduction of points from an assigned perfect score of 100. Moderate and severe disorientation are defined operationally in terms of the attained score.

In a mild case of delirium, only temporal disorientation is present at some time during the waking hours. Disorientation for *place* and *person* usually appears as delirium increases in severity and tends to disappear before temporal disorientation. Assessment of orientation for place involves questions about the name, location, and kind of place the patient is in. It is also important to test the patient's appreciation of direction and distance in regard to places, such as home, with which he or she is familiar (52). As a general rule, in delirium one tends to *mistake the unfamiliar for the familiar* (94). Thus, the hospital may be misidentified as home, or as the patient's place of work, or as a hospital closer to home. The same general rule applies to disorientation for *person*. The patient may misidentify doctors and nurses as friends or relatives. In severe delirium, he or she may fail to recognize family members. Rarely, if ever, does a delirious patient lose awareness of personal identity. *Spatial* disorientation is manifested by the patient's inability to find the way to his or her own room, or to describe how to reach home or some other familiar place, or to follow some normally known route, or to indicate spatial relations of the various components of a familiar place (93).

Some investigators have postulated that disorientation for time and place is a manifestation of denial of illness and a wish to leave the hospital, rather than of disordered memory, perception, and thought (98). This hypothesis fails to distinguish between negative and positive aspects of disorientation. The negative aspects simply mean not knowing the fact as a result of cognitive impairment consequent upon brain dysfunction. The positive aspects include misinterpretation and confabulation that may reflect the patient's wishes to deny and avoid a distressing situation, or wish-fulfilling efforts to minimize the threatening unfamiliarity of the surroundings as well as to reduce anxiety and helplessness.

In summary, disorientation is a diagnostically important feature of delirium, yet one that is not pathognomonic. A patient suffering from dementia, amnestic syndrome, severe anxiety or depression, or schizophrenia, or one who is mentally retarded, may also be disoriented, especially for time, without being delirious. Moreover, disorientation may be absent in mild delirium during much of the daytime, only to become manifest at night or in the dark. As such, it is not diagnostic of delirium.

Noncognitive psychological disorders

In the preceding sections of this chapter, the core psychopathology of delirium, which is essential for its diagnosis, was discussed. Yet the syndrome involves more than cognitive-attentional disturbances. Disordered *psychomotor activity* and disturbed *emotional state* are inseparably linked with the above disturbances. Moreover, delirium is not just a clinical syndrome but an altered state of awareness of self and environment that constitutes a *subjective experience,* one usually unpleasant and even frightening for the affected individual. Of these three aspects, only psychomotor activity (behavior) is included among the diagnostic criteria for delirium in the current official classification of mental disorders (16). Emotional disturbances are listed under the rubric of "associated features," yet they are essential from the patient's point of view, as they determine the subjective quality of a delirious episode, as well as influence cognitive functioning and behavior. Complications of delirium, such as self-injury, may result from high emotional arousal manifested as panic or rage, for example. The emotional and behavioral disturbances can also complicate the differential diagnosis because the patient may be mistakenly thought to suffer from a functional mental disorder such as mania, depression, or schizophrenia. For these reasons, the noncognitive disorders in delirium need to be included in a comprehensive account of its psychopathology.

Disorders of psychomotor behavior

"Psychomotor activity" refers to a person's observable behavior, verbal and nonverbal, in a given situation. It includes such factors as *reaction time* (speed of initiating movement or speech), *speed* of movement, *flow of speech, involuntary movements,* and *handwriting.*

It was pointed out in Chapter 4 that a delirious patient tends to be either *hyperactive* or *hypoactive* compared to his or her premorbid behavioral characteristics. A hyperactive patient's reaction time is short; activity rate is increased; motor response is prompt; overall motility is heightened; and vocalization is frequent, often loud, and uttered under pressure. The patient shows ceaseless, if mostly semipurposeful, activity that may lead to collapse. By contrast, a hypoactive patient displays slow reaction time; reduced activity rate and flow of speech; slow motor response; reduced motility; and general inertia. Either the hyperactive or the hypoactive mode of psychomotor behavior may predominate, or the same patient may shift from one extreme to the other in the course of a single episode of delirium or even during a single day. This is well illustrated by the following description of delirious uremic patients: "The entire course of the illness may shift rapidly from states of overactivity with aggressiveness, crying, laughing, singing, dancing, and swearing to states of lethargy" (99, p 685). Some etiological factors usually give rise to either increased or decreased psychomotor activity. Withdrawal from alcohol or sedative-hypnotics, as well as intoxication with certain drugs, such as trihexyphenidyl hydrochloride (Artane), are typically accompanied by hyperactivity. The same is reported to apply after infarction in the right middle cerebral artery territory associated with damage to the right middle temporal gyrus (100).

Some authors include hyperactivity in their definition of delirium (100,101). In my opinion this is misleading, as discussed in Chapter 4. Psychomotor behavior is but *one* feature of delirium, and the syndrome, as defined in the current American classification of mental disorders (16), comprises *both* extremes of it. Engel and Romano (88) emphasize in their classical paper that while many delirious patients display overactivity and excitement, many more show varying degrees of somnolence, lethargy, and hypoactivity. It is obvious, however, that if an investigator includes psychomotor overactivity among the essential features of delirium, all hypoactive patients will be excluded from the study. Moreover, if a clinical sample consists mostly of, say, patients with delirium tremens, the reported frequency of hyperactivity is liable to be close to 100%. Wolff and Curran (56), for example, state that restlessness was present in all their patients, but their clinical sample was skewed in that it included a large proportion of alcoholics. Their otherwise meticulous study has been uncritically quoted by many authors for the past 50 years and has helped to perpetuate a one-sided view of delirium. In many metabolic encephalopathies and after infarction in the right middle cerebral artery territory, delirium tends to be hypoactive, especially in elderly patients (100,102).

Hypoactivity

Hypoactivity may range from general slowness of motor response and reduced frequency of spontaneous movements and speech to stupor. A few patients are catatonic or mute. Those suffering from encephalitis lethargica, for example, display lethargy, catatonia, catalepsy, and marked slowing of motor responses (103). By contrast, other encephalitic patients are hyperactive, or show unpredictable shifts from overactivity to lethargy and vice versa (103). These observations on patients suffering from the same disease provide a compelling argument in favor of a unitary concept of delirium, regardless of the type of psychomotor behavior displayed. The majority of hypoactive patients are somnolent, indifferent, and generally slow rather than akinetic or catatonic. They may be difficult to rouse and communicate with. Their responses and movements, spontaneous or on command, are slow, and their speech is hesitant. Even though such patients may appear to be lethargic and indifferent, however, they may still experience intense emotions and hallucinations (55). In other words, a lethargic appearance does not necessarily mean that the patient is totally inattentive to the surroundings or devoid of a lively inner mentation. Hypoactive patients are often unrecognized as being delirious by the clinical staff. As a result, their cognitive impairment may go undetected, their anguish is not appreciated, and their ability to hear and understand what is being said about them is not even surmised.

Hyperactivity

This is manifested by increased speed of motor responses and by a heightened frequency and tempo of movements and speech. Such responses, movements, and verbalizations, however, tend to be poorly modulated and controlled.

The increased frequency and speed of spontaneous movements may range in complexity from aimless tossing about (jactitation) to relatively purposeful, goal-directed motor activity that may result in the patient's leaving the ward and wandering away. Groping, flapping, tossing, squirming, grasping or picking at bedclothes (carphology), flailing the arms, searching under the bed, and other such activities are often observed. At a more purposeful and organized level, the patient may dress or undress, get out of bed, explore the surroundings, and so forth. Some patients mimic their usual familiar or occupational activities. Thus, a barman may repeatedly make the gestures of filling a glass, or an avid fisherman may throw an imaginary fishing line again and again. If such activities are relatively well organized and repetitive and reflect the patient's work, one speaks of an "occupational delirium." A hyperactive, agitated delirious patient may be violent and destructive at times. Speech tends to be accelerated, pressed, and incoherent. Shouted commands, calling relatives, screaming, wailing, swearing, and loud singing may all be observed, notably at night. All such vocalizations may be repeated, in a low or loud voice, for hours on end.

Speech, language and writing

Verbal behavior has already been mentioned. The speed, frequency, and loudness of vocalizations are often either increased or decreased in delirium. Speech is absent on occasion, and the patient is mute. At the other extreme, a ceaseless flow of speech, often repetition of the same words or phrases, tends to be part of general overactivity. The pitch of the speech also varies from whispering or low muttering to loud vocalizations. Some patients display multiple abnormalities of speech such as hesitation, repetition, circumlocution, frequent slips of the tongue, and paraphasias (inappropriate substitutions of words or misnaming) (104,105). Some writers (105) assert that language impairment is not usually a prominent feature in delirium and, when present, varies and should be differentiated from aphasia. Reading comprehension, writing to dictation, and relevance (degree of association between the stimulus and the response) tend to be impaired (105). These deficits have been blamed on attention disorders and difficulty in concentrating (105). Finally, writing is usually defective; deficits may include poorly drawn letters, neographisms, improper spatial alignment of letters, and spelling errors (106). *Dysgraphia* is claimed to be the most common linguistic disorder in confusional states (106).

Perseveration

A common feature of the delirious patient's psychomotor behavior is a tendency to perseverate (107). Perseveration, that is, the continuation of a response after it is no longer appropriate, may be tested by asking the patient to copy and maintain alternating letters or repetitive sequential patterns of hand movements, or to give the days of the week forward and then backward (52). The perseverating patient will carry out the first request correctly but, when asked to switch to the next task, will continue to perform the preceding one. An observer may suspect perseveration if a patient spontaneously repeats certain words, phrases, or gestures without rhyme or reason.

Motivation

A discussion of psychomotor behavior and of performance generally would be incomplete without a reference to motivation. This aspect of delirium appears to have been overlooked in clinical accounts published to date. Lezak (52) speaks of "executive functions" in this context, namely, those capacities that enable a person to initiate and sustain goal-directed, purposeful actions successfully. Delirious patients have impaired ability to engage in and sustain such actions. They may be apathetic and easily fatigued, and hence lack motivation to initiate and carry out any activity, even if potentially able to do so. Such reduced or absent motivation (anergy) is typically seen in hypoactive-hypoalert patients and is liable to affect not only their spontaneous behavior, but also their overall performance in response to questions or commands, as in the course of a mental status examination. Hyperactive-hyperalert patients, by contrast, show increased readiness to initiate action and respond to stimuli, but their behavior is disorganized, impulsive, and erratic. Such indiscriminate, poorly modulated, and poorly sustained motivation is bound to make their behavior and performance ineffective in terms of reaching specific goals. These motivational disturbances, combined with the global cognitive-attentional abnormalities, render patients incapable of self-care. Moreover, they can make patients appear more cognitively impaired that they really are—a possibility to consider in conducting an examination.

In summary, the presence of either increased or decreased psychomotor activity constitutes one of the essential features of delirium. A delirious patient may display either hyperactivity or hypoactivity in regard to verbal and nonverbal behavior. It is a fallacy to define delirium as a syndrome characterized by psychomotor hyperactivity, as some writers are wont to do. A whole range of abnormalities involving reaction time, motor response, speed and frequency of spontaneous movements, flow of speech, and writing may occur. Motivation is usually impaired, as is the ability to engage in planned, goal-directed behavior.

Disorders of emotions and mood

Emotional disturbances are very often observed in delirious patients (2,16,55–57). They run the gamut of mostly dysphoric emotions such as fear, anxiety, depression, anger, and apathy. Euphoria has been stressed by some observers (32) but is uncommon. Some patients maintain the same type of emotional state throughout, while others display emotional *lability*. Some investigators have found *fear* to be the most common emotional disturbance (56), while in other series of patients *depression* prevailed (57,88). Many patients appear to be simply *apathetic,* i.e., lacking a distinct emotional tone. For example, in one study 30% of the subjects were reported to exhibit a "shallow, constricted or flattened feeling tone" (57, p 297). Thus, emotional arousal in delirium may range in intensity from apathy to panic, rage, and elation. The emotions are predominantly unpleasant and may vary in quality and intensity not only in the course of a single episode of delirium, but also throughout the day. Many patients are irritable, impulsive, and show poor control and modulation of emotional expression. Verbal and nonverbal concomitants of emotions, including facial expression, may provide clues to the patient's subjective feeling tone and experience. Moreover, autonomic nervous system arousal usually accompanies intense emotions such as fear or anger. One may thus observe dilated pupils, pallor or flushing of the face, sweating, tachycardia, and elevated blood pressure. These signs may, of course, represent manifestations of an intoxication with a substance, such as an anticholinergic drug, that has caused the delirium.

On the whole, intense emotions, mostly fear and anger, tend to accompany the hyperactive-hyperalert variant of delirium, and are often associated with hallucinations and delusions. By contrast, a hypoactive-hypoalert patient is more likely to be apathetic or depressed and not to hallucinate. There are, of course, exceptions to these general trends. Some mildly delirious patients may exhibit *shame* at being confused.

Emotional disturbances in delirium have multiple potential *determinants.* They may reflect the patient's personality; awareness of and concern about being ill and cognitively impaired; content of experienced thoughts, images, and misperceptions; the characteristics of the sensory environment in the treatment setting; and direct involvement of the limbic system (2). Cognitive impairment, with the resulting subjective sense of confusion and helplessness, tends to be highly threatening and stressful in persons for whom maintenance of intellectual and perceptual clarity is crucial for a feeling of security and self-esteem. Paranoid personality traits are readily enhanced by subjective awareness of being less in control of the environment, relatively helpless, and dependent on others. Persecutory delusions and related intense emotions may be elicited in a basically mistrustful and insecure person, but they are sometimes also displayed by one who is normally placid and self-confident.

In addition to personality, factors related to the illness itself influence the patient's emotional state. If, as often happens, delirium results from a traumatic event, such as severe burns or a head injury, or if it complicates a serious, painful, or terminal illness, the aroused emotions are likely to be both unpleasant and intense (108). They reflect the patient's justified sense of being in danger or of having lost something of value, as well as the resulting anguish and distress. If the illness sets in at an otherwise stressful time, it is liable to intensify the already experienced anxiety or depression, or both. Delirium and confusion may augment such emotions even further to the point of despair or panic. Moreover, the content of the delirious patient's thoughts, imagery, dreams, and hallucinations is influenced by his or her emotional state and is liable to have a positive feedback effect on it. Such content may reflect not only the recent stressful life events and related concerns, but also the patient's long-standing unconscious conflicts, guilt feelings, and fears. If hallucination is occurring, that fact alone may frighten the patient on account of its association in our culture with insanity.

The sensory quality of the *environment* in which the patient is being treated is also relevant. Its very unfamiliarity may be frightening, especially in an intensive care unit (109). The sight of strange apparatus and people, the perception of strange and disturbing sounds, or the sight of other patients being resuscitated or dying can all have this effect. Darkness, shadows, glaring lights, and other such features of the surroundings tend to add to the patient's sense of unfamiliarity, danger, and fear. Separation from close, familiar people compounds the feeling of distress. These aspects of a delirious patient's experience tend to be ignored by those in attendance, yet they may result in avoidable crises on the ward, injuries to the patient or others, and possible medicolegal complications.

Apart from the above psychosocial and environmental factors, one other set of variables may influence the patient's emotional state. One may postulate that pathological conditions that involve direct stimulation of the *limbic structures* constituting the anatomical substrate of emotions, or their release from cortical inhibition, or both, can co-determine a delirious patient's emotional state.

Emotional disturbances in delirium are important both for the patient and for those in attendance. High emotional arousal, together with related heightened sympathetic nervous sytem activity and increased catecholamine levels, can have an adverse effect on the patient's prognosis. An intensely fearful and agitated delirious patient who has just suffered a myocardial infarction may develop a lethal cardiac arrhythmia, for example. Depression may lead to attempted suicide. Panic or rage may result in injury to the self or others if the patient tries to run away or fight. An apathetic and quiet delirious patient may gradually slip into stupor and coma without being noticed. Clearly, the emotional state in delirium should be assessed and monitored by the staff in order to prevent the possible complications mentioned above. Failure to do so could result in injury or even death of the patient.

In summary, emotional disturbances in delirium are very common and variable in quality and intensity. Fear, anxiety, depression, and anger, i.e., dysphoric emotions, predominate, but many patients are mostly apathetic and indifferent. These emotional states may shift rapidly and unpredictably, and may be accompanied by congruous verbal and nonverbal behavior. Emotional lability is common. Autonomic nervous system hyperactivity is associated with intense emotional arousal. The quality and intensity of the displayed emotions are co-determined by the patient's personality, illness experience, features of the sensory environment, and other factors. The emotions color the patient's subjective experience, may result in serious complications, and should be assessed for proper management.

Delirium as subjective experience

In the preceding sections, delirium was dissected into its constituent parts. This is necessary for the purpose of clinical research and diagnosis, and ultimately for understanding the pathophysiological mechanisms involved. This analytical approach, however, leaves out one essential element: the quality of the subjective experience of that altered state of awareness that we call "delirium." This point was raised by Fothergill (110) a century ago: "Very few care to analyse their sensations or their remembrances of a delirious past, and consequently there is but little in our literature which tells us of the attitude of delirium *from the patient's point of view"* (p 402), (italics added). A search of the literature has uncovered only a handful of such personal accounts.

An early account can be found in Armstrong's (111) treatise on typhus. He described his own delirium, which was ushered in by a "state of strange confusion" and the "most horrible dreams." Visual hallucinations followed: "As the evening advanced, whenever I closed my eyes I was harassed with a succession of human figures; but it was remarkable, that none of these were representations of the persons who had visited me, all having faces, with one exception, which I had never before seen" (111, p 118).

The most detailed and elaborate personal account of delirium that I could find was given by Mickle (112) in his Presidential Address to the Neurological Society of London in 1901. He referred to what appears to have been his own experience of delirium as "mental wandering" lived through in the course of typhoid fever. He described a wide range of abnormal experiences, including confusion about his own identity; vivid visual illusions and hallucinations; total insomnia; fluctuations in the level of awareness, with periods of relatively lucid thinking; and changes of mood from a predominant state of exaltation to profound, if transient, depression. Particularly interesting are his remarks about the merging of dreams with waking mentation once he was able to sleep: "The phenomena of dreaming on the one hand; the illusory and hallucinatory elements of delirium on the other; have some close resemblances when viewed apart. And in the sleeping state of deliriants, such as it is, the delirium and dreams seem to fuse into one. . . . Then we may speak of delirious dreaming (or of dreamy delirium)" (p 13). Under such influence of "sleep-dream," he wrote, "the illusory and hallucinatory phenomena assumed a greater sensual vivacity." Mickle ended his account on a philosophical note: "When we ponder on the basis of mind, it must, for us, be a lesson in humility. . . . A slight change in the chemical constituents of the blood can raise us to the height of bliss, plunge us into the depth of despair, or, as in our case tonight, with light delirious touch strike many a note in the scale of morbid mind" (p 23).

It is remarkable that Mickle could remember his delirium in such detail. He pointed out, however, that it was rather mild and quiet, and this may be why he was able to retain in memory so many impressions. Several other accounts can be found in the more recent literature. Levin (113), the author of many clinical papers on delirium, has published his own encounter with it in the course of bacterial meningitis. Throughout his delirious episode, he was preoccupied with his professional work; it was, he stated, an "occupational delirium." Guttman (66) experienced an "oneiric delirium" while suffering from typhus and described reliving in a picture-like, panoramic mode a sequence of his personally meaningful life events. Thomson (114), a nurse, described vividly her experiences during delirium: "Birds and stars floated around my head. I was in the bottom of a whirlpool, peering out at the faces of the doctors and nurses calling to me at the top. I whirled and whirled, wanting to call out, to tell them I was coming, but I couldn't." Wilbourn (115), a young physician, delirious during an attack of meningoencephalitis, reported seeing the outside world through a haze and being generally hypersensitive. He summed up his subjective experience as an "unpleasant twilight state between sleep and wakefulness."

As these few and necessarily rather fragmentary personal accounts by physicians and a nurse suggest, the subjective experience of delirium tends to be highly variable, dream-like, and mostly disturbing. It may be rich in personally meaningful thoughts and imagery, which the patient can remember and be distressed by long after the delirium is over (53,116). Indeed, the whole episode is likely to be highly stressful (116). Not all patients, however, experience a vivid, dream-like delirium. For many, it appears to be mainly a drowsy, dull, and vaguely remembered state. Some may have experienced disturbing hallucinations and thoughts, but repressed them upon recovery and hence have mostly an amnesia for these events. Wolff and Curran (56) assert that all of the patients in their study experienced various combinations of uncertainty, perplexity, strangeness, mistrust, fear, and depression. Moreover, patients tends to have similar experiences from one delirious episode to another. I can confirm this from my own repeated childhood experiences of delirium in the course of febrile illnesses. At the height of the fever I hallucinated a large, transparent bubble that seemed to be very heavy, despite its deceptively light appearance, and moved slowly toward me as if about to crush me. It was a distinctly unpleasant and frightening experience.

In summary, from the subjective point of view, delirium is likely to be an unpleasant, disturbing, and often frightening experience, a stressful life event superimposed on the usually already distressing symptoms of the underlying medical condition. This fact should be taken into account by those in attendance, as the patient's state calls for empathic understanding of his or her distress. For some patients, delirium is a disturbing dream-like state of altered awareness of self and environment. For others, it is a period of drowsy and dull lethargy.

References

1. Bleuler M.: Acute mental concomitants of physical diseases, in Benson D. F., Blumer D. (eds): *Psychiatric Aspects of Neurological Disease.* New York, Grune & Stratton, 1975, pp 37–61.
2. Lipowski Z. J.: Delirium, clouding of consciousness and confusion. *J. Nerv. Ment. Dis.* 1967;145:227–225.
3. Ey H.: Disorders of consciousness in psychiatry, in Vinken P. J., Bruyn G. W. (eds): *Handbook of Clinical Neurology,* Vol. 3. Amsterdam, North-Holland, 1969, pp 112–136.
4. Hirsch W.: A study of delirium. *N.Y. Med. J.* 1899;70:109–115.
5. Hoch H.: A study of some cases of delirium produced by drugs. *Studies Psychiatry* 1912;1:75–93.
6. Oakley D. A.: Animal awareness, consciousness and self-image, in Oakley D. A. (ed): *Brain and Mind.* London, Methuen, 1985, pp 132–151.
7. Natsoulas T.: Concepts of consciousness. *J. Mind Behav.* 1983;4:13–59.
8. Frederiks J. A. M.: Consciousness, in Vinken P. J., Bruyn G. W. (eds): *Handbook of Clinical Neurology,* Vol. 3. Amsterdam, North-Holland, 1969, pp 48–61.
9. Broughton R.: Human consciousness and sleep/waking rhythms: A review and some neuro-psychological considerations. *J. Clin. Neuropsychol.* 1982;4:193–218.
10. Davidson J. M., Davidson R. J. (eds): *The Psychobiology of Consciousness.* New York, Plenum Press, 1980.
11. Gloor P.: Consciousness as a neurological concept in epileptology: A critical review. *Epilepsia* (Suppl 2) 1986;27:14–26.
12. Hilgard E. R.: Consciousness in contemporary psychology. *Ann. Rev. Psychol.* 1980;31:1–26.
13. Witelson S. F., Kristofferson A. B. (eds): *McMaster-Bauer Symposium on Consciousness.* Ottawa, Canadian Psychological Association, 1986.
14. Tulving E.: Memory and consciousness. *Can. Psychol.* 1985;26:1–12.
15. Webb A. C.: Consciousness and the cerebral cortex. *Br. J. Anaesth.* 1983;55:209–219.
16. *Diagnostic and Statistical Manual of Mental Disorders,* ed 3 revised. Washington, DC, American Psychiatric Association, 1987.

17. Harré R., Lamb R. (eds): *The Encyclopedic Dictionary of Psychology.* Cambridge, Mass., MIT Press, 1983.
18. Hebb D. O.: *Textbook of Psychology,* ed 3. Philadelphia, WB Saunders Co., 1972.
19. Kleitman N.: *Sleep and Wakefulness.* Chicago, University of Chicago Press, 1963.
20. Lipowski Z. J.: *Delirium. Acute Brain Failure in Man.* Springfield, Ill, Charles C Thomas, 1980.
21. Purkinje J. E.: Wachen, Schlaf, Traum und verwandte Zustände, in Wagner R. (ed): *Handwörterbuch der Physiologie,* Vol 3. Braunschweig, Vieweg, 1846, pp 413–480.
22. Luria A. R.: The quantitative assessment of levels of wakefulness. *Soviet Psychology* 1973;12:73–84.
23. Heinroth A.: *De Delirio Inter Somnum et Vigiliam.* Lipsiae, Typis Guil Staritzii, 1842.
24. Koella W. P.: A modern neurobiological concept of vigilance. *Experientia* 1982;38:1426–1437.
25. Bastiji H., Jouvet M.: Interet de l'agenda de sommeil pour l'etude des troubles de la vigilance. *Electroenceph. Clin. Neurophysiol.* 1985;60:299–305.
26. Feinberg I.: Sleep in organic conditions, in Kales A. (ed): *Sleep Physiology and Pathology.* Philadelphia, J.B. Lippincott, 1969, pp 131–147.
27. Gaillord J. M.: Neurochemical regulation of the states of alertness. *Ann. Clin. Res.* 1985;17:175–184.
28. Okawa M., Matousek M., Petersen I.: Spontaneous vigilance fluctuations in the daytime. *Psychophysiology* 1984;21:207–211.
29. Kripke D. F., Sonnenschein D.: A biologic rhythm in waking fantasy, in Pope K. S., Singer R. L. (ed): *The Stream of Consciousness.* New York, Pleum Press, 1978, pp 323–332.
30. Wollman M. C., Antrobus J. S.: Sleeping and waking thought: Effects of external stimulation. *Sleep* 1986;9:438–448.
31. Ey H., Lairy G. C., de Barros-Ferreira M., et al: *Psychophysiologie du Sommeil et Psychiatrie.* Paris, Masson, 1975.
32. Geschwind N.: Disorders of attention: A frontier in neuropsychology. *Philos. Trans. R. Soc. Lond. Biol.* 1982;298:173–185.
33. Swift H. M.: Delirium and delirious states. *Boston Med. Surg. J.* 1907;157:687–692.
34. Allport D. A.: Selection for action: Some behavioral and neurophysiological considerations of attention and action, in Heuer H., Sanders A. F. (eds): *Perspectives on Perception and Action.* Hillsdale, NJ, Erlbaum, 1987, pp 395–419.
35. Bourne L.E., Dominowski R. L., Loftus E. F.: *Cognitive Processes.* Englewood Cliffs, NJ, Prentice-Hall, 1979.
36. Luria A. R.: *Higher Cortical Functions in Man.* New York, Basic Books, 1966.
37. Luria A. R.: *The Working Brain.* London, Penguin Books, 1973.
38. Mountcastle V. B.: Brain systems for directed attention. *J. R. Soc. Med. (Lond.)* 1978;71:14–27.
39. Posner M. I., Boies S. J.: Components of attention. *Psychol. Rev.* 1971;5:391–408.
40. Posner M. I., Inhoff A. W., Friedrich F. J.: Isolating attentional systems: A cognitive-anatomical analysis. *Psychobiology* 1987;15:107–121.

41. Posner M. I., Rafal R. D.: Cognitive theories of attention and the rehabilitation of attentional deficits, in Meier M. J., Benton A. L. (eds): *Neuropsychological Rehabilitation.* Edinburgh, Churchill Livingstone, 1987, pp 182–201.
42. White A. R.: *Attention.* Oxford, Basil Blackwell, 1964.
43. Pribram K. H.: Mind, brain, and consciousness: The organization of competence and conduct, in Davidson J. M., Davidson R. J. (eds): *The Psychobiology of Consciousness.* New York, Plenum Press, 1980, pp 47–63.
44. Hernandez-Peon R.: Physiological mechanisms in attention, in Russell R. W. (ed): *Frontiers in Physiological Psychology.* New York, Academic Press, 1966, pp 121–147.
45. Hilgard E. R.: Atkinson R. L., Atkinson R. C.: *Introduction to Psychology,* ed 7. New York, Harcourt Brace Jovanovich, 1979.
46. Loftus E. L., Schooler J. W.: Information processing conceptualizations of human cognition: Past, present, and future, in Ruben B. D. (ed): *Information and Behavior,* Vol. 1. New Brunswick, NJ, Transaction Books, 1985, pp 225–250.
47. Barrough P.: *The Method of Physick,* ed 3. London, Field, 1596.
48. Jaspers K.: *General Psychopathology.* Chicago, University of Chicago Press, 1963.
49. Pope K. S., Singer J. L.: The waking stream of consciousness, in Davidson J. M., Davidson R. J. (eds): *The Psychobiology of Consciousness.* New York, Plenum Press, 1980, pp 169–191.
50. Singer J. L.: Navigating the stream of consciousness. *Am. Psychol.* 1975;30:727–738.
51. Levin M.: Thinking disturbances in delirium. *A.M.A. Arch. Neurol. Psychiatry* 1956;75:62–66.
52. Lezak M. D.: *Neuropsychological Assessment,* ed 2. New York, Oxford University Press, 1983.
53. Blank K., Perry S.: Relationship of psychological processes during delirium to outcome. *Am. J. Psychiatry* 1984;141:843–847.
54. Kramer M., Roth T., Arand D., et al: Waking and dreaming mentation: A test of their relationship. *Neurosci. Lett.* 1981;22:83–86.
55. Bleuler M., Willi J., Buhler H. R.: *Akute Psychische Begleiter scheinungen körperlicher Krankheiten.* Stuttgart, Thieme, 1966.
56. Wolff H. G., Curran D.: Nature of delirium and allied states. *A.M.A. Arch. Neurol. Psychiatry* 1935;33:1175–1215.
57. Farber I. J.: Acute brain syndrome. *Dis. Nerv. System.* 1959;20:296–299.
58. Simon A., Cahan R. B.: The acute brain syndrome in geriatric patients. *Psychiatr. Res. Rep.* 1963;16:8–21.
59. Morris G. O., Singer M. T.: Sleep deprivation: The content of consciousness. *J. Nerv. Ment. Dis.* 1966;143:291–304.
60. Lunn V.: On body hallucinations. *Acta Psychiatr. Scand.* 1965;41:387–399.
61. Dewhurst K., Pearson J.: Visual hallucinations of the self in organic disease. *J. Neurol. Neurosurg. Psychiatry* 1955;18:43–57.
62. Lunn V.: Autoscopic phenomena. *Acta Psychiatr. Scand. 46* Suppl 1970;219:118–125.
63. Willanger R., Klee A.: Metamorphopsia and other visual disturbances with latency occurring in patients with diffuse cerebral lesions. *Acta Neurol. Scand.* 1966;42:1–18.

64. Asaad G., Shapiro B.: Hallucinations: Theoretical and clinical overview. *Am. J. Psychiatry* 1986;143:1088–1097.
65. Frieske D. A., Wilson W. P.: Formal qualities of hallucinations: A comparative study of the visual hallucinations in patients with schizophrenic, organic and affective psychoses, in Hoch P. H., Zubin J. (eds): *Psychopathology of Schizophrenia.* New York, Grune & Stratton, 1966, pp 49–62.
66. Guttman O.: Psychic disturbances in typhus fever. *Psychiatr. Q.* 1952;26:478–491.
67. Mendelson J., Solomon P., Lindemann E.: Hallucinations of poliomyelitis patients during treatment in a respirator. *J. Nerv. Ment. Dis.* 1958;126:421–428.
68. Lewis D. J.: Lilliputian hallucinations in the functional psychoses. *Can. Psychiatr. Assoc. J.* 1961;6:177–201.
69. Mavromatis A.: *Hypnagogia.* London, Routledge & Kegan Paul, 1987.
70. Lowe G. R.: The phenomenology of hallucinations as an aid to differential diagnosis. *Br. J. Psychiatry* 1973;123:621–633.
71. Head H.: Certain mental changes that accompany visceral disease. *Brain* 1901;24:344–356.
72. Bender L.: The maturation process and hallucinations in children, in Keup W. (ed): *Origins and Mechanisms of Hallucinations.* New York, Plenum Press, 1970, pp 95–101.
73. Cummings J. L., Miller B. L.: Visual hallucinations. *West. J. Med.* 1987;146:46–51.
74. Dement W., Halper C., Pivik T., et al: Hallucinations and dreaming, in Hamburg D. (ed): *Perception and Its Disorders.* Baltimore, Williams & Wilkins, 1970, pp 335–359.
75. Goodwin D. W., Alderson P., Rosenthal R.: Clinical significance of hallucinations in psychiatric disorders. *Arch. Gen. Psychiatry* 1971;24:76–80.
76. Jacobs B. L.: Dreams and hallucinations: A common neurochemical mechanism mediating their phenomenological similarities. *Neurosci. Biobehav. Rev.* 1978;2:59–69.
77. Keup W. (ed): *Origin and Mechanisms of Hallucinations.* New York, Plenum Press, 1970.
78. Siegel R. K., West L. J. (eds): *Hallucinations: Behavior, Experience, and Theory.* New York, Wiley, 1975.
79. Klüver H.: Neurobiology of normal and abnormal perception, in Hoch P. H., Zubin J. (eds): *Psychopathology of Perception.* New York, Grune & Stratton, 1965, pp 1–40.
80. Gabel S.: Information processing in rapid eye movement sleep. *J. Nerv Ment. Dis.* 1987;175:193–200.
81. Smith R. C.: Do dreams reflect a biological state? *J. Nerv. Ment. Dis.* 1987;175:201–207.
82. Foulkes D., Fleisher S., Trupin E.: Thought-sampling in relaxed wakefulness, in Levin P., Koella W. P. (eds): *Sleep 1974.* Basel, Karger, 1975, pp 142–145.
83. Ribstein M.: Hypnagogic hallucinations. *Adv. Sleep Res.* 1976;3:145–160.
84. Vogel G. W.: Mentation reported from naps of narcoleptics. *Adv. Sleep Res.* 1976;3:161–166.
85. Tachibana M., Tanaka K., Hishikawa Y., et al: A sleep study of acute psychotic states due to alcohol and meprobamate addiction. *Adv. Sleep Res.* 1975;2:177–205.

86. Horowitz M. J.: Hallucinations: An information-processing approach, in Siegel R. K., West L. J. (eds): *Hallucinations: Behavior, Experience, and Theory*. New York, Wiley, 1975, pp 163–195.
87. Squire L. R.: *Memory and Brain*. New York, Oxford University Press, 1987.
88. Engel G. L., Romano J.: Delirium, a syndrome of cerebral insufficiency. *J. Chronic Dis.* 1959;9:260–277.
89. Parkin A. J.: *Memory and Amnesia*. Oxford, Basil Blackwell, 1987.
90. Mercer B., Wagner W., Gardner H., et al: A study of confabulation. *Arch. Neurol.* 1977;34:429–433.
91. Berrios G. E.: Orientation failures in medicine and psychiatry: Discussion paper. *J. R. Coll. Med.* 1983;76:379–385.
92. Koriat A., Fischhoft B.: What day is today? An inquiry into the process of time orientation. *Memory Cognition* 1974;2:201–205.
93. Levin M.: Spatial disorientation in delirium. *Am. J. Psychiatry* 1956;113:174–175.
94. Levin M.: Varieties of disorientation. *J. Ment. Sci.* 1956;102:619–623.
95. Levin H. S., Benton A. L.: Temporal orientation in patients with brain disease. *Appl. Neurophysiol.* 1975;38:56–60.
96. Natelson B. H., Haupt E. J., Fleischer E. J., et al: Temporal orientation and education. *Arch. Neurol.* 1979;36:444–446.
97. Pinsker H.: The implications of OX 3. *Compr. Psychiatry* 1984;25:473–477.
98. Weinstein E. A., Kahn R. L.: *Denial of Illness*. Springfield, Ill, Charles C Thomas, 1955.
99. Baker A. B., Knutson J.: Psychiatric aspects of uremia. *Am. J. Psychiatry* 1946;102:683–687.
100. Mori E., Yamadori A.: Acute confusional state and acute agitated delirium. *Arch. Neurol.* 1987;44:1139–1143.
101. Victor M., Adams R. D.: Confusion, delirium, amnesia, and dementia, in Braunwald E., Isselbacher K. J., Petersdorf R. G., et al. (eds): *Harrison's Principles of Internal Medicine*, ed 11. New York, McGraw-Hill, 1987, pp 127–133.
102. Blass J. P., Plum F.: Metabolic encephalopathies in older adults, in Katzman R., Terry R. D. (eds): *The Neurology of Aging*. Philadelphia, FA Davis, 1983, pp 189–220.
103. Walters J. H.: Encephalitis lethargica revisited. *J. Oper. Psychiatry* 1977;8:37–46.
104. Chedru F., Geschwind N.: Disorders of higher cortical functions in acute confusional states. *Cortex* 1972;8:395–411.
105. Kitselman K.: Language impairment in aphasia, delirium, dementia, and schizophrenia, in Darby J. K. (ed): *Speech Evaluation in Medicine*. New York, Grune & Stratton, 1981, pp 199–214.
106. Chédru F., Geschwind N.: Writing disturbances in acute confusional states. *Neuropsychologia* 1972;10:343–353.
107. Levin M.: Perseveration at various levels of complexity, with comments on delirium. *A.M.A. Arch. Neurol. Psychiatry* 1955;73:439–444.
108. Blank K., Perry S.: Relationship of psychological processes during delirium to outcome. *Am. J. Psychiatry* 1984;141:843–847.
109. Hackett T. P., Cassem N. H., Wishnie H. A.: The coronary-care unit: An appraisal of its psychologic hazards. *N. Engl. J. Med* 1968;279:1365–1370.
110. Fothergill J. M.: The management of delirium. *The Practitioner* 1874;13:400–408.

111. Armstrong J.: *Practical Illustrations of Typhus Fever.* New York, Duyckinck, Long, Collins & Co., 1824.
112. Mickle W. M. J.: Mental wandering. *Brain* 1901;24:1–26.
113. Levin M.: Delirium: An experience and some reflections. *Am. J. Psychiatry* 1968;124:1120–1123.
114. Thomson L. R.: Sensory deprivation: A personal experience. *Am. J. Nurs.* 1973;73:266–268.
115. Wilbourn A. J.: A report on infection inside my head. *Hosp. Phys.* 1972;3:38–64.
115. Mackenzie T. B., Popkin M. K.: Stress response syndrome occurring after delirium. *Am. J. Psychiatry* 1980;137:1433–1435.

6

Etiology

Delirium is, by definition, an organic mental syndrome. This implies that demonstrable brain dysfunction is a necessary condition for its occurrence. Such dysfunction, in turn, may be caused by one or more of a wide range of potential organic etiological factors originating in the brain itself, or elsewhere in the body, or introduced into the body in the form of toxic substances. Delirium may thus be regarded as a nonspecific psychopathological manifestation of disordered cerebral function brought about by one or more toxic, infectious, metabolic, neoplastic, and other pathogenic factors that disrupt the highest integrative functions of the brain. The nonspecificity of the syndrome implies that its occurrence and features do not allow identification of a specific causative agent or disease. Delirium is postulated to constitute the final common path for a large variety of possible etiological factors that cause a widespread disorder of cerebral metabolism, one affecting a whole spectrum of psychological functions, especially the cognitive-attentional ones.

Although the presence of one or more organic etiological factors is necessary for the occurrence of delirium, it may not be sufficient. Clinical observation suggests that the probability of developing the syndrome is increased if certain predisposing and facilitating or contributory factors are also present. These factors render an individual more vulnerable to the development of delirium. Consequently, a discussion of the etiology of delirium should include three classes of causative factors: *predisposing, facilitating,* and *precipitating (organic)* (1).

Predisposing factors

Delirium is a mental disorder to which everyone is potentially susceptible. One writer has aptly referred to this syndrome as "everyman's psychosis" to highlight the universal susceptibility to it (2). Clinical observation indicates, however, that not everyone is equally prone to develop it in the presence of the same etiological factor. For example, Ebaugh et al. (3) studied the incidence of delirium in 200 patients undergoing courses of pyretotherapy, i.e., the induction of fever in a hypertherm heated to 130°–150°F. Each patient's rectal temperature had to reach 104°–107°F in 1 hour. Fifty-four percent of the subjects developed delirium at least once. Forty percent of those who developed it did so on only one occasion, usually during the first treatment, even though they had several exposures to what seemed to have been identical conditions.

As this study suggests, *individual differences* in susceptibility to delirium in response to any given etiological agent probably exist. Some persons become delirious in the course of even a mild infection or after the intake of a small amount of a particular drug or other chemical substance. This readiness to develop the syndrome may be either *selective* or *general.* In the former case, the person is liable to develop it on the basis of a selective, or specific, vulnerability to the effects of a particular drug, or to hypoxia or hypoglycemia, for example. Such differential susceptibility to the deliriogenic potential of a given substance or other etiological factor may reflect a genetic or acquired predisposition. For example, acute porphyria with delirium may be precipitated in a predisposed person by the intake of barbiturates, steroids, and other drugs. Alcohol idiosyncratic intoxication is more likely to occur in a person who has suffered damage to a temporal lobe. Idiosyncrasy to a specific drug, such as acetylsalicylic acid, may underlie susceptibility to delirium on taking a therapeutic dose of it.

By contrast, general susceptibility implies that the person has a higher than average likelihood of becoming delirious in response to a wide range of causative agents. Aging, chronic cerebral disease, and damage of the brain are the most important factors. There is no conclusive evidence that hereditary factors or personality variables influence general susceptibility to delirium (4). Moreover, having a severe mental illness, such as schizophrenia, does not seem to increase the predisposition to develop delirium in the course of a physical illness, for example. One study failed to find a higher than expected incidence of delirium in schizophrenic patients and their relatives or an excessive frequency of schizophrenia among relatives of individuals who became delirious (4). Some anecdotal evidence suggests that patients who have experienced an episode of delirium in the past are more likely to develop it again in the presence of an appropriate deliriogenic factor (5). As mentioned earlier, only three general predisposing factors have been established so far:

1. Age of 60 years or over.
2. Brain damage.
3. Chronic brain disease, such as Alzheimer's disease.

Age is the most important predisposing factor in delirium (6–8). This implies that an elderly person is more likely to develop it in response to a mild infection or to a therapeutic dose of a medical drug, for example, that would not cause delirium in a younger individual. Such heightened general susceptibility to delirium in later life is the result of several factors. They include aging processes in the brain, notably those involving the central cholinergic system; increased vulnerability of the aging brain to hypoxia; reduced efficiency of the homeostatic and immune mechanisms, rendering an elderly person less resistant to disease as well as to stress of any origin; changes in circadian rhythms, including the sleep-wake cycle; a high prevalence of chronic diseases and an increased incidence of acute illnesses, especially respiratory and urinary tract infections; frequent impairment of vision and hearing; and impaired mechanisms of drug metabolism. All these changes combine to render an aging person progressively more prone to the occurrence of delirium. This topic is discussed in more detail in Chapter 18.

Damage to and *chronic, especially degenerative, disease* of the brain are also postulated to increase general susceptibility to delirium. It is a common clinical observation that elderly patients suffering from Alzheimer's disease tend to become delirious more readily than those not so afflicted. For example, a recent study of 2,000 patients aged 55 years and older admitted to medical wards indicated that 41.4% of those with evidence of dementia also suffered from delirium (9). It appears that a *demented elderly individual has the highest general susceptibility* to delirium, which increases with advancing age and progression of the dementing process.

One other predisposing factor should be mentioned in this context, although it is not known whether it increases general rather than specific susceptibility to delirium. *Alcohol and drug addiction* render the person abusing one or both of these substances more prone to delirium as a result of the toxic effects on the brain of the gradually increased quantity of the abused drug, such as cocaine or meperidine, or due to withdrawal of alcohol or a sedative-hypnotic agent in a person who has developed physical dependence on either.

Facilitating factors

A common causal condition in human morbidity is neither necessary nor sufficient for its occurrence, but only contributory (10). This statement applies to delirium in that several psychobiological and environmental variables appear to represent contributory or facilitating rather than necessary etiological factors. It is not clear at this time whether any of these factors can induce the syndrome in the absence of a precipitating organic factor, but this possibility has been suggested and cannot be ruled out. Some evidence shows, however, that the following conditions can facilitate the onset of delirium, increase its severity, and perhaps help prolong its course:

1. Psychosocial stress.
2. Sleep deprivation.
3. Sensory underload or overload.
4. Immobilization.

Psychosocial stress

"Psychosocial stress" refers to information inputs that are personally meaningful and emotionally distressing for the individual, and hence elicit physiological changes in body systems and organs that impose a strain on homeostatic mechanisms (11). Some writers have proposed that such stress may facilitate, and even precipitate, the onset of delirium in an elderly person (12–15). The elderly, these authors argue, have a reduced capacity for homeostatic regulation and hence for resistance to stress due to age-related changes in hypothalamic nuclei, and tend to show an abnormally high and sustained elevation of plasma cortisol levels in response to stress (13,14). Hypercortisolemia so induced results in brain dysfunction and delirium (13,14). *Bereavement* and *relocation* to an unfamiliar environment have been cited as primary examples of psychosocial stress with deliriogenic potential for an elderly person (12). Hart (16) speculated over 50 years ago that "emotional stress" could be associated with chemical changes in the body that might bring about a delirious state.

The above hypotheses are plausible and based on some empirical evidence (13,14). Whether a healthy elderly person can become delirious in response to psychosocial stress alone remains an open question that can be investigated and answered. It seems more likely, however, that this development can occur in an individual with some brain damage but compensated cognitive functioning (17). In the case of younger persons, some investigators have claimed that prolonged stress and related *anxiety* result in significant impairment of the highest integrative functions (17,18). Social isolation, sleep loss, and fatigue may have an additional effect in increasing the degree of brain dysfunction and consequently of cognition (18). Intense emotional arousal, notably anxiety, may be an intervening variable between psychosocial stress on the one hand, and impaired cognitive functioning and possibly delirium on the other. Intense anxiety is accompanied by a catecholamine-mediated increase in blood flow to and energy consumption by the brain (19). One may postulate that this heightened demand for energy by the brain in response to psychosocial stress, one coupled with a reduced capacity of cerebral neurons to produce energy, could facilitate the onset of delirium. However, a recent study has found no relationship between preoperative anxiety and delirium after hip surgery in elderly patients (20). This negative result suggests caution in proposing that psychosocial stress and anxiety may facilitate, not to say induce, delirium in a person with an intact brain.

In the present stage of our knowledge, or rather ignorance, the question of whether psychosocial stress facilitates delirium remains open. Only future research may provide an answer. The inclusion of such stress among the facilitating or contributory factors in delirium is designed to keep this question alive and to encourage appropriate studies. One may tentatively propose that psychosocial stress and the concomitant intense anxiety may facilitate cognitive disorganization and delirium in a person with brain damage or chronic cerebral disease. Hyperventilation, which is commonly associated with anxiety, as well as sleep deprivation and fatigue, may enhance this effect. Moreover, it is reasonable to hypothesize that psychosocial stress and anxiety may increase the severity and duration of delirium due to any organic etiology.

Sleep deprivation and disorders

Since the earliest writings on the subject, disturbed sleep has been noted to precede and follow the onset of delirium. As an eighteenth-century medical dictionary concisely put it, "a Delirium is always attended with want of Sleep, and both proceed from the same Cause." Moreover, "sleeps which are tumultous and disturb'd, as also those unsound Slumbers, during which the Patient is, as it were, half awake, or cries out, and starts up, are the Forerunners of a future Delirium" (21). By contrast, prolonged, sound sleep has been regarded, from Hippocrates on, as a welcome sign of recovery from delirium. Delirious patients typically suffer from more or less severe insomnia, which is also a common prodromal symptom of the incipient onset of the syndrome. Some researchers have concluded that sleep deprivation's principal effects center on the brain, while general homeostasis, with the exception of thermoregulation, is relatively unaffected (22). Considering their practical and theoretical importance for the student of delirium, experimental and clinical studies on sleep deprivation need to be reviewed so far as they are relevant to the syndrome.

EXPERIMENTAL STUDIES

Patrick and Gilbert (23) carried out the first known experimental study of sleep deprivation (SD) in 1896. Most of this research, however, has been done in the past 30 years, having been stimulated by the introduction of electrooculography by Aserinsky and Kleitman (24) in 1953. Several reviews summarize the findings of those studies (22,25–28).

Research on SD has had three foci: loss of all sleep (total SD), reduction of total sleep time (partial SD), and differential sleep deprivation (sleep-stage deprivation). The earlier work involved mostly *total* SD. Tyler (29) studied 350 men deprived of sleep for up to 112 hours. Seventy percent of them reported hallucinations, and 2% developed transient psychotic disorganization resembling schizophrenia. Some writers concluded that prolonged SD could produce a model psychosis (30), but subsequent studies failed to confirm this prediction. For example, a 17-year-old volunteer was studied during 264 hours of SD and at no time displayed psychotic behavior (31). He did, however, experience transient disorientation for time, "waking dreams," lapses of memory, an occasional illusion, irritability, and suspiciousness. At no time was there evidence of hallucinations, delusions, or delirium. A study of four men deprived of sleep for 205 hours likewise failed to find psychosis (32). The subjects experienced episodes of disorientation for time, visual illusions and hallucinations, and some degree of cognitive disorganization. These psychopathological manifestations occurred episodically and seemed to coincide with periods of drowsiness and brief lapses into sleep with the eyes open (microsleeps). Seven medical student volunteers were studied during 72 hours of SD (33). Once again, no psychosis developed, but the subjects experienced visual misperceptions, feelings of depersonalization, disturbances in time perception, and mild intellectual impairment. These changes were ascribed to "hypnagogic states." Four of the volunteers received lysergic acid diethylamide (LSD)-25 during SD, and all developed hallucinations. The investigators proposed that SD seemed to increase the ego-disruptive effects of the hallucinogen.

Two interesting studies focused on disorientation and other cognitive abnormalities related to *drowsiness* during SD (34,35). The researchers asserted that each level of drowsiness—light, moderate, or severe—was accompanied by primary changes in attention, thinking, and interest and by secondary changes in memory, perception, orientation, and emotional expression (34). Yet not all drowsy subjects experienced the secondary changes. Visual, but not auditory, hallucinations, as well as illogical thinking or reverie, occurred readily during drowsiness. The degree of cognitive impairment increased with the duration of SD and the concomitant drowsiness. The sleep-deprived subjects exhibited prolonged episodes of drowsiness punctuated by microsleeps lasting for several seconds each. Impairment of focal attention appeared to be the main disorder during the drowsy state. Illusions and hallucinations experienced in that state seemed to be identical to dreams and resulted from a failure to tell apart images from veridical percepts. The investigators suggested that the cognitive changes observed in drowsiness resemble those seen in narcolepsy and sensory deprivation (34). One might tentatively conclude that they amount to a mild delirium. Thus, it appears that the abnormal mental phenomena encountered in total SD are, at least in part, the result of drowsiness and microsleeps. The latter might represent sleep-onset REM with related dreams or hypnagogic hallucinations (36).

EEG changes accompany total SD. There is a decrease in voltage and the percentage of waking alpha activity, as well as an increase in the percentage of delta and theta waves (25). Even short periods of total SD may evoke EEG abnormalities in epileptic patients (25). On the whole, however, EEG changes during and after SD are slight or moderate in extent.

Some authors point out that many studies of total SD were conducted under constant environmental conditions that amounted to partial perceptual deprivation, and this factor alone could be responsible for the reported visual illusions and hallucinations (22). Horne (22) asserts that true hallucinations are actually quite rare even during prolonged total SD. Moreover, subjects exhibit heightened suggestibility during total SD and may experience visual misperceptions if they have been led to expect them (22). Johnson (26) points out that the response to SD depends on the person's age, physical condition, mental health, experimental situation, environmental support, and the use of drugs to stay awake. Chronic schizophrenics exposed to total SD for 100 hours exhibited reactivation of acute psychotic symptoms (37). Healthy older subjects tended to show greater decrements in performance on cognitive and auditory vigilance tasks during the second night of total SD than younger ones (38). Individual differences have been reported in the decline in performance during repeated exposure to total SD (39). One may hypothesize that the elderly, the brain-damaged, and those suffering from a physical illness are more vulnerable to the cognitively impairing effects of total SD than young, healthy persons. Moreover, the duration of the deprivation appears to be an important variable: the longer the exposure, the higher the probability and severity of impaired cognitive performance. Sleep loss of less than 40 hours does not impair cognitive functions in healthy subjects (27).

In conclusion, experimental total SD does impair cerebral and cognitive functions, as indicated by the EEG changes and decrements in performance on cognitive tasks. The appearance in some cases of misperceptions, disorientation, reduced selective attention, illogical thinking, and other abnormalities of cognitive function and attention could be partly accounted for by the concomitant effects of drowsiness and sensory understimulation.

Partial SD involves abrupt or gradual restriction of the person's habitual sleep time within a 24-hour period. Thus, if the normal sleep period is seven hours and is restricted in the laboratory to 3 hours, the person is exposed to partial SD. This experimental procedure has not produced results relevant to delirium (40).

Differential or sleep stage SD involves preventing the subject selectively from obtaining REM or stage 4 sleep (40). Early workers in this area of SD research postulated that REM deprivation, and thus dream deprivation, would result in intrusion of the dream contents into wakeful awareness, leading to the development of delusions, hallucinations, and other psychotic symptoms (41,42). This interesting hypothesis has not been validated. Dement (42) provided an anticlimax for his earlier statements in this regard when he wrote that "the behavioral change induced by deprivation is trivial compared to the massive effort required to eliminate REM's for long periods of time" (p 343).

It is generally recognized that REM sleep deprivation is not coterminous with dream deprivation, since mental activity, mostly visual in character, is reported from non-REM sleep as well (28). Frequent dreaming occurs during sleep onset in the absence of REM sleep (28,43). Dreams occurring during stage 1 sleep are indistinguishable from those reported on awakening from REM sleep (28). Dreaming takes place to some extent in all stages of sleep, and REM deprivation neither prevents dreaming nor causes marked changes in waking behavior (40). It appears that only total SD can result in elimination of dreaming, and even this possibility is questionable, since mental activity either similar to or identical to dreaming occurs throughout the sleep-wake cycle (28). Links, similarities, and transitions seem to exist among waking imagery, hypnagogic phenomena, and dreaming. On the whole, studies of even prolonged REM deprivation have failed to show any marked behavioral effects (27,28,40); they have not thrown any new light on delirium.

Two studies involving REM deprivation and drug-induced delirium are of interest. Cartwright (44) induced a dream-like state in wakefulness by administering a small dose (3.5 mg intramuscularly) of piperidyl benzilate (Ditran) to a group of young, healthy volunteers. She hypothesized that the subjects who were high dream producers (high REM percentage) would also be high producers of hallucinations under the effects of the experimental drug; that the content of dreams and of drug-induced hallucinations would be similar in their degree of "imaginativeness"; that the EEG and behavioral features of the two states would differ; and that the themes of the drug-induced fantasy and the dream fantasy in the same subject would be similar. The first two of these hypotheses were not supported; the last two were. EEG characteristics of the drug-induced state were different from both the waking and sleep records of the same subjects. The EEG showed slow wave activity, resembling stage 2 or 3 sleep, with superimposed fast wave activity. Thus, under the drug, the EEG records showed signs of wakefulness, as well as those of stage 1, 2, and 3 of sleep. The subjects reported amnesia for most of the drug experience.

They were hyperactive at first, and while later some appeared stuporous, the majority entered a hallucinatory state. Their hallucinations bore a marked similarity to dreams and were referred to as such by the subjects. Total REM time after the drug session was significantly reduced. Cartwright concluded that dream fantasy and drug-induced fantasy were similar. Piperidyl benzoate seemed to elicit a neurophysiological state analogous to that of REM sleep. Cartwright et al. (45) found that the REM sleep–deprived subjects who responded with repeated attempts to regain it and with much EEG disturbance (many intrusions of stage 2 signs into stage 1 REM on the first recovery night) were the same ones who were much disturbed in response to Ditran. They were distinguished by high anxiety levels and a low tolerance for changes in normal brain function.

The above two studies are interesting in that they suggest similarities between delirium and dreaming, since Ditran is an anticholinergic and deliriogenic agent. They also indicate that this drug may cause delirium by bringing about an intermediate state between wakefulness and sleep that also facilitates hallucinatory activity. These studies provide some evidence that individual differences exist in susceptibility to delirium, or at least to hallucinations in that syndrome, and to disruptive effects of REM deprivation. Field dependence, a personality trait, and trait anxiety seem to be the relevant variables.

Some animal studies have found that REM sleep deprivation results in memory impairment (46). This effect can be enhanced by scopolamine and prevented by physostigmine, suggesting interrelationships among the cholinergic system, REM sleep, and memory (46). Like Ditran, scopolamine is an anticholinergic agent that may also induce delirium (47). Greenberg et al. (48) proposed that REM sleep deprivation results in impairment of only emotionally charged memories.

Deprivation of *slow-wave sleep* has been less fully explored than that of REM sleep. Studies have not shown any adverse behavioral effects (27,40,49). It has been suggested that it is the *fragmentation* of sleep, rather than the decrease in slow-wave sleep, that is related to sleepiness and performance deficits during wakefulness (49). Such fragmentation probably occurs in delirium. Johnson (50) proposes that the *disruption* of the sleep-wake cycle may prove more important for waking behavior than the time spent in specific sleep stages. In a delirious patient the sleep-wake cycle is usually disrupted, which may facilitate and increase the cognitive disorganization in delirium.

CLINICAL STUDIES

In contrast to experimental studies, clinical studies have focused on "experiments of nature" in the form of established pathological conditions. In some cases, however, a pathogenic agent has been introduced deliberately in an attempt to replicate a spontaneously occurring disorder and to study its effects on sleep patterns as a dependent variable. For example, fever has been induced by administering a pyrogen and delirium by administering an anticholinergic agent.

Clinical sleep research relevant to delirium has focused mostly on alcohol and drug withdrawal syndromes. Gross et al. (51) hypothesized that alcohol suppresses REM sleep and that during withdrawal of alcohol in heavy drinkers REM rebound would take place, manifested clinically by dream-like hallucinatory activity. These investigators were intrigued by alcoholics' complaints of nightmares after heavy drinking at bedtime and of having difficulty in distinguishing sleeping and dreaming from wakefulness and hallucinating. If an alcoholic stopped or reduced the alcohol intake at this stage, insomnia and hallucinations resulted. They typically occurred at night, when the patient lay awake in the dark with the eyes closed. These subjective reports suggested to Gross and his coworkers that the patients suffered REM deprivation followed by REM rebound. This hypothesis seemed to be supported by the finding of Gresham et al. (52) that a reduction of REM sleep could result from a single bedtime dose of alcohol. Consequently, Gross and his colleagues embarked on a series of pioneering studies in an attempt to throw new light on the putative role of sleep disturbances in the alcohol withdrawal syndrome (53). Initially, they reported striking elevations of REM sleep and almost complete absence of slow-wave sleep in four patients suffering from an acute alcoholic psychosis (51). The patients described vivid dreams that continued as waking hallucinations. Gross et al. postulated that heavy alcohol intake had a dual effect: it enhanced the need for REM sleep and blocked its discharge. When alcohol was withdrawn, a massive rebound of REM sleep occurred and was manifested, in part, as waking hallucinations. These researchers concluded, however, that neither REM sleep deprivation nor rebound could adequately account for alcohol withdrawal delirium. By contrast, Greenberg and Pearlman (54) asserted that such indeed was the case. They reported that alcohol withdrawal from an alcoholic resulted in an increase in stage 1 REM sleep, which reached 100% of total sleep time just before delirium tremens developed. These researchers concluded that heavy alcohol intake led to dream deprivation and that withdrawal of alcohol resulted in an "overflow of stage 1-REM into the waking state"; such "overflow" was manifested clinically as delirium tremens.

The above research attracted considerable attention, as it pointed to a pathogenic role of sleep disturbances in alcohol withdrawal delirium. More than 100 years ago, Lasegue (55) claimed that delirium tremens was nothing but a waking dream. Subsequent studies, however, cast doubt on that attractive hypothesis. Johnson et al. (56) studied chronic alcoholics during both intake of and withdrawal of alcohol. They found that *fragmentation* of sleep and *absence of slow-wave sleep* were the most prominent features. There were frequent awakenings and sleep stage shifts. The percentage of REM sleep was reduced during two nights of alcohol intake but soon returned to normal levels. Slow-wave (stage 4) remained absent in most patients over 10 days of withdrawal. The investigators proposed that changes in sleep characteristics represented the result, *not* the cause, of disturbed behavior, yet it is not clear how they reached that conclusion. In fact, the only patient in their study who developed delirium showed sleep patterns almost identical to those observed by Gross et al. (51) and Greenberg and Pearlman (54). They consisted primarily of stage 1 sleep and showed disruption of REM sleep by frequent awakenings. The relationship between these changes and delirium remains unresolved.

Vogel (57) has criticized some of the early studies linking the rebound of REM sleep with hallucinations and other features of withdrawal delirium. He pointed out that what some of the investigators regarded as REM sleep could have been a confusional state with visual hallucinations occurring during wakefulness. According to Vogel, there was insufficient evidence to claim that the reported hallucinations represented intrusion of REM sleep into a waking state because of the increased pressure of such sleep. He proposed that total sleep deprivation was a more likely explanation for the observed behavioral abnormalities. Wolin and Mello (58) conducted carefully designed studies of alcoholics in states of both intoxication and withdrawal. They concluded that it was premature to assume a predictable relationship between hallucinatory experiences and REM sleep in alcohol withdrawal. No consistent sequence of alcohol-induced suppression of REM sleep, followed by its rebound during withdrawal from alcohol, could be demonstrated. Wolin and Mello asserted that their data failed to support unequivocally the hypothesis that hallucinations represented waking dreams.

More recent work by Japanese researchers (59) cast more doubt on the REM rebound and intrusion hypothesis as originally formulated by the workers quoted above. Summarized by Hishikawa et al. (59), this research indicates that the hypothesis needs to be modified. These authors propose that a characteristic feature of alcohol withdrawal delirium is the intrusion of the rapid eye movements, i.e., the phasic events of REM sleep, into stage 1 sleep, resulting in what they call "stage 1-REM" and "excited stage 1-REM." These two REM stages are devoid of the muscle atonia of REM sleep. Hishikawa et al. argue that increased neural activity, especially hyperexcitation in the reticular activating system and in the neural structure responsible for the rapid eye movements of REM sleep, causes a marked increase in REM density during REM sleep, as well as rapid eye movements during stage 1-REM and excited stage 1-REM. Such increased neural activity, reflected in a low-voltage, mixed-frequency EEG, results in the appearance of dream-like hallucinations in delirium tremens and in transient withdrawal hallucinations. Moreover, the Japanese workers postulate that the occurrence of stage 1-REM or excited stage 1-REM plays an important role in the development of delirium due to a variety of organic factors, such as withdrawal from sedative-hypnotics, brain tumors involving the pons, and intoxication with an anticholinergic agent (biperiden). Demented elderly patients subject to nocturnal delirium often display it as they awaken from stage 1-REM. While rebound hyperexcitation in the central nervous system contributes to the alcohol and drug withdrawal delirium, destruction of the locus ceruleus could result in REM sleep without atonia and consequent nocturnal delirium in the demented elderly. Disinhibition of the neural structure responsible for rapid eye movements could also have this effect (59). Thus, rebound hyperexcitation during abrupt alcohol withdrawal results not in an increase in the amount of REM sleep but rather in the occurrence of stage 1-REM and excited stage 1-REM.

The nature of the relationship between sleep disturbances and delirium of alcohol withdrawal is a complex and unresolved issue (60). As Gross and Hastey (53) point out, in alcoholics *all aspects of sleep may be disrupted.* The symptoms may include insomnia, hypersomnia, naps during the day, frequent awakenings during the night, and nightmares. Instability of the circadian and ultradian sleep rhythms, increasing reduction in the amount of REM sleep with increasing blood alcohol levels, and an increase followed by a reduction of slow-wave sleep, have all been observed. During acute withdrawal from alcohol severe insomnia usually occurs, resulting from difficulty in staying asleep; total lack of sleep may occur. During the first week of withdrawal the patient may display several disturbances of REM sleep: sleep-onset REM, reduced time of REM onset, and fragmentation of the individual REM periods. Moreover, EEG studies during acute withdrawal show a reduced percentage of slow wave sleep which appears to increase the severity of the symptoms. Alcoholics with a history of several episodes of alcohol withdrawal syndrome show more persistent decrements of slow wave sleep and fragmentation of REM sleep (60). Such persistent abnormalities during prolonged abstinence periods seem to indicate the presence of an underlying abnormality in the regulation of sleep and other biological rhythms (60). *Fragmentation* or dissolution of normal circadian and ultradian body and sleep rhythms may prove to be a key factor in precipitating an alcohol withdrawal syndrome.

While delirium due to withdrawal of alcohol and sedative-hypnotics has attracted the attention of sleep researchers, sleep disturbances associated with delirium due to other causes have been relatively little explored. Karacan et al. (61) studied the effects of experimentally induced *fever* on sleep and dreaming. They injected a pyrogen, either etiocholanolone or Lipexal, into male student volunteers, and recorded their body temperature and sleep patterns for four consecutive nights before the injection and two nights after it. The highest mean body temperature so induced was 38.9°C. After the injection, the latency of the onset of stages 1 and 1-REM, as well as of stage 4 sleep, was markedly increased, there were more awakenings, and the amount of stage 1-REM was reduced. Both stage 4 and stage 1-REM were suppressed compared to the baseline nights. These changes were ascribed to the effects of the fever. There was no rebound of REM sleep during the recovery nights. The researchers speculated that with higher and more prolonged fever, the suppression of the two sleep stages would be even more marked. This study might be relevant to delirium, which may accompany fever of any origin. Yet caution is indicated in drawing such a conclusion. Recent studies suggest that fever is the result of the action of interleukin-1 on the thermoregulatory center in the brain; this substance is also able to induce slow-wave sleep (62). It has been suggested that the sleep so induced could reduce the host's energy demands and enhance the efficiency of defense and repair mechanisms (62). The relevance of interleukin-1 effects to febrile delirium, if any, is unclear.

Total loss of sleep has been reported in delirium due to insoluble salts of *bismuth* (bismuth encephalopathy) (63). Studies of sleep disturbances in *metabolic encephalopathies* are relevant to delirium, which often accompanies them. Marked sleep abnormalities have been reported in hepatic encephalopathy (64), renal insufficiency (65), and cardiac decompensation (66). These sleep disturbances typically consist of a reduction of total sleep time, frequent awakenings, disorganization of sleep cycles, and reduction of slow-wave sleep. The observed abnormalities tend to increase in severity as the encephalopathy worsens and diurnal EEG disturbances become more profound.

Studies of sleep disturbances after *open heart surgery* have been prompted by claims that delirium, which may follow this type of operation, might be due in part to sleep deprivation occasioned by frequent awakenings in intensive care units (66–68). Johns et al. (68) reported that two of the patients studied by them developed delirium after open heart surgery, while two did not. The severity of sleep deprivation during the first two postoperative days did not distinguish the patients who later developed delirium from those who did not. The delirium was accompanied by absence of REM sleep and marked reduction of slow-wave sleep. There were prolonged periods of drowsiness and stage 1 sleep, which may have contributed to the delirium. The sleep-wake cycle as a whole was disrupted. Orr and Stahl (69) have reported similar findings. They found evidence of sleep deprivation and fragmentation in their patients, yet none of them became delirious. It appears that sleep deprivation is not a cause of delirium after open heart surgery, but this does not rule out the possibility that it may be a contributory factor. The same statement may hold for noncardiac *major surgery,* which has been reported to be followed by severe sleep deprivation recorded in the surgical intensive care unit (70). Not only was there marked sleep loss, but also severe suppression, or even absence, of stages 3 and 4 and REM sleep. Yet only one patient of the nine studied had a brief delirium; he had a history of heavy drinking (70).

The *elderly,* those aged 65 years and older, are especially prone to develop delirium, as pointed out earlier in this chapter. Recent interest in all aspects of aging has included the sleep-wake cycle (71,72). Webb (72) argues that aging is "associated with a greater amount of sleep disturbance than any or all other aspects of life" (72, p 10). Nearly half of a group of healthy older individuals showed evidence of disturbed sleep in his study. He noted a marked diminution in the amplitude of slow-wave sleep, more labile REM sleep, a modified frequency of sleep stages, longer average sleep latencies, and high awake times. Reynolds et al. (73) have observed a virtual absence of stage 4 sleep in both elderly men and women. Sleep in demented elderly persons is even more disturbed than in geriatric patients without dementia (74). Severely demented patients spend less time asleep and have a more broken sleep (74). Moreover, they show a reduced REM sleep percentage and increased loss of spindles and K-complexes (75). Sleep apnea occurs in about one-quarter to one-third of the healthy elderly, and its prevalence is even higher in those of them who are demented (76,77). The resulting nocturnal hypoxia may worsen the cognitive impairment of a demented individual but not necessarily that of a nondemented one (76–78). Hospitalized, physically ill elderly patients are reported to have a higher prevalence of sleep disorders than their healthy counterparts (79). All these recent findings converge to underscore the high prevalence of sleep pathology in the elderly. It is plausible to postulate that the observed sleep disturbances may facilitate the development of delirium in later life.

Not only sleep loss and fragmentation, but also *hypersomnia* and *parasomnia,* may be associated with behavioral pathology similar to, if not identical to, delirium. Roth et al. (80) described "sleep drunkenness" occurring in some hypersomniacs and associated with confusion, disorientation, and slow responsivity. This state may last for periods ranging from about 15 minutes to several hours and can occur on awakening in an individual suffering from hypersomnia. Guilleminault et al. (81) observed "altered states of consciousness" associated with that syndrome and related to excessive drowsiness and microsleeps. The patients had an abnormally low amount of slow-wave sleep at night and tended to have episodes of automatic behavior, apparently accompanying microsleeps. It is unclear whether these episodes represent delirium. Sleep drunkenness may also be associated with awakening after too little sleep, especially in unfamiliar surroundings, or following the intake of hypnotics, tranquilizers, or alcohol. In some cases, it has been associated with violent behavior and even homicide. A recently identified *parasomnia,* REM sleep behavior disorder (RBD), resembles delirium but is said to be distinct from it (82,83). Patients display hyperactive and even violent behavior that occurs during REM sleep, which is normally accompanied by atonia. It is interesting to note that the Japanese researchers quoted earlier (59) view REM sleep without atonia, or stage 1-REM sleep, as a characteristic sleep disturbance in alcohol and drug withdrawal delirium. RBD differs from delirium in that it occurs during REM sleep, not in the waking state. Yet the difference may be only one of degree of arousal. Feinberg (84) proposed that nocturnal delirium in demented patients could represent intrusion of REM sleep, or rather of dreaming activity associated with that sleep stage, into wakefulness. Clearly, this old hypothesis, namely, that delirium represents, at least in part, a breakthrough of REM sleep and dreams into the waking state, persists and clamors for more research to test it. It is amazing that delirium, a common mental disorder routinely associated with sleep pathology, has been almost totally ignored by sleep researchers.

In summary, experimental and clinical studies indicate a relationship between sleep disturbances and delirium but fail to clarify its exact nature. Total sleep deprivation probably induces mild delirium, or a delirium-like state, in some subjects. Clinical studies confirm the ancient observation that sleep disturbances regularly accompany delirium. These disturbances include sleep loss and fragmentation, changes in sleep stages, and disruption of the circadian sleep-wake cycle. While slow-wave sleep appears to be reduced or absent, REM sleep may be increased, reduced, or lacking atonia. Interpenetration of wakefulness and sleep, with transitions between these two states, seems to be a common feature. One may postulate that sleep disturbances are related to delirium in several possible ways: 1. they may be a *pathogenetic mechanism* that mediates between the impact of a given organic etiological agent on the brain and the onset of delirium; 2. they may be an *independent consequence* of a pathological condition of the brain that also underlies the cognitive-attentional abnormalities referred to as "delirium" and *increase the severity* of the latter; 3. they may determine the occurrence and form of *misperceptions* in delirium; and 4. they may, on occasion, actually *bring about* the cognitive-attentional disturbances characteristic of delirium. Only future research can help clarify this issue. In the meantime, one may tentatively conclude that sleep disturbances can facilitate the onset of delirium.

The relationship between *dreaming* and delirium also remains unclear. Not all delirious patients hallucinate; hence, it is inaccurate to speak of delirium as a waking dream. It is conceivable that hallucinations, when present, represent an intrusion of dreams into wakefulness. Some delirious patients have difficulty in telling apart hallucinations, dreams, imagery, and veridical perceptions. Regis (85) coined the term "délire onirique" (óneiros-dream) to describe the dream-like mental activity experienced by patients delirious as a result of an infection or intoxication. Oneirism has been viewed by some writers as dream-like, hallucinatory activity superimposed on simple confusion.

It was proposed in Chapter 5 that delirium represents, in part, a *disorder of wakefulness.* The discussion in this section offers some support for this contention. An alternative, and perhaps more accurate, formulation is to suggest that delirium is a disorder of the sleep-wake cycle characterized by the irregular appearance of the elements of sleep during wakefulness and those of the waking state during sleep. In other words, *fragmentation* and *disorganization* of the sleep-wake cycle are manifested clinically as delirium.

Sensory deprivation and overload

Sensory deprivation and overload have been reported to impair cognitive-perceptual functions, especially in the elderly and the demented. I have proposed that they may facilitate the onset of delirium (86). It is therefore appropriate to review some of the experimental and clinical studies on these two environmental conditions insofar as they pertain to this syndrome.

EXPERIMENTAL SENSORY DEPRIVATION

In 1951, Hebb and his coworkers at McGill University in Montreal introduced an experimental technique that marked the beginning of studies on the psychophysiological effects of sensory deprivation (87,88). Volunteer subjects were confined to bed, their eyes covered with translucent goggles allowing only formless light to pass through; they carried earphones through which a constant buzzing sound was presented; and their arms and hands were covered with cardboard cuffs and cotton gloves, reducing tactile stimulation. After varying periods of confinement, the subjects displayed such phenomena as decreased intellectual efficiency, vivid imagery, visual and auditory hallucinations, mood shifts, increased suggestibility, impaired directed thinking, and delusions. Most subject could not tolerate the experiment for more than 72 hours; those who remained in confinement for longer periods usually developed complex hallucinations and delusions. These widely publicized early sensory deprivation experiments inaugurated two decades of intensive studies using three different techniques: 1. confinement to bed in a soundproof room; 2. confinement in a tank-type respirator; and 3. suspension in a water tank. A distinction should be made between *sensory deprivation,* in which the experimental environment provided total reduction in sensory inputs, and *perceptual deprivation,* in which the sensory input was homogeneous and unpattered (white noise, diffuse light) (88). Hebb's original method exemplified the perceptual deprivation technique. However, this whole area of research came to be designated "sensory deprivation."

Hebb, after reading my first article on delirium (86), commented: "The hallucinatory activity (which I call hallucinatory because the subjects reported that if they didn't know that they were wearing goggles they would have thought that they were looking at a movie screen) in these nonpsychiatric subjects is obviously closely related to delirium" (89). This impression seemed to be supported by reports that even relatively brief exposure to sensory deprivation (one-hour session) included EEG slowing manifested by a decrease in occipital alpha wave frequency (90). Yet, as in SD experiments, the dramatic behavioral symptoms reported in the early studies on sensory deprivation were not found in the later experiments. Suedfeld (91) has suggested that variables other than sensory deprivation as such could have confounded many of the earlier studies and resulted in reports of *psychological stress* in reponse to a strange, novel experimental situation. This, combined with suggestion, could have contributed to the psychopathological effects of sensory deprivation reported by the early investigators. The question of whether hallucinations occur in SD has never been answered. Suedfeld (91) asserts that it is extremely rare for a subject exposed to sensory deprivation to report hallucinations of the type observed in psychotic patients. Rather, illusions and vivid imagery seem to have been mislabeled by some investigators as "hallucinations." Ziskind (92) reviewed the phenomena of sensory deprivation and proposed that immobilization as well as social isolation were confounding variables in sensory deprivation experiments and contributed to their reported effects. Moreover, reduced awareness and wakefulness, or a *hypnagogic state,* occurring in sensory-deprived subjects, could account for misperceptions, confusion, and anxiety. This "hypnoid syndrome" appears to be identical to that exhibited by subjects of sleep deprivation studies, ascribed to drowsiness and microsleeps (34). What hallucinations do occur in sensory deprivation experiments are mostly visual, simple, and transient (88).

Cognitive abnormalities have been observed in sensory deprivation experiments (88). Performance of complex cognitive tasks is impaired, but on simple tasks, such as digit span and rote learning, performance is seldom defective and may actually improve (93). Other cognitive abnormalities include impaired directed thinking, distractibility, short attention span, increased suggestibility, and disorientation for time (88).

Studies of sensory deprivation showed a meteoric rise and fall: hardly any have been reported in the past 15 years after a flurry of activity in the 1960s. One interesting recent study, however, is worthy of mention in this context. Mazziotta and Phelps (94) have carried out a series of studies using positron emission tomography (PET) on normal subjects exposed to audiovisual sensory deprivation. In response to having their eyes closed and patched, and their ears plugged at the same time, the subjects showed a significant *reduction* in right hemisphere glucose metabolism. The reduction was most marked in the inferior prefrontal cortex, posterior temporal cortex, and lateral occipital cortex. These findings are intriguing, as they indicate that cerebral glucose metabolism, especially in the right hemisphere, may be affected by partial sensory deprivation even in normal subjects. As discussed in Chapter 7, reduction in cerebral oxidative metabolism is the main proposed pathogenetic mechanism in delirium. One may speculate that the effects on such metabolism in an elderly individual, especially a demented one exposed to some degree of sensory deprivation as a result of visual impairment, for example, could facilitate the onset of delirium.

In summary, experimental sensory deprivation studies have shown that subjects exposed to reduced or monotonous sensory inputs exhibit a variety of cognitive and perceptual abnormalities, as well as mild slowing of the EEG. These abnormalities resemble but do not seem to amount to delirium. The latter involves some degree of memory impairment, for example, yet sensory deprived subjects did not display consistent deficits of registration, retention, or recall. Their digit span was usually intact, in contrast to that of delirious patients. One may conclude that sensory deprivation does not induce delirium in a young, healthy subject. This does not, however, rule out the possibility that sensory deprivation may *faciliate* delirium in the aged, the brain-damaged, and the physically ill. The PET studies mentioned here, as well as the clinical ones about to be reviewed, indicate that this may be so.

CLINICAL STUDIES

Clinical observations on patients subjected to various forms of sensory and perceptual deprivation suggest that these factors can contribute to the onset of delirium and possibly increase its severity. In 1863, Sichel (95) reported delirium in patients aged 60 years and older who had undergone cataract extraction. He noted that the delirium occurring in blindfolded patients after such surgery usually took place during the night. Schmidt-Rimpler (96) extended these observations and postulated that a predisposed patient might become delirious after cataract surgery as a result of a sudden deprivation of familiar visual stimulation. However, his patients had received atropine, a potentially deliriogenic drug.

The above anecdotal reports were probably the first to link reduced visual sensory input with delirium. Jackson (97), in his review of the syndrome in hospitalized eye surgery patients, concluded cautiously that "the evidence for sensory deprivation has been mixed, and the issue has not been resolved" (p 372). An early, partly experimental, study was carried out by Cameron (98).

His subjects were elderly patients suffering from dementia and nocturnal delirious episodes. He wondered if the latter were due to fatigue or darkness. In an attempt to resolve this issue, Cameron blindfolded the patients early in the day and noted that within 1 hour of the start of the experiment they were unable to find various objects in the room whose location they had been able to point out with the eyes open. The majority of the patients confabulated and, while blindfolded, described the location of nonexistent objects such as windows. Cameron concluded that the senile patients could not maintain the "spatial image" once darkness had cut off proper visual cues. Such loss of spatial orientation could trigger anxiety and confusion. Cameron hypothesized that nocturnal delirium in a senile patient could result from the inability to maintain spatial orientation without the aid of repeated visualization. This hypothesis is further discussed in Chapter 18.

Sensory deprivation has been invoked to account for such events as the "break-off phenomena" of pilots at high altitude (99); delirium in intensive care units (100) and tank-type respirators (101); and psychological disturbances in patients treated in germ-free isolator units (102). Sensory monotony has been claimed to contribute to delirium in surgical intensive care units (100). A report by Mendelson et al. (101) on the occurrence of hallucinations, delusions, and confusion in patients with poliomyelitis treated in a respirator stimulated interest in the hypothesis that the findings of experimental sensory deprivation studies could be applied to clinical situations to account for delirium and similar mental disturbances occurring in a variety of settings (103). Not only sensory deprivation but also social isolation has been postulated to contribute to the "isolation stress" thought to play a role in some cases of delirium, especially in the elderly (104).

As mentioned above, two clinical settings attracted attention as potential harbingers of sensory deprivation: *intensive care units* and *germ-free isolators.* One author proposed the label "intensive care syndrome" for what he proclaimed to be a "new disease of medical progress" (105). That "new disease" was really delirium, neither a "new" condition nor a "disease." Holland et al. (106) called it a "myth." These investigators found no significant difference in the incidence of delirium between the patients admitted to a general medical intensive care unit and a matched group of patients admitted to a general medical ward. Of the intensive care unit patients, 12.5% became delirious; in each case, the delirium could be adequately accounted for by the underlying physical illness. Sensory deprivation or monotony did not seem to play a role in the development of the syndrome in the intensive care unit. Reports from surgical intensive care units seemed to provide some support for the hypothesis that sensory deprivation might play a contributory role in the delirium encountered there. For example, Wilson (107) found the incidence of postoperative delirium to be more than twice as high in a windowless intensive care unit as in one with windows. The incidence was 40% in the former and 18% in the latter. In another study, only 7 of 322 patients treated in a surgical intensive care unit were diagnosed as suffering from an organic brain syndrome (108). Other investigators failed to implicate sensory deprivation in their study of delirium in a surgical intensive care unit and concluded that the occurrence of the syndrome could be adequately explained by organic factors (109). Despite these equivocal findings, a recent review of psychiatric complications after surgery states flatly that "isolation, sensory deprivation, monotony, and loss of orienting cues all promote delirium" (110, p 52).

Studies of *coronary care units* have not provided unequivocal support for the postulated role of sensory deprivation in delirium either (111–113). Delirium has been reported to occur in 2% to 12% of patients (111–114). One report refers vaguely to the probable contributory role of "sensory monotony" (113). Other authors speak of "violent fluctuations" in sensory input and marvel at the low incidence of delirium in this unattractive environment (111). Some writers suggest that the intensive care units actually feature *both* sensory deprivation and overload (115).

A number of studies, reviewed by Lesko et al. (102), have focused on the psychological effects of *germ-free isolation.* Germ-free units are used for conditions such as severe aplastic anemia, leukemia, radiation injury, and severe combined immunodeficiency disease. Patients placed in these units are exposed to prolonged social isolation and are reported to suffer not from sensory deprivation but rather from "touch deprivation," i.e., they miss physical human contact (116). On the whole, patients tend to tolerate this environment surprisingly well, and if delirium does occur, it does not seem to be related to isolation or sensory deprivation. (102,116).

In summary, clinical studies provide some support for the putative contribution to delirium of reduced sensory input or sensory monotony. Such an effect is most likely to occur in the elderly and the brain-damaged individual, especially if other conditions that may impair cognitive functioning, such as sleep loss, coexist. There is no evidence that sensory deprivation alone can cause delirium.

SENSORY OVERLOAD

The environmental condition opposite to sensory deprivation is sensory overload. Several experimental studies of sensory overload have found that it may result in cognitive impairment, illusions, hallucinations, disturbances in time sense, distortions of body image, and delusions (117). In clinical situations, sensory overload may be produced, especially in intensive care units, by auditory and visual stimuli originating from monitoring apparatus, fans, oxygen equipment, and conversatons among the staff (115). Studies of hospital noise show that high levels of it exist in recovery rooms and acute care units, and may be sufficiently intense to stimulate patients' hypophyseal-adrenocortical axis, as well as causing sleep loss (115,118). It appears that sensory overload is more prevalent than sensory deprivation in intensive care units and more likely to facilitate delirium (115). Levels of sensory stimulation needed for optimal cognitive activity appear to decline with age, rendering the elderly susceptible to the disorganizing effects of sensory overload on cognition (7). One could postulate that sensory overload may be more likely to facilitate delirium in an elderly person.

UNFAMILIARITY

One other aspect of the environment that has been linked to delirium, especially in the elderly, is its unfamiliarity (119,120). Some anecdotal accounts indicate that an elderly patient may develop delirium on transfer to an unfamiliar environment, such as a hospital (119,120). It is likely that these patients suffer from unrecognized dementia and decompensate cognitively when deprived of familiar sensory cues. For centuries it has been common to encourage relatives to stay with delirious patients, as well as provide them with familiar objects to reduce their anxiety and confusion.

Immobilization

The last factor that may facilitate the onset of delirium is immobilization. A series of studies by Zubek and his associates (121) found that immobilized subjects displayed impaired performance on intelligence tests and those of perceptual-motor functions. Some subjects exhibited "visual experience of hallucinatory-like nature," vivid imagery and dreams, inability to concentrate, and difficulty in logical thinking. Moreover, their EEG featured a slowing of the frequencies in the occipital region. Thus, the effects of immobilization on healthy subjects were not unlike those of sensory deprivation, and led the investigators to suggest that the former condition involved a reduction in the level of kinesthetic and proprioceptive stimulation and hence represented a form of partial sensory deprivation.

Ryback et al. (122) investigated the effects of prolonged bed rest (5 weeks) on the psychological functioning, sleep, and EEG of healthy volunteers. No significant cognitive impairment was detected, even though the subjects complained of mental sluggishness. EEG changes were similar to those found in severe sensory deprivation. Sleep was affected: an increase in deep sleep and a decrease of stages 1 and 2 were observed.

Clinical implications of this experiment have been suggested for patients with orthopedic, neurological, cardiac, pulmonary, and other disorders requiring prolonged immobilization and recumbency (123). In particular, some authors have postulated that immobilization is one of the risk factors for the development of delirium in an elderly patient with hip fracture (124). Otherwise, the role of this factor in facilitating the syndrome remains equivocal.

One could argue cogently that conditions such as immobilization, unfamiliarity of the environment, social isolation, and sensory deprivation and overload are forms of *stress* that may induce nonspecific psychophysiological and neuroendocrine stress responses (11). If this indeed is the case, such responses could help to precipitate delirium because of their deleterious effects on cerebral function, notably in an elderly, brain-damaged individual.

Organic causes (precipitating factors)

The causative organic factors in delirium may be grouped into four general classes (125):

1. Primary cerebral disease (focal, widespread, or both).
2. Systemic diseases affecting the brain secondarily.
3. Intoxication with exogenous substances; i.e., medical and recreational drugs, and poisons of industrial, plant, and animal origin.
4. Withdrawal from substances of abuse, generally alcohol and sedative-hypnotic drugs.

The presence of cerebral dysfunction due to one or more of the above organic factors is a necessary condition for the occurrence of delirium. The mere presence of a given pathogenic factor need not, however, be a *sufficient* condition for the syndrome to occur. Certain characteristics of the organic etiological factors, as well as those of the host and the environment, are postulated to co-determine the onset, severity, and duration of delirium. The putative predisposing and facilitating host and environmental factors were discussed in the preceding sections of this chapter. The following characteristics of the organic factors are deemed to facilitate the occurrence of delirium in an individual exposed to them (126).

Absolute strength of the pathogenic factor

This variable refers to the quantitative or intensity dimension of the given etiological factor. It is assumed that the degree of deviation from the dynamic steady state of the organism, i.e., from homeostasis, tends to determine the probability that a given noxious agent responsible for it will affect cerebral oxidative metabolism and hence result in delirium. Examples include the degree of hypoxia or hypoglycemia; the concentration of the various electrolytes in the body fluids; hypothermia and hyperthermia; the quantity of the ingested toxic agent; the extent of burns; and the force of impact of trauma to the head. As a general rule, the greater the amount or strength of a toxic or other noxious factor, and the greater the consequent deviation from normal homeostasis and cerebral metabolism, the higher the probability that delirium will develop.

Concurrence of two or more pathogenic factors

If more than one etiological factor is present at a given time, the probability of delirium increases, even if each of them individually would not suffice to bring it about. This situation is commonly observed in the elderly (6,7). In many cases of postoperative delirium, one finds a combination of several pathogenic factors, such as administration of anesthetic, narcotic, and anticholinergic agents; electrolyte imbalance; infection; and hypoxia, which have an additive adverse effect on cerebral metabolism and thus increase the probability of delirium. Other common examples of such multifactorial deliriogenic conditions include severe burns and systemic infections. One may propose that the larger the number of coexisting pathogenic factors, the greater the risk that delirium will occur and will be severe.

Rate of change in the physicochemical milieu

The higher the rate of such change, the more likely is delirium to develop. A rapidly rising intracranial pressure, a sudden drop in the blood glucose or calcium level, rapid withdrawal of alcohol or sedative from an addicted person, rapid onset of hypoxia or hypercapnia—all of these conditions increase the probability of delirium due to the short time span in which homeostasis has been disturbed. Moreover, a rapid rise in the serum calcium or sodium level from an initially abnormally low level may have the same result, even though the final concentration would not suffice to induce delirium. By contrast, patients suffering from a chronic disease, such as pulmonary or hepatic insufficiency, have time to adapt to the changes in blood oxygen and ammonia levels, and may show no cognitive dysfunction with levels of either substance that would have been high enough to induce it had the disease developed rapidly.

Duration of exposure to the etiological factor

It appears that, other conditions being equal, a critical duration of exposure to a given pathogenic factor is needed for delirium to develop. If the duration is too brief, the syndrome may not take place; if it is too long, a subacute or chronic organic mental syndrome such as a reversible dementia is more likely to be diagnosed.

Degree of spread and site of brain dysfunction

Some pathological conditions, such as the metabolic encephalopathies, bring about *widespread* reduction of cerebral oxidative metabolism and of the synthesis of certain neurotransmitters. Such conditions are particularly apt to cause delirium. On the other hand, certain *focal* brain lesions, notably those involving the right hemisphere, may cause the syndrome as a result of damage to the presumed anatomical substrate of attention (127). Moreover, a focal lesion of the brain, such as a rapidly growing neoplasm, may exert a widespread effect on cerebral metabolism, either because it precipitates increased intracranial pressure or because it suppresses the function of the reticular activating system or of other brain structures whose dysfunction can reduce the metabolism of the whole brain.

Pharmacological properties of toxic substances

Certain drugs, notably the anticholinergic agents, exert an effect on the brain that facilitates the occurrence of delirium. Cholinergic blockade brought about by a wide range of anticholinergic drugs provides a classic example of pharmacological action on the central nervous system that makes a given agent potentially deliriogenic.

In clinical practice, the most common organic causes of delirium include *intoxication by medical, notably anticholinergic, drugs; metabolic encephalopathies; systemic infections; withdrawal from substances of abuse; head trauma; vascular disorders; and cancer.* These and other organic causes are listed in Table 6–1 and are discussed in specific detail in Part II.

The etiology of delirium is seen as *multifactorial.* While one or more organic factors causing cerebral dysfunction are necessary for the syndrome to occur, certain characteristics of the host and of the host's social and nonhuman environment predispose to and facilitate its onset in response to an organic factor. An age of 60 years and over, brain damage, chronic cerebral disease resulting in dementia, and possibly addiction to alcohol predipose to the development of delirium. Sleep loss and fragmentaion, as well as disruption of the circadian sleep-wake cycle, psychosocial stress, sensory under- and overstimulation, and immobilization are all putative facilitating factors. They are postulated to elicit stress responses as one possible aspect of their contributory role in delirium. Ultimately, all these facilitating factors are thought to contribute to the brain dysfunction manifested clinically as delirium. The elderly, especially those suffering from dementia, are generally considered to be more vulnerable to delirium than any other population.

TABLE 6–1 Organic Causes of Delirium

1. INTOXICATION BY DRUGS AND POISONS
   a. Drugs: aminophylline, antiarrhythmic agents, antibiotics, anticholinergic agents, anticonvulsants, antihypertensive drugs, antineoplastic drugs, antiparkinsonian agents, bismuth salts, cimetidine, corticosteroids, digitalis derivatives, disulfiram, indomethacin, interferon, lithium, metrizamide, opiates, ranitidine, salicylates, sedative-hypnotics, etc.
   b. Alcohol: ethyl and methyl
   c. Illicit drugs: cocaine, phencyclidine
   d. Addictive inhalants: ether, gasoline, glue, nitrites, nitrous oxide
   e. Industrial poisons: carbon disulfide, carbon monoxide, heavy metals, methyl chloride and methyl bromide, organic solvents, organophosphate insecticides
   f. Poisons of animal, plant, and mushroom origin
2. WITHDRAWAL SYNDROMES
   a. Alcohol
   b. Sedatives and hypnotics: barbiturates, benzodiazepines, bromides, chloral hydrate, ethchlorvynol, glutethimide, meprobamate, methyprylon, paraldehyde
   c. Amphetamines (?)
3. METABOLIC ENCEPHALOPATHIES
   a. Hypoxia
   b. Hypoglycemia
   c. Hepatic, pancreatic, pulmonary, or renal insufficiency (encephalopathy)
   d. Avitaminosis: cyanocobalamin (vitamin B_{12}), folate, nicotinic acid, pyridoxine (?), thiamine
   e. Hypervitaminosis: intoxication by vitamins A and D
   f. Endocrinopathies: hyperinsulinism, hyperosmolar nonketotic hyperglycemia, hyperthyroidism, hypothyroidism, hypopituitarism, Addison's disease, Cushing's syndrome, hypoparathyroidism, hyperparathyroidism
   g. Disorders of fluid and electrolyte metabolism
      i. Dehydration, water intoxication
      ii. Acidosis, alkalosis
      iii. Hypercalcemia, hypocalcemia, hyperkalemia, hypokalemia, hypernatremia, hyponatremia, hypermagnesemia, hypomagnesemia
   h. Errors of metabolism
      i. Porphyria
      ii. Carcinoid syndrome
      iii. Hepatolenticular degeneration (Wilson's disease)
4. INFECTIONS
   a. Intracranial
      i. Bacterial meningitis—meningococcal, pneumococcal, *Hemophilus influenzae,* tuberculous, etc.
      ii. Viral encephalitis: herpes simplex virus and zoster virus, acquired immune deficiency syndrome (AIDS)
      iii. Fungal infections: cryptococcosis, coccidioidomycosis, histoplasmosis, moniliasis, mucormycosis
      iv. Protozoal infections: cerebral malaria, toxoplasmosis
      v. Trichinosis
      vi. Neurosyphilis
      vii. Postinfectious and postvaccinial encephalomyelitis
   b. Systemic: acute rheumatic fever, bacteremia, brucellosis, diphtheria, infectious mononucleosis, influenza, legionnaires' disease, malaria, mumps, pneumonia, psittacosis, toxic shock syndrome, Rocky Mountain spotted fever, septicemia, subacute bacterial endocarditis, typhoid, typhus
5. HEAD TRAUMA: concussion, contusion
6. EPILEPSY: ictal, interictal, postictal

TABLE 6–1 Organic Causes of Delirium *Continued*

7. NEOPLASM: extracranial, remote effects of
8. VASCULAR DISORDERS
   a. Cerebrovascular
      i. Transient ischemic attacks
      ii. Hypertensive encephalopathy
      iii. Thrombosis, embolism, subarachnoid hemorrhage
      iv. Cerebral vasculitis
      v. Multi-infarct dementia
      vi. Migraine
   b. Cardiovascular
      i. Myocardial infarction
      ii. Congestive heart failure
      iii. Cardiac arrhythmias
      iv. Endocarditis
      v. Pulmonary embolism
9. INTRACRANIAL SPACE-OCCUPYING LESIONS
   a. Abscess
   b. Aneurysm
   c. Neoplasm, primary or secondary
   d. Parasitic cyst
   e. Subdural hematoma
10. DISORDERS OF THE HEMATOPOIETIC SYSTEM
   a. Severe anemia of any type
   b. Erythremia
   c. Thrombotic thrombocytopenic purpura
   d. Macroglobulinemia
11. DISORDERS DUE TO HYPERSENSITIVITY
   a. Serum sickness
   b. Food allergy (?)
12. INJURY BY PHYSICAL AGENTS
   a. Heat stroke (hyperthermia)
   b. Hypothermia
   c. Radiation damage
   d. Electrocution

References

1. Lipowski Z. J.: Delirium (acute confusional state), in Frederiks J.A.M. (ed): *Handbook of Clinical Neurology,* Vol. 2 (No. 46): *Neurobehavioural Disorders.* Amsterdam, Elsevier, pp 523–559.
2. Aita J. A.: Everyman's psychosis—the delirium. *Nebr. Med. J.* 1968;10:424–427.
3. Ebaugh F. G., Barnacle C. H., Ewalt J. R.: Delirious episodes associated with artificial fever: A study of 200 cases. *Am. J. Psychiatry* 1936;23:191–217.
4. Bleuler M., Willi J., Buehler H. R.: *Akute psychische Begleiterscheinungen körperlicher Krank heiten.* Stuttgart, Thieme, 1966.
5. Morse R. M., Litin E. M.: Postoperative delirium: A study of etiologic factors. *Am. J. Psychiatry* 1969;126:388–395.

6. Lipowski Z. J.: Acute confusional states (delirium) in the elderly, in Albert M. L. (ed): *Clinical Neurology of Aging.* New York, Oxford University Press, 1984, pp 277–297.
7. Lipowski Z. J.: Transient cognitive disorders (delirium, acute confusional states) in the elderly. *Am. J. Psychiatry* 1983;140:1426–1436.
8. Liston E. H.: Delirium in the aged. *Psychiatr. Clin. North. Am.* 1982;5:49–66.
9. Erkinjuntti T., Wikstrom J., Palo J., et al: Dementia among medical inpatients. *Arch. Intern. Med.* 1986;146:1923–1926.
10. Susser M.: *Causal Thinking in the Health Sciences.* London, Oxford University Press, 1973.
11. Lipowski Z. J.: Psychosomatic medicine: Past and present. Part II. Current state. *Can. J. Psychiatry* 1986;31:8–13.
12. Kennedy A.: Psychological factors in confusional states in the elderly. *Gerontol. Clin.* 1959;1:71–82.
13. Kral V. A.: Confusional states: Description and management, in Howells J. G. (ed): *Modern Perspectives in the Psychiatry of Old Age.* New York, Brunner/Mazel, 1975, pp 356–362.
14. Kral V. A.: Stress and mental disorders of the senium. *Med. Serv. J. Canada* 1962;18:363–370.
15. Wolanin M. O., Phillips L. R. F.: *Confusion.* St. Louis, C. V. Mosby, 1981.
16. Hart B.: Delirious states. *Br. Med. J.* 1936;2:745–749.
17. Chapman L. F., Thetford W. N., Berlin L., et al: Highest integrative functions in man during stress. *Proc. Assoc. Res. Nerv. Ment. Dis.* 1958;36:491–534.
18. Hinkle L. E.: The physiological state of the interrogation subject as it affects brain function, in Biderman A. D., Zimmer H. (eds): *The Manipulation of Human Behavior.* New York, Wiley, 1961, pp 19–50.
19. Siesjö B. K., Carlsson C., Hagerdal M., et al: Brain metabolism in the critically ill. *Crit. Care Med.* 1976;4:283–294.
20. Simpson C. J., Kellett J. M.: The relationship between pre-operative anxiety and post-operative delirium. *J. Psychosom. Res.* 1987;31:491–497.
21. James R.: *A Medicinal Dictionary.* Vol. 2. London, T. Osborne, 1745.
22. Horne J. A.: Sleep function, with particular reference to sleep deprivation. *Ann. Clin. Res.* 1985;17:199–208.
23. Patrick G. T. W., Gilbert J. A.: On effects of loss of sleep. *Psychol. Rev.* 1896;3:469–483.
24. Aserinsky E., Kleitman N.: Regularly occurring periods of eye motility, and concomitant phenomena, during sleep. *Science* 1953;118:273–274.
25. Horne J. A.: A review of the biological effects of total sleep deprivation in man. *Biol. Psychol.* 1978;7:55–102.
26. Johnson L. C.: Sleep deprivation and performance, in Webb W. B. (ed): *Biological Rhythms, Sleep and Performance.* New York, Wiley, 1982, pp 111–141.
27. Naitoh P.: Sleep deprivation in human subjects: A reappraisal. *Waking Sleeping* 1976;1:53–60.
28. Vogel G. W.: A review of REM sleep deprivation. *Arch. Gen. Psychiatry* 1975;32:749–761.
29. Tyler D.: Psychological changes during experimental sleep deprivation. *Dis. Nerv. Syst.* 1955;16:293–299.
30. West L. J., Janszen H., Lester B., et al: The psychosis of sleep deprivation. *Ann. N.Y. Acad. Sci.* 1962;96:66–70.

31. Gulevich G., Dement W., Johnson L.: Psychiatric and EEG observations on a case of prolonged (264 hours) wakefulness. *Arch. Gen. Psychiatry* 1966;15:29–35.
32. Pasnau R. O., Naitoh P., Stier S., et al: The psychological effects of 205 hours of sleep deprivation. *Arch. Gen. Psychiatry* 1968;18:496–505.
33. Bliss E. L., Clark L. D., West C. D.: Studies of sleep deprivation—relationship to schizophrenia. *A.M.A. Arch. Neurol. Psychiatry.* 1959;81:348–359.
34. Morris G. O., Singer M. T.: Sleep deprivation: The content of consciousness. *J. Nerv. Ment. Dis.* 1966;143:291–304.
35. Morris G. O., Williams H. L., Lubin A.: Misperception and disorientation during sleep deprivation. *Arch. Gen. Psychiatry* 1960;2:247–254.
36. Slap J. W.: On dreaming at sleep onset. *Psychoanal. Q.* 1977;46:71–81.
37. Koranyi E. K., Lehmann H. E.: Experimental sleep deprivation in schizophrenic patients. *Arch. Gen. Psychiatry* 1960;2:534–544.
38. Webb W. B., Levy C. M.: Age, sleep deprivation, and performance. *Psychophysiology* 1982;19:272–276.
39. Webb W. B., Levy C. M.: Effects of spaced and repeated total sleep deprivation. *Ergonomics* 1984;27:45–48.
40. Johnson L. C.: The effect of total, partial, and stage sleep deprivation on EEG patterns and performance, in Burch N., Altschuler H. L. (eds): *Behavior and Brain Electrical Activity.* New York, Plenum, 1974, pp 1–30.
41. Dement W. C.: The effect of dream deprivation. Science 1960;131:1705–1707.
42. Dement W. C.: Sleep deprivation and the organization of the behavioral states, in Clement C., Purpura D., Mayer F. (eds): *Sleep and Maturing Nervous System.* New York, Academic Press, 1972, pp 319–361.
43. Vogel G., Foulkes D., Trosman H.: Ego functions and dreaming during sleep onset. *Arch. Gen. Psychiatry* 1966;14:238–248.
44. Cartwright R. D.: Dream and drug-induced fantasy behavior. *Arch. Gen. Psychiatry* 1966;15:7–15.
45. Cartwright R. D., Monroe L. J., Palmer C.: Individual differences in response to REM deprivation. *Arch. Gen. Psychiatry* 1967;16:297–303.
46. Skinner D. M., Overstreet D. H., Orbach J.: Reversal of the memory-disruptive effects of REM sleep deprivation by physostigmine. *Behav. Biol.* 1976;18:189–198.
47. Ketchum J. S., Sidell F. R., Crowell E. B., et al: Atropine, scopolamine, and Ditran: Comparative pharmacology and antagonists in man. *Psychopharmacology (Berl.)* 1973;28:121–145.
48. Greenberg R., Schwartz W. R., Pearlman C., et al: Memory, emotion, and REM sleep. *J. Abnorm. Psychol.* 1983;92:378–381.
49. Bonnet M. H.: Performance and sleepiness following moderate sleep disruption and slow wave sleep deprivation. *Physiol. Behav.* 1986;37:915–918.
50. Johnson L. C.: Are stages of sleep related to waking behavior? *Am. Scientist* 1973;61:326–338.
51. Gross M. M., Goodenough D., Tobin M., et al: Sleep disturbances and hallucinations in the acute alcoholic psychoses. *J. Nerv. Ment. Dis.* 1966;142:493–514.
52. Gresham S. C., Webb W. B., Williams R. L.: Alcohol and caffeine: Effects on inferred visual dreaming. *Science* 1963;140:1226–1227.
53. Gross M. M., Hastey J. M.: Sleep disturbances in alcoholiam, in Tarter R. E., Sugarman H. H. (eds): *Alcoholism: Interdisciplinary Approaches to an Enduring Problem.* Reading, Mass, Addison-Wesley, 1977, pp 1–42.

54. Greenberg R., Pearlman C.: Delirium tremens and dreaming. *Am. J. Psychiatry* 1967;124:133–142.
55. Lasegue C.: Le délire alcoolique ńest pas un délire, mais un réve. *Arch. Gen. Med.* 1881;88:326–338.
56. Johnson L. C., Burdick J. A., Smith J.: Sleep during alcohol intake and withdrawal in the chronic alcoholic. *Arch. Gen. Psychiatry* 1970;22:406–418.
57. Vogel G. W.: REM deprivation. III. Dreaming and psychosis. *Arch. Gen. Psychiatry* 1968;18:312–329.
58. Wolin S. J., Mello N. K.: The effects of alcohol on dreams and hallucinations in alcohol addicts. *Ann. N.Y. Acad. Sci.* 1973;215:266–302.
59. Hishikawa Y., Sugita Y., Teshima Y., et al: Sleep disorders in alcoholic patients with delirium tremens and transient withdrawal: Reevaluation of the REM rebound and intrusion theory, in Karacan I. (ed): *Psychophysiological Aspects of Sleep.* Park Ridge, NJ, Noyes Publishers, 1981, pp 109–122.
60. Zarcone V. P.: Sleep and alcoholism, in Chase M., Weitzman E. D. (eds): *Sleep Disorders. Basic and Clinical Research.* New York, SP Medical and Scientific Books, 1983, pp 319–325.
61. Karacan I., Wolff S. M., Williams R. L., et al: The effects of fever on sleep and dream patterns. *Psychosomatics* 1968;9:331–339.
62. Dinarello C. A.: Interleukin-1 and the pathogenesis of the acute-phase response. *N. Engl. J. Med.* 1984;311:1413–1418.
63. Billiard M., Besset A., Renaud B., et al: L'insomnie de l'encephalopathie bismutique. *Electroencephalogr. Clin. Neurophysiol.* 1977;7:147–152.
64. Kurtz D., Zenglein J. P., Imler M., et al: L'etude du sommeil nocturne au cours de l'encephalopathie porto-cave. *Electroencephalogr. Clin. Neurophysiol.* 1972;33:167–178.
65. Passouant P., Cadilhac J., Baldy-Moulinier M., et al: L'etude de sommeil nocturne chez des uremiques chroniques soumis à une épuration extrarenale. *Electroencephalogr. Clin. Neurophysiol.* 1970;29:441–449.
66. Blachley P. H., Starr A.: Post-cardiotomy delirium. *Am. J. Psychiatry* 1964;121:371–375.
67. Dein B. M., Rosen H., Dickstein K., et al: The problems of sleep and rest in the intensive care unit. *Psychosomatics* 1971;12:155–163.
68. Johns M. W., Large A. A., Masterton J. P., et al: Sleep and delirium after open heart surgery. *Br. J. Surg.* 1974;61:377–381.
69. Orr W. C., Stahl M. L.: Sleep disturbances after open heart surgery. *Am. J. Cardiol.* 1977;39:196–201.
70. Aurell J., Elmqvist D.: Sleep in the surgical intensive care unit: Continuous polygraphic recording of sleep in nine patients receiving postoperative care. *Br. Med. J.* 1985;290:1029–1032.
71. Emser W., Kurtz D., Webb W. B. (eds): *Sleep, Aging and Related Disorders.* Basal, Karger, 1987.
72. Webb W. B.: Disorders of aging sleep. *Interdiscipl. Topics Gerontol.* ›87;22:1–12.
73. Reynolds C. F., Kupfer D. J., Taska L. S., et al.: Sleep of healthy seniors: A revisit. *Sleep* 1985;8:20–29.
74. Allen S. R., Seiler W. O., Stähelin H. B., et al: Seventy-two hour polygraphic and behavioral recordings of wakefulness and sleep in a hospital geriatric unit. Comparison between demented and nondemented patients. *Sleep* 1987;10:143–159.

75. Reynolds C. F., Kupfer D. J., Taska L. S., et al: EEG sleep in elderly depressed, demented, and healthy subjects. *Biol. Psychiatry* 1985;20:431–442.
76. Berry D. T. R., Phillips B. A., Cook Y. R., et al: Sleep-disordered breathing in healthy aged persons: Possible daytime sequelae. *J. Gerontol.* 1987;42:620–626.
77. Erkinjuntti T., Partineau M., Sulkava R., et al: Sleep apnea in multiinfact dementia and Alzheimer's disease. *Sleep* 1987;10:419–425.
78. Knight H., Millman R. P., Gur R. C., et al: Clinical significance of sleep apnea in the elderly. *Am. Rev. Respir. Dis.* 1987;136:845–850.
79. Lucas E. A., Wooten V., Anderson-Brakhop C., et al: The polysomnographic diagnosis of sleep disorders in elderly medical patients. *Ala. J. Med. Sci.* 1986;23:140–145.
80. Roth B., Nevsimalova S., Rechtschaffen A.: Hypersomnia with "sleep drunkenness." *Arch. Gen. Psychiatry* 1972;26:256–262.
81. Guilleminault C., Phillips R., Dement W. C.: A syndrome of hypersomnia with automatic behavior. *Electroenceph. Clin. Neurophysiol.* 1975;38:403–413.
82. Schenck C. H., Bundlie S. R., Ettinger M. G., et al: Chronic behavioral disorders of human REM sleep: A new category of parasomnia. *Sleep* 1986;9:293–308.
83. Schenck C. H., Bundlie S. R., Patterson A. L., et al: Rapid eye movement sleep behavior disorder. *J.A.M.A.* 1987;257:1786–1789.
84. Feinberg I.: Sleep in organic brain conditions, in Kales A. (ed): *Sleep. Physiology and Pathology.* Philadelphia, Lippincott, 1969, pp 131–147.
85. Regis E.: *Précis de Psychiatrie.* Paris, Doin, 1923, pp 345–387.
86. Lipowski Z. J.: Delirium, clouding of consciousness and confusion. *J. Nerv. Ment. Dis.* 1967;145:227–255.
87. Bexton W. H., Heron W., Scott T. H.: Effects of decreased variation in the sensory environment. *Can. J. Psychol.* 1954;8:70–76.
88. Zubek J. P. (ed): *Sensory Deprivation: Fifteeen Years of Research.* New York, Appleton-Century-Crofts, 1969.
89. Hebb D. O.: Personal communication, February 2, 1968.
90. Marjerrison G., Keogh R. P.: Electroencephalographic changes during brief periods of perceptual deprivation. *Percept. Motor Skills* 1967;24:611–615.
91. Suedfeld P.: The benefits of boredom: Sensory deprivation reconsidered. *Am. Scientist* 1975;63:60–69.
92. Ziskind E.: A second look at sensory deprivation. *J. Nerv. Ment. Dis.* 1964;138:223–232.
93. Zubek J. P.: Behavioral and physiological effects of prolonged sensory and perceptual deprivation: A review, in Rasmussen J. (ed): *Man in Isolation and Confinement.* New York, Aldine, 1973, pp 9–83.
94. Mazziotta J. C., Phelps M. E.: Human sensory stimulation and deprivation: Positron emission tomographic results and strategies. *Ann. Neurol.* (Suppl) 1984;15:50–60.
95. Sichel A.: Sur une espece particulière de délire senile qui survient quelque fois aprés l'extraction de la cataracte. *Ann. Oculistique* 1863;49:154–168.
96. Schmidt-Rimpler H.: Delirien nach Verschluss der Augen und in Dunkel-Zimmern. *Arch. Psychiatr.* 1879;9:233–243.
97. Jackson C. W. Jr.: Clinical sensory deprivation: A review of hospitalized eye-surgery patients, in Zubek J. P. (ed): *Sensory Deprivation: Fifteen Years of Research.* New York, Appleton-Century-Crofts, 1969, pp 332–373.
98. Cameron D. E.: Studies in nocturnal delirium. *Psychiatr. Q.* 1941;15:47–53.

99. Clark B., Graybiel A.: The break-off phenomenon: A feeling of separation from the earth experienced by pilots at high altitudes. *J. Aviation Med.* 1957;28:121–126.
100. Kornfeld D. S.: The hospital environment: Its impact on the patient. *Adv. Psychosom. Res.* 1972;8:252–270.
101. Mendelson J., Solomon P., Lindemann E.: Hallucinations of poliomyelitis patients during treatment in a respirator. *J. Nerv. Ment. Dis.* 1958;126:421–428.
102. Lesko L. M., Kern J., Hawkins D. R.: Psychological aspects of patients in germ-free isolation: A review of child, adult, and patient management literature. *Med. Pediatr. Oncol.* 1984;12:43–49.
103. Leiderman P. H., Mendelson J., Wexler D., et al: Sensory deprivation: Clinical aspects. *Arch. Intern. Med.* 1958;101:389–396.
104. Oster C.: Sensory deprivation in geriatric patients. *J. Am. Geriatr. Soc.* 1977;24:461–464.
105. McKegney F. P.: The intensive care syndrome. *Conn. Med.* 1966;30:633–636.
106. Holland M., Koss N., Kerstein M., et al: The ICU syndrome: Fact or fancy? *Psychiatry Med.* 1973;4:241–249.
107. Wilson L. M.: Intensive care delirium. *Arch. Intern. Med.* 1972;130:225–226.
108. Hale M., Koss N., Kerstein M., et al: Psychiatric complications in a surgical ICU. *Crit. Care. Med.* 1977;5:199–203.
109. Katz N. M., Agle D. P., De Palma R. G., et al: Delirium in surgical patients under intensive care. *Arch. Surg.* 1972;104:310–313.
110. Seiberg C. P.: Recognition, management, and prevention of neuropsychological dysfunction after operation. *Int. Anesthesiol. Clin.* 1986;24:39–58.
111. Hackett T. P., Cassem N. H., Wishnie H. A.: The coronary-care unit: An appraisal of its psychological hazards. *N. Engl. J. Med.* 1968;279:1365–1370.
112. Cay E. L., Vetter N., Philip A. E., et al: Psychological reactions to a coronary care unit. *J. Psychosom. Res.* 1972;16:437–447.
113. Parker D. L., Hodge J. R.: Delirium in a coronary care unit. *J.A.M.A.* 1967;201:702–703.
114. Tesar G. E., Stern T. A.: Evaluation and treatment of agitation in the intensive care unit. *J. Intensive Care Med.* 1986;1:137–148.
115. Hansell H. N.: The behavioral effects of noise on man: The patient with "intensive care unit psychosis." *Heart Lung* 1984;13:59–65.
116. Holland J., Plumb M., Yates J., et al: Psychological response of patients with acute leukemia to germ-free environments. *Cancer* 1977;40:871–879.
117. Lipowski Z. J.: Sensory and information inputs overload: Behavioral effects, in Lipowski Z. J.: *Psychosomatic Medicine and Liaison Psychiatry. Selected Papers.* New York, Plenum Medical Book Co, 1985, pp 47–69.
118. Falk S. A., Woods N. F.: Hospital noise-levels and potential health hazards. *N. Engl. J. Med.* 1973;289:774–781.
119. Litin E. M.: Mental reaction to trauma and hospitalization in the aged. *N. Engl. J. Med.* 1956;162:1522–1524.
120. Levin M.: Toxic delirium precipitated by admission to hospital. *J. Nerv. Ment. Dis.* 1952;116:210–214.
121. Zubek J. P., MacNeill M.: Effects of immobilization: Behavioral and EEG changes. *Can. J. Psychol.* 1966;20:316–366.
122. Ryback R. S., Lewis O. F., Lessard C. S.: Psychobiologic effects of prolonged bed rests (weightlessness) in young healthy volunteers (study II). *Aerospace Med.* 1971;42:529–535.

123. Steinberg F. V.: *The Immobilized Patient.* New York, Plenum Medical Book Co, 1980.
124. Williams M. A., Campbell E. B., Raynor W. J., et al: Predictors of acute confusional states in hospitalized elderly patients. *Res. Nurs. Health* 1985;8:31–40.
125. Lipowski Z. J.: Delirium (acute confusional states). *J.A.M.A.* 1987;258:1789–1792.
126. Lipowski Z. J.: Organic brain syndromes: Overview and classification, in Benson D. F., Blumer D. (eds): *Psychiatric Aspects of Neurologic Disease.* New York, Grune & Stratton, 1975, pp 11–35.
127. Mori E., Yamadori A.: Acute confusional state and acute agitated delirium. *Arch. Neurol.* 1987;44:1139–1143.

7

Pathogenesis and Pathophysiology

"Pathogenesis" refers to the events that occur between the impact of a noxious agent on the host and the outcome (1). This chapter will focus on the putative pathophysiological mechanisms and processes that intervene between the impact of a disease or a toxic agent on the brain and the onset of delirium. Our knowledge of this area is fragmentary, and much remains to be elucidated. What Hart (2) wrote more than 50 years ago is still largely true today: "Of the precise processes by which delirium is mediated we know nothing. In discussing at the present time the possible pathogenesis of delirium we have therefore to leave the sphere of knowledge and enter that of hypothesis and speculation" (p 747). Hart postulated that the impairment of cerebral function underlying delirium could be produced by a wide range of factors whose connection to the syndrome might be no more specific than that between hemiplegia and its various causes. This nonspecific relationship, namely, one in which a large number of determinants and intervening pathophysiological mechanisms may result in a relatively circumscribed set of clinical manifestations, almost certainly occurs in delirium. The fact that relatively little is still known about these mechanisms despite the recent rapid progress in the neurosciences is surprising, and highlights the neglect of this common syndrome by researchers.

The best-documented pathogenetic hypothesis views delirium as a psychopathological and behavioral manifestation of widespread reduction of cerebral oxidative metabolism and imbalance of neurotransmission (3). The pathophysiological mechanisms are likely to involve one or more of the following disturbances (3):

1. Reduction of cerebral oxidative metabolism.
2. Impairment of mechanisms for the liberation or conservation of chemical energy stored in the fuels.
3. Deficient synthesis, blockade, or imbalance of certain neurotransmitters, notably acetylcholine, in the brain.
4. Increased central noradrenergic activity (in alcohol withdrawal delirium).
5. Disruption of synaptic transmission.
6. Presence of false neurotransmitters.
7. Disturbances in the normal ionic passage through excitable membranes.
8. Gross alterations in the electrolyte and water content, osmolality, and pH of the internal milieu.
9. Impaired synthesis of macromolecules needed for renewal of the structural and functional elements of the neuron.

Delirium as disturbance of cerebral metabolism and neurotransmission

Engel and Romano (4) have developed a concept of delirium as a "syndrome of cerebral insufficiency" and have postulated that a reduction of cerebral metabolism underlies all cases of it. This reduction is manifested both psychologically and physiologically. Psychologically, cerebral insufficiency is reflected in an impairment of cognitive function, i.e., in deficits and disturbances in the areas of attention, consciousness, thinking, memory, perception, and spatiotemporal orientation. Physiologically, cerebral insufficiency is indicated by a generalized slowing of the EEG background activity, which roughly parallels changes in the functional metabolism of cerebral neurons. Engel and Romano observed that the level of cognitive functioning correlated closely with changes in EEG frequency. Progressive reduction in the level of cognition was accompanied by progressive slowing of the EEG, while improvement in such functioning was associated with faster EEG background activity. Cerebral metabolic insufficiency may involve such factors as a deficient supply of substrates, mostly glucose and oxygen, to the brain; damage to the enzyme systems necessary for proper utilization of the substrates; disruption of synaptic transmission; and damage to cell membranes.

Engel and Romano (4) have marshaled impressive evidence from both clinical and experimental studies in support of their hypothesis of the pathogenesis of delirium. Yet studies of cerebral metabolism in this syndrome using such modern techniques as positron emission tomography (PET) have not been carried out; hence, validation of the hypothesis must await future research. Engel and Romano have based their conclusions on the EEG findings to be reviewed in a later section. Otherwise, the results of the studies on the biochemical and neurophysiological disturbances that underlie coma have been applied to delirium on the assumption that this syndrome represents a transitional state between waking consciousness on the one hand, and stupor and coma on the other. The generality of this assumption is, however, open to question. It may apply to many cases of delirium but not to all. A wide range of disorders, best exemplified by metabolic and toxic encephalopathies, may cause both delirium and coma. On the other hand, alcohol and sedative-hypnotic withdrawal syndromes often feature delirium that does not progress to coma unless complications, such as infection, seizures, or cardiovascular failure, alter their course. Engel and Romano (4) have proposed that delirium tremens represents a variant of delirium, one more closely related to organic mental disorders produced by lysergic acid diethylamide (LSD) or quinacrine, for example, and not associated with the slowing of the EEG background activity. This issue will be discussed later. It is brought up at this point to underscore the likelihood that delirium, as defined in this book, involves more than one pathophysiological mechanism (5–8).

Numerous experimental studies of delirium induced by anticholinergic agents were carried out in the 1960s and led to the conclusion that an imbalance of central cholinergic and adrenergic neurotransmitters, involving both the medial ascending reticular activating system and the medial thalamic diffuse projections systems, represented a major pathogenetic mechanism in delirium (9). These studies are discussed in detail in a later section. More recently, Blass et al. (10) proposed that impairment of oxidative metabolism in the brain results in reduced synthesis of neurotransmitters, especially acetylcholine, whose relative deficiency in the brain is a common denominator in metabolic-toxic encephalopathies. Acetylcholine metabolism decreases in hypoxia and thiamine deficiency, for example (11,12). Hypoxia impairs acetylcholine synthesis and brings about changes in mental function at levels that do not alter common measures of energy metabolism (12,13). The inhibition of acetylcholine metabolism may be due to calcium-dependent release of this neurotransmitter (13).

This interesting hypothesis provides a link between Engel and Romano's (4) claim that reduced oxidative metabolism in the brain underlies delirium and the experimental observation showing that the syndrome can be readily induced by anticholinergic drugs. Moreover, physostigmine salicylate, a cholinesterase inhibitor, has been used successfully to reverse delirium caused not only by such drugs but also by other agents (see Chapter 10). Cholinergic mechanisms appear to be involved in memory, attention, arousal, and REM sleep (8,14,15). Administration of scopolamine to human subjects impairs alertness, selection and evaluation of information from the environment, and ability to recall or recognize the received information (15). Scopolamine reduces global cerebral blood flow, with a predominantly frontal deficit (16). All these observations suggest that deficient acetylcholine synthesis or cholinergic blockade, or both, may bring about cognitive-attentional and sleep-wake cycle disturbances, the essential features of delirium. This empirical evidence strongly indicates that central cholinergic deficiency plays an important pathogenetic role in this syndrome but does not rule out the possibility that other mechanisms may be involved in at least some cases of it (see Chapter 10 for further discussion).

Most studies of delirium that have a bearing on its pathogenesis have used the EEG as a laboratory indicator of cerebral dysfunction. A few investigators have measured cerebral blood flow (17–19). One group of researchers employed computed tomography (20). Magnetic resonance imaging and PET have not been used to study delirium to date. As a result of this meager data base, the pathogenesis of the syndrome is largely a matter of speculation and inference from studies of brain function and its disturbances that appear to be relevant to it. Recent work that may have a bearing on this subject will be briefly reviewed in the hope that it will generate hypotheses and research. Because a reduction of *cerebral metabolism* has been postulated to be a basic pathophysiological mechanism in delirium, recent research on this topic will be reviewed first. *Cerebral blood flow* is believed to be intimately related to the metabolism of the brain, and techniques currently used to measure it have already been applied in the studies of alcohol withdrawal delirium (17,19). Both brain metabolism and cerebral blood flow are reflected in the *electroencephalogram*. As mentioned earlier, EEG studies of delirium have so far been the main source of data on the brain dysfunction that accompanies it. Disturbances in *neurotransmission* have already been mentioned in this context, and experimental work on delirium induced by anticholinergic agents must be reviewed in some detail. Finally, mechanisms thought to underlie *consciousness* and the *sleep-wake cycle* are highly relevant to the syndrome and call for a brief discussion.

Cerebral metabolism and delirium

As mentioned earlier, direct studies of cerebral metabolism in delirious patients have not been reported to date. It is usually assumed, however, that the cognitive-attentional disturbances that constitute the core psychopathology of delirium reflect a reduction or derangement of oxidative metabolism in the brain. Indirect support for this contention is provided by studies of conditions such as hypoxia and hypoglycemia, which can lead to both delirium and coma. Siesjö et al. (21) assert that many clincial disorders associated with transient psychological manifestations of cerebral dysfunction share a common feature: an abnormal alteration of brain metabolism. In addition to hypoglycemia and hypoxia-ischemia, conditions such as hyperthermia, acidosis, and anxiety may adversely affect cerebral metabolic rate (CMR) and cognitive functioning. Cerebral function and energy metabolism are closely linked; hence, an appreciation of modern concepts of the latter is basic to the understanding of metabolic encephalopathies (22).

The brain constitutes only about 2% of total body weight, but its energy expenditure and oxygen consumption are disproportionately high for its size. The brain of a normal, conscious, young adult consumes about 20% of the total body basal oxygen (23). This high level of oxidative metabolism is used almost entirely for the oxidation of glucose and the production of energy. The central nervous system has very little endogenous fuel (22). Consequently, a steady supply of glucose to the brain is essential. Glucose, however, is not the only source of cerebral energy; ketone bodies and lactate, for example, may be used as fuels in some circumstances (22). Adenosine triphosphate (ATP) serves as the immediate source of energy for the work of the neuronal cell. Anaerobic glycolysis normally yields only about 5% of the ATP produced, and hence cannot replace the aerobic oxidation of glucose as an adequate source of energy for the brain. It follows that continuous delivery of oxygen is crucial because there is hardly any reserve of this element, and the central nervous system (CNS) extracts about one-third of the total blood oxygen (22). Complete cessation of cerebral blood flow results in loss of consciousness within about 6 seconds (23). Yet even if cerebral blood flow (CBF) continues at a normal or higher than normal rate, the supply of substrates may be insufficient if the arterial contents of oxygen or glucose fall below critical levels. A fall of arterial oxygen tension (PaO_2) to below 60 torr may impair certain tal functions, such as short-term memory (21). The brain is less vulnerable to glucose deprivation than to oxygen deprivation, since its glycogen content, though low, is relatively higher; also, ketone bodies may be utilized instead of glucose, as occurs in starvation or diabetes. In these conditions, glucose may constitute less than one-half of the oxidizable substrate, yet brain function remains normal (21). Despite this substitution, however, severe or prolonged hypoglycemia leads to irreversible neuronal damage (24). In hepatic encephalopathy, the transport of ketone bodies is sharply reduced and the brain appears to be incapable of utilizing these substrates (22). Thus, a low blood glucose level in this condition is particularly detrimental.

A breakthrough in the study of cerebral metabolism occurred with the introduction of PET (25,26). This technique involves injection of radionuclides with an excess positive charge that decay by emitting a positron. PET has enabled researchers to study cerebral glucose and oxygen metabolism, receptor distribution and affinity, drug metabolism, CBF, and tissue pH (25). Natural isotopes of carbon, nitrogen, and oxygen are replaced with short-lived isotopes ^{11}C, ^{13}N, ^{15}O, and ^{18}F. (as a substitute for hydrogen). Sokoloff et al. (27) developed a technique to measure the local cerebral glucose metabolic rate (LCMR glu) autoradiographically in animals, using ^{14}C-labeled deoxyglucose (DG). Based on this technique, ^{18}F fluorodeoxyglucose (FDG) and ^{11}C deoxyglucose have been used with PET to measure LCMR glu in humans (25,26). This method has been used to study both normal cerebral function and the biochemical processes underlying neuropsychiatric disturbances (25,26,28). It allows imaging of neurotransmitter systems that are of particular importance in understanding mental disorders such as schizophrenia and dementia (25,26,28). Unfortunately, this superior research technique has not yet been used to study delirium and to elucidate its pathophysiology.

Increased neuronal activity is accompanied by increased oxygen consumption and energy utilization by brain cells. The latter require energy for two principal tasks: biosynthesis and transport (21,22). "Biosynthesis," which occurs mostly in cell bodies or in nerve terminals, refers to resynthesis of the constantly degraded macromolecules, membranes, and cell organelles. Active transport processes include axoplasmic transport, the acquisition of essential nutrients, reuptake of neurotransmitters, and the transport of ions responsible for the maintenance of transmembrane electrical potentials (22). A great deal of energy appears to be used for ion transport, i.e., mostly extrusion of sodium ions and accumulation of potassium ions in order to restore concentration gradients for these ions across the excitable membranes following depolarization. Both biosynthesis and transport utilize energy provided by high-energy phosphates, i.e., ATP or other nucleoside triphosphates such as phosphocreatine.

A very close correlation has been established between LCMR glu and local CBF (22,29). This coupling between brain function and cerebral perfusion appears to hold in most, but not all, situations (29). For example, cholinergic blockade with scopolamine abolishes the CBF increase, but not the increase in the cerebral metabolic rate for oxygen ($CMRO_2$) during transition from high-voltage to low-voltage sleep (29). On the whole, however, there is a coupling of neuronal activity, metabolic rate, and blood flow in the brain. On the basis of studies of local cerebral glucose utilization, Sokoloff (30) has proposed that the changes in local metabolic rate may provide chemical mechanisms for the regulation and adjustment of regional CBF. The nature of these mechanisms is still a matter of speculation. It has been suggested that increased metabolic demand of cerebral tissue brings about a focal and neurally governed vasodilatation, which may be mediated by adrenergic, dopaminergic, cholinergic, and serotonergic nerves (29). Whatever the coupling mechanisms may eventually prove to be, increased neuronal activity is usually accompanied by an elevated metabolic rate and increased blood flow. By contrast, when the rate of neuronal firing decreases, both CMR and CBF decline. In some circumstances, however, a disproportionate increase in flow occurs (29).

Of particular interest for the student of delirium is the relationships between mental activity, normal and abnormal, and cerebral metabolism. In the past, it was assumed that such metabolism remains constant in different types of mental activity, with the possible exception of anxiety, and that a relatively close correlation exists between CMR and the level of consciousness (23). Both of these time-honored assumptions have been challenged in recent years. PET has provided a technique with which to study local sensory, motor, memory, and cognitive functions in human subjects (25,26). For example, when a subject is faced with a specific task rather than the passive perception of stimuli, frontal cortical zones show increased glucose utilization (26). Subjects asked to recall specific aspects of auditory stimuli display activation of the hippocampus and parahippocampus that was not observed when auditory perception without memory tasks was required (26). Moreover, when damage occurs to one cerebral structure or its interconnecting fiber bundles, functional effects can be found at multiple sites through a given network (26). Metabolic changes in one site may affect metabolic measurements in both adjacent and distant regions. One may hypothesize that such interconnectedness of brain structures could account for the fact that delirium can follow infarction in the distribution of the middle cerebral artery in the nondominant hemisphere or of the posterior cerebral artery, for example (see Chapter 16). Thus, a focal lesion can result in widespread metabolic effects throughout the brain and hence in delirium.

The relationship between the level of consciousness and the CMR appears to be relatively close (23). Cerebral oxygen consumption in the normal alert state has been found to be 3.5 ml/100 g/min; in confusion, 2.8 ml/100 g/min; and in coma, 2.0 ml/100 g/min (23). Thus, depressed levels of awareness are accompanied by parallel decrements in CMR. The generality of this finding is open to question, however. Some drugs, such as ketamine or diazepam, may produce anesthesia or unconsciousness, or both, without causing a concurrent decrease in oxygen consumption by the brain (31). Bachelard (32) asserts that coma is due not to energy failure but rather to sensitivity of specialized processes in the brain that are not necessarily involved in energy metabolism. Psychological symptoms and EEG changes tend to precede any detectable failure in energy metabolism and appear to result from biochemical changes other than reduced energy production. Hypoxia, hypoglycemia, hepatic encephalopathy, and other encephalopathies leading to coma seem to share certain common features but also display differences in their biological mechanisms (24). An impairment of brain function, manifested by EEG slowing and behavioral changes, occurs before any demonstrable cell damage or failure of energy, as assessed by concentrations of ATP and creatine phosphate. Oxidative metabolism may be maintained even when the supply of substrates is reduced. The energy state is maintained, but there is derangement of intermediary metabolism. It is apparently incorrect to assume that a failure in energy metabolism is a necessary condition for delirium (21,32). For further discussion of metabolic encephalopathies see Chapter 14.

Certain conditions that increase or decrease functional activity of the brain alter its energy demands correspondingly and are accompanied by parallel variations in energy production. These conditions are relevant to delirium. Amphetamine intoxication, anxiety, hyperthermia, and epileptic seizures increase cerebral functional activity, oxygen consumption, CBF, and CMR. During focal or generalized epileptic seizures, both brain metabolism and blood flow are significantly elevated; both are reduced in the postictal and interictal states (25). *Anxiety* is particularly important in regard to delirium. Betz (33) found an increase in CBF in human subjects in response to anxiety-provoking stimuli. The amount of bodily movement, and the intensity as well as the duration of anxiety, appeared to be the main variables. In patients with a panic disorder, metabolic hyperactivity has been found in the right parahippocampal gyrus (28). Increased secretion of catecholamines leads to increased CBF and brain oxygen consumption in experimental animals (34). One may postulate that anxiety could heighten cerebral metabolic demands and reduce oxygen tension, facilitating the onset of or exacerbating delirium. Anxiety and stress could increase cerebral energy consumption, and relief of anxiety by sedation is indicated in patients with abnormally compromised cerebral energy production, such as occurs in hypoglycemia, hypoxia, and ischemia (21).

Hyperthermia increases cerebral energy requirements. Animal studies have shown that $CMRO_2$ increases by about 5% for each 1° C increase in temperature (21). These findings may be relevant to febrile delirium, since hyperthermia has been known to induce it even in the absence of an acute infection.

Also relevant to delirium are findings of the studies on cerebral metabolism in *sensory deprivation* and the *sleep-wake cycle.* LCMR glu was measured using FDG and PET in normal volunteers in states of selective and combined visual and auditory deprivation (35). There was a progressive decline in overall glucose metabolism as sensory inputs were increasingly reduced. This study demonstrated how sensitive cerebral activity is to changes in environmental stimulation. Relative increases in frontal LCMR glu were observed in all the tested states, i.e., selective or combined auditory or visual deprivation. Right greater than left decreases in LCMR were found in specific regions during combined audiovisual stimulation. The researchers concluded that it was difficult to define a stable resting state of the human brain. This study suggests that sensory deprivation could contribute to delirium by reducing cerebral metabolism (see Chapter 5).

Studies of cerebral blood flow and metabolism in the *sleep-wake cycle* are important in the present context, since disturbances of this cycle regularly accompany and are actually viewed as part of the syndrome (see Chapter 5). CMR is relatively high during alert wakefulness. Any factor that increases alertness, such as pain or anxiety, will increase the work of the brain (36). Frontal and prefrontal areas of the cerebral cortex have the highest CBF and CMR during wakefulness, the "hyperfrontal pattern" (37). There is thus strong evidence that increased cerebral activity during wakefulness and alert awareness of the environment is associated with increased CBF and CMR. During sleep, CBF and CMR progressively decrease from wakefulness to stage 4 sleep, especially in the frontal and central areas of the brain (36). During REM sleep, an increase in CBF and CMR glu occurs, notably in the visual cortex and in parts of the temporal and frontal lobes (36,38). These changes are thought to be secondary to the metabolic changes in the brain. In this regard, it is interesting that delirium has often been referred to as a "waking dream" (see Chapters 1 and 5), yet there appear to be differences in both CMR and CBF between the syndrome and REM sleep.

Engel and Romano (4) have asserted that advances in the knowledge of cerebral metabolism are essential for further progress in understanding the pathogenesis and pathophysiology of delirium. In the 30 years since the publication of their seminal paper, remarkable advances in the measurement of brain metabolism under various normal and pathological conditions have occurred; unfortunately, they have thrown little light on the pathogenesis of the syndrome. Delirium does not represent a manifestation of the *failure* of cerebral energy metabolism and actually precedes it. CBF during delirium tremens is increased and correlates significantly with visual hallucinations and psychomotor hyperactivity (17). Alcohol withdrawal delirium, however, may be viewed as a variant, and not a prototype, of delirium generally as the syndrome is currently defined (see Chapter 13, Ref. 4). The metabolism of cerebrospinal fluid (CSF) has been studied in patients with clouded consciousness (39). Significantly higher levels of uncompensated metabolic (lactate) acidosis have been found in these patients compared to normally conscious control subjects. Disturbances of consciousness due to various causes correlate with pH, lactate concentraion, and HCO_3 level in the CSF. These findings indicate reduced functional activity of cerebral neurons and alteration of cerebral metabolism in the direction of enhanced anaerobic glycolysis. Increased CSF acidosis may, in turn, result in a further disturbance of brain metabolism; hence, a vicious circle appears to be created. Measuring the lactate concentration in the CSF could have prognostic value in evaluating patients with clouded consciousness (39).

Cerebral blood flow

Measurement of CBF has played an important role in attempts to correlate CMR with different levels of consciousness and with various forms of mental activity in both normal and brain-damaged subjects (16–19,21,29,31,33, 37,40–44). Recent refinements in the technique of measuring CBF (42) have provided a useful investigative tool that may throw new light on the pathogenesis of delirium. Patterns of behavior are more likely to be adequately reflected in the CBF and CMR in individual structural and functional units than in the brain as a whole (45). Since 1961, the development of methods to measure regional cerebral blood flow (rCBF) has allowed a remarkable increase in information about regional cerebral hemodynamics under various normal and morbid conditions.

Measurement of total CBF in humans became feasible with the introduction of the nitrous oxide technique by Kety and Schmidt (45) in 1945. The refinement of this method by Lassen and Ingvar (46) has made it possible to measure rCBF in humans. The new method initially involved injection into the common carotid artery of radioactive ^{85}Kr and later of ^{133}Xe. Later, these radioactive tracers were applied by inhalation. ^{133}Xe is the tracer used at present. The most recent technique involves the ^{133}Xe inhalation method coupled with single photon emission computed tomography (SPECT) (42).

As mentioned earlier, in normal, resting, conscious subjects, CBF and CMR are considerably higher in frontal and prefrontal areas of the cerebral cortex than in postcentral, notably temporal, areas (37,41). This resting hyperfrontal pattern is asymmetrical; CBF in the right prefrontal region is somewhat higher than in the left (41). Ingvar (41) hypothesizes that the frontal/prefrontal cortex provides the substrate for the *temporal* organization of behavior and cognition in terms of the past, present, and future. This intact organization appears to be an essential precondition for conscious awareness, as well as for selection and making sense of incoming information. In delirium, the impairment of such selection and grasp of sensory stimulation from the patient's own body and environment is a crucial psychopathological feature. It follows that the frontal and prefrontal regions are likely to be dysfunctional in this syndrome. A study of CBF in a patient suffering from bromide delirium found that the normal hyperfrontal pattern was lacking (18). However, CBF was not significantly correlated with confusion in patients with delirium tremens (17). These contradictory findings call for more studies of CBF in delirium of various etiologies. It is interesting to note that in a patient with acute amphetamine intoxication, with paranoid features and clear orientation, CBF was elevated by about 30% compared to the preintoxicated state, and the maximum increase occurred in the left hemisphere and the frontal regions (47). In Alzheimer's disease, CBF is generally decreased, notably in the temporo-parieto-occipital regions (43,48). Risberg (43) reports that the Lund group of investigators attempted to differentiate dementia from acute organic mental syndromes with the aid of rCBF studies. In schizophrenia, hypofrontality, i.e., reduction in rCBF in the frontal and prefrontal regions of the cortex, has been demonstrated (49). Such hypofrontality is not specific to schizophrenia; it may be observed in other brain disorders as well (49). Reduced frontal/prefrontal cortical function may lead to a diminished ability to produce and maintain stable cognitive and behavioral sets, which in turn leads to general cognitive disturbances including confusion (49). Final elucidation of this issue must await more studies of rCBF in delirium.

CBF has been shown to correlate with EEG frequency (50). Decreased CBF is associated with a slow-wave EEG, and vice versa. There are exceptions to this general rule, however. During slow-wave sleep, CBF is only slightly reduced in the presence of a large proportion of slow waves in the EEG. In children, CBF is high, while the EEG tends to be slow. Another exception is provided by cerebral hypoxia, which induces lactacidosis in the brain and thus disrupts the normal regulation and autoregulation of CBF (50). Following cerebral anoxic lesions, a high CBF may exist despite the presence of a slow-wave EEG. Finally, reduced CBF in the presence of a normal EEG has been reported (7).

In summary, functional neuronal activity and CMR generally correlate well with CBF. These variables also correlate, with some exceptions, with level of consciousness. When CBF is significantly reduced, the level of consciousness tends to be correspondingly lower (23). When arterial blood is deficient in oxygen or glucose, or both, even normal or increased CBF may be found in the presence of confusion. Reduced level of consciousness is usually, if not invariably, associated with reduced CMR and CBF. CBF and substrate supplies may be adequate, yet CMR may be reduced and the level of consciousness lowered. In the latter case, a reduction in neuronal activity and a corresponding drop in energy demand are likely to occur. Anesthesia with halothane, methoxyflurane, and nitrous oxide in a subject with a normal brain exemplifies this type of condition (51).

Studies of rCBF in delirium have been few to date and are clearly needed. It appears that the syndrome may occur in association with either reduced or increased (delirium tremens, hyperthermia) CBF. Ingvar's (41) hypotheses regarding the role of frontal and prefrontal cortical regions in normal consciousness appear to be relevant to delirium. One should keep in mind, however, Sokoloff's (52) comment that "the mechanisms of behavior are far too subtle to be reflected in blood flow or metabolic rate, even if measured at the most minute level" (p 250).

Electroencephalographic studies

Studies of delirium employing the EEG have provided most of the meager information we have about the pathophysiology and pathogenesis of this syndrome. With the exceptions noted in the preceding section, the EEG reflects the functional and metabolic activity of the brain. Neuronal activity determines $CMRO_2$, which in turn influences CBF and the frequency of EEG background activity. In particular, there appears to be a definite relationship between rCBF and low-frequency rhythms over a wide range of rCBF levels (53). On the whole, reduced cerebral function, $CMRO_2$, and CBF tend to be accompanied by a slowing of the EEG. With progressive reduction of the level of consciousness, there is a diffuse slowing of background rhythms from alpha to theta and delta activity (54,55). Three major pathophysiological mechanisms can result in alteration of consciousness: (1) metabolic encephalopathy; supratentorial mass lesions compressing the diencephalic and mesencephalic reticular formation; and infratentorial mass or destructive lesions (6,54). Delirium and coma can be brought about by all three of these mechanisms.

Pioneering studies of the EEG in delirium were carried out by Engel, Romano, and their co-workers in the 1940s (56–61). Engel et al. (56) developed a quantitative method for the expression of frequency distribution in the EEG. They made a count of complete waves in 300 one-second intervals and expressed the distribution of frequencies per second as a percentage of the whole. This method yielded a spectrum of frequencies ranging from 1 to 12 per second, together with some low-voltage activity. The distribution of waves per second, rather than that of individual wavelengths, was thus determined. The investigators found their method adequate to detect the magnitude of shifts in frequency under various conditions in which such shifts were diffuse rather than paroxysmal.

Romano and Engel (57) reported their major findings in 1944. They had studied 53 patients suffering from a broad range of cardiovascular, respiratory, cerebral, metabolic, infectious, and toxic diseases. All of their subjects displayed evidence of delirium, characterized by an increased fluctuation in the level of awareness, loss of ability to do abstract thinking, attentional deficits, and impairment of memory and calculation. All the patients showed EEG abnormalities, which the investigators classified arbitrarily into five stages, ranked in the order of increasing severity, as follows (57):

Stage I: Appearance of a small amount of regular and irregular slow frequencies (5–7 c/sec)

Stage II: Further decrease in the regularity of the tracing and an increase in both low-voltage fast activity and regular and irregular theta waves

Stage III: Low-voltage activity and some regular and irregular slow frequencies (3–6 c/sec) predominant

Stage IV: Irregular, disorganized record, no recognizable alpha activity (8–12 c/sec), and predominance of slow frequency (2–7 c/sec), with small amounts of low-voltage fast activity

Stage V: Normal frequencies few or absent; predominance of fairly regular, moderately high-voltage slow activity (3–7 c/sec).

The EEG abnormalities reversed completely, or almost so, to a normal pattern in most patients. The investigators concluded that delirium, as defined by them, was associated with an electrical disturbance of the brain, which was reversible to the extent that the clinical features of delirium were reversible. The EEG abnormalities included a decrease in frequency, disorganization, and, in the last stage, reorganization at a lower energy level. The researchers hypothesized that the decrease in frequency reflected reduced levels of, or reduced responses to, cortical excitation; the latter was likely caused by a reduced metabolic rate of the neurons or a decrease in the arousing effect of afferent impulses to the cortex. The abnormal electrical activity, as demonstrated by the EEG, was postulated to arise from damaged or dying cells. The EEG abnormalities were *nonspecific* in terms of the etiology of delirium. They showed a correlation with the psychological deficits and abnormalities that define delirium as a clinical syndrome. The character of the EEG changes appeared to be independent of the specific underlying cerebral disorder but was related to the intensity, duration, and reversibility of the implicated noxious factors.

In subsequent papers (59–61), Engel, Romano, and their collaborators extended their original observations summarized above. They demonstrated that measures taken to correct a major physiological derangement underlying delirium in a given patient could lead to a reversal of the syndrome and its associated EEG abnormalities (59). For example, administration of 100% oxygen to delirious patients with congestive heart failure or pulmonary decompensation frequently resulted in an improvement of the EEG record.

Engel and his co-workers initiated studies on experimentally induced delirium (59,61). For example, they induced the syndrome by oral administration of ethanol to healthy volunteers and chronic alcoholics (59). As intoxication developed, progressive slowing of the EEG background rhythms correlated with changes in the level of awareness. The degree of change in frequency rather than the appearance of any particular frequency appeared to be the significant variable. In cases where the record obtained prior to the experimental intoxication was fast or fast normal, the tracing taken during gross intoxication had a frequency distribution within the normal range (8–12 c/

sec). Experimental induction of delirium by exposure to simulated high altitudes in a decompression chamber, and hence hypoxia, showed results similar to those of experimental alcohol intoxication and hypoglycemia (61).

Engel and Romano summarized their findings in two review articles (4,62). They interpreted their results as demonstrating that the core psychological disturbance in delirium results from alteration of cerebral cortical metabolism secondary to disease or intoxication (61). They proposed that this metabolic derangement underlies all instances of delirium, and is reflected in concurrent cognitive abnormalities and the relatively generalized slowing of the EEG (4). Combined, these two abnormalities are essential features of the syndrome. Moreover, the EEG may be viewed as the most sensitive and reliable indicator of the underlying cerebral insufficiency. The otherwise nonspecific EEG changes, coupled with the presence of increased fluctuation in the level of awareness, as manifested by a fluctuating impairment of cognitive functions, provide a basis for the differentiation of delirium from other mental disorders. A single normal EEG does not mean, however, that delirium is absent, since the particular patient's premorbid record may have been faster. The slowing of the EEG in delirium is thus relative to the individual's premorbid tracing and may fall within the statistically normal range. Only serial recordings can clarify this issue in some cases. Those delirious patients whose EEG fails to show slow activity will be found to have either a fast normal or a faster than statistically normal (more than 12 c/sec) record on recovery.

The generalizability of the findings and conclusions reported by Engel and Romano (4) has been a subject of some controversy. Their critics, notably Adams and Victor (63), contend that in milder degrees of delirium there is no EEG abnormality at all, and that in some cases of the syndrome only activity in the fast beta frequency is present. The latter statement holds for some drug intoxications and withdrawal syndromes (54). Engel and Romano (4), however, consider the alcohol withdrawal delirium to be a variant of delirium generally, one that is closer in its clinical features to mental disorders induced by such drugs as lysergic acid, mescaline, and quinacrine. This whole issue appears to turn on semantics and will finally be resolved when PET studies are carried out and help to establish whether alcohol and drug withdrawal deliria involve different metabolic processes from the much more common deliria due to metabolic disorders, infections, and drug intoxications.

No one has yet attempted to replicate the studies and findings of Engel, Romano, and their collaborators. There is general agreement, however, that in most cases of delirium the EEG is slowed, as those investigators have observed (54,55,64–66). Yet exceptions have been reported (67). Some very abnormal tracings may be found on occasion in patients who fail to show manifestations of reduced consciousness, while normal tracings have been observed when consciousness is reduced (67). Diffuse alpha-like EEG activity may occur in patients who are comatose due to cerebral anoxia, focal brain stem lesions, and some drug intoxications (68). Such alpha coma is rare, however (68). Seizure activity has been observed in structures such as the hippocampus and brain stem in the presence of clouding or loss of consciousness and a normal scalp EEG. A corticogram does not always reflect the pathology of the midbrain, brain stem, or limbic structures, despite the presence of reduced consciousness (68,69). In delirium due to sedative-hypnotic or alcohol withdrawal, the background rhythms are often normal or may show low-amplitude, fast activity (68). These exceptions are theoretically and practically important, and suggest that clinical delirium may result from different brain processes.

The finding of diffuse slowing of the background frequencies in most delirious patients raises the question of the psychological correlates of such slowing in other situations. Changes in theta activity are most consistently related to various components of attention (69). A review of studies of the relation between theta waves and various psychological variables indicates that theta activity accompanies the state of reduced alertness, i.e., receptivity to external stimuli (69). However, theta activity has also been observed to accompany active problem-solving and perceptual processing tasks (69). This discrepancy cannot be accounted for at this time. In general, diffuse slowing of the background EEG activity in a normal awake person tends to correlate positively with reduced attention span and impaired cognitive functioning (69–71).

Experimental delirium and the EEG

Delirium induced experimentally by anticholinergic agents has been studied by EEG. These studies have yielded observations that throw some light on the pathophysiology of the syndrome and deserve a separate discussion.

In the late 1950s, Czech workers began to experiment with benactyzine, a strong anticholinergic agent (72). They noted that when this drug was administered in a dose of 15 to 70 mg, it caused delirium in healthy volunteers. The delirium lasted for 3 to 5 hours and featured gross impairment of intellectual performance and memory, thinking disturbances, visual hallucinations, and disordered psychomotor activity. Physostigmine failed to reverse these symptoms. Excretion of 5-hydroxy-indolacetic acid was found to be reduced and correlated with the appearance of delirious symptomatology. This finding led researchers to hypothesize that the deliriogenic potential of benactyzine depended on the drug's capacity to interfere with both acetylcholine and serotonin metabolism. The EEG records taken during the induced delirium showed a breakdown of the background alpha activity and a predominance of delta waves.

Abood and Meduna (73) studied deliriogenic properties of synthetic anticholinergic agents, namely, various congeners of the piperidyl benzilates. One compound, designated JB-329, when administered to healthy volunteers in doses of 5 to 10 mg orally, caused auditory and visual hallucinations and delirium. JB-329, or Ditran, was actually a mixture of two isomers: *N*-ethyl-2-pyrrolidyl-methyl-cyclopentylphenyl glycolate (70%) and *N*-ethyl-3-piperidyl-cyclopentylphenyl glycolate (30%) (74). Other researchers reported that Ditran could induce delirium in patients with a history of delirium tremens that was quite similar to the latter (75). Deliriogenic effects of this drug could be counteracted by tetrahydroaminacrin, a compound with potent anticholinesterase activity. These early observations stimulated a sizable body of research on the behavioral and EEG effects of Ditran, and have contributed to the understanding of the pathogenesis of delirium (74–82). It is interesting to note at this point that tetrahydroaminoacridine has recently been reported to show some promise in the treatment of Alzheimer's disease (83).

Itil (80–82) and Itil and Fink (9,84) have reported on their extensive investigations of the behavioral and EEG changes induced by Ditran in humans. Three main behavioral responses to the drug were observed (9). With a low dose (0.01–0.02 mg/kg), the changes consisted of slight fluctuations in attention and consciousness, and were accompanied by low-voltage theta and delta activity. Used in higher doses (0.04–0.25 mg/kg), Ditran provoked in some subjects a stupor-like state. High doses of the drug (0.10–0.25 mg/kg) elicited a reduction in and fluctuation of awareness, perceptual distortions, thought disturbances, severe anxiety, and restlessness. These behavioral effects were accompanied by a reduction of alpha activity and the appearance on the EEG of high-voltage theta and delta waves, with superimposed 20–40 c/sec fast beta activity. Both the behavioral and the EEG changes induced by Ditran were modified by administering various drugs during the experimental delirium. Intravenous chlorpromazine interrupted the delirium and induced coma and increased slowing of the EEG, with decreased fast beta activity. Administration of tetrahydroaminacrin resulted in a reversal of the delirium in 10 to 20 minutes, as well as decreased delta waves and fast beta activity. Intravenous LSD (0.001–0.002 mg/kg) produced increased alertness, as well as psychomotor hyperactivity. The investigators hypothesized that, in delirium, changes occur in the central cholinergic and adrenergic mechanisms that affect the medial ascending reticular activating system and the medial thalamic diffuse projection systems. The former exercises mainly a cortical inhibitory function (reflected in the appearance of slow waves on the EEG), while the latter have a predominantly facilitatory effect on the cortex (reflected in fast activity in the EEG). Thus, a relative increase in either central inhibitory or stimulatory function, subserved by one or the other of these systems, may determine the type of delirium, i.e. whether it is hyperactive or hypoactive. This interesting hypothesis seems to be supported by the finding of increased CBF and central noradrenergic activity in alcohol withdrawal delirium that is typically hyperactive (17,85).

Atropine (0.04–0.30 mg/kg) induced more slow waves but less fast activity in experimental subjects than Ditran (84). The relative proportion of slow or fast activity was related to the clinical manifestations induced by either drug, especially the degree of psychomotor activity and the presence of hallucinations. An earlier study had shown that atropine administered to healthy volunteers in a dose of 10 mg orally impaired recent memory and attention span but did not induce illusions, hallucinations, delusions, or disorientation (86). The EEG showed a consistent shift toward lower-amplitude and slow activity. Itil (81) observed that high doses of atropine and Ditran induced in some subjects a sleep-like state that differed significantly in both its clinical and EEG features from normal sleep. In a later paper, Itil (82) reported on the digital computer–analyzed EEG records during REM sleep, as well as following Ditran and LSD administration. He found that an EEG pattern characterized by both very slow and very fast activity occurred in both REM sleep and anticholinergic delirium. Itil hypothesized that both REM sleep and delirium depended on inhibition of the central cholinergic mechanism.

In an interesting study, Cartwright (79) noted that Ditran gave rise to EEG tracings markedly different from the experimental subjects' normal waking and sleep records. The EEG taken during Ditran-induced delirium displayed features of both wakefulness and stages 1, 2, and 3 sleep. REM periods were both persistent and of high amplitude. Mean total REM time the night following Ditran administration was significantly reduced in comparison to the predrug night. The content of dreams obtained from the subjects on a night 1 to 2 weeks prior to or after the drug experience was quite similar to that of Ditran-induced hallucinations. This led Cartwright to postulate that the fantasies produced under dreaming and drug conditions were derived from the same substrate of ongoing mental life. She proposed that Ditran appeared to create a neurophysiological state different from, and yet analogous to, that of REM sleep and dreaming. It is interesting to note in this regard that Jacobs (87) has proposed that the similarity between dreams and drug-induced hallucinations reflects a common neurochemical mechanism, i.e., inactivation of the brain serotonin system.

Behavioral and EEG effects of atropine, scopolamine, and Ditran are qualitatively similar (74). All three drugs induce delirium in normal volunteers when given in equivalent intramuscular doses. Subjects pass through an initial stage of drowsiness and "stupor," and then progress to a "pseudowakeful" state characterized by disordered attention, impaired recent memory, defective abstract thinking and judgment, and disturbed time perception (74). Lucid intervals are observed in even the most severely delirious subjects. Illusions and hallucinations, most often visual, are commonly present. Ditran delirium has been found to be similar to alcohol withdrawal delirium (76,77) but different from LSD psychosis (88). It is associated with marked changes in somatosensory and visual evoked potentials (78). The earlier portions of the evoked responses tend to be augmented or speeded up by Ditran, while the later portions are reduced or slowed by it. These changes have been interpreted as pointing to reduced activity of central information processing coupled with lowered inhibitory activity and thus increased responsiveness of the brain during Ditran delirium (78).

A number of other anticholinergic compounds, including amitriptyline, have been applied to induce experimental delirium (89–91). Scopolamine produces an increased deliriogenic effect after only 1 night of sleep deprivation (92). This drug appears to decrease the amount of REM sleep and to postpone its onset. Physostigmine reverses the impairment of wakefulness caused by anticholinergic agents and by sleep loss (92). In recent years, scopolamine has been used experimentally not to induce delirium but to study its effects on cognition and attention (93,94). When administered transdermally to healthy volunteers, the drug caused impairment on tasks requiring sustained attention (93). When injected subcutaneously to healthy volunteers, it produced marked decrements in selection and evaluation of environmental information, as well as impairment of immediate recall, delayed recall, recognition, and memory scanning (94). Alertness was reduced. Interestingly, as noted in an earlier section, scopolamine reduces frontal cortex perfusion (16). All these findings suggest that central cholinergic blockade elicits cognitive-attentional deficits and abnormalities that are essential clinical features of delirium. Unfortunately, the experimental work on anticholinergic delirium that flourished in the 1960s and produced important observations and hypotheses faded away in the early 1970s. Thus, this information clamors for synthesis and further research. There are, for example, intriguing analogies between the deliriogenic effects of central cholinergic blockade and the putative contributory role of cholinergic deficiency in Alzheimer's disease (95,96). Patients suffering from this disease show a behavioral supersensitivity to scopolamine relative to elderly controls (96). Physostigmine and other cholinesterase inhibitors tend to reverse the cognitive deficits brought about by scopolamine and have been used, with varying success, as replacement therapy in Alzheimer's disease (95,96). However, the specificity of the scopolamine model for a cholinergic deficiency state is open to question (95). Dementia of Alzheimer's disease and delirium appear to involve reduction in cholinergic input, as well as deficiencies in other neurotransmitters and neuromodulators.

In summary, studies of delirium induced experimentally by anticholinergic drugs indicate strongly that the elicited psychopathological and EEG changes reflect, in part, the pathogenetic role of cholinergic blockade in this syndrome. The concomitant EEG changes tend to correlate with the reduced level of awareness and the cognitive impairment. When EEG changes involve a preponderance of diffuse slow background activity, the behavioral alterations are likely to include sedation, drowsiness, memory impairment, and psychomotor hypoactivity. If a considerable amount of fast EEG activity is superimposed on slow background activity, one observes increased psychomotor activity, perceptual abnormalities, and delusional misinterpretations of internal and external information inputs. There is an analogy between the deliriogenic effects of experimentally induced cholinergic blockage and the contributory pathogenetic role of cholinergic deficiency in the dementia of Alzheimer's disease and several other diseases. Patients suffering from one of these dementias are highly sensitive to cholinergic blockage, and this may account, in part, for their vulnerability to delirium. (For further discussion of anticholinergic delirium and its reversal by physostigmine, see Chapter 11).

Summary of the EEG findings in delirium

Bilateral, diffuse abnormality, notably slowing of the EEG background activity, is a usual, if not an invariable, feature of delirium. Fast activity may or may not be superimposed on the slow background rhythms. Its relative preponderance is usually associated with the hyperactive variant of delirium. Increased variability of the EEG frequencies and wave amplitudes tends to be associated with greater alertness, wakefulness, psychomotor activity, and perceptual distortions. In alcohol withdrawal delirium, the EEG is either normal or shows low-voltage and relatively fast dysrhythmia. Slowing of the EEG found in most cases of delirium due to metabolic, infectious, and toxic factors tends to correlate with reduced alertness, consciousness, and wakefulness on the one hand, and with diminished cerebral blood flow, oxygen consumption, and metabolic rate, on the other. The EEG features of hyperactive delirium show some resemblance to those of REM sleep. In hypoactive delirium, relatively slow background activity tends to predominate and resembles the EEG tracings taken in the period of transition from wakefulness to sleep. The assorted changes of the EEG in delirium have been explained by altered function of the reticular activating system and the medial thalamic diffuse projection systems. In one study, EEG patterns in patients with deep midline brain lesions could not be distinguished from those seen with diffuse cortical and subcortical encephalopathies (97). On occasion, generalized, bilaterally synchronous bursts of slow waves and essentially normal background activity have been observed in patients with diffuse encephalopathies and altered consciousness (98).

The EEG changes in delirium are *nonspecific*. An increase in slow waves can occur physiologically during sleep, as well as in pathological states such as metabolic encephalopathies, space-occupying lesions of the brain, head trauma, cerebrovascular accidents, and dementia. Moreover, all drugs producing sedation give rise to significant slowing of the EEG (99). The EEG is a highly useful aid in the diagnosis of delirium (see Chapters 8 and 9). Like any other laboratory test, however, the EEG must always be viewed in conjunction with pertinent psychological and other clinical findings. Moreover, a single recording carried out during delirium may be interpreted as being normal and yet may be relatively abnormal if one uses the patient as his or her own standard for comparison. In such a case, only serial recordings can disclose pathological changes. The EEG abnormalities may, in some cases, antedate or outlast delirium, or both.

Recent advances in the techniques of EEG recording and quantification of its background activity should be applied to the study of delirium, as they may help advance our knowledge of the EEG alterations in this syndrome. Changes in the amplitude and frequency of the EEG rhythms in states of diffuse cerebral pathology can be quantified and displayed graphically with the application of computer methods (99). Digital spectral analysis represents an advance in recording and monitoring EEG background activity. Compression and graphic display of the EEG data is already being used to monitor cerebral activity in medical and surgical settings (see Chapter 18). However, computerized spectral analysis offered only a modest advantage over visual EEG analysis in a study of patients with Alzheimer's disease (100). Magnetoencephalography has been applied in epilepsy research and could be used in studies of delirium (101). The somnogram and comagram are useful additions to the techniques of monitoring electrophysiological changes in the brain during sleep and loss of consciousness (102). One looks forward to an extension of these techniques to delirium in the form of a "deliriogram" that can be used to record EEG background activity and other rhythms during delirium. Mobile, long-term monitoring of the EEG has been used in the study of epilepsy and could be applied to that of delirium as well (103,104). Finally, another technical advance used in the differential diagnosis of cerebral dysfunction, neurometrics, could be applied to delirious patients (105). Application of these technological advances to the study of delirium will help to clarify its relationship to the EEG changes.

The association between abnormal EEG records and most cases of delirium raises a question: Does this finding throw any light on the pathophysiology of delirium? The EEG reflects the activity of the cerebral cortex modulated in varying degree by afferent impulses (106). Electrical potentials recorded from the scalp are summated synaptic potentials originating in the pyramidal cells of the cortex. Rhythmic discharges generated in the thalamic nuclei elicit responses in the cortical cells that are recorded as the electrical potentials. The frequencies of these potentials, as well as those of the thalamic discharges, are determined by the thalamic cells. Desynchronization of the cortical potentials during activation is brought about by impulses originating in the reticular formation that abolish the rhythmic discharges in the thalamic nuclei (106). The EEG changes that accompany delirium indicate an interference with the above mechanisms. These changes suggest a derangement of the processes subserving normal arousal, attention, wakefulness, and sleep. Acute brain disorders of any etiology tend to disorganize the circadian sleep-wake cycle. Such disorganization appears to be an invariable concomitant of delirium. Except in severe brain damage, the quantitative EEG reflects cerebral metabolism and blood flow. The EEG changes in delirium indicate alterations in these two parameters of brain function. Moreover, they suggest an inquiry into the neurophysiological and neurochemical mechanisms underlying arousal, wakefulness, sleep, and consciousness.

Cerebral substrates of arousal, attention, consciousness, and the sleep-wake cycle in relation to delirium

Delirium is often referred to as a disorder of consciousness, attention, or wakefulness. Therefore, it seems logical to review briefly some of the current views on the putative neuroanatomical and neurochemical bases of these behavioral constructs. The literature on this subject is large, and full of controversy and open ends, no doubt related partly to the notorious ambiguity of terms such as "consciousness," "arousal," "awareness," and "attention" (see Chapter 6). As Robbins and Everitt (107) point out, for example, "monolithic terms such as 'attention' and 'memory' are in danger of becoming as empty as old concepts of arousal" (p 1450). One author has actually proclaimed the death of the old arousal theory and written its obituary (108).

Despite its many different connotations, the concept of *arousal* is still considered essential for understanding how the monoaminergic and cholinergic systems affect psychological functions (107). Since the discovery, in 1949, of the ascending reticular activating system (ARAS) by Moruzzi and Magoun (109), it has traditionally been assumed that cerebral activation, indicated by the presence of low-voltage fast activity in the neocortex and rhythmic, slow activity in the hippocampus, is correlated with arousal, while deactivation, indicated by the presence of large-amplitude, irregular slow waves or spindles in both the neocortex and the hippocampus, is correlated with sleep or coma (110). High levels of activity in the ARAS produce low-voltage fast activity in the neocortex, while low levels of activity in this system give rise to slow waves or spindles in the neocortex. Slow waves or spindles may also occur as a consequence of increased activity in an ascending reticulocortical slow wave–inducing system that seems to act as an antagonist to the ARAS (110). The state of wakefulness in humans is believed to depend on a continuous inflow of ascending impulses from the ARAS that maintain the central tone of the forebrain (111). The initial experiments of Moruzzi and Magoun (109) involved the ARAS of the lower brain stem. Later investigators included additional structures, so that the ARAS has come to be viewed as stretching throughout the brain stem and extending to the diencephalon and the basal regions of the telencephalon.

This traditional theory of arousal has been challenged on the grounds that neocortical slow-wave activity is not well correlated with either the level of arousal or consciousness, and that the states of sleep and wakefulness do not depend on the integrity of the cerebral cortex or of ARAS-cortical projections (110). In recent years, the concept of arousal has undergone a revision and become fractionated (107). Evidence indicates that the ARAS has many components, including the ascending noradrenergic, dopaminergic, serotoninergic, and cholinergic systems, whose action seems to mediate different aspects of arousal (107).

A number of diffuse projection systems from the brain stem and basal forebrain to the cortex appear to be involved in the modulation of cortical arousal, as well as attention and motivation (112). They include both thalamic nuclei and nonthalamic subcortical systems. Ojemann (113) has proposed that the thalamocortical ARAS and its interaction with the language cortex of the dominant hemisphere are an essential part of the brain mechanism for *conscious experience.* Luria (114) asserts that the medial zones of the hemispheres may be viewed as a system superimposed upon the ARAS. Patients with lesions in those zones display disturbances of consciousness and memory that in some cases resemble those of delirium (114). Lesions of the upper part of the brain stem and the walls of the third ventricle may produce sleep or an oneiroid, drowsy state accompanied by reduced cortical activation (114). Lesions of the hippocampal structures produce attentional deficits such as increased distractibility, inability to sustain attention, and frequent intrusion of irrelevant associations. Distinction between past and present, and between dream and waking perception, becomes confused. All these abnormalities strongly resemble those encountered in delirium.

There is a close connection between arousal and *attention* (107). A distinction is made between divided and selective attention (107). The former involves the capacity to perform more than one task simultaneously, while the latter refers to resistance to distraction (107). In recent years, progress has been made in identifying the neuronal structures and pathways that constitute the neuroanatomical substrate of attention (115,116). Three brain areas for visual attention have been identified: the posterior parietal lobe, a portion of the thalamus (part of the pulvinar), and areas of the midbrain related to eye movements (115). The lateral left frontal lobe is involved in semantic operations, while the anterior cingulate is involved in selecting language and other types of information for action (115). As Posner et al. (115) emphasize, visual imagery, word reading, and shifting visual attention are not performed by a single brain area; each of these tasks involves a large number of component computations that must be brought into play in order to perform the cognitive task. The reticular afferents to the posterior parietal lobe from the intralaminar thalamic nuclei, nucleus locus ceruleus, and raphe nuclei provide the activation (arousal) necessary for attentional performance (116). PET studies have shown that subjects attending to visual stimuli showed significantly higher right hemispheric metabolic rates (116).

Geschwind (117) has proposed that confusional states represent "global disorders of attention." He writes that "the disturbances in attention as a result of a disorder of the nervous system go under many different names, e.g. delirium, confusion, or even the acute brain syndrome, a barbaric nomenclature that has become widely used, especially among American psychiatrists" (p 175). "Barbaric" or not, the term "delirium" has been used for 2,000 years. Geschwind proceeds to give a rather skewed account of the clinical features of the confusional state. For example, he states that a "dramatic feature" of this state is playful behavior and facetiousness. This remark suggests that he had contact with a rather selected sample of delirious patients, most of whom show apathy, depression, or fear rather than facile jocularity. Geschwind asserts that confusional states frequently occur in association with lesions of the right hemisphere, such as infarctions, and reflect its dominance for attention. He offers no other evidence to support his contention that confusional states in general are focal rather than global cerebral disorders. Considering that the vast majority of the cases of delirium are due to toxic, metabolic, and infectious factors, Geschwind's simplistic localizationism sounds unconvincing. There is general agreement that the syndrome typically features attentional disturbances (see Chapter 6), but it does not follow logically from this fact that its pathogenesis involves primarily the putative attentional network of the brain. Delirium involves not only disorders of attention but also impairment of information processing and memory, sleep-wake cycle disruption, and abnormal psychomotor behavior. These widespread abnormalities point to a widespread involvement of both cortical and subcortical structures and their assorted functions, rather than to a single neural network.

Delirium has been traditionally viewed as a disorder of *consciousness* interposed between normal wakeful and alert state on the one hand, and stupor and coma on the other (6). The proposed key role of the diffuse corticothalamic projection systems in conscious experience has already been referred to (113). Subcortical structures, notably the brain stem, are essential for maintaining consciousness because of their role in regulating cortical arousal and wakefulness, both of which are necessary conditions for conscious awareness and alertness. Ingvar (41), quoted earlier, argues persuasively that the frontal/prefrontal cortex is essential for conscious awareness. Other authors argue that changes in EEG activity, in level of consciousness, and in degree of responsiveness to incoming information are independent expressions of the same basic pathological process, and the presence of delirium indicates a generalized impairment of cerebral functions or at least bilateral lesions of limbic structures (6). The degree of abnormality of each of these three parameters is claimed to vary according to the etiology and the site of the responsible lesion (6). Global impairment of consciousness may result from mesodiencephalic, deep hemispheric, and bilateral and diffuse hemispheric lesions. Brain stem lesions tend to produce akinetic mutism or coma rather than delirium. Extensive tumors of the brain stem may occasionally fail to result in impaired consciousness, while coma may be produced without any apparent involvement of the ARAS. All types of EEG changes may be found with every degree of coma (6). Lesions in the pons or pontomesencephalic area may be accompanied by alpha activity in the EEG even in deep coma. On the whole, however, both coma and delirium are positively correlated with the presence of diffuse slow background activity in the EEG.

The above observations underscore the complexity of brain mechanisms underlying consciousness and its disorders. Since conscious awareness requires full wakefulness, and since delirium may be regarded, in part, as its disorder, one that is invariably accompanied by disturbances of the *sleep-wake cycle,* it seems appropriate to review briefly the current views on the brain structures and neurochemistry involved in its regulation.

Morgane (118) points out that it has become necessary to regard wakefulness and the states of sleep as the outcome of complex neurophysiological interactions that involve many regions of the brain. Early attempts to account for the alteration of the sleep-wake cycle resulted in the formulation of the "monoaminergic theory," which posited the essential role of the monoamine-containing neurons for both the induction and the maintenance of the various components of the sleep-wake cycle. Localized and more or less discrete sleep centers, such as nuclei or specific cell groups, were believed to control sleep and wakefulness (118,119). More recently, these concepts have been revised and modified.

Hobson et al. (119) have proposed that the sleep cycle is generated by the interaction of multiple neuronal populations rather than by localized sleep centers. Generation of the ultradian sleep cycle cannot be accounted for by one nuclear group or neurotransmitter. This revision of the views of sleep regulation does not seem to be generally accepted, yet it reflects the need to account for the growing complexity of the neurophysiology and neurochemistry of the distinct behavioral states of wakefulness and sleep (118–121). As one writer modestly states, "Because of technological limitations, we still know little of what is going on inside the human brain during SWS, or, for that matter, during any other form of sleep. All we can do, metaphorically speaking, is to scratch the surface" (36, p 165).

Wakefulness consists of two different states: phasic and tonic (120). The former is responsible for arousal, the latter for the maintenance of wakefulness for a certain period. A number of putative neurotransmitters have been proposed to play a role in the regulation of the state of vigilance. They include acetylcholine, noradrenaline, serotonin, dopamine, gamma-aminobutyric acid (GABA), histamine, adenosine, and several neuropeptides (120). The role of the first of these neurotransmitters has been most firmly established to date (118–121). Initially, serotonin was viewed as the active inducer and maintainer of slow-wave sleep, while noradrenaline was believed to play a similar role in REM sleep (118). Interactions of serotonergic neurons of the raphe system and catecholaminergic neurons of the locus coeruleus were thought to play a key role in the regulation of the sleep-wake cycle. More recently, the monoamine theory has undergone a revision. Neurons in the locus coeruleus actually appear to inhibit REM sleep via noradrenergic neurotransmission (125). The noradrenaline-containing cells of the locus coeruleus stop firing during REM sleep but are continuously active in wakefulness and non-REM sleep (125). Apparently, a key function of REM sleep is to reduce activity in the noradrenaline-containing cells in the locus coeruleus (125). Only during REM sleep are postsynaptic cells free of noradrenergic activity. Serotonin-containing raphe nuclei also stop discharging in REM sleep and thus represent, along with the locus coeruleus, REM-off cells (119,125). These nuclei discharge most rapidly during wakefulness, and their activity is markedly reduced or ceases during both non-REM and REM sleep (125,126). These neurons seem to have a "hypnotonic" effect. It has been observed, however, that parachlorophenylalanine, which decreases the synthesis of serotonin, reduces the amount of REM but not of non-REM sleep (14). There is a discrepancy in this respect between human pharmacological and animal studies (14). The former tend to point to a relation between serotonin and REM sleep, while the latter suggest a role for this neurotransmitter in both REM and non-REM sleep. Some investigators assert that available evidence does not support a significant role of serotonergic nuclei in the regulation of REM sleep (125). Cholinergic mechanisms are involved in the induction of REM sleep, in addition to their arousing and awakening effects (11,120,122–125). The role of dopamine in the regulation of the sleep-wake cycle remains ambiguous. Agents that tend to enhance dopamine activity, such as methylphenidate, decrease total sleep time (14). GABA is a major cortical inhibitory transmitter system that appears to participate in the regulation of the sleep-wake cycle (120). Elevation of the GABA concentration tends to promote sleep.

In summary, available information indicates that the regulation of the sleep-wake cycle involves the interaction of multiple sets of neurons and a number of neurotransmitters (119). A reciprocal interaction of cholinergic, serotonergic, and noradrenergic systems appears to play a major, if not the only, role in the regulation of the sleep-wake cycle. Given the paucity of sleep studies in delirium (see Chapter 5) and the growing complexity of the hypotheses concerning the generation and maintenance of both wakefulness and the sleep stages, it is impossible at this time to draw any conclusions about the relationship between disorders of the sleep-wake cycle and delirium. The syndrome is most readily induced by cholinergic deficiency and blockade, i.e., conditions in which wakefulness is likely to be reduced and REM sleep decreased. By contrast to anticholinergic agents, anticholinesterases increase REM sleep and, at higher doses, elicit wakefulness when administered during sleep. One may speculate, therefore, that acetylcholine deficiency results in both a disorder of consciousness and a disturbance of the normal sleep cycle, which together comprise the syndrome of delirium. Moreover, the cholinergic deficiency is likely to disturb the delicate balance between the cholinergic, serotonergic, and noradrenergic neuronal networks and neurotransmission, which may lead to a marked disorganization of the whole sleep-wake cycle in a delirious patient. There is an obvious need for sleep researchers to finally address the issue of the disturbances of this cycle in delirium.

Miscellaneous pathogenetic mechanisms

Several pathogenetic mechanisms operating in the induction of delirium have been hypothesized by various authors in addition to those already discussed. They include *hypercortisolemia, beta-endorphinergic dysfunction,* and changes in the transmission functions of *glutamate.*

Kral (127) hypothesized that delirium in the elderly represents a reaction to acute stress mediated by abnormally high levels of circulating corticosteroids, or by increased vulnerability of the hypothalamus to their effects, or by both (see Chapter 18). Other investigators have observed a significant and unusually prolonged postoperative increase in circulating levels of cortisol in patients who become delirious following elective surgery (128; Chapter 19, this volume). This change was absent in the patients who did not develop delirium after an operation. The circadian rhythm of cortisol was totally disrupted only in those patients recovering in an intensive care unit who were delirious. Serum cortisol levels were markedly elevated after open heart surgery, but they did not differ in psychotic and nonpsychotic patients (129). The pathogenetic role of hypercortisolemia in delirium remains hypothetical and calls for more research to clarify it.

Koponen et al. (130) studied elderly delirious patients and found a significant reduction in CSF beta-endorphin-like immunoreactivity compared with controls. These researchers suggest that dysfunction in the beta-endorphinergic neurons may increase susceptibility to delirium. On the other hand, other investigators have found increased and prolonged plasma beta-endorphin levels in postoperative delirium (130,131); however, in one study, such elevated levels were no different in delirious and nondelirious patients (129). Thus, the putative pathogenetic role of beta-endorphins in delirium remains intriguing but unresolved.

Finally, some researchers have implicated altered transmitter functions of glutamate in the clinical symptomatology of some metabolic and toxic encephalopathies (131). So far, no one has studied the glutamate levels in the central nervous system in delirium.

In summary, both direct and indirect evidence indicates that delirium, as currently defined, represents the final common pathway for a variety of pathophysiological processes and mechanisms involving both cortical and subcortical structures and their interconnections whose integrated activity subserves normal wakefulness, alertness, information processing, attention, memory, and the sleep-wake cycle. Delirium results from some disintegration of these processes that is manifested both behaviorally and electrophysiologically. The best-established hypothesis at this time proposes that delirium may result from any factor that reduces cerebral oxidative metabolism and synthesis of acetylcholine, or brings about cholinergic blockade, or both. Other neurotransmitters, notably serotonin and noradrenaline, may also be involved. Thus, an imbalance in normal neurotransmission probably involving the ARAS, the medial thalamic projection systems, the frontal/prefrontal cortex, the right parietal lobe, and the limbic system appears to be necessary for delirium. Other brain areas may prove to be involved as well. There is little evidence to support the notion that a relatively focal brain lesion alone may produce the syndrome, unless it causes a widespread disturbance of cerebral metabolism and neurotransmission.

The EEG has been the most frequently used indicator of cerebral dysfunction in delirium. It shows a range of abnormalities, including diffuse slowing of background activity—the most common abnormality—as well as mixed slow and fast activity, and predominantly fast activity. The degree of alertness, psychomotor activity, and perceptual abnormalities present in a given case of delirium tends to be reflected in the EEG background activity, which in turn reflects CMR and CBF. It has been hypothesized that relative involvement of the medial reticular activating system and the medial thalamic projection systems determines, via imbalance of cholinergic and adrenergic neurotransmission, the level of consciousness and psychomotor activity in a delirious patient, as well as the nature of the alteration in the EEG background activity. The spectrum of alertness and the EEG background frequency appear to parallel the level of cerebral cortical excitability and arousal, one analogous to slow-wave sleep and REM sleep, respectively. The delirium of alcohol and drug withdrawal states represents that end of the spectrum marked by increased arousal, alertness, psychomotor activity, and fast EEG background activity, occurring in the presence of impaired information processing and reduced capacity for selective and sustained attention. Thus various patterns of imbalance of normal noradrenergic, serotonergic, and cholinergic neurotransmission appear to underlie all cases of delirium. Additional neurotransmitters, as well as some neuropeptides, may prove to be involved as well. Studies of cerebral metabolism and neurotransmission in delirium employing the latest techniques, such as PET, SPECT, and magnetic resonance imaging, are overdue and may finally help elucidate the pathophysiology and pathogenesis of this syndrome and its clinical variants.

References

1. Susser M.: *Causal Thinking in the Health Sciences.* New York. Oxford University Press, 1973.
2. Hart B.: Delirious states. *Br. Med. J.* 1936;2:745–749.
3. Lipowski, Z. J.: Delirium (acute confusional state), in Frederiks J. A. M. (ed): *Handbook of Clinical Neurology.* Vol 2 (No 46): *Neurobehavioral Disorders.* Amsterdam, Elsevier, pp 523–559.
4. Engel G. L., Romano J.: Delirium, a syndrome of cerebral insufficiency. *J. Chronic Dis.* 1959;9:260–277.
5. McCandless D. W. (ed): *Cerebral Energy Metabolism and Metabolic Encephalopathy.* New York, Plenum Press, 1985.
6. Plum F., Posner J. B.: *The Diagnosis of Stupor and Coma,* ed 3. Philadelphia, F. A. Davis, 1980.
7. Siesjö B. K.: *Brain Energy Metabolism.* New York, Wiley, 1978.
8. Stahl S. M., Iversen S. D., Goodman E. C. (eds): *Cognitive Neurochemistry.* Oxford, Oxford University Press, 1987.
9. Itil T., Fink M.: Anticholinergic drug-induced delirium: Experimental modification, quantitative EEG and behavioral correlations. *J. Nerv. Ment. Dis.* 1966; 143:492–507.
10. Blass J. P., Gibson G. E., Duffy T. E., et al: Cholinergic dysfunction: A common denominator in metabolic encephalopathies, Pepeu G., Ladinsky H. (eds): *Cholinergic Mechanisms.* New York, Plenum Press, 1981, pp 921–928.
11. Barclay L. L., Gibson G. E., Blass J. P.: Impairment of behavior and acetylcholine metabolism in thiamine deficiency. *J. Pharmacol. Exp. Ther.* 1981;217:537–543.
12. Gibson G. E., Peterson C., Sansone J.: Decreases in amino acid and acetylcholine metabolism during hypoxia. *J. Neurochem.* 1981;37:192–201.

13. Gibson G. E.: Hypoxia, in McCandless D. W. (ed): *Cerebral Energy Metabolism and Metabolic Encephalopathy.* New York, Plenum Press, 1985, pp 43–78.
14. Mendelson W. B.: *Human Sleep.* Research and Clinical Care. New York, Plenum, 1987.
15. Wesnes K., Simpson P., Kidd A.: An investigation of the range of cognitive impairments induced by scopolamine 0.6 mg s.c. *Human Psychopharmacol.* 1988;3:27–41.
16. Honer W. G., Prohovnik I., Smith G., et al: Scopolamine reduces frontal cortex perfusion. *J. Cereb. Blood. Flow. Metab.* 1988;8:635–641.
17. Hemmingsen R., Vorstrup S., Clemmesen L., et al: Cerebral blood flow during delirium tremens and related clinical states studied with xenon-133 inhalation tomography. *Am. J. Psychiatry* 1988;145:1384–1390.
18. Berglund M., Nielsen S., Risberg J.: Regional cerebral blood flow in a case of bromide psychosis. *Arch. Psychiatr. Nervenkr.* 1977;223:197–201.
19. Berglund M., Risberg J.: Regional cerebral blood flow during alcohol withdrawal related to consumption and clinical symptomatology. *Acta Neurol. Scan.* 1977;56(Suppl 64):480–481.
20. Koponen H., Hurri L., Stenback U., et al: Acute confusional states in the elderly: A radiological evaluation. *Acta Psychiatr. Scand.* 1987;76:726–731.
21. Siesjö B. K., Carlsson C., Hagerdal M., et al: Brain metabolism in the critically ill. *Crit. Care Med.* 1976;4:283–294.
22. Hawkins R.: Cerebral energy metabolism, in McCandless D. W. (ed): *Cerebral Energy Metabolism and Metabolic Encephalopathy.* New York, Plenum Press, 1985, pp 3–23.
23. Sokoloff L.: Neurophysiology and neurochemistry of coma. *Exp. Biol. Med.* 1971;4:15–33.
24. Auer R. N., Siesjö B. K.: Biological differences between ischemia, hypoglycemia, and epilepsy. *Ann. Neurol.* 1988;24:699–707.
25. Jamieson D., Alavi A., Jolles P., et al: Positron emission tomography in the investigation of central nervous system disorders. *Radiol. Clin. North Am.* 1988;26:1075–1088.
26. Phelps M. E., Mazziotta J. C.: Positron emission tomography: Human brain function and biochemistry. *Science* 1985;228:799–809.
27. Sokoloff L., Reivich M., Kennedy C., et al: The [^{14}C]deoxyglucose method for the measurement of local cerebral glucose utilization: Theory, procedure and normal values in the conscious and anesthetized albino rat. *J. Neurochem.* 1977;28:897–916.
28. Andreasen N. C.: Brain imaging: Applications in psychiatry. *Science* 1988; 239:1381–1388.
29. Lou H. C., Edvinsson L., MacKenzie E. T.: The concept of coupling blood flow to brain function: Revision required? *Ann. Neurol.* 1987;22:289–297.
30. Sokoloff L.: Relation between physiological function and energy metabolism in the central nervous system. *J. Neurochem.* 1977;29:13–26.
31. Siesjö B. K.: Physiological aspects of brain energy metabolism, in Davison A. N. (ed): *Biochemical Correlates of Brain Structure and Function.* London, Academic Press, 1977, pp 175–213.
32. Bachelard H. S.: Biochemistry of coma, in Davison A. N. (ed): *Biochemistry and Neurological Disease.* Oxford, Blackwell, 1976, pp 228–277.

33. Betz E.: CBF during emotional stimuli, in Ingvar D. H., Lassen N. A. (eds): *Brain Work.* Copenhagen, Munksgaard, 1975, pp 366–370.
34. Carlsson C., Hagerdal M., Kaasi A. E., et al: A catecholamine mediated increase in cerebral oxygen uptake during immobilization stress in rats. *Brain Res.* 1977;119:223–231.
35. Mazziotta J. C., Phelps M. E., Carson R. E., et al: Tomographic mapping of human cerebral metabolism: Sensory deprivation. *Ann. Neurol.* 1982;12:435–444.
36. Horne J.: *Why We Sleep.* Oxford, Oxford University Press, 1988.
37. Ingvar D. H.: Functional landscapes of the brain pertaining to mentation. *Human Neurobiol.* 1983;2:1–4.
38. Heiss W. D., Beil C., Herholz K., et al: Determination of regional glucose metabolism in the brain. *Neurol. Neurobiol.* 1986;21:49–64.
39. Schnaberth G., Schubert H.: Bewusstseinsstörung und Liquormetabolismus. *Arch. Psychiatr. Nervenkr.* 1974;218:211–222.
40. Berne R. M., Winn H. R., Rubio R.: The local regulation of cerebral blood flow. *Progr. Cardiovasc. Dis.* 1981;24:243–260.
41. Ingvar D. H.: "Memory of the future": An essay on the temporal organization of conscious awareness. *Human Neurobiol.* 1985;4:127–136.
42. Lassen N. A.: Cerebral blood flow by SPECT using xenon-133. *Neurol. Neurobiol.* 1986;21:173–189.
43. Risberg J.: Regional cerebral blood flow measurements by 133 Xe-inhalation: Methodology and applications in neuropsychology and psychiatry. *Brain Lang.* 1980;9:9–34.
44. Ryding E., Bradvik B., Ingvar D. H.: Changes of regional cerebral blood flow measured simultaneously in the right and left hemisphere during automatic speech and humming. *Brain* 1987;110:1345–1358.
45. Kety S. S., Schmidt C. F.: The nitrous oxide method for the quantitative determination of cerebral blood flow in man: Theory, procedure, and normal values. *J. Clin. Invest.* 1948;27:476–483.
46. Lassen N. A., Ingvar D. H.: The blood flow of the cerebral cortex determined by radioactive krypton-85. *Experientia* 1961;17:42–43.
47. Berglund M., Risberg J.: Regional cerebral blood flow in a case of amphetamine intoxication. *Psychopharmacology* 1980;70:219–221.
48. Gemmell H. G., Sharp P. F., Besson J. A. O., et al: Differential diagnosis in dementia using the cerebral blood flow agent ^{99m}Tc HM-PAO: A SPECT study. *J. Comput. Assist. Tomogr.* 1987;11:398–402.
49. Ingvar D. H.: Evidence for frontal/prefrontal cortical dysfunction in chronic schizophrenia: The phenomenon of "hypofrontality" reconsidered, in Helmchen H., Henn F. A. (eds): *Biological Perspectives of Schizophrenia.* New York, Wiley, 1987, pp 201–211.
50. Ingvar D. H.: Cerebral blood flow and metabolism related to EEG and cerebral function. *Acta Anaesth. Scand.* 1971;45:110–114.
51. Lassen N. A., Christensen M. A.: Physiology of cerebral blood flow. *Br. J. Anaesth.* 1976;48:719–734.
52. Sokoloff L.: Cerebral circulation and behavior in man: Strategy and findings, in Mandell A. J., Mandell M. P. (eds): *Psychochemical Research in Man.* New York, Academic Press, 1969, pp 237–252.
53. Menon D., Koles Z., Dobbs A.: The relationship between cerebral blood flow and the EEG in normals. *Can. J. Neurol. Sci.* 1980;7:195–198.

54. Brenner R. P.: The electroencephalogram in altered states of consciousness. *Neurol. Clin.* 1985;3:615–631.
55. Markand O. N.: Electroencephalography in diffuse encephalopathies. *J. Clin. Neurophysiol.* 1984;1:357–407.
56. Engel G. L., Romano J., Ferris E. B., et al: A simple method of determining frequency spectrums in the electroencephalogram. *A.M.A. Arch. Neurol. Psychiatry* 1944;51:134–146.
57. Romano J., Engel G. L.: Delirium. I. Electroencephalographic data. *A. M. A. Arch. Neurol. Psychiatry* 1944;51:356–377.
58. Engel G. L., Romano J.: Delirium. II. Reversibility of the electroencephalogram with experimental procedures. *A.M.A. Arch. Neurol. Psychiatry* 1944;51:378–392.
59. Engel G. L., Rosenbaum M.: Delirium. III. Electroencephalographic changes associated with acute alcoholic intoxication. *A.M.A. Arch. Neurol. Psychiatry* 1945;53:44–50.
60. Engel G. L., Romano J., Goldman L.: Delirium. IV. Quantitative electroencephalographic study of a case of acute arsenical encephalopathy. *A.M.A. Arch Neurol. Psychiatry* 1946;56:659–664.
61. Engel G. L., Webb J. P., Ferris E. B.: Quantitative electroencephalographic studies of anoxia in humans; comparison with acute alcoholic intoxication and hypoglycemia. *J. Clin. Invest.* 1945;24:691–697.
62. Romano J., Engel G. L.: Physiologic and psychologic considerations of delirium. *Med. Clin. North Am.* 1944;28:629–638.
63. Adams R. D., Victor M.: *Principles of Neurology,* ed 2. New York, McGraw-Hill, 1981, p 281.
64. Flügel K. A.: *Die Elektroenzephalographie der Funktionspsychosen.* Stuttgart, Thieme, 1974.
65. Obrecht R., Okhomina F. O. A., Scott D. F.: Value of EEG in acute confusional states. *J. Neurol Neurosurg. Psychiatry* 1979;42:75–77.
66. Pro J. D., Wells C. E.: The use of the electroencephalogram in the diagnosis of delirium. *Dis. Nerv. Syst.* 1977;38:804–808.
67. Cadilhac J., Ribstein M.: The EEG in metabolic disorders. *World Neurol.* 1961; 2:296–308.
68. Ganji S., Peters G., Frazier E.: Alpha-coma: Clinical and evoked potential studies. *Clin. Electroenceph.* 1987;18:103–133.
69. Schacter D. L.: EEG theta waves and psychological phenomena: A review and analysis. *Biol. Psychol.* 1977;5:47–82.
70. Jenkins C. D.: The relation of EEG slowing to selected indices of intellective impairment. *J. Nerv. Ment. Dis.* 1962;135:162–170.
71. Obrist W. D., Busse E. W., Eisdorfer C., et al: Relation of the electroencephalogram to intellectual function in senescence. *J. Geront.* 1962;17:197–206.
72. Vojtechovsky M., Vitek V., Rysanek K.: Experimentelle Psychose nach Verabreichung von Benactyzin. *Arzneimittelforsch* 1966;16:240–242.
73. Abood L. G., Meduna L. J.: Some effects of a new psychotogen in depressive states. *J. Nerv. Ment. Dis.* 1958;127:546–550.
74. Ketchum J. S., Sidell F. R., Crowell E. B., et al: Atropine, scopolamine, and Ditran: Comparative pharmacology and antagonists in man. *Psychopharmacologia (Berl)* 1973;28:121–145.
75. Gershon S., Olariu J.: JB 329—A new psychotomimetic: Its antagonism by tetrahydroaminacrin and its comparison with LSD, mescaline and sernyl. *J. Neuropsychiatry* 1960;1:283–292.

76. Alpert M., Angrist B., Diamond F., et al: Comparison of Ditran intoxication and acute alcohol psychoses, in Keup W. (ed): *Origins and Mechanisms of Hallucinations.* New York, Plenum Press, 1970, pp 245–259.
77. Angrist B., Urcuyo L., Gershon S.: Response to incremental doses of Ditran in abstinent alcoholics and drug users. *Compr. Psychiatry* 1974;15:201–204.
78. Brown J. C. N., Shagass C., Schwartz M.: Cerebral evoked potential changes associated with the Ditran delirium and its reversal in man. *Rec. Adv. Biol. Psychiatry* 1965;7:223–234.
79. Cartwright R. D.: Dream and drug-induced fantasy behavior. *Arch. Gen. Psychiatry* 1966;15:7–15.
80. Itil T. M.: Quantitative EEG changes induced by anticholinergic drugs and their behavioral correlates in man. *Recent Adv. Biol. Psychiatry* 1966; 8:151–173.
81. Itil T. M.: Anticholinergic drug-induced sleep-like EEG pattern in man. *Psychopharmacologia (Berl)* 1969;14:383–393.
82. Itil T. M.: Changes in digital computer analyzed EEG during "dreams" and experimentally induced hallucinations, in Keup W. (ed): *Origins and Mechanisms of Hallucinations.* New York, Plenum Press, 1970, pp 71–91.
83. Summers W. K., Majovski L. V., Marsch G. M., et al: Oral tetrahydroaminoacridine in long-term treatment of senile dementia, Alzheimer type. *N. Engl. J. Med.* 1986;315:1241–1245.
84. Itil T., Fink M.: EEG and behavioral aspects of the interaction of anticholinergic hallucinogens with centrally active compounds. *Prog. Brain Res.* 1969;28:149–168.
85. Linnoila M., moderator: Alcohol withdrawal and noradrenergic function. *Ann. Intern. Med.* 1987;107:875–889.
86. Ostfeld A. M., Machne X, Unna K. R.: The effects of atropine on the electroencephalogram and behavior in man. *J. Pharmacol. Exper. Ther.* 1960;128:265–272.
87. Jacobs B. L.: Dreams and hallucinations: A common neurochemical mechanism mediating their phenomenological similarities. *Neurosci. Biobehav. Rev.* 1978; 2:59–69.
88. Wilson R. E., Shagass C.: Comparison of two drugs with psychotomimetic effects (LSD and Ditran). *J. Nerv. Ment. Dis.* 1964;138:277–286.
89. Arnold O. H., Kryspin-Exner K.: Das experimentelle Delir. *Wien. Z. Nervenheilk.* 1965;22:73–93.
90. Bente D., Stoerger R., Tautz N. A.: Weitere klinische-experimentelle Untersuchungen zur Frage der durch zentrale Anticholinergica erzeugten Verwirrtheitszustände. *Arzneimittelforsch.* 1966;16:231–233.
91. Bauer A.: Verlaufsanalyse der durch zentral anticholinergisch wirkenden Substanzen erzeugten Psychosen an Hand von 70 Fallen. *Arzneimittelforsch.* 1966;16:233–234.
92. Safer D. J., Allen R. P.: The central effects of scopolamine in man. *Biol. Psychiatry* 1971;3:347–355.
93. Parrott A. C.: Transdermal scopolamine: Effects upon psychological performance and visual functioning at sea. *Human Psychopharmacol.* 1988;3:119–125.
94. Wesnes K., Simpson P., Kidd A.: An investigation of the range of cognitive impairments induced by scopolamine 0.6 mg s.c. *Human Psychopharmacol.* 1988;3:27–41.

95. Cummings J. L., Benson D. F.: The role of the nucleus basalis of Meynert in dementia: Review and reconsideration. *Alzheim. Dis. Assoc. Disord.* 1987;1:128–145.
96. Smith G.: Animal models of Alzheimer's disease: Experimental cholinergic denervation. *Brain Res. Rev.* 1988;13:103–118.
97. Schaul N., Gloor P., Gotman J.: The EEG in deep midline lesions. *Neurology* 1981;31:157–167.
98. Schaul N., Lueders H., Sachdev K.: Generalized bilaterally synchronous bursts of slow waves in the EEG. *Arch. Neurol.* 1981;38:690–692.
99. Itil T. M., Itil K. Z.: Memory, drugs and dynamic brain mapping of computerized EEG, in: Bes A et al (eds): *Memory, Drugs and Dynamic Brain Mapping of Computerized EEG.* New York, J. Libbey Eurotext, 1986, pp 311–328.
100. Brenner R. P., Reynolds C. F., Ulrich R. F.: Diagnostic efficacy of computerized spectral versus visual EEG analysis in elderly normal, demented and depressed subjects. *Electroenceph. Clin. Neurophysiol.* 1988;69:110–117.
101. Rose D. F., Smith P. D., Sato S.: Magneto-encephalography and epilepsy research. *Science* 1987;238:329–335.
102. Bickford R: Computer analysis of background activity, in Remond A. (ed): *EEG Informatics.* Amsterdam, Elsevier/North Holland, 1977, pp 215–242.
103. Bridgers S. L., Ebersole J. S.: The clinical utility of ambulatory cassette EEG. *Neurology* 1985;35:166–173.
104. Stefan H., Burr W. (eds): *Mobile Long-term EEG Monitoring.* Stuttgart, Fischer, 1982.
105. John E. R., Prichep L. S., Fridman J., et al: Neurometrics: Computer-assisted differential diagnosis of brain dysfunction. *Science* 1988;239:162–169.
106. Kiloh L. H., McComas H. J., Osselton J. W., et al: *Clinical Electroencephalography,* ed 4. London, Butterworths, 1981.
107. Robbins T. W., Everitt B. J.: Psychopharmacological studies of arousal and attention, in Stahl S. M., Iversen S. D., Goodman E. C. (eds): *Cognitive Neurochemistry.* Oxford, Oxford University Press, 1987, pp 135–170.
108. Ranck J. B.: An obituary for old arousal theory. *Behav. Brain Sci.* 1981;4:487–488.
109. Moruzzi G., Magoun H. W.: Brain stem reticular formation and activation of the EEG. *Electroencephal. Clin. Neurophysiol.* 1949;1:455–473.
110. Vanderwolf C. H., Robinson T. E.: Reticulo-cortical activity and behavior: A critique of the arousal theory and a new synthesis. *Behav. Brain. Sci.* 1981; 4:459–514.
111. Bremer F.: Cerebral hypnogenic centers. *Ann. Neurol.* 1977;2:1–6.
112. Saper C. B.: Diffuse cortical projection systems: Anatomical organization and role in cortical function, in *Handbook of Physiology,* Section I, *The Nervous System,* Vol. 5. Bethesda, MD, American Physiological Society, 1987, pp 169–210.
113. Ojemann G.: Brain mechanisms for consciousness and conscious experience. *Can. J. Psychol.* 1986;27:158–167.
114. Luria A. R.: *The Working Brain.* London, Penguin Books, 1973.
115. Posner M. I., Petersen S. E., Fox P. T., et al: Localization of cognitive operations in the human brain. *Science* 1988;240:1627–1631.
116. Reivich M., Alavi A., Fieschi C., et al: Cerebral metabolic and hemodynamic effects of sensory and cognitive stimuli in normal subjects. *Neurol Neurobiol.* 1986; 21:65–81.

117. Geschwind N.: Disorders of attention: a frontier in neuropsychology. *Philos. Trans. R. Soc. Lond. Biol.* 1982;298:173–185.
118. Morgane P. F.: Amine pathways and sleep regulation. *Brain Res. Bull.* 1982; 9:743–749.
119. Hobson J. A., Lydic R., Baghodoyan H. A.: Evolving concepts of sleep cycle generation: From brain centers to neuronal populations. *Behav. Brain Sci.* 1986; 9:371–448.
120. Gaillard J. M.: Neurochemical regulation of the states of alertness. *Ann. Clin. Res.* 1985;17:175–184.
121. McGinty D. J., Morrison A., Drucker-Colin R., et al (eds): *Brain Mechanisms of Sleep.* New York, Raven Press, 1985.
122. Gillin J. C., Sitaram N.: Rapid eye movement (REM) sleep: Cholinergic mechanisms. *Psychol. Med.* 1984;14:501–506.
123. Riemann D., Joy D., Hochli D., et al: Influence of the cholinergic agonist RS 96 on normal sleep: Sex and age effects. *Psychiatry Res.* 1988;24:137–147.
124. Shiromani P. J., Armstrong D. M., Berkowitz A., et al: Distribution of choline acetyltransferase immunoreaction somata in the feline brainstem: Implications for REM sleep generation. *Sleep* 1988;11:1–16.
125. Siegel J. M., Rogawski M. A.: A function for REM sleep: Regulation of noradrenergic receptor sensitivity. *Brain Res. Rev.* 1988;13:213–233.
126. Morgane P. J.: Monoamine theories of sleep: The role of serotonin—a review. *Psychopharmacol. Bull.* 1981;17:13–17.
127. Kral V. A.: Confusional states: Description and management, in Howells J. G. (ed): *Modern Perspectives in the Psychiatry of Old Age.* New York, Brunner/Mazel, 1975, pp 356–362.
128. McIntosh T. K., Bush H. L., Yeston N. S., et al: Beta-endorphin, cortisol and postoperative delirium: A preliminary report. *Psychoneuroendocrinology* 1985; 10:303–313.
129. Naber D., Bullinger M.: Neuroendocrine and psychological variables relating to post-operative psychosis after open-heart surgery. *Psychoneuroendocrinology* 1985;10:315–324.
130. Koponen H., Stenback U., Mattila E., et al: CSF beta-endorphin immunoreactivity in delirium. *Biol. Psychiatry* 1989; 25:938–944.
131. Engelsen B.: Neurotransmitter glutamate: Its clinical importance. *Acta Neurol. Scand.* 1986;74:337–355.

8

Diagnosis

General remarks

Diagnosis of delirium involves *two essential steps:* first, the syndrome has to be recognized on the basis of its characteristic clinical features; and second, the underlying organic etiological factor (or factors) must be identified by means of a general medical history, physical examination, and appropriate laboratory tests. These two steps will be discussed in this chapter.

A physician wrote that delirium was a syndrome that "no doctor likes to miss" (1). Like it or not, he or she often does miss it, especially in its early stage or mild form, as well as in a demented elderly patient (2–6). Several factors appear to be responsible for the reportedly frequent nonrecognition of delirium by physicians. Its clinical manifestations are protean, as was pointed out in Chapters 4 and 5, and may at times mimic other mental disorders such as mania, depression, or schizophrenia. Its early or prodromal symptoms seem to be often overlooked or ignored by the medical staff. There is continuing disagreement and confusion in the medical literature in regard to the proper definition of and diagnostic criteria for the syndrome. The existence and the diagnostic criteria, as well as the clinical importance of delirium, have not been sufficiently emphasized in the teaching of medical students and residents. All of these factors contribute to the common failure to diagnose the syndrome in the medical setting. Yet to diagnose it is relatively easy, especially once its symptoms have reached a certain degree of severity, and provided, of course, that the clinician is familiar with them. Moreover, it is important to make the diagnosis *early* in order to initiate a search for the underlying etiological factor (or factors), to start appropriate, cause-related treatment, and to forestall a crisis on the ward occasioned by the disturbed behavior and its possible serious consequences for the patient. As no specific diagnostic test or scale for the syndrome has yet been developed, or at least generally accepted, its diagnosis must be made primarily on *clinical grounds,* according to the diagnostic criteria listed in Chapter 4 and further elaborated in Chapter 5. There is no need to repeat that material here, and only some selected points that may aid in the timely diagnosis of the syndrome will be highlighted in the section to follow.

Clinical diagnosis

Clinical diagnosis of delirium is based on several overlapping sources of relevant information: *history, observation, clinical interview,* and *mental status examination.*

Crucial to the diagnosis of delirium is a *history* of a relatively recent (i.e., hours to days) *change* in the patient's observable behavior and cognitive functioning. Such a change is usually brought to the physician's attention by the patient's family, the nurses, the family doctor, or some other observer. Less often, the patient may complain of being "confused." It is important to be familiar with and pay attention to the *prodromal* symptoms of delirium, such as insomnia, vivid dreams or nightmares, restlessness, irritability, distractibility, hypersensitivity to light and sounds, anxiety, and a subjective sense of difficulty in marshaling one's thoughts. Fleeting illusions and hallucinations. especially visual ones, may also occur at this stage and be reported by the patient. These symptoms are often frightening, indicating impending loss of the normal sense of control over thinking, grasp, and perception. It is such relative loss of control over one's cognitive processes that is usually referred to as "confusion" by both patients and clinical staff. Moreover, the patient may complain of having difficulty concentrating, keeping track of the date and time of the day, and telling apart dreaming from waking imagery and true perceptions. Alternatively, no complaints at all may be voiced, but an alert observer may notice that the patient has suddenly started to behave in a strange fashion and to display unusual hyperactivity or lethargy, drowsiness during the day, bewilderment, distractibility, and lapses of memory and judgment. A relatively acute appearance of such unaccustomed behavior in a person known to be physically ill, or who is receiving medications, or is in a postoperative period, or is known or suspected to abuse alcohol or other substances should lead at once to a systematic inquiry to rule out delirium. In a person aged 60 years or older, the acute onset of confusion may be the first indication of a physical illness, such as a myocardial infarction or pneumonia; hence, its early recognition is vitally important.

In the case of a hospitalized patient, *observations* made by the nursing staff may play a key role in the diagnosis of delirium. The syndrome often becomes manifest first, and is usually most conspicuous, *during the night.* Consequently, observations by the night nurses are especially useful in drawing attention to a change in the patient's mental state. In the author's experience, notes in the chart made by nurses, who see the patient frequently both by day and by night, provide the most useful diagnostic clues to delirium. Notes recorded by the night nursing staff are particularly valuable. It is important for a night nurse to report such observations verbally and record them in the patient's chart before the delirium becomes florid and creates an emergency situation on the ward. The nurse may note that the patient wakes up after just a few hours of sleep and displays bewilderment, disorientation, anxiety, and restlessness. Such a patient may report vivid dreams or hallucinations, or both, and may be uncertain if he or she has been dreaming, hallucinating, or watching actual events. Such nocturnal confusion is quite characteristic of delirium. The patient may be seen trying to get out of bed, fumbling with the bedclothes, and apparently frightened. A few questions asked at this point may suffice to elicit disorientation for time and place, misidentification of people, and distractibility. Of course, observation by the nursing staff should continue during the daytime as well. It follows that nurses should be trained to recognize symptoms of delirium, including the prodromal ones, and report them without delay to the physician in charge of the patient. All too often, however, in my experience, either the nurse fails to pay attention to the more subtle changes in the patient's behavior or the physician ignores what the nurse has reported. As a result, the patient's mental disorder is liable to progress and becomes noticed only when its manifestations become all too obvious. Psychiatric consultants are frequently asked to see at once a patient who has just attempted to leave the ward in the middle of the night, struck a nurse or another patient, or pulled out his or her intravenous line, for example. Such crises should be avoidable, since a patient seldom becomes severely disturbed and grossly delirious without any premonitory signs, which are usually manifest over the course of a few days or nights. Reading nurses' notes in the chart should be a matter of routine, as they may reveal that the patient's behavior has changed and suggests an incipient delirium. The medical staff should take note of such information and initiate proper action before the full-blown syndrome becomes obvious and creates a crisis.

A patient may give a history and display symptoms suggestive of delirium on admission to the hospital or develop the syndrome at any time during hospitalization. In the former case, the diagnosis should be made positively or tentatively in the course of taking the admission history, i.e., during the initial *clinical interview.* The examiner may observe cognitive and attentional deficits in the process of taking the patient's history. Memory gaps, inconsistencies in reporting events immediately preceding the admission and since arrival in the hospital, distractibility, more or less disorganized thinking, deficits in orientation, and bewilderment may all be observed at this early stage; they should prompt further inquiry into the patient's mental state. The patient may or may not be willing to report an awareness of being confused and may attempt to conceal it from the examiner. To elicit a history and evidence of cognitive impairment, one must proceed tactfully and unobtrusively. Before asking a formal set of questions to test the patient's mental status, the examiner may ask if the patient has noticed any recent change in memory, concentration, alertness, and sleep pattern. Has he or she experienced some forgetfulness, difficulty in concentrating, sleep disturbance, nightmares, unaccustomed daytime drowsiness, irritability, or nervousness? The patient may be told that such symptoms are common in the course of any physical illness, and that it is important for the doctor to be aware of them in order to take proper measures to prevent worsening of the psychological difficulties. This informal, nonthreatening initial approach is more likely to elicit diagnostically important information from a mildly delirious patient than an instant barrage of formal questions to test his or her mental status. It may be useful to ask if the patient has ever experienced delirium in the past, perhaps in the course of a febrile illness in childhood or after an operation. If the answer is positive, it suggests that the patient may be prone to delirium or is at least familiar with it and its transient nature. Once reassured that he or she is not going insane and is not regarded by the doctor as "crazy"—a common fear—the patient is liable to become more willing to report changes in mental functioning and to cooperate in the mental status examination.

The majority of delirious patients develop the full syndrome *after* admission to the hospital. An elderly patient especially may be, or may appear to be, cognitively intact when admitted, only to become delirious on the first night in the unfamiliar hospital environment. In this event, the nurses are usually the first to observe the behavioral change and must report it at once. It is then up to the physician to pursue the appropriate diagnostic inquiry. In general, the following features indicate the presence of an incipient or a fully developed delirium:

1. A relatively acute change in the patient's behavior and mental functioning.
2. Appearance of symptoms suggestive of impaired thinking, recent memory, perceptual clarity, and orientation for time and place.

3. Observable evidence of distractibility, i.e., difficulty in mobilizing, shifting, maintaining, and focusing attention in response to questions.
4. Irregular and unpredictable *fluctuation* of the above cognitive and attentional deficits during the daytime and their worsening during a sleepless night.
5. Reduced accessibility of the patient to verbal communication as a result of reduced or abnormally heightened alertness, i.e., impaired readiness to respond.
6. Appearance of visual illusions and hallucinations to which the patient tends to respond with fear or anger and agitation.
7. Markedly increased or reduced psychomotor, i.e., both verbal and nonverbal behavior, with a tendency to display incoherent speech.
8. Appearance of fleeting, mostly persecutory, delusions that tend to accompany hallucinations and shift in content in response to environmental stimuli.
9. Disrupted sleep-wake cycle, with insomnia at night and excessive drowsiness during the day, or complete sleep loss, or reversal of the circadian sleep-wake cycle.
10. A tendency to exhibit at any time so-called *lucid intervals,* marked by improved accessibility, attention, and grasp of the situation.

The above features allow one to make a presumptive diagnosis of delirium in most cases. In general, *acute onset of cognitive and attentional deficits and abnormalities, whose severity fluctuates during the day and tends to increase at night, is practically diagnostic* (7). The relevant symptoms are elicited by the history and confirmed by direct observation. The presence and severity of cognitive deficits and attentional disturbances should be further established by a systematic *mental status examination* and selected psychological tests at the bedside, to be discussed in the next section.

It is important to keep in mind several common *sources of error* in diagnosing delirium, or rather, errors in diagnostic reasoning that may result in missing the diagnosis (3–6). First, a patient experiencing prodromal or early symptoms is likely to look normal and behave appropriately on superficial contact. It is only in the course of an interview that he or she may voice diagnostically suggestive complaints or display cognitive-attentional deficits. Second, many even severly cognitively impaired patients are quiet, listless, or just drowsy. It is a common error, aided and abetted by misleading descriptions of the syndrome in the medical literature, to believe that a delirious patient is invariably restless, agitated, noisy, and hallucinating. Such a skewed conception of delirium is liable to result in a missed diagnosis in a quiet, undisturbing, and inconspicuous patient (8). Third, the severity of psychological disturbance in the form of psychotic features, i.e., delusions, hallucinations, and inappropriate behavior, does not correlate positively with the severity of the cognitive-attentional deficits and with objective indices of cerebral dysfunction, such as the EEG abnormality. In other words, conspicuously disturbed and disturbing behavior does not necessarily indicate that the patient's brain function is severly disordered. Fourth, the presence of psychotic features or abnormal emotions neither increases nor decreases the probability that the patient is suffering from delirium. The latter is diagnosed on the basis of the criteria listed earlier, regardless of whether the patient is psychotic, or emotionally disturbed, or not. And finally, delirium may feature either reduced or abnormally increased alertness, i.e., readiness to respond to external stimuli. In both of these instances, however, the patient's ability to respond in a selective, directed, and sustained manner is compromised.

Mental status examination

Assessment of the mental state, including cognitive functions, should be an integral part of the initial evaluation of every medical patient, especially one admitted to the hospital. A bedside cognitive examination is particularly important in detecting impairment suggestive of delirium, dementia, and other mental disorders in which cognitive performance is globally or selectively affected. Elaborate psychological tests that take an hour or more to complete have no place in the diagnosis of delirium. A delirious patient is usually too ill, distractible, easily tired, and uncooperative to sustain prolonged psychological testing. Nor is such testing necessary in order to make a diagnosis. A mental status (including cognitive) examination must be carried out at the bedside, be relatively simple, and take no more than 20 or 30 minutes to complete. The examiner may wish to use one of the several rating scales designed to assess cognitive performance. The recorded level of cognitive functioning on admission to the hospital can serve as a baseline for comparison with the results of later assessment during hospitalization. This approach has the advantage of allowing one to establish whether the patient's cognitive performance has improved or deteriorated during the hospital stay (9–12). Moreover, an apparently sudden decline in a patient's cognitive functioning, suggestive of an incipient delirium, can be more readily ascertained if the results of the admission cognitive test are available, in a quantified form, for comparison.

Some authors maintain that a formal cognitive examination is not necessary for the diagnosis of delirium. Cameron et al. (2), for example, assert that clinicians have difficulty in diagnosing delirium because they encounter problems in administering and interpreting cognitive tests. These authors studied patients admitted to an acute medical ward and concluded that the *DSM-III* diagnositc criteria for delirium are both reliable and sufficient for screening hospitalized patients; no rating scales are needed. While this study is provocative, one may argue that a rating scale is a screening instrument that allows a *quantified* assessment of a patient's performance, one that is less arbitrary than a purely clinical diagnostic judgment and better suited for monitoring cognitive functioning over time.

Several rating scales for the bedside testing of cognitive functioning have been developed (10–15), some of them specifically designed for diagnosing delirium (16–19). Probably the most often used screening test has been the Mini-Mental State (MMS) examination (10,20,21). It is brief and easily scored, but it does not distinguish between delirium and dementia and is of little value in patients aged 60 years and older, as well as those with less than an eighth-grade education (20). Moreover, the MMS has been criticized for its substantial false-negative rate, notably in patients with focal brain lesions and those with mild diffuse cognitive dysfunction (13,15). The more recent Neurobehavioral Cognitive Status Examination (NCSE) is claimed to have greater sensitivity and to permit a more precise differential assessment of cognitive functions (12,15). The NCSE assesses attention, level of consciousness, and orientation, as well as five areas of cognition: language, memory, construction ability, calculation, and reasoning (12). Its proponents claim that its greater sensitivity compared to the other bedside rating scales makes it more suitable for the detection of delirium, dementia, and circumscribed cognitive deficits. This claim will need to be reappraised in the light of future clinical studies.

Lowy et al. (18) have devised the Delirium Scale (D-Scale) for the diagnosis of delirium and for research on the syndrome. It consists of 58 items in 13 categories and takes about 40 minutes to administer. The scale allows scoring and offers a comprehensive, quantified assessment of the patient's cognitive, psychomotor, and emotional functioning. Its validity and reliability, however, have not been tested to date, and it has been criticized for not being specific for delirium (19). The recently published Symptom Rating Scale for Delirium (DRS) is claimed to be a screening instrument for the diagnosis of delirium and quantification of its severity (19). It is a 10-item rating scale scored by the examiner on the basis of information about the patient derived from a clinical interview, mental status examination, medical history, and so forth. The scale is comprehensive and likely to prove of value for research purposes rather than for routine clinical use.

Bedside testing of cognition has been critically reviewed in recent years (12,13,22,23), and the reliability and validity of certain time-honored tests has been questioned. For example, the validity of the subtraction of serial 7s as a test of attention, strongly recommended in the earlier literature on delirium (8), has been challenged (22,23). The test is now said to be of no value in differentiating patients with an organic mental disorder from those without it if education and other demographic variables are controlled for (23). The digit span test is often used to examine level of awareness, even though it has been shown to be of little value in discriminating organic from functional mental disorders (24). Despite these criticisms, however, the advantage of the assorted screening tests is that they provide standardized methods of data collection and interpretation (13). They do help to detect moderate to severe delirium, but they tend to miss more mild and subtle cognitive impairment, and it is questionable whether they enhance the diagnostic accuracy of a careful clinical interview (13). There is little doubt that no scale available today can substitute for a discerning clinical evaluation of the patient's history and observed verbal and nonverbal behavior. Such an assessment should take into account the patient's age, level of education, and ethnic background (does the patient know enough English to understand the questions?). The diagnosis of delirium is made by an appraisal of all the information obtained from the history and direct observation of the patient, as well as from a mental status examination, with or without a standardarized rating scale. The mental status examination should include the patient's cognitive performance and attention (accessibility). The following test items may serve this purpose:

1. Attention — Subtraction of serial 3s from 100; counting from 20 backward; reversing days of the week or months of the year
2. Orientation — Date, day of week, and time of day; ability to name and locate the place the patient is in (usually the hospital); identification of familiar persons by name and by relationship to the patient
3. Memory — Ability to recall three words and three objects after 5 minutes; to repeat digits forward and backward; and to describe the circumstances of the hospitalization and to give the date and reasons for it
4. Abstract thinking — Difference between a lake and a river; commonality between an orange and a banana; definitions of a few common words; interpretation of a simple proverb
5. Speed and dynamics of thought — Word fluency test, i.e., asking the patient to say as many single words as possible within 1 minute (the norm is about 30 words)

In summary, the diagnosis of delirium rests on the history of an acute onset of characteristic symptoms reflecting global disturbance of cognition and attention that tends to fluctuate in severity in the daytime and to be most marked at night. A disturbed sleep-wake cycle and either increased or reduced psychomotor activity strengthen the diagnostic impression. Illusions and hallucinations, if present, are typically visual or both visual and auditory. Evidence of impaired information processing and disordered attention is obtained through direct observation of the patient during the clinical interview, and may be confirmed and quantified by the use of a bedside rating scale. Once the diagnosis of delirium has been made it is imperative to look for the etiological factors involved.

Etiological diagnosis

The second and crucial step in the diagnosis of delirium is to determine its etiology. Many organic factors, listed in Chapter 6, can cause it, either singly or in combination. If the patient is known to suffer from a physical illness, such as pneumonia or hepatic encephalopathy, the situation is clear and extensive laboratory investigations are not usually needed. In some cases, however, the etiology may be obscure and the causative factor, or factors, must be sought at once. It goes without saying that a thorough medical history has been taken, a physical examination, including a neurological one, performed, routine laboratory tests done, and the patient's medications carefully scrutinized before additional laboratory investigations are ordered. This task may be facilitated if one knows the most common reported causes of delirium. Three recently published reports, comprising a total of 300 patients, offer some guidance (25–27). Intoxication, systemic infection, metabolic encephalopathy, and circulatory disorders were among the most frequently identified causes of delirium.

Medical history

To focus the diagnostic inquiry and use diagnostic tests more discriminately, the clinician may find it helpful to address the following questions:

1. What is the patient's age? The most likely causes of delirium tend to differ for each age group:
   A. Childhood (3 through 16 years)
      Infection: measles, scarlet fever, mumps, influenza, meningitis, encephalitis
      Intoxication with medical or recreational drugs, poisonous plants
      Head trauma

Epilepsy
Migraine
Hypoglycemia
Acute glomerulonephritis

B. Adolescence and young adulthood (17–40 years)
Intoxication (as above)
Withdrawal from alcohol and sedative-hypnotics
Infection: influenza, pneumonia, acquired immune deficiency syndrome, infectious mononucleosis, meningitis, encephalitis, hepatitis
Metabolic encephalopathy
Epilepsy
Head trauma

C. Middle age (41–64 years)
Intoxication (as above)
Metabolic encephalopathy
Systemic infection
Head trauma
Alcohol and sedative-hypnotic withdrawal
Circulatory disease

D. Old age (65 years and older)
Intoxication with medical, especially anticholinergic, drugs
Systemic infection: pneumonia, urinary tract infection
Neoplasm, intra- or extracranial
Metabolic encephalopathy
Myocardial infarction
Cerebrovascular accident, disease
Head trauma

2. Does the patient abuse alcohol, sedative-hypnotics, or both?
3. Is the patient known to suffer from a chronic disease, either cerebral or systemic, that could predispose him or her to delirium?
4. Is the patient taking any potentially deliriogenic medications, especially anticholinergics?
5. Is there a history of recent head injury, and hence a possibility of subdural hematoma?
6. Is there a history of intellectual decline, personality change, loss of consciousness, or episodes of inappropriate or confused behavior in the recent past? A positive answer would direct the inquiry to rule out an *insidious* intracranial or systemic disease affecting brain function and thus capable of inducing delirium.
7. What is the patient's occupation? Is there a possibility of exposure to industrial poisons?

8. Is there a possibility of foul play in the form of poisoning with agents such as arsenic or insulin?
9. Is the patient surreptitiously taking potentially deliriogenic drugs such as meperidine, cocaine, insulin, digoxin, or steroids?
10. Does the patient suffer from a chronic mental illness accompanied by self-neglect and nutritional (including vitamin) deficiency?
11. Has the patient had recent exposure to intense heat or cold?
12. Is the patient known to be allergic to specific drugs or foods? If so, this could point to an allergic encephalopathy or autoimmune disease.
13. Is the patient known to suffer from an error of metabolism, such as porphyria?
14. Has the patient traveled recently to areas where certain infections and infestations are known to be endemic, such as malaria, typhoid, yellow fever, or rickettsial infections?
15. Is the patient at increased risk for acquired immune deficiency syndrome?

Answers to the above questions should be sought in a patient who develops delirium in the absence of an obvious cause, as they may provide clues to guide laboratory investigations. The latter must be selected *discriminately* on the basis of sound clinical judgment.

Laboratory investigations

1. Blood chemistries
   A. Serum levels of sodium, potassium, chloride, bicarbonate, phosphate, magnesium, blood urea nitrogen, hepatic enzymes, vitamins B_{12} and folate, glucose
   B. Blood screen for specific drugs and poisons
   C. Levels of thyroid hormone and cortisol
2. Hemogram
3. Urinalysis
4. Serum protein electrophoresis
5. Lupus erythematosus cell preparation and antinuclear antibody levels
6. Serum serological test for syphilis
7. Human immune deficiency virus serology
8. Electrocardiogram
9. Chest x-ray film
10. Cerebrospinal fluid examination, including serology, culture, protein electrophoresis, glutamine
11. EEG
12. Computed tomography
13. Magnetic resonance imaging

It must be emphasized that in most cases only some of the above laboratory tests will be needed. There is no reason, for example, to order an expensive test, such as a computed tomography scan unless the physical examination discloses abnormal neurological findings or an EEG indicates the presence of a focal brain lesion (28).

The electroencephalogram

The role of the EEG in the diagnosis of delirium is discussed in Chapter 7 and need not be repeated. This test can be of considerable value in the differential diagnosis of delirium (8,29–32), but its routine use is not warranted. The diagnosis of the syndrome is made primarily on clinical grounds, as emphasized in the earlier sections of this chapter. The EEG is useful only if there is reason to suspect that primary cerebral disease is responsible for delirium in a given case, or when doubt exists about whether the patient suffers from delirium rather than a different form of psychopathology. The differential diagnosis is discussed in Chapter 9. What must be emphasized at this point is that slowing of the background activity, with or without superimposed fast waves, is the single most important EEG abnormality indicative of delirium. Such slowing, however, also commonly occurs in Alzheimer's disease (33) and is absent in alcohol and drug withdrawal delirium (29,32). Like any other laboratory test, the EEG must always be viewed in conjunction with pertinent clinical findings, both psychological and from other sources. Serial rather than single recordings may be of special value in a diagnostic dilemma.

The more common causes of delirium are considered in Part II. Their discussion should aid the clinician in making an etiological diagnosis in a given patient. Differentiation of the syndrome from other mental disorders is the subject of the next chapter.

References

1. Stead E. A.: Reversible madness. *Med. Times* 1966:94:1403–1406.
2. Cameron D. J., Thomas R. I., Mulvihill M., et al: Delirium: A test of the *Diagnostic Statistical Manual* criteria on medical inpatients. *J. Am. Geriatr. Soc.* 1987;35:1007–1010.
3. Daniel D. G., Rabin P. L.: Disguises of delirium: *South. Med. J.* 1985;78:666–672.
4. Dubin N. R., Weiss K. J., Zeccardi J. A.: Organic brain syndrome: The psychiatric imposter. *J.A.M.A.* 1983;249:60–62.
5. Perez E. L., Silverman M.: Delirium: The often overlooked diagnosis. *Int. J. Psychiatry M.* 1984;14:181–189.
6. Trzepacz P. T., Teague G. B., Lipowski Z. J.: Delirium and other organic mental disorders in a general hospital. *Gen. Hosp. Psychiatry* 1985;7:101–106.

7. Lipowski Z. J.: Delirium (acute confusional states). *J.A.M.A.* 1987;258:1789–1792.
8. Engel G. L., Romano J.: Delirium, a syndrome of cerebral insufficiency. *J. Chronic Dis.* 1959; 9:260–277.
9. Fields S. D., MacKenzie C. R., Charlson M. E., et al: Reversibility of cognitive impairment in medical inpatients. *Arch. Intern. Med.* 1986;146:1593–1596.
10. Folstein M. F., Folstein S. E., McHugh P. R.: "Mini-Mental State." *J. Psychiatr. Res.* 1975;12:189–198.
11. Jacobs J. W., Bernhard M. R., Delgado A., et al: Screening for organic mental syndromes in the medically ill. *Ann. Intern. Med.* 1977;86:40–46.
12. Kiernan R. J., Mueller J., Langston J.W., et al: The neurobehavioral cognitive status examination: A brief but differential approach to cognitive assessment. *Ann. Intern. Med.* 1987;107:481–485.
13. Nelson A., Fogel B.S., Faust D.: Bedside cognitive screening instruments: A critical assessment. *J. Nerv. Ment. Dis.* 1986;174:73–83.
14. Roca R. P.: Bedside cognitive examination. *Psychosomatics* 1987;28:71–76.
15. Schwamm L. H., Van Dyke C., Kiernan R. J., et al: The neurobehavioral cognitive status examination: Comparison with the cognitive capacity screening examination and the mini-mental state examination in a neurosurgical population. *Ann. Intern. Med.* 1987;107:486–491.
16. Anthony J. C., LeResche L.A., Von Korff M. R., et al: Screening for delirium on a general medical ward: The tachistoscope and a global accessibility rating. *Gen. Hosp. Psychiatry* 1985;7:36–42.
17. Kitchen A. D., Wakefield P. L., Woolsey R. M.: Development of a screening instrument to discriminate between delirium and dementia. *Psychosom. Med.* 1983;45:81–82.
18. Lowy F. H., Engelsmann F., Lipowski Z. J.: Study of cognitive functioning in a medical population. *Compr. Psychiatry* 1973;14:331–338.
19. Trzepacz P. T., Baker R. W., Greenhouse J.: A symptom rating scale for delirium. *Psychiatry Res.* 1988;23:89–97.
20. Anthony J. C., Le Resche L., Niaz U., et al: Limits of the "Mini-Mental State" as a screening test for dementia and delirium among hospital patients. *Psychol. Med.* 1982;12:397–408.
21. Rabins P. V., Folstein M. R.: Delirium and dementia: Diagnostic criteria and fatality rates. *Br. J. Psychiatry.* 1982;140:149–153.
22. Keller M. B., Manschreck T. C.: The bedside mental status examination—reliability and validity. *Compr. Psychiatry* 1981;22:500–511.
23. Rosen A. M., Fox H. A.: Tests of cognition and their relationship to psychiatric diagnosis and demographic variables. *J. Clin. Psychiatry* 1986;47:495–498.
24. Hinton J., Withers E.: The usefulness of the clinical tests of the sensorium. *Br. J. Psychiatry* 1971;119:9–18.
25. Newton N. L., Janata A.: Delirium, a study of 100 cases. *Stress Med.* 1986;2:267–270.
26. Purdie F. R., Honigman B., Rosen P.: Acute organic brain syndrome: A review of 100 cases. *Ann. Emerg. Med.* 1981;10:455–461.
27. Sirois F.: Delirium: 100 cases. *Can. J. Psychiatry* 1988;33:375–378.
28. Rosenberg C. E., Anderson D. C., Mahowald M. W., et al: Computed tomography and EEG in patients without focal neurologic findings. *Arch. Neurol.* 1982;39:291–292.
29. Brenner R. P.: The electroencephalogram in altered states of consciousness. *Neurol. Clin.* 1985;2:615–631.

30. Markand O. N.: Electroencephalography in diffuse encephalopathies. *J. Clin. Neurophysiol.* 1984;1:357–407.
31. Obrecht R., Okhomina F. O. A., Scott D. F.: Value of EEG in acute confusional states. *J. Neurol. Neurosurg. Psychiatry* 1979;42:75–77.
32. Pro J. D., Wells C. E.: The use of the electroencephalogram in the diagnosis of delirium. *Dis. Nerv. Syst.* 1977;38:804–808.
33. Rae-Grant A., Blume W., Lau C., et al: The electroencephalogram in Alzheimer-type dementia. *Arch. Neurol.* 1987;44:50–54.

9

Differential Diagnosis

The clinical features of delirium, listed in Chapter 8, are usually sufficiently characteristic to enable its diagnosis in most cases. The global cognitive-attentional deficits and abnormalities, the acute onset and diurnally fluctuating course, and the relatively brief duration render the syndrome readily distinguishable. The issue of a differential diagnosis does come up at times, however, especially in the elderly, in whom a distinction from dementia may be difficult, as well as in an occasional younger patient suffering from an acute functional or a nondelirious toxic psychosis or a dissociative state. Such differential diagnostic problems will be discussed in this chapter.

Differentiation from other organic mental syndromes

Delirium versus dementia

These two syndromes not only share global impairment of cognitive functions but may also coexist in the same patient especially an elderly one. These two facts have created problems for clinicians, as the following quotation from a medical editorial highlights: "In epidemiological surveys acute confusional states are less prevalent, but in the hospital service acute confusion is all too often equated with dementia" (1, p 1559). Hodkinson (2) asserts that the distinction between dementia and an acute confusional state is difficult to make in clinical practice, since the psychiatric symptomatology of these two syndromes shows no difference. This last statement is open to question, as no studies systematically comparing the symptoms of delirium and dementia have been published to date. One cannot deny, however, that those symptoms do overlap and are not sharply delineated (3–6).

As defined in *DSM-III-R* (7), dementia implies impairment in short- and long-term memory associated with impaired thinking and judgment, with other disturbances of higher cortical functions, or with personality change. These impairments and disturbances must be sufficiently severe to interfere with the individual's occupational performance, or social functioning, or both. As in all organic mental syndromes, in dementia the etiology is assumed to be "organic," i.e., a primary or secondary brain disease. As currently defined, dementia does not imply irreversibility. On the contrary, its course may be progressive, static, or remitting (7). This concept is a noteworthy departure from the traditional view of dementia as irreversible and usually progressive. By the same token, its distinction from delirium on the basis of irreversibility has been abolished, and the concept of reversible dementia has become widely accepted (8–11). Consequently, the boundary between delirium and dementia has become even more blurred and, to some extent, an arbitrary distinction. Some authors have proposed that confusional states lasting for weeks to months should be classified as dementias (9), but there is no agreement on this point. As a general rule, delirium is, by definition, a *transient* disorder that seldom lasts for more than a month (7), while dementia is a clinical state that endures for months or years (11). Clearly, the issue of diagnostic boundaries in this area of psychopathology is still ambiguous and controversial, and must be resolved. Despite these definitional problems, however, it is vitally important to distinguish delirium from the most common dementias of later life, namely, the progressive ones such as Alzheimer's disease and multi-infarct dementia. The practical importance of this differential diagnosis is obvious: the diagnosis of delirium suggests that an acute medical condition, or an acute exacerbation of a chronic physical illness, or drug toxicity, is present, and calls for immediate investigation and appropriate management whether the patient is demented or not (3–12).

The *history* is the most important single source of information in the differential diagnosis of delirium from dementia. Typically, the most common dementias are insidious, by contrast to the acute onset of delirium, although at times dementia may set in suddenly, as after head trauma or cardiac arrest. As a general rule, however, a patient who by all available accounts functions well intellectually, and then suddenly develops a cognitive-attentional disorder that fluctuates in severity over the course of a day and becomes most marked at night, is suffering from delirium unless proven otherwise (6). Similarly, a patient who has displayed intellectual impairment, say impaired memory, with or without a personality change, for months or years, and who suddenly develops the symptoms just mentioned, may also be suffering from delirium and deserves immediate medical attention. Because information about the mode of onset of the cognitive disorder (i.e., whether abrupt or insidious) is so important for the differential diagnosis, the history must be sought from all available sources.

At times, the history may not be obtainable, since the patient is often a poor historian, or may live alone or with a demented spouse. In this case, direct observation of the patient's *symptoms* and behavior, as well as cognitive performance at the time of examination, must be relied on for the diagnosis. The prominent disturbances of *attention* that render the patient's *accessibility* precarious and tend to fluctuate over 24 hours point to delirium. In other words, a reduced level of *consciousness,* or awareness, regardless of whether the patient is hypo- or hyperalert and hypo- or hyperactive, tends to distinguish delirium from dementia even though, in both of these conditions, cognitive functions are globally impaired. Moreover, a demented patient is liable to display both short- and long-term *memory* impairment, while a delirious one is more likely to exhibit deficits of short-term memory only. He or she is less likely, for example, to forget commonly known facts and dates. *Thinking* in delirium, as revealed by the patient's verbal communications, is typically incoherent and disorganized, while that in dementia tends to be impoverished. Moreover, fleeting persecutory delusions, often associated with predominantly visual hallucinations and illusions, are more likely to be observed in delirium than in dementia. Similarly, confusion between imagery, dreams, and true perceptions is more common in a delirious than in a demented patient. Rapid shifts in the level of *psychomotor activity* during the day, coupled with predominant hyperactivity and restlessness during the night, are also features of delirium rather than dementia. While the speech of a delirious patient is often incoherent, hesitant, and either slow or pressured, that of a demented individual is more likely to feature difficulty in finding words. Disruption of the *sleep-wake cycle,* with insomnia at night and daytime drowsiness, is more common of delirium than of dementia. Finally, a delirious patient is more likely to show signs of a *physical illness,* such as fever, tachycardia, or asterixis.

Table 9–1 summarizes the distinctions between delirium and dementia. It should be emphasized that a differential diagnosis on the basis of symptoms alone may sometimes be impossible. As stated earlier, there is no sharp dividing line between the psychopathological manifestations of these two syndromes; they shade over into each other and overlap. They may be viewed as a continuum of pathological states due to relatively widespread cerebral dysfunction, which may be completely or partly reversible, or irreversible and progressive. By definition, the diagnosis of delirium presupposes a reversible dysfunction, yet one that may be, and in an elderly patient often is, super-

TABLE 9–1 Differential Diagnosis of Delirium and Dementia

Feature	Delirium	Dementia
Onset	Acute, often at night	Insidious
Course	Fluctuating, with lucid intervals during the day; worse at night	Stable over the course of the day
Duration	Hours to weeks	Months or years
Awareness	Reduced	Clear
Alertness	Abnormally low or high	Usually normal
Attention	Lacks direction and selectivity; distractibility; fluctuation over the course of the day	Relatively unaffected
Orientation	Usually impaired for time; tendency to mistake unfamiliar for familiar places and persons	Often impaired
Memory	Immediate and recent impaired	Recent and remote impaired
Thinking	Disorganized	Impoverished
Perception	Illusions and hallucinations, usually visual and common	Often absent
Speech	Incoherent, hesitant, slow or rapid	Difficulty in finding words
Sleep-wake cycle	Always disrupted	Fragmented sleep
Physical illness or drug toxicity	Either or both present	Often absent, especially in Alzheimer's disease

imposed upon more chronic and either irreversible or only partially reversible brain pathology. To agonize over the diagnosis of delirium versus a *reversible* dementia seems futile, as in both cases a thorough search for a treatable cause is mandatory. Moreover, if the condition diagnosed as delirium persists unabated for over *1 month,* the diagnosis may be changed to dementia, since such a change in diagnostic label no longer implies a hopeless prognosis.

The EEG may be of some value in the differential diagnosis of delirium and dementia. In the former, the EEG is usually abnormal and features a generalized slowing of the background acitivity (13–16). This statement does not hold for delirium due to sedative-hypnotic drug and alcohol withdrawal, in which excessive low-amplitude fast activity tends to predominate (13). In one study, diffuse slowing of the EEG was helpful in distinguishing delirium from dementia in medically ill patients (17). The EEG in Alzheimer's disease and multi-infarct dementia tends to show increased slowing (18,19), making its value for the differentiation of dementia due to these diseases from delirium problematic. Serial EEG recordings may be helpful occasionally, since in delirium normalization of the tracing tends to accompany improvement in cognitive functioning (14).

Delirium versus organic mental syndromes other than dementia

Differentiation of delirium from other organic mental syndromes, those that, unlike dementia, do not feature global cognitive impairment, does not usually present serious problems.

Amnestic syndrome features short- and long-term memory impairment, with relative preservation of other cognitive functions (7). While disorientation and impaired concept formation may be present, it is the memory pathology that dominates the clinical picture. Occasionally, amnestic syndrome and delirium may coexist, as in Wernicke's encephalopathy. In delirium, impairment involves mostly short-term memory, and the clinical picture invariably includes other cognitive abnormalities, as well as a disorder of awareness.

Organic hallucinosis is characterized by prominent, persistent, or recurrent hallucinations (7). As such, it represents a relatively limited form of psychopathology that is clearly different from delirium, as it lacks global cognitive-attentional disturbances. Generalized EEG slowing is absent.

Organic delusional syndrome involves prominent delusions, which may be associated with mild cognitive impairment, hallucinations, and symptoms suggestive of schizophrenia (7). This disorder may be caused by drugs, such as amphetamines and hallucinogens, or may accompany temporal lobe epilepsy. It differs from delirium by the absence of attentional disturbances and reduced level of awareness. Generalized EEG slowing is absent.

Organic mood syndrome features symptoms suggestive of mania or a major depressive episode (7). Even though mild cognitive impairment is said to be often observed (7), this syndrome lacks the characteristic disturbances of attention and consciousness that distinguish delirium. Generalized EEG slowing is absent.

Organic anxiety syndrome is marked by prominent, recurrent panic attacks or generalized anxiety (7). It may be due to endocrine disorders, such as hyperthyroidism or pheochromocytoma, or may be caused by intoxication with cocaine or amphetamines, for example. Although mild cognitive impairment and some difficulty in sustaining attention are present (7), the clinical picture resembles a panic or a generalized anxiety disorder rather than delirium. EEG slowing is absent.

Organic personality syndrome is characterized by a persistent personality disturbance that typically involves impaired capacity for the controlled and appropriate expression of emotions and impulses, for planning action, and for exercising adequate social judgment. Some patients display general lack of motivation and drive. Global congnitive-attentional disturbances are absent, and by contrast to delirium, this syndrome is usually chronic.

Intoxication is a residual category in the official classification that refers to maladaptive behavior after the use of a psychoactive substance (7). Its diagnosis is otherwise made by exclusion of other organic mental syndromes, including delirium.

Withdrawal is another residual diagnostic category for a mental disorder that follows cessation of, or reduction in, the use of a psychoactive substance, such as alcohol or corticosteroids (7). As in the case of intoxication, there are no distinguishing essential features, and the distinction from withdrawal delirium is made by exclusion.

In summary, organic mental syndromes other than delirium lack impaired level of awareness combined with global cognitive-attentional deficits and disturbances. Dementia involves relatively persistent and sustained rather than transient, brief, and irregularly fluctuating cognitive impairment, and lacks the reduction in the level of awareness, except in its most advanced stage. Amnestic syndrome and organic hallucinosis are relatively selective, or limited, rather than global cognitive deficits and abnormalities. Organic delusional, mood, and anxiety syndromes do not feature global cognitive impairment either, nor is the EEG background activity diffusely slowed in any of them. This does not mean that the EEG is necessarily normal. Depending on the etiological factors involved, it may show a focal abnormality, or epileptiform potentials, or a low-voltage fast activity, for example. When caused by drugs and severe, organic delusional, mood, and anxiety syndromes are often referred to as "toxic psychoses." They are *not* coterminous with delirium. Such "psychoses" include those caused by amphetamines, methylphenidate, cocaine, LSD-25, atabrine, beta-blocking agents, mescaline, and a host of other substances. They are distinct from delirium both symptomatically and in terms of EEG abnormalities, if any. The same applies to the organic personality syndrome. Intoxication and withdrawal are residual categories that, by definition, must lack the features of delirium (7).

Differentiation from functional psychiatric disorders

Schizophrenia and schizophreniform disorder

The diagnostic criteria for schizophrenia given in *DSM-III-R* (7) make the differential diagnosis between that disorder and delirium a relatively simple matter. To diagnose schizophrenia, continuous signs of the disturbance should last for at least 6 months; this requirement clearly distinguishes this disorder from delirium. The 6-month period must comprise an active phase, featuring a combination of characteristic psychotic symptoms that include delusions, hallucinations, a thought disorder (incoherence or marked loosening of associations), catatonic behavior, and flat or inappropriate affect (7). If one follows this currently accepted definition of the phenomenology of schizophrenia, any problem in distinguishing it from delirium could arise only in the case of a patient seen in the active phase of the schizophrenic psychosis, and only when the history of the prodromal symptoms is unavailable. In such a case, the differential diagnosis must rely on an analysis of the patient's current acute symptoms. *DSM-III-R* (7) states that in delirium, as well as in schizophrenia and the schizophreniform disorder, the clinical picture may include hallucinations, delusions, and disordered thinking; however, in delirium, such psychotic symptoms are stated to be "extremely random and haphazard, without evidence of systematization" (7, p 102). This distinction is, of course, relative. It does apply to delusions, which in delirium, by contrast to schizophrenia, tend to be fleeting, unsystematized, and shifting in content in response to environmental stimuli. Hallucinations in delirium, if present, are predominantly visual, or visual and auditory; in schizophrenia, by contrast, the most common hallucinations are auditory, usually consisting of single or multiple voices (7). Purely auditory hallucinations, especially of voices keeping up a running commentary on the patient's experiences and conduct, are unusual in delirium but common in schizophrenia. A formal thought disorder, exemplified by loosening of associations, is not a feature of delirium. The thinking disorder in this syndrome is characterized by difficulty in controlling the train of thought, thus rendering it disorganized and inefficient in problem solving. Moreover, thinking in delirium tends to be less autistic and bizarre than in schizophrenia. Schizophrenic patients do not usually display global impairment of cognitive functions. Recent memory and orientation are both disordered in delirium, but not in schizophrenia. A schizophrenic may appear to be disoriented and claim to be on the planet Venus, or may state the date grossly incorrectly, for example, but such disorientation is usually delusional rather than spatiotemporal (20). A delirious patient typically mistakes unfamiliar surroundings and persons for familiar ones. The severity of the symptoms in delirium characteristically fluctuates in the course of a day, with lucid intervals interspersed among periods of increased confusion and attentional disturbances. A schizophrenic patient does not usually display such striking oscillations of psychopathology over the course of a day. Catatonic symptoms are much more often a feature of schizophrenia than of delirium. Finally, the EEG in delirium is characterized by slowing of the background activity, an abnormality that is absent in schizophrenia.

Thus, if one follows the diagnostic criteria for schizophrenia presented in *DSM-III-R*, differentiating it from delirium should not present a major problem. A review of the recent literature on schizophrenia suggests, however, that the situation may not always be that simple. Schizophrenia is a complex, heterogeneous disorder that includes abnormalities in perception, attention, communication, volition, affective modulation, cognition, and psychomotor behavior (21).

Abnormalities of the same aspects of psychological functioning are also involved in delirium. This calls for more specific delineation of the differences between the two disorders. The present requirement that symptoms have to be present for 6 months for a diagnosis of schizophrenia has not gone unchallenged, and is viewed by some observers as being too narrow and arbitrary (21). Recent studies on the biological aspects of this disorder indicate the presence of several subtypes, one of which is marked by cognitive impairment and evidence of structural abnormality of the brain (22–24). A substantial minority of patients with the clinical picture of schizophrenia have some type of organic brain disorder (25), notably epilepsy and neurosyphilis (26). The phenomenology of acute organic psychosis differs from that of schizophrenia, however; visual hallucinations, misidentification of others, and different content of delusions set the two disorders apart (27). On the other hand, recent studies on attentional performance in schizophrenic patients have found that those of them who display positive symptoms show a deficit in selective attention, as demonstrated by a digit-span task (28,29). Moreover, some recent authors speak of the disorder of consciousness in schizophrenia and point out that acutely symptomatic schizophrenic patients have difficulty in sustaining attention (30). Because the current diagnostic criteria for delirium rely so heavily on the patient's reduced ability to maintain and shift attention, convergence with acute schizophrenia in this regard is noteworthy and calls for comparative studies of attentional disturbances in both disorders.

The *schizophreniform disorder* is currently classified outside the spectrum of schizophrenia, even though the essential features of both are identical, except that the duration of schizophreniform disorder is less than 6 months (7). Consequently, the guidelines for its differential diagnosis from delirium are the same as those for schizophrenia. The schizophreniform disorder, however, tends to feature emotional turmoil, fear, confusion, and vivid hallucinations more often than schizophrenia (7), and this may at times create a problem in differentiating it from delirium. "Confusion" in this context, according to some investigators, contains features of delirium and is a favorable prognostic sign (31). In one study, disorientation to place, time, and person was found in 18%, 16%, and 7%, respectively, of 112 schizophrenics (32). When an acute schizophreniform disorder occurs in response to marked psychological stress, the level of consciousness may be reduced during the first few days or weeks of the illness (33). On the whole, the concept of the schizophreniform disorder is relatively new, and its nosological status is unclear. It does appear to have a better prognosis than schizophrenia (34) but its clinical features are still poorly differentiated. *DSM-III-R* includes "confusion, disorientation, or perplexity at the height of the psychotic episode" among the prognostically favorable symptoms of the schizophreniform disorders but does not explain what these symptoms really mean. They do suggest some overlap with those of delirium, and a comparative study of these two disorders is highly desirable.

Brief reactive psychosis

This form of mental disorder is more likely to cause difficulties in differentiation from delirium than any other currently recognized psychosis. Its essential feature is a sudden onset of psychotic symptoms of at least 1 hour's, but no more than 1 month's, duration, occurring in response to major stress (7). Symptoms of this psychosis may include delusions, hallucinations, catatonic behavior, incoherent thinking, and emotional turmoil (7). The patient may confabulate, be disoriented, and display impairment in recent memory. Perplexity or confusion is a common feature. According to *DSM-III-R* (7), delirium can be distinguished from this disorder only if the history or laboratory tests indicate the presence of an organic factor that is deemed to be causally related to the symptoms.

This gray area of psychiatric nosology has been poorly delineated and inadequately studied to date. Scandinavian psychiatrists have long separated from the class of schizophrenic disorders a group of psychoses that are similar but characterized by an acute onset in response to psychological trauma, transient character, and the frequent presence of confusion (35–37). The Scandinavians refer to these disorders as "reactive" or "psychogenic" psychoses (35–37). There appears to be no agreement about the operational criteria for, and hence the boundary of, these psychoses (36). They seem to share some common symptomatic features with delirium, but their etiology is, by definition, nonorganic, which alone sets them apart from this syndrome. A similar concept in French psychiatry has existed for a century under the designation "bouffée délirante," but its popularity appears to be waning (38). In Norway, reactive psychoses featuring a disturbance of consciousness have been labeled "hysteric psychoses" (39). A similar concept was advanced by Levin (40), who called it "psychogenic delirium" and asserted that it occurred in cases of hysteria and dementia praecox. It differed from "organic" delirium in that consciousness in it did not fluctuate and the patient was oriented. More recently, the term "pseudo-delirium" has been proposed for delirium-like functional psychoses (6,41). A medley of acute psychoses, including the organic ones, has at times been given the generic label "transient psychosis" (42).

As this confusing terminology suggests, this area of psychiatry has been badly neglected. It clamors for research and for an end to the prevailing nosological and semantic muddle. Psychoses falling into this vague borderland between acute schizophrenia and delirium have been described since the early nineteenth century. A review of the English-language medical literature of the past 150 years reveals a host of designations for and numerous accounts of such psychoses, including "acute delirium" (43), "delirium of collapse" (44), "Bell's mania" (45), "acute confusional insanity" (46), "oneirophrenia" (47), and "acute exhaustive psychoses" (48). The proposed etiology of these assorted disorders differs widely. Connolly (46), for example, claimed that what he called "acute confusional insanity," a condition closely resembling delirium, could arise from various causes, including puerperium, tuberculosis, nostagia, emotional shock, and sexual excess. More recently, similar transient psychoses have often been reported in developing countries, supposedly reflecting cultural factors (42). In the developed countries, such syndromes are typically precipitated by a catastrophic event, such as a natural disaster or bereavement. Their clinical features include severe restlessness and excitement, vivid and often terrifying hallucinations, "confusion," and panic. Overactivity, insomnia, dehydration, and nutritional deficiencies that are commonly present may complicate the clinical picture and give rise to delirium (49,50). Clinical diagnostic differentiation may then become impossible, and the overriding concern should be to correct the complicating medical disorder and to treat the excitement, overactivity, and insomnia. A closely related condition is *lethal catatonia,* a relatively rare, life-threatening psychosis associated with fever (49–51). This syndrome may occur in the course of both organic and functional disorders. It features severe excitement, which may give rise to stupor; catatonic symptoms; auditory and visual hallucinations; delusions; clouding of consciousness; and hyperthermia (51). The relationship between lethal catatonia and delirium is unclear. No EEG studies of this condition seem to have been carried out to date.

As the preceding discussion suggests, a variety of transient psychoses may display some, if not all, of the clinical manifestations of delirium in the absence of a demonstrable brain disorder or an identifiable organic cause. As pointed out earlier, the classification of these reactive and atypical psychoses leaves much to be desired. Their nosological status remains unclear, as does their relationship to delirium and to some of the other organic mental syndromes. Psychiatric researchers, at least in the United States, have largely ignored this important area of psychopathology, one whose elucidation is long overdue.

Differential diagnosis between the assorted reactive and atypical psychoses on the one hand, and delirium on the other, should include an EEG and other investigations, such as a computed tomography scan, to establish whether demonstrable cerebral dysfunction is present. A thorough medical evaluation is, of course, necessary. If the EEG is normal despite symptoms suggestive of delirium, the diagnosis of a reactive psychosis should be entertained. An interview with the use of intravenous sodium amylobarbitone may be helpful in the differential diagnosis (52–54). Global cognitive deficits due to cerebral dysfunction, an essential feature of delirium, become accentuated by the drug. By contrast, if such deficits are a manifestation of a functional psychosis in the absence of brain pathology, they tend to clear up under the influence of the drug.

Mood disorders

Manic episodes and major depressive episodes may on occasion present a problem in the differential diagnosis of delirium. The essential feature of a manic episode is an abnormally and persistently elevated, expansive, or irritable mood (7). The symptoms that occur in such mood may include decreased need for sleep, distractibility, psychomotor agitation, delusions, hallucinations, and catatonic symptoms (7). Confusion has often been reported in manic patients (55–59). In one study, confusion was reported in about one-third and visual hallucinations in about one-quarter of manic patients (58). Presumably "confusion" in this context referred to spatiotemporal disorientation and other cognitive deficits, but this is not clear. Global cognitive impairment was reported in nearly one-half of 30 manic patients (60). In 1849, Bell (45) described a series of patients with clinical features of both mania and delirium; he concluded that this was a new mental disorder. Later in the nineteenth century, that disorder came to be known as "Bell's" or "delirious mania" and is currently viewed as a variant of a manic episode (55,57). It features sudden onset, manic symptoms, and some characteristics of delirium. The patient is incoherent, hyperactive or lethargic, and disoriented (55,57). Despite these features resembling delirium, however, evidence of an organic causal factor is absent and the EEG does not show slowing of the background activity (57,59,61). These last two features allow one to differentiate delirious mania from delirium. Moreover, manic patients do not display global cognitive impairment that fluctuates in the course of a day and tends to be most marked at night. Some investigators claim that confusional states resembling delirium occur in about 5% of patients with manic-depressive disorders, but that on closer inquiry these states can be distinguished from delirium on clinical grounds (62). Even though the patients may appear to be disoriented, they are likely to be either disinterested in giving correct answers to questions about orientation or just playful. They tend to misidentify people for important persons in their own lives and may display loss of awareness of personal identity (55)—a very unusual symptom in delirium.

Major depressive episode is not likely to cause difficulty in the differential diagnosis from delirium, except in an elderly patient displaying such cognitive symptoms as disorientation, memory loss, and distractibility. These features characterize depressive *pseudodementia* and may create difficulties in differentiating it from both dementia and delirium (6). "Pseudodementia" has no precise meaning and has been reported in association with depressive illness, mania, hysteria, and delirium (63). The term implies the presence of cognitive impairment that is suggestive of dementia but cannot be accounted for by a relevant organic disorder. It occurs most often in the course of a major depressive episode in later life (64). In 5% to 20% of elderly patients with apparent delirium, no organic factor can be detected, and the diagnosis of depressive pseudodementia (or pseudodelirium) should be entertained (6). Disorientation, bewilderment, incoherent thinking, memory impairment, and perceptual and psychomotor disturbances of relatively rapid onset appear to characterize this disorder. Depressed mood is usually present and tends to antedate the onset of cognitive deficits. The patient may have a history of mood disorder, either bipolar or unipolar. Persistent questioning may reveal that the patient is cognitively more or less intact but is too preoccupied with personal thoughts, too agitated, or too psychomotorically retarded to perform on request. The person may give a clear account of the illness and past history in response to open-ended questions but will reply "I don't know" to direct questions. Moreover, such patients tend to complain vocally of being forgetful: "I can't remember anything" is a common complaint. Responses on cognitive examination tend to be inconsistent; patients may claim not to recognize their whereabouts yet are fully oriented for time and have no difficulty finding their way around. Cognitive impairment does not fluctuate irregularly during the day, and the patient does not display the marked attentional disturbances characteristic of delirium. Laboratory evidence of diffuse cerebral dysfunction is absent, and the EEG is not diffusely slowed. In an occasional case, if doubt persists about whether delirium is present, the sodium amobarbital interview may be helpful, as in the case of manic episode (52–54).

Dissociative and factitious disorders

The essential feature of *dissociative disorders* is a disturbance or alteration of memory, the sense of one's own identity, or consciousness (7). These disorders often develop rapidly and their course is transient, as is the case in delirium. The dissociative disorders that may occasionally present a problem in the differential diagnosis with this syndrome include *psychogenic fugue* and *psychogenic amnesia* (7,65,66). Psychogenic fugue features an abrupt loss of personal ("episodic") memory, a loss of the sense of personal identity and assumption of a new one, and a period of wandering or travel. The episode usually lasts for some hours or days and is followed by amnesia for the period of the fugue. A severe precipitating stress, such as combat in wartime, is always present, and a period of depressed mood usually occurs just before the onset of the fugue (66). Perplexity and disorientation may occur. The essential feature of psychogenic amnesia is sudden inability to recall important personal information. There is often a history of organic amnesia due to a head injury, for example. Psychogenic amnesia is usually limited but in a rare case may extend to the person's entire life (7). The patient may display perplexity and disorientation and may wander aimlessly. In many if not all cases, semantic (conceptual) memory and memory of skills remain intact (66). A common form of psychogenic amnesia is that for a criminal act (66). Delirium can be readily distinguished from these dissociative disorders by its global cognitive-attentional disturbances rather than by predominantly selective memory impairment; loss of the sense of personal identity occurs rarely, if at all, in delirium. The EEG in dissociative states is normal. An interview with the aid of intravenous sodium amobarbital is usually successful in restoring memory function in a dissociative state (52,67).

Listed among the dissociative disorders not otherwise specified is *Ganser syndrome,* associated with giving "approximate answers" ("vorbeireden") to questions, amnesia, disorientation, perceptual disturbances, and conversion symptoms (7,68,69). The nosological status of this rare syndrome has been a subject of some controversy. Its etiology appears to be varied. It has been reported in association with schizophrenia, hysteria, and a host of organic conditions (68). Some authors regard it as a disorder of consciousness, while others consider it to be a hysterical or an atypical dissociative state, or a form of factitious disorder with psychological symptoms (68,69). The EEG is normal in most cases (70). Ganser, who described the syndrome in 1897, viewed this disorder as a hysterical twilight state featuring a fluctuating level of consciousness; defective memory; inability to answer correctly the simplest questions, with a tendency to give only approximately correct answers; visual and auditory hallucinations; conversion symptoms; rather abrupt recovery; and amnesia for the disorder after recovery (71). This rare condition may be difficult to differentiate from delirium on account of the disturbance of consciousness. However, the degree of inconsistency in the patient's cognitive performance and the tendency to give grotesquely inaccurate answers—for example, that a bird has three legs or that $2 + 2 = 5$, are highly suggestive of Ganser syndrome and are not encountered in delirium. Also, as already stated, the EEG is usually normal in that syndrome.

The essential feature of a *factitious disorder with psychological symptoms* is intentional simulation of symptoms (often psychotic) suggestive of mental disorder (7). The manner in which the patient presents the symptoms reflects his or her conception of mental disorder. These patients may complain of memory impairment or confusion but never try to simulate delirium—a virtually impossible task to accomplish with any success. On the other hand, a patient with a factitious disorder with physical symptoms (Munchausen syndrome) may develop true delirium as a consequence of self-induced infection and associated high fever (72).

In summary, the differential diagnosis of delirium includes its distinction from other organic mental syndromes, schizophrenia, manic and major depressive episodes, brief reactive psychosis, dissociative disorders, and factitious disorder with psychological symptoms. In most cases the syndrome can be distinguished clinically by its unique set of symptoms, its acute onset, and its fluctuating and transient course. In the case of a clinically similar disorder, the EEG and a sodium amobarbital (Amytal) interview may be of diagnostic value.

References

1. Millard P. H.: Last scene of all. *Br. Med. J.* 1981;283:1559–1560.
2. Hodkinson H. M.: Confusional states in the elderly, in Barbagallo-Sangiorgi G., Exton-Smith A. N. (eds): *The Aging Brain.* New York, Plenum Press, 1980, pp. 155–159.
3. Lipowski Z. J.: Acute confusional states (delirium), in Albert M. L. (ed): *Clinical Neurology of Old Age.* New York, Oxford University Press, 1984, pp 277–297.
4. Lipowski Z. J.: Delirium (acute confusional states). *J.A.M.A.* 1987;258:1789–1792.
5. Lipowski Z. J.: Differentiating delirium from dementia in the elderly. *Clin. Gerontol.* 1982;1:3–10.
6. Lipowski Z. J: Transient cognitive disorders (delirium, acute confusional states) in the elderly. *Am. J. Psychiatry* 1983;140:1426–1436.
7. *Diagnostic and Statistical Manual of Mental Disorders,* ed 3 revised. Washington, DC, American Psychiatric Association, 1987.
8. Byrne E. J.: Reversible dementia. *Int. J. Geriatr. Psychiatry* 1987;2:73–81.
9. Mahler M. E., Cummings J. L., Benson F.: Treatable dementias. *West. J. Med.* 1987;146:705–712.
10. Council on Scientifc Affairs: Dementia. *J.A.M.A.* 1986;256:2234–2238.
11. Differential diagnosis of dementing diseases. National Institutes of Health Consensus Development Conference Statement, Vol 6, No 11. July 6–8, 1987.
12. Larson E. B., Reifler B. V., Sumi S. M., et al: Diagnostic evaluation of 200 elderly outpatients with suspected dementia. *J. Gerontol.* 1985;40:536–543.
13. Brenner R. P.: The electroencephalogram in altered states of consciousness. *Neurol. Clin.* 1985;3:615–631.
14. Engel G. L., Romano J: Delirium, a syndrome of cerebral insufficiency. *J. Chronic Dis.* 1959;9:260–277.
15. Obrecht R., Okhomina F. O. A., Scott D. F.: Value of EEG in acute confusional states. *J. Neurol. Neurosurg. Psychiatry* 1979;42:75–77.
16. Pro J. D., Wells C. E.: The use of the electroencephalogram in the diagnosis of delirium. *Dis. Nerv. Syst.* 1977;38:804–808.
17. Rabins, P. V., Folstein M. F.: Delirium and dementia: Diagnostic criteria and fatality rates. *Br. J. Psychiatry* 1982;140:149–153.

18. Leuchter F. A., Spar J. E., Walter D. O., et al: Electroencephalographic spectra and coherence in the diagnosis of Alzheimer's-type and multi-infarct dementia. *Arch. Gen. Psychiatry* 1987;44:993–998.
19. Rae-Grant A., Blume W., Lau C., et al: The electroencephalogram in Alzheimer-type dementia. *Arch. Neurol.* 1987;44:50–54.
20. Levin M.: Varieties of disorientation. *J. Ment. Sci.* 1956;102:619–623.
21. Andreasen N. C.: The diagnosis of schizophrenia. *Schizophr. Bull.* 1987;13:9–22.
22. Murray R. M., Lewis S. W., Reveley A. M.: Towards an aetiological classification of schizophrenia. *Lancet* 1985;2:1023–1026.
23. Seidman L. J.: Schizophrenia and brain dysfunction: An integration of recent neurodiagnostic findings. *Psychol. Bull.* 1983;94:195–238.
24. Wokin A., Jaeger J., Brodie J. D., et al: Persistence of cerebral metabolic abnormalities in chronic schizophrenia as determined by positron emission tomography. *Am. J. Psychiatry* 1985;142:564–571.
25. Davison K.: Schizophrenia-like psychoses associated with organic cerebral disorders. A review. *Psychiatr. Dev.* 1983;1:1–34.
26. Editorial: Schizophrenia and organic disease. *Lancet* 1987;2:776–777.
27. Cutting J.: The phenomenology of acute organic psychosis: Comparison with acute schizophrenia. *Br. J. Psychiatry* 1987;151:324–332.
28. Green M., Walker E.: Attentional performance in postive- and negative-symptom schizophrenia. *J. Nerv. Ment. Dis.* 1986;174:208–213.
29. Walker E, Harvey P.: Positive and negative symptoms in schizophrenia: Attentional performance correlates. *Psychopathology 1986;19:294–302.*
30. Anscombe R.: The disorder of consciousness in schizophrenia. *Schizophr. Bull.* 1987;13:241–260.
31. Vaillant G. E.: Prospective prediction of schizophrenic remission. *Arch. Gen. Psychiatry* 1964;11:509–518.
32. Newmark C. S., Raft D., Toomey T., et al: Diagnosis of schizophrenia: Pathognomonic signs or symptom clusters. *Compr. Psychiatry* 1975;16:155–163.
33. Van Praag G. E.: About the impossible concept of schizophrenia. *Compr. Psychiatry* 1976;17:481–497.
34. Coryell W., Tsuang M. T.: Outcome after 40 years in *DSM-III* schizophreniform disorder. *Arch. Gen. Psychiatry* 1986;43:324–328.
35. Jauch D. A., Carpenter W. T.: Reactive psychosis 1 and 11. *J. Nerv. Ment. Dis.* 1988;176:72–86.
36. Retterstol N.: Present state of reactive psychoses in Scandinavia. *Psychopathology* 1987;20:68–71.
37. Stromgren E.: The development of the concept of reactive psychoses. *Psychopathology* 1986;20:62–67.
38. Johnson-Sabine E. C., Mann A. H., Jacoby R. J., et al: Bouffée délirante: An examination of its current status. *Psychol. Med. 1983;13:771–778.*
39. Refsum H. E., Astrup C.: Hysteric reactive psychoses: A follow-up. *Neuropsychobiology* 1982;8:172–181.
40. Levin H. L.: Organic and psychogenic delirium. *N.Y. Med. J.* 1914;99:631–633.
41. Goldney R., Lander H.: Pseudodelirium. *Med. J. Aust.* 1979;1:630.
42. Tuppin J. P., Halbreich U., Pena J. J.: *Transient Psychosis: Diagnosis, Management and Evaluation.* New York, Brunner/Mazel, 1984.
43. Editorial: Acute delirium in 1845 and 1860. *Am J. Insanity* 1864;21:181–200.
44. Weber H.: On delirium or acute insanity. *Med. Chir. Trans. (Lond.)* 1865;30:135–159.

45. Bell L. V.: On a form of disease resembling some advanced stages of mania and fever. *Am. J. Insanity* 1849;6:97–127.
46. Connolly N.: Acute confusional insanity. *Dubl. J. Med. Sci.* 1890;89:506–518.
47. Meduna L. J.: Oneirophrenia: *The Confused State.* Urbana, University of Illinois Press, 1950.
48. Adland M. L.: Review, case studies, therapy, and interpretation of the acute exhaustive psychoses. *Psychiatr. Q.* 1947;21:38–69.
49. Christoffels J., Thiel J. H.: Delirium acutum, a potentially fatal condition in the psychiatric hospital. *Psychiatr. Neurol. Neurochir.* 1970;73:177–187.
50. Tolsma F. J.: The syndrome of acute pernicious psychosis. *Psychiatr. Neurol. Neurochir.* 1967;70:1–21.
51. Mann S. C., Caroff S. N., Bleier H. R., et al: Lethal catatonia. *Am. J. Psychiatry* 1986;143:1374–1381.
52. Perry J. C., Jacobs D.: Overview: Clinical applications of the amytal interview in psychiatric emergency settings. *Am. J. Psychiatry* 1982;139:552–559.
53. Santos A. B., Manning D. E., Waldrop W. M.: Delirium or psychosis? Diagnostic use of the sodium amobarbital interview. *Psychosomatics* 1980;21:863–864.
54. Ward N. G., Rowlett D. B., Burke P.: Sodium amylobarbitone in the differential diagnosis of confusion. *Am. J. Psychiatry* 1978;135:75–78.
55. Bond T. C.: Recognition of acute delirious mania. *Arch Gen. Psychiatry* 1980;37:553–554.
56. Carlson G. A., Goodwin F. K.: The stages of mania: A longitudinal analysis of the manic episode. *Arch. Gen. Psychiatry* 1973;28:221–228.
57. Swartz M. S., Henschen G. M., Cavenar J. O., et al: A case of intermittent delirious mania. *Am. J. Psychiatry* 1982;139:1357–1358.
58. Taylor M. A., Abrams R.: The phenomenology of mania. *Arch. Gen. Psychiatry* 1973;29:520–522.
59. Thase M. E., Reynolds C. F.: Manic pseudodementia. *Psychosomatics* 1984;25:256–260.
60. Taylor M. A., Abrams R.: Cognitive dysfunction in mania. *Compr. Psychiatry* 1986;27:186–191.
61. Van Sweden B.: Disturbed vigilance in mania. *Biol. Psychiatry* 1986;21:311–313.
62. Mentzos S., Lyrakos A., Tsiolis A.: Akute Verwirrtheitszustande, *Nervenarzt* 1971;42:10–17.
63. Bulbena A., Berrios G. E.: Pseudodementia: Facts and figures. *Br. J. Psychiatry* 1986;148:87–94.
64. La Rue A., Spar J., Hill C. D.: Cognitive impairment in late-life depression: Clinical correlates and treatment implications. *J. Affect. Dis.* 1986;11:179–184.
65. Akhtar S., Brenner I.: Differential diagnosis of fugue-like states. *J. Clin. Psychiatry* 1979;40:381–385.
66. Kopelman M. D.: Amnesia: Organic and psychogenic. *Br. J. Psychiatry* 1987;150:428–442.
67. Ruedrich S. L., Chu C. C., Wadle C. V.: The amytal interview in the treatment of psychogenic amnesia. *Hosp. Community Psychiatry* 1985;36:1045–1046.
68. Carney M. W. P., Chary T. K. N., Robotis P., et al: Ganser syndrome and its management. *Br. J. Psychiatry* 1987;151:697–700.
69. Cocores J. A., Santa W. G., Patel M. D.: The Ganser syndrome: Evidence suggesting its classification as a dissociative disorder. *Int. J. Psychiatry Med.* 1984;14:47–56.

70. Cocores J. A., Schlesinger L. B., Gold M. S.: A review of the EEG literature on Ganser's syndrome. *Int. J. Psychiatry Med.* 1986–87;16:59–65.
71. Schorer C. E.: The Ganser syndrome. *Br. J. Criminol.* 1965;41:120–131.
72. Aduan R. P., Fauci A. S., Dale D. C., et al: Factitious fever and self-induced infection. *Ann. Intern. Med.* 1979;90:230–242.

10

Treatment

Treatment of delirium has concerned physicians since antiquity, as documented in Chapter 1. Therapeutic methods have varied, reflecting changes in the state of knowledge of the syndrome, as well as changing views of its etiology and pathophysiology. However, certain general management principles have prevailed since antiquity and are still applied today. These include providing a relaxing environment, emotional support, sedation in case of agitation, and ensuring rest, sleep, and good nutrition. The following brief historical account of the therapy of delirium will serve as an introduction to a discussion of its modern management.

Historical evolution of treatment

Some of the cardinal rules of the management of delirium had been clearly spelled out by the beginning of the Common Era. Roman medical writers, such as Aretaeus, Soranus, and Galen, active in the second century A.D., formulated therapeutic guidelines that in general are still applicable. Aretaeus (1) taught that a phrenitic (delirious) patient should be placed in a dark room if he was disturbed by the light and in a bright one if he was afraid of the dark. Rest and sleep were to be aided by administering poppy boiled in oil. Soranus of Ephesus (2) recommended that a delirious patient should be treated in a quiet, well-lit room without pictures on the walls, as these might lead to visual hallucinations. At times, the patient would have to be physically restrained in order to prevent self-injury from jumping out of the window, for example. Venesection and cupping were recommended. Galen (3) taught that fever delirium was secondary to and symptomatic of many systemic diseases that affected the brain by "consensus" or "sympathetically." Consequently, treatment had to focus on the underlying condition. This seemed to be the first time in history that the crucial need for etiological treatment of delirium was explicated.

In later centuries, medical writers modified and added specific details to the above general principles but basically did not change them until the nineteenth century, when bloodletting, a traditional key component of the treatment of delirium from the time of Galen on, was gradually abandoned. This mode of therapy was based on the prevailing views on the pathophysiology of the syndrome. Avicenna (3), among others, viewed delirium as a symptom of brain disease caused by black, yellow, or red bile, or by hot, burning blood rushing to the brain. Treatment therefore had to involve diversion of the disturbing humors from the brain by removal or cooling of the overheated blood. Bleeding was carried out by phlebotomy or cupping glasses, or by leeches. Gatinaria (4), a fifteenth-century writer, recommended bleeding from the legs, while Riviére (4), writing in the seventeenth century, urged that blood be removed from the veins of the head. He also advised that the whole body of the patient be cooled, yet cautioned against the use of cooling medicines such as the oil of roses, violets, or water lilies.

Bloodletting continued to be a popular treatment for mental illnesses, including delirium, well into the nineteenth century. Benjamin Rush (5), for example, was a prominent advocate of it on the assumption that the cause of mental diseases originated in the blood vessels. Esquirol (6), in his famous treatise on mental disorders published in 1835, deplored the abuse of this treatment and recommended that it be applied only to plethoric patients "when the head is strongly congested." In such cases, leeches should be applied to the jugular vein and temporal arteries and cups to the base of the head. A century earlier, Frings (7) expressed similar views in regard to phrenitis (delirium) and criticized Galenists for advocating bleeding as the treatment of choice for this condition. He referred to them in this context as being the "most expert in the Art of Killing." In 1813 Sutton (8) published his famous treatise on delirium tremens, a condition he distinguished from other forms of delirium on the basis of an adverse response to bloodletting but a favorable response to opium. Gallway (9) inveighed against bloodletting, especially if applied to delirious patients with "low or adynamic symptoms." He asserted that a physician who bled such a patient using "various instruments of professional torture to the head" would soon find that he had "dealt his patient a knock-down blow." By the late nineteenth century, bloodletting had gradually faded away as a treatment for delirium. It was replaced by the application of evaporating lotions or an ice bag to the head, cold baths, and other such methods designed to lower fever and reduce the presumed hyperemia of the brain and the raised intracranial pressure (10,11). Yet, as late as 1899, Hirsch (12) found it necessary to condemn venesection as a treatment for delirium.

During the nineteenth century, several major aspects of the treatment of delirium were expanded or modified: first, treatment of the underlying medical condition was stressed; second, sedation and therapy for insomnia were modified; and third, general supportive measures were expanded. Salter (13), an eminent English surgeon, wrote in 1850 that it was essential to understand the underlying cause of delirium in a given patient in order to treat the individual effectively. This general guideline was echoed by Verco (11): "In the treatment of delirium the best results will follow prescriptions according to causal indications" (p 340). Hirsch (12) reaffirmed this precept but also stressed the need for symptomatic treatment of the syndrome, regardless of its cause. Thus, the key concept of treating the pathological condition deemed responsible for delirium in a given patient was unequivocally stated. Progress in medical knowledge and therapy during the nineteenth century made feasible this important advance.

Sedation has been used to treat agitated, delirious patients since antiquity. Opium was by far the most popular drug. During the nineteenth century, several new drugs were introduced to enrich the clinician's armamentarium. Graves (14), the famous Dublin physician, announced in 1836 that he had achieved remarkable success in treating delirium in the course of typhus with frequent doses of tartar emetic. He pointed out that its remarkable effectiveness had nothing to do with its emetic action. During the second half of the nineteenth century, a number of drugs came into use for the management of agitation and insomnia associated with delirium: bromides, chloral hydrate, chloroform, hyoscine, hyoscyamine, morphine, and paraldehyde (10–12). Barbiturates were introduced in 1903 and became the leading sedative-hypnotics for decades. All these drugs had been used, to varying degrees, for the symptomatic treatment of delirium until the introduction of the major and minor tranquilizers in the 1950s. From then on, these new drugs entirely replaced the old ones in the management of delirium.

General supportive and nursing measures became increasingly sophisticated and comprehensive. Greiner (15), the author of a remarkable book on delirium published in 1817, discussed these measures with impressive sensitivity for the patient's psychological predicament and needs. Details of his unusually humane therapeutic approach can be found in Chapter 1. At about the same time, Rees's (16) encyclopedia was published, containing these guidelines for the general management of a delirious patient: "Every source of irritation whatever, such as strong light, noises, conversation of visitors, motion or exertion of the body, etc. should be studiously avoided." Moreover, one should pay attention to the patient's state of nutrition, fluid intake, and bladder and bowel function. These guidelines, formulated over 170 years ago, could hardly be improved upon today. Fothergill (10) recommended that delirious patients be kept in their own room with a close relative in attendance, since unfamiliar surroundings and persons were likely to provoke frightening fantasies and hence attempts at escape. Attendants should try to restrain an agitated and fearful delirious patient by appealing to "what is left of his reason," rather than by using physical force. Phillips (17) emphasized that management of such a patient called for both careful nursing care and close attention on the part of the physician: "It requires tact, careful observation of details and infinite patience," he wrote. The patient might sustain self-injury and attempt suicide as a result of the disturbed mental state; hence, the windows should be barred and the patient never left unattended. Hawley (18), a nurse, drew attention to the common worsening of delirium during the night and described symptoms that could help nurses to recognize deterioration of the patient's mental condition.

By the beginning of this century, the basic principles of the treatment of delirium had been clearly spelled out. The therapeutic advice offered by many of the early writers on the subject is impressive for its remarkable sensitivity to the patient's emotional suffering and needs. It is sobering to note that in many modern hospitals these time-honored therapeutic principles seem to be ignored, reflecting the depersonalized approach to patient care in recent decades. In the remainder of this chapter, the guidelines for modern treatment are outlined. They combine old precepts with more recently introduced therapeutic techniques.

General principles of modern treatment

The modern management of delirium comprises *two main aspects:* first, elimination or correction of the underlying causal factor (or factors) by appropriate medical or surgical intervention; and second, general symptomatic and supportive measures aimed at securing adequate rest, sleep, nutrition, fluid and electrolyte balance, and overall optimal comfort and protection against self-injury for the patient (19–21). These two key aspects of treatment, the etiological and the symptomatic, obviously overlap, since malnutrition, dehydration, electrolyte imbalance, and vitamin deficiency may contribute to the onset, continuation, and severity of delirium. Treatment of the causes of the syndrome must follow the currently accepted therapeutic measures described in the medical literature and falls mostly outside the scope of this book. Some of these measures will be referred to in Part II. Only the general guidelines will be discussed in the sections to follow, with special emphasis on symptomatic and supportive treatment.

Identification and adequate treatment of the underlying cause

As soon as delirium has been diagnosed on clinical grounds, its etiology must be sought. In many cases, especially in older patients, more than one factor is likely to exist; all of these factors must be identified and either eliminated or adequately treated. A given patient may, for example, suffer from hypoxia, dehydration, electrolyte imbalance, infection, and drug toxicity. Unless all of these etiological factors are identified and properly dealt with, the delirium is liable to continue.

It is most important to obtain a detailed history of the patient's recent and current intake of medical and recreational drugs and alcohol. Elderly patients, in particular, are notoriously sensitive to even therapeutic doses of the commonly used medical drugs and may become delirious as a result of intoxication. Rapid withdrawal of sedative-hypnotic agents or alcohol, or both, from an abuser may lead to withdrawal delirium. Such a patient may sometimes conceal the history of substance abuse and thus create a diagnostic puzzle. A drug screen may be of value in some cases, and a history of otherwise unexplained seizures can provide a diagnostic clue. Virtually every known drug may cause delirium as a consequence of overdosage; or age-related changes in drug action, metabolism and elimination; or due to individual idiosyncrasy. It follows that any medications are potentially suspect and should be withheld or their dosage reduced, if possible. Etiological factors in delirium are discussed in general terms and listed in Chapter 8, and are considered in more specific detail in Part II.

Maintenance of Fluid and Electrolyte Balance and Nutrition

An agitated, overactive delirious patient can readily develop dehydration and sodium depletion, as well as exhaust the body stores of vitamins, especially those of the B complex. As a result, the severity of the delirium may increase. Many elderly delirious patients suffer from depression or dementia, or both, prior to the development of delirium, and their food and fluid intake may have been inadequate for some time. Consequently, such patients may show signs of malnutrition, dehydration, and avitaminosis. Clearly, these deficits need to be corrected, and proper fluid and electrolyte balance, as well as nutrition and vitamins, provided.

Sedation and Sleep

Not every delirious patient needs to be sedated. In fact, many patients are lethargic, hypoactive, and have difficulty staying awake during the day; they hardly require sedatives. On the other hand, an agitated, restless, excited, and hyperactive patient does need sedation in order to avoid serious, even lethal, complications resulting from self-injury or from worsening of the physical condition, as in severe coronary heart disease, for example. An agitated, confused delirious patient may tear open sutures, or pull out arterial or intravenous catheters, or try to escape and sustain a fracture. Adequate sedation is necessary in order to prevent such serious complications.

The choice and dosage of the sedative or tranquilizer to sedate a delirious patient must be based on several considerations. First, the *etiology* of the delirium must be taken into account. For example, a patient suffering from hepatic encephalopathy could pass into coma if given chlorpromazine to control agitation. The same drug could precipitate hypothermia in a myxedematous patient (22). The presence of hypertension or coronary heart disease contraindicates the use of a tranquilizer likely to induce hypotension or a cardiac arrhythmia. If delirium is known or suspected to be caused by an anticholinergic agent, one should obviously avoid using tranquilizers with marked anticholinergic side effects. Second, the patient's *age* is important; the dosage of a psychotropic drug must be reduced in an elderly individual. Third, the *effectiveness* of the drug in reducing agitation and excitement without causing undesirable side effects on cardiovascular, respiratory, hepatic, renal, and central nervous functions needs to be considered. Not only the choice and dosage of the drug are important, but also the route of administration in order to achieve an optimal therapeutic effect.

Not one psychotropic drug available today is ideally suited and safe for all cases of delirium. The following discussion of the advantages and disadvantages of the commonly used tranquilizers and sedatives may help the reader make the optimal choice in a given case. Drug treatment of delirium due to various specific causes will be discussed further in Part II. The following classes of sedatives and tranquilizers have been recommended by various writers.

BARBITURATES

There is no place for the use of these drugs in delirium other than that due to barbiturate and, possibly, benzodiazepine withdrawal. They are liable to make a delirious patient unduly obtunded or, in some cases, paradoxically agitated; their cumulative effect could precipitate coma; and they have no remedial effect on delusions and hallucinations (23,24).

PARALDEHYDE

This drug was often recommended for the treatment of delirium in the past (25). Its disadvantages include the possible development of a sterile abscess with intramuscular injection, pulmonary edema after intravenous injection, and difficulty in adjusting the dosage with rectal administration (26). This drug is not recommended.

BENZODIAZEPINES

These drugs are effective anxiolytic agents as well as sedative-hypnotics (27). In the treatment of alcohol withdrawal syndrome and hepatic encephalopathy, they are the drugs of choice (23,28). Otherwise, their usefulness in the treatment of delirium is limited. Some writers recommend the use of intravenous lorazepam, in conjunction with intravenous haloperidol, for the management of acutely agitated, delirious cancer patients (29). Midazolam, a benzodiazepine with a rapid onset of action and a short elimination half-life, has been recommended for sedation in the intensive care unit (30). Benzodiazepines are generally ineffective against the severe agitation, hallucinations, and delusions of a delirious patient (23). In the elderly, they may induce excessive sedation, confusion, and paradoxical excitement (31). The benzodiazepines with longer half-lives, such as flurazepam hydrochloride and diazepam, undergo hepatic oxidation. As hepatic blood flow decreases with age, they tend to have increased half-lives in the elderly and hence are not recommended for such patients (32). Shorter-acting agents, including lorazepam, midazolam, and oxazepam, are definitely preferred to induce sleep in an elderly delirious patient (33). It is also important to determine whether such a patient had taken a benzodiazepine drug prior to hospitalization, since its rapid withdrawal on admission could itself give rise to delirium (34).

PHENOTHIAZINES

Some writers recommend the use of one of the phenothiazine tranquilizers, such as chlorpromazine (35) or thioridazine (33), for the treatment of agitation in a delirious patient. In my opinion, the side effects of these drugs militate against their use in delirium, especially in the elderly. Chlorpromazine and thioridazine are potent alpha blockers and hence carry a serious risk of hypotension, especially when administered parenterally (36). Adverse reactions were reported in 12.2% of 556 medical patients treated with chlorpromazine, including hypotension, tachycardia, cardiac arrest, drowsiness, coma, extrapyramidal symptoms, convulsions, hepatitis, and respiratory depression (37). Postural hypotension was observed in 41% of patients receiving psychotropic drugs, mostly phenothiazines (38). They may be hazardous in geriatric, cardiac, hypertensive, and myxedematous patients and those with hepatic disease. Strongly antimuscarinic agents, such as chlorpromazine and thioridazine, can produce confusion and may thus worsen the condition of a delirious patient (39). The elderly are especially sensitive to sedation and orthostatic hypotension (40). Oversedated elderly patients may become more confused and agitated (40). Falls resulting from hypotension tend to have more serious consequences in such patients than in younger ones (40). There is a general consensus that high-potency neuroleptics, such as haloperidol, are less likely to induce hypotension and excessive sedation in an elderly delirious patient and are thus preferred (40).

As Greenblatt et al. caution, "Psychotropic drug treatment in medically ill patients should not be undertaken lightly" (41). In my opinion, if delirious patients are sufficiently agitated, restless, fearful, and overactive either to endanger their health and life or to make their medical management impossible, an effective antipsychotic agent should be administered in an adequate dose. Because of their cardiovascular and other side effects, phenothiazines are generally unsuitable for this purpose, and their use is not recommended.

BUTYROPHENONES

Haloperidol, a member of this class of drugs, may be considered the *drug of choice* for the treatment of agitation in delirium (23,29,39,40,42–49). Since its introduction in 1958, haloperidol has conclusively shown marked antipsychotic, anxiolytic, and antiemetic properties. It is a high-potency neuroleptic with beneficial effects on hallucinations, delusions, aggressivity, psychomotor hyperactivity, and agitation (45). The main advantages of this drug in the management of delirium include its effectiveness against all the above symptoms, its high potency, and its relatively low toxicity (45). For these reasons, haloperidol is currently the drug of choice for the management of hyperactive delirium at any age. It is more effective and less toxic than chlorpromazine in the elderly patient (40). It is generally preferred for the physically ill patient for the following reasons: it seldom causes marked hypotension; has negligible cardiotoxic effects; has relatively low anticholinergic, antiadrenergic, and autonomic nervous system effects; has no undesirable interaction with digitalis, diuretics, and other cardiovascular drugs; has a wide margin of safety; and seldom, if ever, causes delirium (23,29,39,40,42–49).

Haloperidol does have adverse effects, including extrapyramidal reactions, orthostatic hypotension, dyskinesia, neuroleptic malignant syndrome, catatonia, laryngeal spasm, cardiac arrhythmia, and liver disease (45,50–53). It must be stressed, however, that with the exception of extrapyramidal reactions, mild hypotension, and acute dyskinesia and akathisia, these side effects are rare. The highest incidence of extrapyramidal effects has been observed in the elderly, in women, and with doses of 4 to 20 mg daily (54). Parenteral, especially intravenous, administration of haloperidol, even in high doses, is less likely to induce extrapyramidal effects than oral dosage (55). The drug is devoid of hypnotic effects but may indirectly facilitate sleep by calming an agitated patient.

The detoxification and inactivation of haloperidol take place largely in the liver and are accomplished by oxydative dealkylation (56). No psychoactive metabolites are produced, which helps define the relation between the serum concentration of the drug and its antipsychotic effect (57). Traces of unmetabolized haloperidol can be found in the urine. Pharmacokinetic studies suggest that a serum haloperidol concentration of 9 to 15 ng/ml is associated with an optimal reduction of psychotic symptoms (57). The bioavailability of oral haloperidol is about 60% to 70%, which means that the oral dose should be 1.4–1.7 times higher than the intramuscular dose to produce an equivalent serum concentration of the drug (58). Elderly patients may respond well to small doses (58). Barbiturates and diphenylhydantoin induce metabolism of haloperidol and hence depress its serum concentration (58). Oral haloperidol appears in the serum within about 60–90 minutes, followed by peak levels in 4–6 hours (45). Intramuscular haloperidol is rapidly absorbed, with peak serum levels in 20–40 minutes (45). After intravenous administration, the action of the drug is rapid—5–20 minutes—and its serum concentration falls equally rapidly for about 1 hour during the distribution phase (45). Parenteral administration achieves almost 100% bioavailability (45). Oral administration twice daily is usually sufficient. The extrapyramidal effects tend to appear after 12–16 hours (59). Dystonic reactions may be relieved rapidly by parenteral administration of 1–2 mg of benztropine mesylate or 1–2 mg of biperiden (54). Subsequently, either of these drugs should be given in the same dosage orally every 4–6 hours for a total of about four doses.

Haloperidol can be administered orally in tablet form or as a liquid concentrate, intramuscularly, or intravenously. All of these routes have been used in the treatment of delirious patients, and the dosage of the drug has varied greatly (23,29,30,44,46–49). The route of administration depends on the patient's age, the degree of agitation, and, to some extent, the treatment setting, i.e., an emergency department or an intensive care unit, for example. No dogmatic or rigid dose schedule should be followed, but rather a flexible regimen adjusted according to the variables just mentioned, as well as to the individual patient's response.

For a mildly or moderately agitated, restless, and fearful delirious patient under the age of 60 years, lower doses are recommended. Haloperidol in oral doses of 5–10 mg in the morning and at bedtime is usually sufficient. An alternative treatment schedule can involve an initial dose of 5–10 mg intramuscularly, followed by a repeated injection 1 hour later if the patient fails to respond. Otherwise, the injection may be given twice daily for a day or two; once adequate symptomatic control has been achieved, the patient should receive 5–15 mg orally twice a day. Of course, intramuscular administration may have to be used if the patient relapses or refuses oral medication. The oral dosage should be continued and gradually decreased over the course of several days. If the systolic blood pressure falls below 100 mmHg, treatment should be stopped.

For a severely agitated delirious adult under 60 years of age and free of hepatic disease, *rapid tranquilization* is the method of choice (23,29,42,44–47,49). The preferred route of administration is intramuscular (23,42,44), although some writers have recommended the intravenous one (29,46,49). The drug is usually given in doses of 5–10 mg every 30–60 minutes until tranquilization is achieved, usually after four to six injections. Subsequently, the drug is administered orally in doses one-half to two times higher than the parenteral dose. Some authors assert that rapid tranquilization may also be achieved with the concentrate administered orally and recommend it as a primary approach (23). Several writers have reported the use of large intravenous doses of haloperidol for the management of severe agitation in cancer (29), cardiac (49), and postoperative (46) patients. Doses as high as 240 mg of intravenous haloperidol have been used (29). The starting dose was usually 3–5 mg and was rapidly increased to single doses of 10–75 mg (29,46,49). The authors assert that this form of rapid tranquilization is effective, safe, and possibly lifesaving (29,46,49). It has been pointed out, however, that no controlled studies of the efficacy of intravenous administration of haloperidol have been reported to date; hence, whether this procedure is more effective than intramuscular treatment, and equally safe, remains an open question (23). Haloperidol is not formally approved for intravenous use by the U.S. Food and Drug Administration (23). The patients most suitable for this type of haloperidol administration are those hospitalized in well-controlled medical environments (45). I have not had personal experience with it and cannot comment, except to state that I have generally found intramuscular therapy in moderate doses quite efficacious in most cases of delirium encountered on the medical and surgical wards.

A patient aged 60 years or older should receive lower doses of haloperidol under most circumstances (21,32,40,47). If the patient is severely agitated, rapid tranquilization may be induced with doses as low as 0.5 mg intramuscularly given every hour (47). Alternatively, an initial dose of 3–5 mg intramuscularly may be administered and repeated after 30–60 minutes if no response has been observed. For milder delirium, liquid concentrate in doses of 0.25–3 mg twice daily may be sufficient. Extrapyramidal side effects are common in the elderly and may be controlled with benztropine mesylate, 1–2 mg at bedtime.

No absolute contraindications to haloperidol have been established. The drug should be avoided in hepatic encephalopathy and anticholinergic delirium. The above guidelines for its use in an agitated, delirious patient are to be viewed as just that. No single regimen is appropriate for all patients; the clinician must use good judgment.

A note on *sleep* is helpful. As mentioned earlier, a patient sedated with haloperidol is likely to sleep adequately, even though this drug is not a hypnotic; on occasion, sleep onset is delayed. In such a case, a benzodiazepine with relatively short elimination half-life, such as lorazepam, midazolam, or temazepam, may be used. On the whole, however, it is preferable to avoid hypnotics in delirium. I have occasionally used hydroxyzine, in doses of 25–100 mg at bedtime. An antihistamine, this drug is safe and free of undesirable side effects other than drowsiness.

Provision of an optimal sensory and social environment

The quality of the environment influences the onset, severity, and duration of delirium. Physicians have been aware of this fact since antiquity and have provided guidelines on how to modify environmental stimuli in order to minimize their potentially adverse effects on the delirious patient. Some of these precepts were discussed earlier in this chapter, and should be recapitulated and expanded in the light of current knowledge and practice. Proper attention to the quality of the sensory and social environments, of delirious patients, is important not only for the adequate management of delirium but also for the *prevention* of its avoidable features and complications, such as marked restlessness, panic, self-injury, attacks on others, and excessive autonomic nervous system arousal. Aspects of the environment that are believed to facilitate the development of these undesirable features, and possibly of delirium itself, were discussed in Chapter 5. They include excessive and deficient sensory stimulation and information inputs, disruption of sleep, and provocation of anxiety and anger.

The patient is best cared for in a quiet, well-lighted room, with a dimmed light at night. A single room is usually preferable. Excessive noise and confusing sounds, such as the messages broadcast on the hospital intercom system or a loud television, should be avoided. The patient needs to be protected against exposure to the bustle of a busy ward, with its unfamiliar and, hence, confusing sounds and sights. Delirious patients tend to misinterpret these stimuli as threats to their well-being and respond to them with fear. On the other hand, a patient left alone for long periods, especially in a dark room, or one exposed to the monotonous sounds of various apparatus, is liable to be understimulated. This may facilitate the onset of hallucinations, interfere with spatiotemporal orientation, and foster agitated and disturbing behavior. To counteract such sensory and information deprivation, the patient should be provided with an adequate flow of orienting, reassuring, and calming sensory and information inputs. A radio or televison set may be helpful, but good judgment is essential. For example, letting the patient watch a noisy, violent television show is more likely to disturb than to calm. Music has a therapeutic and soothing effect on many people and may help calm an agitated patient. On the other hand, a lethargic patient who has difficulty staying awake may become more alert and responsive when allowed to watch a reasonably quiet and amusing television show. Clearly, staff members have to pay attention to these details and use their judgment in adjusting the level of stimulation to the patient's needs.

Familiarity is another aspect of the environment important for a person with compromised cerebral function. The hospital environment is unfamiliar for most patients, and hence tends to be confusing and frightening for many of them. Its cognitively disorganizing and threatening effects may be alleviated by letting a trusted relative or friend stay with the patient outside of routine visiting hours to provide a familiar, and hence reassuring and calming, social stimulation. The relative should be told that the patient is delirious, i.e., suffering from a temporary mental disturbance due to a physical illness. This explanation avoids creating the fear that the patient has permanently lost his or her mind. A family member should be asked to orient the patient, i.e., state the date, and the names of the hospital and of the doctors and nurses in attendance, as well as talk calmly about matters that interest the patient. It is generally helpful to involve the family in the care of a delirious patient in order to provide familiarity and emotional support, and to enhance cognitive clarity and counteract the sense of fear and isolation (60). It may be useful to bring a few photographs and other familiar objects from home and display them so that the patient can see them and be reassured.

Weisman and Hackett (61) have offered a good example of the application of these guidelines to the prevention and treatment of delirium after eye surgery. The cornerstone of their approach was a systematic attempt to provide patients with perceptual cues so as to facilitate reality testing, spatiotemporal orientation, and a sense of familiarity. Repeated explanations and encouragement were employed. These and other strategies discussed here are being increasingly applied in caring for patients in intensive care units, where the incidence of delirium tends to be relatively high (62–64).

Having discussed the issues of sensory stimulation and the familiarity of the environment, we need to consider the kind of *information* provided for the delirious patient. It is important to tell the patient that he or she is suffering from a delirium and what this means. The word "delirium" is familiar to many people and is usually associated with fever and childhood ailments; hence, it is not usually perceived and feared as insanity. The patient needs to be told that there may be some difficulty in thinking, understanding, and remembering, and that the staff will help the patient cope with this confusion, which in any case is only transient. The patient who is hallucinating should be reassured similarly that hallucinations are a temporary disturbance akin to waking dreams and induced by the illness. Delusions, if any, should not be directly challenged or ridiculed. Rather, alternative and more realistic explanations should be offered for what the patient tends to misinterpret. For example, if the patient claims that men intent on killing him are waiting outside his room, it may help to let him get up and see what actually goes on there. In addition to verbal information, it is often useful to provide other aids that may enhance the patient's sense of control and hence security. A clock and a calendar should be placed in the patient's field of vision to facilitate orientation. It is preferable to restrict the number of visitors and staff so as to avoid information overload, undue excitement, and fatigue. Finally, interruption of the patient's sleep should be avoided as much as possible. All of these measures tend to reduce a delirious patient's agitation, fear, and psychotic experiences, and hence the need for medication and physical restraints.

Nursing care

Nursing care of a delirious patient is crucially important. After all, the nurses have more contact with the patient than anybody else. The cornerstones of their care include careful observation, timely reporting of behavioral change, emotional support, and reorientation (65–71). It is best if one nurse can have the most contact with the patient throughout each work shift and see him or her frequently and unhurriedly. A nurse is usually the first person to observe early symptoms of delirium, especially at night, and should so alert the physician in charge without delay. Severe agitation and an emergency situation may be prevented by timely diagnostic assessment, sedation, and close supervision of the patient. A nurse should periodically provide reorientation by telling the patient where he or she is and what the date is. If continuous nursing care cannot be provided and the patient is markedly disturbed, special attendants should be ordered to stay in the room around the clock. This admittedly rather expensive measure may help prevent costly medicolegal complications resulting from accidents such as falls and fractures. Physical restraints are best avoided. They tend to increase the patient's agitation, fear, and paranoia. Moreover, they predispose to the development of deep vein thrombosis and pulmonary embolism (72). With close supervision of the patient and adequate and timely sedation, physical restraints should have no place in the management of delirium.

By creating a nonthreatening, supportive, and comfortable environment, nurses not only play a key role in the treatment of a delirious patient but also reduce the incidence of delirium in some cases (70). They can also carry out clinical research and thus contribute to the knowledge about the syndrome (73,74). The ability to recognize the features of the syndrome clinically is, of course, necessary for effective nursing care. Many articles on the care of delirious patients have appeared in nursing journals in recent years, highlighting the profession's awareness of its importance (65–71). A nurse must not only diagnose the syndrome but also assess the personality, coping strategies, and psychological needs of the patient. Every patient has a different personality, education, sociocultural background, mode of coping with the illness, and degree of cognitive dysfunction. Thus, an evaluation of these variables is needed to guide a nurse's approach. These patients also call for patience, forbearance, and understanding on the part of the nursing staff. A nurse's understanding of the patient's condition, a calm attitude toward his or her often irrational talk and behavior, and attention to the patient's safety and comfort are the key elements of good nursing care in delirium. The nurses can help to prevent and alleviate its most disturbing and hazardous aspects. It is usually up to them to bring the patient's mental state to the physician's attention, both verbally and by a written report in the chart, and to make sure that this information is acted upon. Since delirium often becomes manifest for the first time during the night, the role of the night nurse is particularly important.

Psychiatric consultation and psychotherapy

The psychiatric consultant has an important role to play in the diagnosis and management of delirium. This is often the physician most familiar with delirium, its manifestations and disguises, its causes, and its treatment (75–78). About 15% to 20% of patients referred for psychiatric consultation from medical and surgical wards and special units suffer from delirium. This proportion is likely to rise in the years to come as a result of the growing number of elderly patients in general hospitals. The role of the consultant in this context includes several key aspects: assistance with diagnosis; advice on etiological investigations; advice on and supervision of management, including the choice, dosage, and route of administration of psychotropic drugs; teaching medical and nursing staff how to recognize and treat delirium; advice on issues involving a delirious patient's competence; and supportive psychotherapy at the bedside.

To be helpful, a psychiatric consultation should be requested early, i.e., as soon as delirium is suspected. Timely referral may enable the consultant to help prevent the development of florid symptoms and the attendant risk of complications. All too often, however, in my experience, an urgent psychiatric consultation is requested because the patient is already highly disturbed, disrupts the ward routine, threatens others, or has inflicted self-injury. Almost invariably, such an emergency had been preceded by mild delirious symptoms for a few days, but the staff, notably the physicians, had ignored them. Typically, a night nurse had reported that the patient was awake and confused during the night, and duly recorded this observation in the patient's chart, but no action was taken until a crisis arose.

To recognize that a patient is delirious is important not only because of the potential complications that may ensue, but also because the development of delirium in a physically ill patient implies that brain function is disordered. This fact is important for several reasons. In may indicate that the underlying disease is getting worse or that complications, such as an infection or electrolyte imbalance, have developed. It may signify that the patient's medications exert a toxic effect on the brain, either directly or indirectly. It may be a warning sign that the patient is becoming moribund. And finally, it suggests that unless treatment is instituted promptly, the patient may suffer irreversible brain damage. All of these considerations are sufficiently important to underscore the need for an early referral for psychiatric consultation of any patient displaying signs of delirium so as to confirm the diagnosis, plan investigations, and institute proper management.

The role of a psychiatric consultant in this context involves more than assisting in the diagnosis and the choice of a proper psychotropic agent. Often the consultant must also act as a *therapist* to the patient and *adviser* to the staff on proper psychological management. The consultant can add an important dimension to the understanding of a delirious patient that may help the clinical staff provide more sensitive and humane management. This involves an appraisal of the patient's personality, coping style and strategies, fears, and emotional needs. What a patient says and how he or she acts in the course of delirium is not just coincidental. Rather, it is imbued with meaning for the patient, expressed and communicated verbally and nonverbally. To appreciate this fact may make management easier (79). The patient can be approached as an individual with unique concerns, fears, and ways of coping with them. The therapist's aim is to allay the patient's fear or despair and enhance cognitive control and the sense of security (61,79). This involves providing supportive and directive psychotherapy at the bedside (61). Giving information, reorientation, and encouragement to an anxious and bewildered delirious patient may go a long way toward diminishing anxiety, alleviating anguish, and thus reducing the need for psychotropic drugs or physical restraints. To pay empathetic attention to what the patient says, even if the talk is disjointed and at times incoherent, may provide useful clues in choosing the psychotherapeutic approach. The patient may fear death, or be worried about his or her family, or relive a past traumatic event, or express longing for a particular person, for example. These concerns should be addressed by the therapist in an attempt to reduce their emotional impact. Such intervention may not only have an immediate beneficial effect but may also help prevent a stress response after the resolution of delirium (80,81).

Some writers have recommended a psychotherapeutic approach referred to as the "confrontation problem-solving technique" (82,83). This involves presenting the patient with a statement about a symptom or disturbed behavior exhibited by him or her, followed by a question: "What do you think or feel about what I told you?" This technique is claimed to enhance the patient's reality testing, cognitive control, capacity for reflection and self-examination, and adaptive coping (83). I have not used this form of therapy, but it appears to be worth trying.

The liaison psychiatrist also plays the traditional role of mediator and interpreter, the *liaison* proper (84). This implies gathering information about the patient from all available sources and mediating between the patient and the clinical staff, as well as his or her family. Clarifying the situation for the patient, explaining his or her utterances and behavior to the staff and family, and advising them on how best to approach the patient and why—these are the elements of the liaison role in these cases. The consultant facilitates communication among all the persons involved and tries to foster understanding of the patient's predicament and behavior. This role is particularly valuable in the case of disturbed and disturbing delirious patients. Skillful liaison may help prevent crises and involve crisis intervention.

Lastly, the psychiatric consultant may become involved in the *legal aspects* of delirium (85). Surprisingly little has been written about this subject. A delirious patient may present legal and ethical problems related to the issue of competence to give informed consent for medical and surgical procedures, including the administration of psychotropic drugs (85). Fogel et al. (85) discuss this subject in their thoughtful and informative article, which is worth summarizing. In a medical emergency situation, a delirious patient can be treated without consent. It is advisable, however, to involve a family member, or a second clinician, or both, in the decision-making process. A psychiatrist may be consulted in such a case and asked whether the patient is suffering from a delirium, a condition due directly to a physical illness, or from a functional mental illness. In the latter case, the patient must be treated according to the mental health laws of the state. In a clear-cut case of delirium, if the patient's condition requires urgent, lifesaving medical or surgical intervention, the physician may proceed with appropriate investigations and treatment on the basis of the doctrine of implied consent. In other words, it is assumed that the patient would give informed consent if he or she were mentally competent to do so. This implies that an individual suffering from delirium lacks the requisite ability to comprehend and evaluate information about the nature, merits, and risks of the proposed procedure, and hence cannot exercise proper judgment and make a valid decision. The situation tends to be legally more ambiguous if the patient requires urgent but nonemergency medical treatment. In this case, involvement of a third party, i.e., a family member or another physician, or both, is advisable. In regard to the administration of a neuroleptic to an agitated delirious patient, this may be done even without the patient's consent in order to carry out medically essential diagnostic or therapeutic procedures. The doctrine of implied consent seems to apply in such a case. It is important for the physician to record in the medical record the need for the urgent medical intervention and the evidence supporting a diagnosis of delirium, as well as its relevance to the lack of informed consent.

Can a delirious patient be considered guilty of assaulting and injuring another person? Probably not, since impaired consciousness would be considered an extenuating circumstance—a case of insane automatism (86).

Electroshock therapy (ECT)

A number of reports published in the psychiatric literature over the past several decades have suggested that ECT may be a useful adjunct to, and on occasion a lifesaving measure in, the treatment of severe delirium (87–91). I have occasionally resorted to ECT in cases where, regardless of the cause, the delirium was accompanied by persistent overactivity that threatened the survival of a patient who failed to respond to tranquilizers. A case in point involved a middle-aged woman with cancer who became psychotic, was given haloperidol, and developed acute liver failure as an apparent adverse effect of this drug. She became delirious and displayed ceaseless restlessness that failed to respond to benzodiazepines. She was given little hope of survival by the attending physician and was left to die. On my advice, she was transferred to the psychiatric ward, where three ECT treatments on consecutive days resulted in remission of her delirium and restlessness. Such cases are admittedly rare but memorable. It appears that two or three ECT treatments, given with proper medical precautions and in the presence of an anesthetist, may be highly effective in controlling the patient's life-threatening restlessness and agitation. ECT is not recommended as a routine treatment of delirium, but it may be considered as a last resort in severe and refractory cases.

Summary

The management of delirium has two key aspects: etiological and symptomatic. Treatment of the underlying cause (or causes) is crucial and presupposes a correct diagnosis of the syndrome and its etiology. Symptomatic management must follow these guidelines:

1. Close monitoring of the patient's mental state and behavior.
2. Ensuring sleep; a benzodiazepine drug with a relatively short half-life, such as lorazepam or temazepam, or hydroxyzine, may be used.
3. Sedation of the restless, agitated, hyperactive, and fearful patient; haloperidol, given orally, intramuscularly, or intravenously, is currently the drug of choice. Its dosage and route of administration should be adjusted to the individual patient's needs.
4. The environment should be structured to avoid extremes of sensory stimulation and information inputs for the patient; social support and adequate sensory stimulation should be provided.
5. Nutrition, fluid intake, electrolyte balance, and vitamin intake should be ensured.
6. General nursing care aimed at reorienting the patient, observing and reporting his or her behavior, and providing emotional support is essential.
7. Psychiatric consultation must be requested before a crisis develops.
8. Supportive psychotherapy at the bedside is valuable to calm the patient and prevent the postdelirium stress syndrome.
9. The issue of informed consent for treatment must be considered.
10. ECT therapy may be used occasionally.

References

1. *The Extant Works of Aretaeus, The Cappadocian,* ed F. Adams. London, Sydenham Society, 1861.
2. Aurelianus C.: *On Acute Diseases and on Chronic Diseases,* ed I. E. Drabklin. Chicago, University of Chicago Press, 1950.
3. Whitwell J. R.: *Historical Notes on Psychiatry.* Philadelphia, Blakiston, 1937.
4. Diethelm O.: *Medical Dissertations of Psychiatric Interest.* Basel, Karger, 1971.
5. Rush B.: *Medical Inquiries and Observations upon the Diseases of the Mind.* Philadelphia, Kimber & Richardson, 1812.
6. Esquirol J. E. D.: *Mental Maladies.* New York, Hafner, 1965.
7. Frings P.: *A Treatise on Phrensy.* London, Gardner, 1746.
8. Sutton T.: *Tracts on Delirium Tremens, on Peritonitis and on Some Other Inflammatory Affections.* London, Underwood, 1813.
9. Gallway M. B.: Nature and treatment of delirium. *Lond. Med. Gaz.* 1838;1:46–49.
10. Fothergill J. M.: The management of delirium. *The Practitioner* 1874;13:400–408.
11. Verco A.: Delirium. *Bart Hosp. Rep. (Lond.)* 1877;13:332–342.
12. Hirsch W.: A study of delirium. *N.Y. Med. J.* 1899;70:109–115.
13. Salter T.: Practical observations on delirium. *Prov. Med. Surg. J.* 1850;1:677–684.
14. Graves R. J.: Cases of violent delirium, occurring at an advanced stage of maculated or typhous fever, and treated successfully by doses of tartar emetic, frequently repeated. *Dubl. J. Med. Sci.* 1836;9:449–466.
15. Greiner F. C.: *Der Traum und das fieberhafte Irreseyn.* Altenburg, Brockhans, 1817.

16. Rees A.: *The Cyclopedia; or Universal Dictionary of Arts, Sciences, and Literature.* Vol 12. First American ed. Philadelphia, S. F. Bradford, 1818.
17. Phillips J.: Delirium. *Cleve. Med. J.* 1909;8:531–542.
18. Hawley E. A.: Manifestations of delirium in the night-time. *Am. J. Nurs.* 1907–8;8:757–761.
19. Lipowski Z. J.: Delirium (acute confusional states) *J.A.M.A.* 1987;258:1789–1792.
20. Lipowski Z. J.: Delirium, clouding of consciousness and confusion. *J. Nerv. Ment. Dis.* 1967;145:227–255.
21. Lipowski Z. J.: Transient cognitive disorders (delirium acute confusional states) in the elderly. *Am. J. Psychiatry* 1983;140:1426–1436.
22. Editorial: Organic psychosis. *Br. Med. J.* 1874;2:214–215.
23. Dubin W. R., Weiss K. J., Dorn J. M.: Pharmacotherapy of psychiatric emergencies. *J. Clin. Psychopharmacol.* 1986;6:210–222.
24. Heller S. S.: The organic patient and medical problems, in Glock R. A., Meyerson A. T., Robbins E., et al (eds): *Psychiatric Emergencies.* New York, G. Brune & Stratton, 1976, pp 135–146.
25. Cohen S.: The toxic psychoses and allied states. *Am. J. Med.* 1953;15:813–828.
26. Thompson W. L., Johnson A. D., Maddrey W. L.: Diazepam and paraldyhyde for treatment of severe delirium tremens. *Ann. Intern. Med.* 1975;82:175–180.
27. Greenblatt D. J., Shader R. I., Abernethy D. R.: Current status of benzodiazepines. Part I. *N. Engl. J. Med.* 1983;309:354–358.
28. Misra P.: Hepatic encephalopathy. *Med. Clin. North. Am.* 1981;65:209–226.
29. Adams F., Fernandez F., Anderson B.: Emergency pharmacotherapy of delirium in the critically ill cancer patient. *Psychosomatics* 1986;27:33–37.
30. Figge H., Huang V., Kaul A. F., et al: The pharmacotherapy of the behavioral manifestations of the ICU syndrome. *J. Crit. Care* 1987;2:199–205.
31. Baldessarini R. J.: *Chemotherapy in Psychiatry. Principles and Practice.* Cambridge, Mass, Harvard University Press, 1985.
32. Everitt D. E., Avorn J.: Drug prescribing for the elderly. *Arch. Intern. Med.* 1986;146:2393–2396.
33. Levkoff S. E., Besdine R. W., Wetle T.: Acute confusional states (delirium) in the hospitalized elderly. *Ann. Rev. Gerontol. Geriatr.* 1986;6:1–26.
34. Foy A., Drinkwater V., March S., et al: Confusion after admission to hospital in elderly patients using benzodiazepines. *Br. Med. J.* 1986;293:1072.
35. Muskin P. R., Mellman L. A., Kornfeld D. S.: A "new" drug for treating agitation and psychosis in the general hospital: Chlorpromazine. *Gen. Hosp. Psychiatry* 1986;8:404–410.
36. Simpson G. M., Pi E. H., Sramek J. J.: Adverse effects of antipsychotic agents. *Drugs* 1981;21:138–151.
37. Swett C.: Adverse reactions to chlorpromazine in medical patients. *Curr. Ther. Res.* 1975;18:199–206.
38. Jefferson J. W.: Hypotension from drugs. *Dis. Nerv. Syst.* 1974;35:66–71.
39. Black J. L., Richelson E., Richardson J. W.: Antipsychotic agents: A clinical update. *Mayo Clin. Proc.* 1985;60:777–789.
40. Salzman C.: Treatment of the elderly agitated patient. *J. Clin. Psychiatry* 1987;48(5, Suppl):19–22.
41. Greenblatt D. J., Shader R. I., Lofgren S.: Rational psychopharmacology for patients with medical disease. *Annu. Rev. Med.* 1976;27:407–420.
42. Clinton J. E., Sterner S., Stelmachers Z., et al: Haloperidol for sedation of disruptive emergency patients. *Ann. Emerg. Med.* 1987;16:319–322.

43. Kiely W. F.: Psychiatric syndromes in critically ill patients. *J.A.M.A.* 1976;245:2759–2761.
44. Moore D. P.: Rapid treatment in critically ill patients. *Am. J. Psychiatry* 1977; 134:1431–1432.
45. Settle E. C., Ayd F. J.: Haloperidol: A quarter century of experience. *J. Clin. Psychiatry* 1983;44:440–448.
46. Sos J., Cassem N. H.: Managing postoperative agitation. *Drug Ther.* 1980;10:103–106.
47. Steinhart M. J.: The use of haloperidol in geriatric patients with organic mental disorder. *Curr. Ther. Res.* 1983;33:132–143.
48. Steinhart M. J.: Treatment of delirium—a reappraisal. *Int. J. Psychiatry Med.* 1978–79;9:191–197.
49. Tesar G. E., Murray G. B., Cassem N. H.: Use of high-dose intravenous haloperidol in the treatment of agitated cardiac patients. *J. Clin. Psychopharmacol.* 1985;5:344–347.
50. Fuller C. M., Yassinger S., Donlon P., et al: Haloperidol induced liver disease. *West. J. Med.* 1977; 127:515–518.
51. Geller B., Greydanus D. E.: Haloperidol-induced comatose state with hyperthermia and rigidity in adolescence: Two case reports with a literature review. *J. Clin. Psychiatry* 1979;40:102–103.
52. Mehta D., Mehta S., Petit J., et al: Cardiac arrhythmia and haloperidol. *Am. J. Psychiatry* 1979;136:1468–1469.
53. Van Putten T., May P. R. A., Marder S. R.: Akathisia with haloperidol and thiothixene. *Arch. Gen. Psychiatry* 1984;41:1036–1039.
54. Ayd F. J.: Haloperidol update: 1975. *Proc. R. Soc. Med.* 1976;69(Suppl 1):14–22.
55. Menza M. A., Murray G. B., Holmes V. F., et al: Decreased extrapyramidal symptoms with intravenous haloperidol. *J. Clin. Psychiatry* 1987;48:278–280.
56. Forsman A., Folsch G., Larson M., et al: On the metabolism of haloperidol in man. *Curr. Ther. Res.* 1977;21:606–617.
57. Perry P. H., Pfohl B. M., Kelly M. W.: The relationship of haloperidol concentrations to therapeutic response. *J. Clin. Psychopharmacol.* 1988;8:38–43.
58. Forsman A., Ohman R.: Applied pharmacokinetics of haloperidol in man. *Curr. Ther. Res.* 1977;21:396–411.
59. Forsman A., Ohman R.: Pharmacokinetic studies on haloperidol in man. *Curr. Ther. Res.* 1976;20:319–336.
60. Rynearson E. K.: The acute brain syndrome: A family affair. *Psychiatric Ann.* 1977;7:77–83.
61. Weisman A. D., Hackett T. P.: Psychosis after eye surgery. *N. Engl. J. Med.* 1958;258:1284–1289.
62. Benzer H., Mutz N., Pauser G.: Psychosocial sequelae of intensive care. *Int. Anesthesiol. Clin.* 1983;21:169–180.
63. Tesar G.E., Stern T. A.: Evaluation and treatment of agitation in the intensive care unit. *J. Intensive Care Med.* 1986;1:137–148.
64. Turner G. O.: *The Cardiovascular Care Unit.* New York, Wiley, 1978.
65. Adams M., Hanson R., Norkool D., et al: Psychological responses in critical care units. *Am. J. Nurs.* 1978;78:1504–1512.
66. Kroner K.: Dealing with the confused patient. *Nurs. 79* 1979;9:71–78.
67. Sullivan N., Fogel B. S.: Could this be delirium? *Am. J. Nurs.* 1986;86:1359–1363.
68. Trockman G.: Caring for the confused or delirious patient. *Am. J. Nurs.* 1978;78:1495–1499.

69. Wilkinson O.: Out of touch with reality. *Am. J. Nurs. 1978;78:1492–1494.*
70. Williams M. A., Campbell E. B., Raynor W. J., et al: Reducing acute confusional states in elderly patients with hip fractures. *Res. Nurs.* 1985;8:329–337.
71. Williams M. A., Ward S. E., Campbell E. B.: Confusion: Testing versus observation. *J. Gerontol. Nurs.* 1988;14:25–30.
72. Gillick M. R., Serrell N. A., Gillick L. S.: Adverse consequences of hospitalization in the elderly. *Soc. Sci. Med.* 1982;16:1033–1038.
73. Evans L. K.: Sundown syndrome in institutionalized elderly. *J. Am. Geriatr. Soc.* 1987;35:101–108.
74. Williams M. A., Campbell E. B., Raynor W. J., et al: Predictors of acute confusional states in elderly hospitalized patients. *Res. Nurs. Health* 1985;8:31–40.
75. Daniel D. G., Rabin P. L.: Disguises of delirium. *South. Med. J.* 1985;78:666–672.
76. Dubin W. R., Weiss K. J., Zoccardi J. A.: Organic brain syndrome. The psychiatric imposter. *J.A.M.A.* 1983;249-60–62.
77. Perez E. L., Silverman M.: Delirium: The often overlooked diagnosis. *Int. J. Psychiatry Med.* 1984;14:181–189.
78. Trzepacz P. T., Teague G. B., Lipowski Z. J.: Delirium and other organic mental disorders in a general hospital. *Gen. Hosp. Psychiatry* 1985;7:101–106.
79. Richeimer S. H.: Psychological intervention in delirium. *Postgrad. Med.* 1987;81:173–180.
80. Blank K., Perry S.: Relationship of psychological processes during delirium to outcome. *Am. J. Psychiatry* 1984;141:843–847.
81. MacKenzie T. B., Popkin M. K.: Stress response syndrome occurring after delirium. *Am. J. Psychiatry* 1980;137:1433–1435.
82. Garner H.: Confrontation technique applied to confusional and delirious states. *Ill. Med. J.* 1970;137:71–73.
83. Godbole A., Falk M.: Confrontation—problem solving therapy in the treatment of confusional and delirious states. *Gerontologist* 1972;12:151–154.
84. Lipowski Z. J.: *Psychosomatic Medicine and Liaison Psychiatry. Selected Papers.* New York, Plenum, 1985.
85. Fogel B. S., Mills M. J., Landen J. E.: Legal aspects of the treatment of delirium. *Hosp. Commun. Psychiatry* 1986;37:154–158.
86. McLay W. D. S.: Impaired consciousness: Some grey areas of responsibility. *J. Forens. Sci. Soc.* 1977;17:113–120.
87. Dudley W. H. C., William J. G.: Electroconvulsive therapy in delirium tremens. *Compreh. Psychiatry* 1972;13:357–360.
88. Kramp P., Bolwig T. G.: Electroconvulsive therapy in acute delirious states. *Compreh. Psychiatry* 1981;22:368–371.
89. Lieser H.: Heilkrampfe als leben-rettende Therapie. *Med. Mschr.* 1957;6:350–358.
90. Roberts A. H.: The value of ECT in delirium. *Br. J. Psychiatry* 1963;109:653-655.
91. Roth M., Rosie J. M.: Use of electroplexy in mental disease with clouding of consciousness. *J. Ment. Sci.* 1953;99:103–110.

Part II

Organic Causes of Delirium

The more common organic causes of delirium are listed in Table 6–1. The purpose of this part is to draw attention to those substances and diseases whose association with the syndrome has been reported in the literature and that must be considered in order to establish its etiology in a given patient. The emphasis throughout is on distinct clinical features, if any, and on pathophysiological mechanisms, if known, as well as on specific aspects of management relevant to delirium associated with various organic factors. It's assumed that the reader is familiar with medical terminology. Consequently, clinical features, diagnosis, and treatment of the various medical conditions that can give rise to the syndrome will not be discussed, and only information directly pertinent to it will be provided. Clearly, this part cannot serve as a mini-textbook of medicine focused on delirium. I have tried to keep the chapters that follow as brief as possible and yet adequate for ready reference to the many organic factors that can cause delirium. Some of these factors cause delirium only rarely, but they may be implicated in an occasional patient and hence are practically important. Rather than overwhelm the reader with a mass of details, I have taken a selective approach and aimed at clarity and clinical usefulness.

11

Intoxication with Medical Drugs

Overdoses as well as therapeutic doses of many currently used drugs can give rise to delirium. These are the most common and important single cause of the syndrome, especially in later life. The elderly are particularly prone to develop delirium in response to even therapeutic doses of the most frequently used drugs. In the sections to follow, the agents that have been reported to cause delirium (listed in Table 6–1) will be discussed. Not all of them have the same deliriogenic potential, and some rarely cause the syndrome. They are included, however, to alert the clinician to the fact that an occasional patient may develop delirium as a result of using one of them, perhaps due to allergy or individual hypersensitivity (idiosyncrasy). Unless such a drug is withheld, the patient may continue to be delirious, and extensive, costly, and even hazardous investigations may be done in a vain attempt to identify the cause of the delirium. By contrast, drugs with anticholinergic properties have a high deliriogenic potential, which has been fully documented experimentally and clinically. These drugs will be discussed first, and in greater detail, because of their practical importance.

Anticholinergic agents

Belladonna alkaloids and synthetic drugs with anticholinergic properties are the single most important group of deliriogenic substances (1). Children and the elderly are particularly prone to develop delirium in response to even therapeutic doses of these drugs. A few scopolamine or atropine eye drops may induce delirium in some cases (2–5). The effectiveness of these agents in precipitating the syndrome has been conclusively documented by studies discussed in Chapter 7. Their clinical importance is related to their many therapeutic uses in medicine, surgery, and psychiatry; the availability of over-the-counter preparations containing anticholinergics; the tendency to abuse some of these drugs as benzhexol hydrochloride (Artane), in order to elicit a hallucinatory altered state of consciousness (6–8); and the widespread tendency to prescribe drugs with anticholinergic properties for the elderly (9–11). Anticholinergic delirium requires special treatment that differs from the treatment recommended for delirium due to most other factors. Neuroleptics, such as butyrophenones and phenothiazines, have anticholinergic effects and are consequently unsuitable for this purpose.

The propensity of belladonna alkaloids to cause delirium has been known since antiquity (12,13). Theophrastus described their deliriogenic potential in the fourth century B.C. as follows: "If you drink two drams, you will induce a greater madness; mind and eyes will see apparitions and startling fantasies. If you give three drams, he will labor under a madness from which he cannot free himself and ceaseless rages will ensue" (13, p 405). The term "belladonna" was introduced into scientific literature in the sixteenth century (13). Belladonna alkaloids were used for centuries for medicinal, religious, cosmetic, and homicidal purposes (12,13).

Belladonna alkaloids occur in plants of the Solanaceae family, which yield a mixture of the alkaloids atropine and scopolamine. Both of them, as well as their methylated derivatives, have had many uses in medicine. In addition, a large number of synthetic drugs with anticholinergic properties are currently available, including antidepressants, antiemetics, antihistamines, antiparkinsonian agents, antispasmodics, cycloplegics, and neurotropics (antipyschotics). All of these drugs have been reported to cause delirium at times.

Delirium induced experimentally by anticholinergic agents was discussed in Chapter 7. With an adequate dose, the syndrome was elicited in all subjects. This does not deny the fact that the effects of these drugs on the central nervous system (CNS) are to some extent variable and unpredictable (12). They cause both stimulation and depression of the CNS and give rise to what Longo (14) has called the "CNS anticholinergic syndrome." This term should not be taken to imply that delirium due to anticholinergic agents has unique psychopathological features that distinguish it from that due to all other etiological factors. This is far from true. There is no evidence for the occurrence of any distinct drug-specific deliria, whose psychopathological manifestations are diagnostic of the implicated agent. Studies of atropine, scopolamine, and Ditran have found that they produce qualitatively similar behavioral effects, but that they differ in their potency and relative central affinity, as well as the duration of their action (15). Scopolamine has central potency eight to nine times that of atropine. All three drugs, given in large doses to normal volunteers, produced initial drowsiness, which progressed to stupor and restlessness. Relatively large doses of atropine and scopolamine are needed to induce delirium in healthy subjects. Intramuscular doses of atropine (175 μg/kg) or scopolamine (25 μg/kg) are usually sufficient (15). Scopolamine, in a dose of 10 μg/kg administered intravenously, can trigger delirium (16). Ambient temperatures higher than the subject's body temperature, sleep loss, and pain all enhance the deliriogenic effect of this drug (15). Doses of atropine higher than 5–10 mg are usually needed to produce marked CNS effects. It is noteworthy, however, that in atropine toxicity therapy for schizophrenia, doses of up to 200 mg intramuscularly were used (17). With such high doses, delirium was induced first, followed by coma. Restlessness appeared within an hour after injection of the drug, accompanied by excitement, confusion, and hallucinations. The restless patients could usually be calmed by reassurance (17). Low to moderate doses of scopolamine (0.3–0.8 mg) produce sedation: restlessness tends to appear only after higher doses (16). In some cases, a paradoxical reaction may occur: a relatively low dose may give rise to excitement and restlessness (12).

Most of the experimental work on anticholinergic delirium has been carried out on healthy young adults, and even some of them displayed a higher than average propensity to develop it. In clinical practice, one must consider that *children* and the *elderly* are especially sensitive to the deliriogenic effects of anticholinergic agents. Even single doses of 1% scopolamine eye drops cause delirium in some patients (5); transdermal scopolamine may have the same effect (18). As few as 15 eye drops of 1% atropine solution, administered topically and containing 0.75 mg of atropine per drop, may give rise to delirium (4). Increased sensitivity to atropine in very young children (under the age of 2 years) and in the elderly has been partly explained by a prolonged elimination phase half-life of the drug (19). Anticholinergic agents tend to impair cognitive functioning in elderly, especially demented, patients (9–11). This is not suprising, since the central cholinergic system is generally affected in later life and even more so in dementia of the Alzheimer type; in addition, the anticholinergics impair both attention and memory in information processing (19, 20). Thus, the combination of altered pharmacokinetics, central cholinergic deficiency, and the effects of anticholinergics on the anatomical substrates of memory and arousal appears to render the elderly particularly vulnerable to delirium in response to even therapeutic doses of these agents. Apart from these age-related effects, elevated plasma anticholinergic activity is postively associated with postoperative delirium (21–23). This observation also implicates the central cholinergic system and its antagonists as important factors in the development of delirium.

The *diagnosis* of delirium due to anticholinergic agents is tentatively established when one or more of these drugs has recently been used and when phsyical examination reveals the presence of peripheral muscarinic blockade (24–26). The latter may suggest such a diagnosis if a history of drug exposure is absent or uncertain. Symptoms of anticholinergic intoxication are both physiological and psychological (26). The former include:

1. Dilated and poorly reactive or unreactive pupils
2. Flushed face
3. Dry skin and mucous membranes
4. Blurred vision
5. Tachycardia
6. Urinary retention
7. Elevated blood pressure
8. Diminished or absent bowel sounds
9. Increased respiratory rate
10. Fever

In addition, some patients display ataxia, dysphagia, dysarthria, muscle twitching, hyperreflexia, and convulsions (12,14–16,24–26). The psychological symptoms are those of an agitated delirium of some severity. In severe intoxication, the patient may develop coma, with hyperreflexia and extensor plantar reflexes. If the patient is an adolescent or an adult, a test dose of physostigmine salicylate may help establish the diagnosis (24,25). The drug is given intramuscularly or slowly (to avoid convulsions) intravenously in a dose of 1–2 mg. If no cholinergic signs appear and there is no change in the clinical picture within 30 minutes, the dose may be repeated. The pulse, bowel motility, and mental state change rapidly in response to physostigmine injection if anticholinergic intoxication is present (24). Thus, physostigmine salicylate offers a useful diagnostic aid in this condition.

Treatment of anticholinergic delirium involves administration of physostigmine salicylate (Antilirium). Kleinwächter (27) treated atropine delirium with Calabar extract, which contains physostigmine, and reported that the response of a severely intoxicated patient was so successful that the extract appeared to be a specific antidote to atropine. This remarkable clinical observation waited almost a century to be rediscovered. In 1949, Forrer (17) developed the so-called atropine toxicity therapy for schizophrenia and found that physostigmine, administered intravenously, could reverse both the central and peripheral effects of very high doses of atropine. In the 1960s, several writers reported excellent results in treating anticholinergic delirium with physostigmine and proposed that this drug could be used as an effective antidote against any drug possessing central anticholinergic activity (28,29).

Several authors (24–26) recommend the following procedure for treatment with physostigmine:

1. Evaluation of the patient, with special attention to vital signs, pupillary size and responsiveness to light, bowel sounds, urinary output, appearance of the skin, electrocardiogram, and mental status.
2. A diagnostic dose if the etiology is unknown and anticholinergic delirium is suspected. Physostigmine salicylate (Antilirium) in a dose of 1–2 mg is given intramuscularly or subcutaneously. If the patient had taken anticholinergic drugs, the peripheral signs of muscarinic blockade will change only slightly or not at all; in the absence of such intake, cholinergic signs should appear in 10–30 minutes, including lacrimation, miosis, sweating, salivation, and bradycardia.
3. Treatment proper begins with 1 or 2 mg of physostigmine given by intramuscular or slow intravenous injection. If no cholinergic signs or clinical changes follow in 15–30 minutes, a second injection of 1 or 2 mg should be given. If toxic signs persist or the patient relapses, further doses of physostigmine should be administered every 30 minutes to 2 hours. Treatment should be continued until the clinical state improves or cholinergic toxicity develops.
4. Monitor changes in pulse, electrocardiogram, temperature, bowel motility, urine output, orientation, and recent memory.
5. Support vital functions and reassure the patient.
6. Diazepam may be given in a mild case of anticholinergic intoxication or if physostigmine is not immediately available. An initial dose of 40 mg orally or 10 mg intramuscularly, to be followed by 10 mg every 4 hours, should provide adequate sedation; physostigmine administration is not always needed.
7. Watch for signs of cholinergic toxicity that may follow excessive or too rapid administration of physostigmine: bradycardia (heart block), respiratory paralysis, bronchospasm, laryngospasm, and (occasionally) seizures.
8. Atropine sulfate must be available to counteract cholinergic crisis and given intravenously in a dose of 0.5–1 mg.
9. Phenothiazines and haloperidol should not be used because of their anticholinergic properties;
10. In children and the elderly, the dosage of physostigmine should be about half of that for an adult: 0.5 mg by slow intravenous injection repeated, if necessary, at intervals of 5–20 minutes for a total of 2 mg (25, 30).

Contraindications to physostigmine include a history of coronary heart disease, asthma, peptic ulcer, diabetes, ulcerative colitis, mechanical obstruction of the bowel or bladder, glaucoma, pregnancy, hypothyroidism, and myotonia congenita and atrophica (25).

Physostigmine has been used not only to treat anticholinergic intoxication but also to reverse delirium, excessive sedation, and coma due to drugs lacking marked, if any, anticholinergic properties, such as amantadine (31), alcohol (32), benzodiazepines (33–36), cimetidine (37), phencyclidine (38), quinidine (39), and ranitidine (40). In a few cases, it has been reported to be effective in the treatment of delirium tremens (41). On the whole, however, physostigmine is recommended primarily in the more severe cases of anticholinergic delirium.

Explanatory hypotheses have been put forward to account for the pathogenesis of anticholinergic delirium and for the effectiveness of physostigmine in reversing it. On the basis of experimental studies carried out in the 1960s, Itil and Fink (42) have hypothesized that anticholinergic substances change the balance of noradrenergic and cholinergic mechanisms in the medial ascending reticular activating system and the medial thalamic diffuse projection systems. According to these authors, concurrent stimulation of these two systems results in a combination of cerebral cortical inhibition and excitation manifested clinically as delirium. The central cholinergic system plays a crucial rôle in learning and memory processes, as well as in attention (19,20,43, 44). Processing of both external and internal information is believed to be modulated by that system, which is activated by the midbrain reticular formation (45). Modifications of the cholinergic system by drugs impair the efficiency of information processing (20). Cholinergic mechanisms appear to be involved in the retention of recent events of transient importance (working memory) and in the retention of information with long-term importance (reference memory) (19). Anticholinergic agents reduce cortical desynchronization and arousal and interfere with acquistion of information (20). Experimental studies with scopolamine have led to the hypothesis that this drug has its primary effects on the retrieval of already stored information and interferes with the transfer of information from short- to long-term memory (46). Moreover, a single intravenous dose of scopolamine impairs psychomotor functions and causes sedation (47). It is possible that central cholinergic blockade by cholinolytic agents affects both the cholinergic neurons in the hippocampal structures involved in memory storage and the ascending cholinergic reticular system involved in cortical arousal. As a result, there is concurrent impairment of memory, as well as of alertness and wakefulness. The cognitive-attentional disturbances induced by cholinergic blockade appear to correspond to those that constitute the core psychopathology of delirium. However, performance tests on immediate memory span are not affected by anticholinergic agents (44), although they usually show impairment in delirium.

Physostigmine, by contrast, appears to improve memory by facilitating information input and by its short-term action on consolidation (20). It reverses the central cholinergic blockade brought about by the anticholinergic agents and has a general analeptic effect in cases of sedation due to substances that do not affect the cholinergic system (28,29,33,44,48). Moreover, physostigmine increases cerebral blood flow and oxygen consumption (35). In normal subjects, intravenous infusion of physostigmine induces a "physostigmine syndrome" marked by difficulty in thinking, decreased speech, psychomotor retardation, and depressed affect (49).

Anticholinergic delirium and its reversal by physostigmine, a cholinesterase inhibitor, are theroretically important, as they indicate a key role of cholinergic deficiency in the pathogenesis of at least some cases of delirium. Blass and Plum (50) hypothesize that a reduced rate of cerebral oxidative metabolism results in reduction of acetylcholine synthesis, and the consequent cholinergic deficiency is a common denominator in metabolic-toxic encephalopathies, one of whose manifestations is delirium.

Drugs with anticholinergic properties include the following major classes:

1. Anticholinergic premedicants
2. Antidepressants
3. Antiemetics
4. Antihistamines
5. Antiparkinsonian agents
6. Antipsychotics (neuroleptics)
7. Antispasmodics
8. Asthma powders
9. Cyclopegics and mydriatics
10. Proprietary hypnotics

Anticholinergic Premedicants

Atropine and scopolamine (hyoscine) have been widely used as part of premedication for reduction of secretions, protection against vagal overactivity, sedation, and amnesia (21–23,48,51,52). Scopolamine has been used since 1902 to produce "twilight sleep," or amnesia, during labor (53). Common doses for premedication are 0.6 mg of atropine and 0.4 mg of scopolamine (hyoscine) (51). The latter, but not the former, drug has been found to have detrimental effects on memory and on motor tasks (52). Delirium has been reported in 20% of patients premedicated with scopolamine (54) and in about 10% of women undergoing obstetric anesthesia (12). Several studies have found an association between plasma anticholinergic activity and postoperative delirium (21–23). Physostigmine has been used to reverse such delirium in surgical patients (48,54).

Antidepressants

Tricyclic antidepressants have anticholinergic properties and have been reported to produce delirium (24,25,55–65). Amitriptyline is particularly likely to do so and has actually been used to induce delirium experimentally. In one study, about 8% of 152 patients treated with this antidepressant became delirious (66). The combination of relatively potent anticholinergic activity and sedative properties is probably responsible for the propensity of this drug to cause delirium. Moreover, the probability of developing delirium appears to increase at higher plasma drug levels, i.e., above 450 ng/ml (62). The reported incidence of delirium in patients treated with tricyclic antidepressants ranges from 1.5% to 20% (60). A recent large-scale epidemiological study has found a lower incidence, i.e., about 1.2% (63). In a study of medically ill patients treated with these drugs, 16% became delirious; this was the most common major side effect (61). The risk of developing tricyclic delirium increases with age and is highest in patients aged 60 years and older (63). This finding underscores the sensitivity to the deliriogenic potential of anticholinergic agents in later life. It has been estimated that about 5% of elderly patients receiving amitriptyline or imipramine become delirious (67). Interestingly, delirium induced by tricyclics shows no signs of peripheral muscarinic blockade such as dilated pupils or urinary retention (6). This observation has led some writers to suggest that mechanisms other than anticholinergic blockade could be involved (67). The prevalent view, however, is that delirium due to tricyclic antidepressants represents central anticholinergic toxicity and can be reversed by physostigmine (24,25,57, 58,64).

In summary, delirium due to tricyclic antidepressants is relatively infrequent and is more likely to occur in the elderly. Both therapeutic doses and overdoses can precipitate it. In a case of overdosage it may precede or follow coma, or it may be the main behavioral manifestation of toxicity. Amitriptyline has the highest antimuscarinic potency, and hence the highest deliriogenic potential, of the tricyclic antidepressants.

Antiemetics

Benzquinamide (68) and meclizine (69) have been reported to produce delirium, which was successfully reversed by physostigmine (68).

Antihistamines

Dimenhydrinate (70,71), diphenhydramine (72–75), promethazine (76), tripelennamine (77), and other antihistamines (12,78) may cause delirium.

Antiparkinsonian agents

Benztropine, biperiden, trihexyphenidyl, and procyclidine have all been used for the treatment of extrapyramidal motor disorders and have been reported to cause delirium in some patients (12,79–88). Persons of all ages are susceptible to this complication and may develop it with therapeutic doses of these drugs (79). Individual hypersensitivity has been blamed in some cases (87). Antiparkinsonian agents have been subject to abuse for pleasurable effects by some patients (6–8,80,85,88). Benztropine mesylate is widely used to control the extrapyramidal side effects of psychotropic drugs, and most cases of delirium occur in patients receiving it in combination with one or more neuroleptics (79,87,88). The incidence of delirium due to benztropine among psychiatric patients is reported to be low (79). The syndrome may appear within several hours of the intake of the first dose and usually clears up within 1 week of drug withdrawal (79). As little as 2 mg of benztropine may precipitate delirium in some patients (79). As expected, the elderly, especially those who are demented, are particularly sensitive to the central anticholinergic effects of antiparkinsonian agents (84). Physostigmine has been used successfully to reverse delirium produced by these drugs (81).

Antipsychotics (neuroleptics)

Delirium induced by chlorpromazine and other phenothiazine derivatives used as antipsychotic agents has been reported since 1955 (89–94). A recent epidemiological study found the incidence of the syndrome to be about 1% in patients treated with these drugs (63). Delirium due to phenothiazine derivatives occurs most often in patients aged 50 years and older and in those who are brain-damaged (89,94). The deliriogenic potential of these drugs reflects their central cholinergic activity and sedative-hypnotic effects. Chlorpromazine, chlorprothixene, and thioridazine are particularly likely to cause delirium. High initial doses, as well as combinations of these drugs with other anticholinergic agents, predispose to its development (89,90). Thus, avoidance of polypharmacy should help prevent delirium in patients treated with neuroleptics. Lower doses of these drugs are generally advisable in the elderly and the demented.

Butyrophenones, the other major class of neuroleptics, appear to cause delirium very rarely. Only a handful of cases have been reported in patients receiving haloperidol (94–96). This drug is liable to induce the *neuroleptic malignant syndrome* more readily than any other neuroleptic (97–99). A potentially fatal complication of psychotropic drug use, this syndrome features hyperthermia and extrapyramidal symptoms; delirium occurs in about half of the cases (98).

Antispasmodics

Anticholinergic drugs are used as spasmolytics in a wide range of gastrointestinal disorders. Despite their widespread use, however, very few cases of delirium are believed to be caused by them (12,82,100,101).

Asthma powders

Belladonna alkaloids were used for the treatment of asthma in the past (12). Atropine sulfate administered by inhalation is still used occasionally and has been reported to cause delirium (102). Asthmador, a nonprescription preparation, contains both atropa and datura herbs, whose active principles are atropine and scopolamine. Other asthma powders containing these alkaloids are available as cigarettes or pipe mixture. While these preparations only occasionally cause delirium on inhalation for the relief of bronchospasm, they have been abused by the young and taken by mouth. One or two teaspoons of asthma powder were usually dissolved in cola drinks or beer or swallowed in capsules (102). In a study of 212 cases, hallucinations were reported in nearly one-half, and disorientation was found in about 20% (102). Delirium induced by Asthmador is similar to that caused by other anticholinergic agents (103).

Cycloplegics and mydriatics

Atropine, scopolamine, and cyclopentolate have been used in eye drops and have caused a number of cases of delirium (2–4,12,15,104). As mentioned earlier, even a small number of drops may induce delirium in children, in the elderly, and in persons who have idiosyncratic reactions to these drugs (2–4,12,15,104). It is believed that delirium due to eye drops occurs when they are swallowed in tears and absorbed from the intestinal tract or absorbed directly into the general circulation through the conjunctiva.

Proprietary hypnotics

Many nonprescription hypnotics contain small quantities of scopolamine (12,26,105,106). The three agents most often implicated in one study were Sominex, Nytol, and Sleepeze (106). All of these drugs can cause delirium if taken in accidental or deliberate overdoses (105).

Various herbal medicines containing atropine and scopolamine can cause delirium (107). Plants and mushrooms that cause anticholinergic toxicity will be discussed in the section on poisons.

Sedative-hypnotics

Sedative-hypnotic drugs are the medications most often prescribed today. The incidence of delirium caused by these drugs is unknown. It appears that intoxication, as defined in the current classification of mental disorders (108), is the most common organic mental syndrome induced. It features disturbances of perception, wakefulness, attention, thinking, judgment, emotional control, and psychomotor behavior (108). These disruptions also characterize delirium, and the boundary between these two syndromes is arbitrary. Hallucinations and delusions are often present in delirium but are not a feature of intoxication. Delirium, as currently defined, is a relatively uncommon complication of either acute or chronic poisoning with sedative-hypnotics and appears to occur most often in the elderly, especially those who are demented. Idiosyncratic reactions to these drugs are more likely to be manifested by paradoxical excitement or rage than by delirium. The latter, however, can result from withdrawal of the drug from an addict. Withdrawal syndromes are discussed in Chapter 12.

Barbiturates

These drugs were introduced in 1903; by 1905, delirium induced by barbital was reported (109). Subsequent reports of both acute and chronic barbital toxicity showed, however, that delirium was a relatively uncommon manifestation (109). Indeed, it is seen only occasionally in patients with chronic barbiturate intoxication (110). Acute poisoning by an overdose of barbiturates, or from hypersensitivity to them, typically results in coma; delirium may precede its onset and usually follows emergence from it. Moreover, delirium is more likely to occur when a barbiturate is taken in combination with alcohol or an anticholinergic agent. A barbiturate may precipitate an attack of acute intermittent porphyria or hepatic encephalopathy, and thus cause delirium indirectly. A similar effect may follow the intake of one of these drugs in a patient with chronic pulmonary or renal insufficiency or hypothyroidism. An elderly patient is particularly likely to become delirious while treated with a barbiturate (111); even a therapeutic dose can have this effect. Barbiturates have been largely displaced by benzodiazepines as the preferred sedative-hypnotics.

Chloral hydrate

This hypnotic was introduced in 1869 and is still widely used. Reports of its abuse appeared in the medical literature not long after its introduction (109).

Some famous men, such as Nietzsche and Rossetti, became addicted to it (112). Drowsiness with optic, often lilliputian, and auditory hallucinations are common features of chloral hydrate delirium (109). Threatening, and hence frightening, voices may be heard.

Paraldehyde

Introduced in 1881, this drug was occassionally abused by alcoholics. Delirium due to it has generally been reported in the German literature (109) and appears to be very rare today.

Bromides

These sedative-hypnotics were introduced in 1840 and were a common cause of delirium. In recent years, however, reports of bromism have been rare (113–115). Bromide delirium is usually preceded by intoxication for days or weeks and tends to last for several days after the drug has been discontinued (116). Occasionally, it may be followed by death or by a prolonged paranoid psychosis (116). A variety of visual symptoms are common in bromide delirium, including photophobia, dysmorphopsia, illusions, hallucinations, and delusions concerning the patient's eyes (117). Pupils are often dilated and react sluggishly to light. Other common neurological symptoms and signs include slurred speech, ataxia, positive Romberg test, absent gag reflex, tremor, nystagmus, extensor plantar reflexes, and ptosis (114,116,118). The EEG shows diffuse slowing of background activity that may persist for weeks or even months after resolution of the delirium (119,120). Cerebral blood flow is reduced (121), and a computed tomogram may show diffuse brain swelling (115). Diagnosis of bromide toxicity rests on measuring the serum bromide level. The normal level varies from 0.1 to 3.7 mg/100 ml (122). Intoxication may occur at levels as low as 60 mg/100 ml, but if delirium is manifest, levels of 150 mg/100 ml or higher are likely to be found (119). Hyperchloremia may be the first indication of bromism and can be demonstrated by autoanalyzer measurement of the serum chloride concentration (123). Treatment of bromide delirium involves administration of ammonium chloride, 6 g/day, and meralluride, 2 ml/day. A large chloride load enhances bromide excretion (114). Hemodialysis is needed only in very severe cases (114). Haloperidol may be used to control agitation. Symptoms often persist for a few weeks after the onset of treatment or recur episodically in response to rebound of serum bromide related to the movements of the bromide ion from intracellular and extracellular compartments as a result of the concentration gradient induced by diuresis (118). The prognosis is generally good.

Benzodiazepines

Introduced in 1960, these drugs are by far the most often used sedatives and hypnotics today (124–126). They have replaced barbiturates for the relief of anxiety and insomnia. Intoxication with these agents features daytime drowsiness, decreased mental acuity, ataxia, and memory impairment (124,125). "Confusion" is mentioned by some writers as a less common manifestation of benzodiazepine toxicity; reports of delirium are few and mostly involve triazolam (127–130). A study of over 1,00 patients seen in emergency wards as a result of benzodiazepine overdosage does not mention delirium as part of the clinical picture (131). The elderly are especially sensitive to the effects of benzodiazepine drugs, which may induce or aggravate global cognitive impairment in later life (132). Long-acting benzodiazepines, such as flurazepam, are particularly likely to have this effect (132,133) and should be avoided (134). Because the elimination half-lives of short- and intermediate-acting benzodiazepines, such as oxazepam, lorazepam, temazepam, alprazolam, and triazolam, are basically unchanged as a consequence of aging processes, their use is preferred in the elderly (133). The incidence of benzodiazepine delirium in older patients is unknown. Intoxication and reversible dementia appear to be the most common organic mental syndromes induced by these agents (132). Delirium due to benzodiazepine withdrawal seems to be more common than that due to their toxicity; it is discussed in Chapter 12.

Miscellaneous sedative-hypnotics

Meprobamate, glutethimide, methyprylon, ethchlorvynol, ethinamate, and methaqualone can all cause both acute and chronic intoxication resembling that due to barbiturates. All of these agents have addictive potential, and an abstinence syndrome, sometimes featuring delirium, may follow their abrupt withdrawal. Intoxication with these drugs is characterized by drowsiness, cognitive impairment, and ataxia. Disorientation, memory impairment, and confusion have been observed in some intoxicated patients (135). Delirium apparently due to glutethimide has been reported (136,137). This drug has some anticholinergic activity, and patients intoxicated with it show signs of peripheral muscarinic blockade (12). The use of these sedative-hypnotics has declined sharply in the past decade.

Antibiotic, antimalarial, antituberculous, antiviral, and antifungal drugs

Antibiotics

Most of the commonly used antibacterial agents, including sulfonamides, penicillin, streptomycin, chloromycetin, tobramycin, and rifampin, have been reported to cause delirium in an occasional patient (138). Delirium, with marked auditory hallucinations and persecutory delusions, in a girl who received penicillin intramuscularly and orally for 10 days was reported in 1948 (139). The patient became delirious 4 days after developing what seemed to be serum sickness. In the past 40 years, a number of reports on delirium in the course of penicillin treatment have been published (140–145). Five clinical syndromes associated with procaine penicillin have been described: 1. cerebral edema of allergic origin; 2. toxic encephalopathy; 3. hypersensitivity to penicillin with fever; 4. paranoid psychosis in patients with general paresis treated with procaine penicillin; and 5. an acute, brief, nonallergic, acute psychotic reaction (140). Penicillin may induce delirium when administered intravenously in very high doses (144). The acute, non-allergic, psychotic reaction (Hoigne's syndrome) is probably due to an effect of procaine on the limbic system (142). *Chloramphenicol* administered orally has induced delirium on occasion (146). Patients with typhoid who received this drug tended to develop the syndrome when they were afebrile and the infection seemed to be under control (146). A hyperanabolic state, like that seen in the early stages of convalescence from infection or trauma, may pre-dispose to chloramphenicol delirium, due either to the drug's inhibitory effect on protein synthesis or to hepatic injury (146). Administration of large doses of vitamins has been recommended to counteract the appearance of chlor-amphenicol neurotoxicity. Delirium in association with ototoxicity has been reported following intravenous administration of *erythromycin* (147). The use of *cephalosporins* in patients with renal insufficiency has produced delir-ium in some cases (138). Isolated cases of the syndrome have occurred in response to *streptomycin* (148), *gentamicin* (149), *cephalexin* (150), *griseo-fulvin* (151), *tobramycin* (152), *rifampin* (153), and *metronidazole* (154).

Antimalarial drugs

Behavioral toxicity has been reported with quinacrine (Atabrine), *chloro-quine,* and other antimalarial drugs (155). Psychotic reactions are said to occur in about 4 per 1,000 patients treated with *quinacrine.* It appears that two distinct syndromes are involved: a paranoid psychosis similar to that observed with sympathomimetic stimulants and delirium (156–159). In the latter, the patients are typically agitated, restless, hallucinated, and delu-sional; convulsions may occur. An agitated paranoid psychosis may be fol-lowed by delirium, whose onset can be rapid or insidious (157).

Chloroquine was initially believed to be less neurotoxic than quinacrine, but this appears not to be so: its effects can be not only deliriogenic but also lethal (160). Seizures and death may follow intoxication with this widely used drug. Delirium produced by it typically features severe anxiety, aggressiveness, and depression with suicidal tendencies, i.e., symptoms that can mask cognitive impairment and lead to the misdiagnosis of a functional psychosis (160).

Antituberculous drugs

Three drugs used for chemotherapy of tuberculosis may cause mental disorders: isoniazid, cycloserine, and ethionamide (12,161). As these drugs are usually administered in combination, it is not easy to identify the offending agent when psychosis develops.

Isoniazid (INH) can give rise to two types of behavioral toxicity: a schizophrenia-like psychosis and delirium (12,162). Pyridoxine, 1 g intravenously, has been used successfully to treat INH overdosage (163). INH competitively inhibits the action of coenzymes produced in the body from pyridoxine; this inhibition is believed to account for the drug's neurotoxicity (161). Delirium due to INH may feature marked persecutory delusions and hence may be mistaken for a paranoid psychosis. It can persist for several weeks after discontinuation of the drug (12). *Cycloserine* may cause nervousness, insomnia, nightmares, difficulty in concentrating, seizures, and delirium (164). *Ethionamide* rarely gives rise to delirium (165).

Antiviral drugs

Acyclovir has occasionally been reported to cause delirium in patients receiving marrow transplants and it those treated for herpesvirus infections (166). The same effect has been observed in patients receiving *vidarabine* (167,168).

Antifungal drugs

Delirium, with diffuse slowing of the EEG, may occur during intrathecal administration of *amphotericin B* for coccidioidomycosis and histoplasmosis (169,170).

Anticonvulsant drugs

All the currently used anticonvulsant drugs can cause behavioral toxicity (171–174). *Carbamazepine* (173), *diphenylhydantoin* (171,172), *ethosuximide* (171,172), *phenobarbitone* (171,172), *primidone* (171,172), and *sodium valproate* (174) may all produce intoxication manifested by some degree of cognitive impairment, drowsiness, bradykinesia, and signs of cerebellar dysfunction. It appears that simple intoxication is the most common organic mental syndrome complicating treatment with these drugs, and one that may merge imperceptibly with a reversible dementia. Delirium seems to be distinctly uncommon. The mental symptoms of both acute and chronic anticonvulsant toxicity are related to the serum levels of the antiepileptic drugs rather than to their actual daily dosage (172). Susceptibility to the toxic effects of these agents shows striking individual differences. Some epileptic patients develop mental symptoms with therapeutic drug serum levels and in the absence of the usual signs of toxicity, such as nystagmus and ataxia. Adverse mental effects of diphenylhydantoin, phenobarbitone, and primidone have been postulated to result from interference with normal folate metabolism (172). Consequently, when a patient taking anticonvulsants develops cognitive impairment, one should check both the serum drug levels and those of folate and vitamin B_{12}.

Antiparkinsonian agents

Drugs with anticholinergic activity that are used in the treatment of Parkinson's disease are discussed in the section on anticholinergic agents. The drugs most commonly used for the control of parkinsonism, i.e., amantadine, bromocriptine, and levodopa, have all been reported to cause delirium (175–186).

Amantadine produces delirium in an occasional patient (175–177). The syndrome is more likely to complicate treatment with *bromocriptine* (178–183). In one series, about 20% of patients treated with this drug developed "mental changes," either delirium or a schizophreniform psychosis (179). Seven of the 10 patients who became delirious had prior evidence of a mild dementia. Even a low dose of bromocriptine can precipitate delirium in a susceptible patient (178). Older patients, especially those with dementia, are more likely to become delirious while taking this drug (179).

Levodopa has been reported to produce delirium in 4% to 13% of parkinsonian patients (12,184). The true incidence of this complication is unknown, however, since the various published reports use undefined terms such as "organic brain syndrome," "psychosis," "delirium," "confusion," or "psychiatric disturbances." A typical statement asserts that the most common mental side effect of levodopa is a set of symptoms resembling an organic brain syndrome, one with "predominance of confusion and disorientation, sometimes progressing to frank delirium" (12, p 156). In one report, delirium was observed to occur in 6 of 45 patients treated with the drug (184). Five of those six patients had shown evidence of a mild chronic organic mental syndrome (presumably dementia) prior to the initiation of levodopa treatment. Delirium developed after about 4 months of therapy, was often associated with dyskinetic movements, and cleared after discontinuation or dose reduction of the drug (184).

Sroka et al. (185) evaluated 93 levodopa-treated parkinsonian patients for the presence of an organic mental syndrome. Transient episodes of confusion occurred in one-third of the patients classified as having "typical" Parkinson's disease. Those episodes were dose dependent and related to the duration of levodopa therapy, and occurred significantly more often in patients with abnormal computed tomography scans. It was suggested that acute confusional states in a patient with "typical" parkinsonism indicate that some degree of cerebral atrophy is present.

Nausieda et al. (186) observed prominent sleep abnormalities in 100 parkinsonian patients. They proposed that fragmentation of the sleep-wake cycle and of sleep architecture, as well as altered dreaming, precede the development of the levodopa delirium. These investigators postulated that chronic administration of levodopa induces depression of central serotonin levels, ultimately resulting in serotonergic supersensitivity and consequent sleep fragmentation and delirium. This interesting hypothesis links sleep pathology with delirium and suggests a possible pathogenetic mechanism for that syndrome. An alternative hypothesis is that elevated dopamine levels in the brain and consequent excessive dopaminergic activity in the limbic structures may result in delirium. This issue remains unresolved and intriguing. Tryptophan has been tried in an effort to treat levodopa delirium, but the results have been unimpressive (187). It is interesting to note that delirium has occurred in patients given tryptophan, especially in combination with monamine oxidase inhibitors (188).

Bismuth salts

Bismuth *subnitrate* and *subgallate* may cause delirium (189–192). In one study, 45 patients developed "encephalopathy" while being treated with bismuth subnitrate for a colonic disorder over periods ranging from 1 month to 30 years (192). All of the patients had bismuth blood levels of about 150 μg/l (normal, less than 20 μg/l). They initially suffered from insomnia, visual hallucinations, anxiety, and depression, followed by a rapid onset of delirium. The EEG showed generalized slowing of the background activity, absence of alpha waves, and low-voltage beta rhythm. The majority of the EEG records returned to normal within 3 months (192).

All bismuth salts may induce the above features, including delirium. Bismuth may be absorbed through the skin when used as a cream (191). In the brain, it inactivates thiol groups of enzymes and induces diminished utilization of oxygen and glucose and increased production of lactate. Bismuth may also damage the blood-brain barrier and thus increase its permeability (191). CBF becomes reduced. In some cases of bismuth delirium, patients displayed total insomnia (189). They experienced vivid visual, auditory, and gustatory hallucinations, especially during the night. Recovery followed within 3 months of the cessation of bismuth therapy.

Cardiac and antihypertensive drugs

Digitalis

Delirium due to digitalis was first reported by Durozier in 1874 and many times since (12). Some authors have questioned whether digitalis as such ever causes the syndrome and suggested that congestive heart failure alone could account for it (12,193). King (194) argued, however, that it was unusual to see agitated delirium in a cardiac patient who was not receiving digitalis. One may tentatively conclude that the drug does produce delirium in some patients. Digitalis is a neuroexcitatory drug whose extracardiac toxic effects, as well as the cardiac arrhythmias induced by it, are likely to reflect activation of the CNS (195). The neuropsychiatric side effects of digitalis occur with doses similar to those that precipitate cardiac arrhythmias, and may precede, accompany, or follow them. In some cases, delirium may occur without any other evidence of digitalis intoxication (196). The latter is strongly associated with the use of diuretics and occurs in 20% to 25% of hospitalized patients treated with digitalis (197). Neurological symptoms develop in 40% to 50% of patients with clinical digitalis intoxication (198). The incidence of delirium in this context is unknown, but the syndrome is most likely to occur in elderly patients (198–201). Psychiatric patients are particularly vulnerable to digitalis toxicity if they receive lithium, have electrolyte imbalance, or show increased autonomic nervous system arousal (202). Both therapeutic doses (199) and overdoses (203) may induce delirium.

Any digitalis preparation may be potentially deliriogenic. Both digoxin and digitoxin have been reported to precipitate delirium. The former drug can pass the blood-brain barrier (12). Serum digoxin levels in excess of 2 ng/ml are liable to be toxic (12). The more common neuropsychiatric symptoms of digitalis toxicity include visual disturbances and formed hallucinations, weakness, drowsiness, dizziness, restlessness, insomnia, nightmares, anxiety, depression, hyperactivity, and seizures (12,198,204,205). The development of such symptoms in a patient receiving digoxin should immediately suggest the possibility that delirium is about to occur or is already present. Serum levels of digoxin must be determined without delay; if they are found to be in the toxic range, the dosage should be reduced or the drug discontinued. Neuropsychiatric symptoms may be the earliest sign of potentially lethal digoxin toxicity. If agitated delirium does develop, haloperidol may be used to control the agitation (202). One should keep in mind that delirium in this context may be partly due to other factors, such as diuretics or antiarrhythmic drugs, hypokalemia, hypoxemia, hypothyroidism, or renal insufficiency (205). These potentially contributory deliriogenic factors must be corrected.

Antiarrhythmic agents

Neuropyschiatric side effects, including delirium, may complicate treatment with virtually all antiarrhythmic agents, both old and new (12,198,206). *Amiodarone* (198,206), *flecainide* (198,206), *lidocaine* (198,206–208), *lorcainide* (209), *mexiletine* (206), *phenytoin* (198), *procainamide* (210), *quinidine* (211,212), and *tocainide* (213) all cause a variety of neuropsychiatric complications, including hallucinations and frank delirium. These side effects reflect drug idiosyncrasy or dose-related toxicity, or both. Delirium is an uncommon complication of antiarrhythmic therapy, with the possible exception of lidocaine therapy (198,206–208). Some 15% of patients treated with this drug develop toxic reactions (198). Fear of impending death or the delusion that death has actually occurred ("doom anxiety") is reportedly a characteristic feature of lidocaine toxicity (208).

Antihypertensive drugs

Neuropsychiatric side effects can complicate therapy with most of the currently used antihypertensive drugs (198,214). These toxic effects are believed to be due to overdosage, chronic effects on the sympathetic nervous system, or drug interaction (198). *Beta-adrenergic receptor blocking agents,* notably *propranolol* and its analogues, have been reported to induce a visual or tactile organic hallucinosis, vivid dreams, depression, and delirium (198,214,215–221). The incidence of neuropsychiatric toxicity from propranolol varies widely in published studies, ranging from one 1% to over 20% (215). The prevalence of depression in patients treated with this drug is no higher than that in control patients (215). Delirium has been reported in isolated cases of propranolol treatment but appears to be rare (216–221). The drug is lipophilic and readily crosses the blood-brain barrier. The mechanism of propranolol-induced delirium is unknown. The drug increases delta and fast activity in the EEG and reduces alpha activity (222). *Timolol,* another beta-adrenergic blocker used topically to reduce intraocular pressure, has been reported to cause "confusion" in 14% of CNS toxicity cases (223–225).

Alpha-adrenergic receptor blocking agents, notably *clonidine,* have also been reported to induce delirium occasionally (226–228). *Methyldopa* stimulates central adrenergic receptors and reduces the sympathetic outflow from the CNS (198). It depletes the brain of noradrenaline and serotonin. Several reports of depression, impairment of cognitive functioning, and delirium have been published (229–231). In one case, the onset of delirium was apparently facilitated by the concurrent administration of *haloperidol* (231). Both of these drugs block central dopamine receptors, and this synergistic activity may produce delirium in an occasional patient.

The calcium channel blockers, such as *nifedipine* and *verapamil,* cause delirium in a few cases (232–234). The same statement applies to *sodium nitroprusside* (214). *Diuretics,* such as *acetazolamide* (235), rarely precipitate delirium, which is probably secondary to metabolic acidosis. Elderly patients and those with hepatic disease are particularly vulnerable.

Contrast agents

Neuropsychiatric adverse effects, including delirium, can occur following the use of radiological contrast agents, notably *metrizamide* (234–243). In two studies, 7% to 10% of patients who had received metrizamide for myelography displayed a "pronounced organic psychosis" (243) or "confusion" (240). Mild impairment of cognition occurs transiently in a substantial proportion of patients given this contrast medium (236) and is less common in those given *iohexol* instead (236,242). Delirium usually appears within 24 hours, occurs more often after cervical and thoracic than lumbar myelography, and clears within several hours to days. A variety of neurological signs, such as asterixis, diplopia, and transient aphasia, may accompany the delirium. The EEG changes occur in about 15% to 35% of patients given metrizamide and feature diffuse slowing and, less often, transient spike activity (235,237,241). It has been postulated that metrizamide brings about the neuropsychiatric side effects by impairing brain glucose metabolism (235). Some patients display an organic hallucinosis rather than delirium (240,243). The latter has also been reported in elderly patients following arteriography with *meglumine iothalamate* (239).

Corticosteriods

Psychotic reactions to corticosteroids were often reported during the decade 1950–1960. Since then, the number of reports has dropped. This decline may reflect the lower incidence of psychosis with the currently used drugs, such as prednisone and prednisolone, compared to cortisone and adrenocorticotropic hormone (ACTH), the drugs used in the 1950s. Prednisone is the most often used corticosteroid drug; the incidence of associated psychosis is about 3% (244). With doses exceeding 80 mg/day, however, psychiatric complications occur in about 18% of patients (244).

The nature of the steroid psychoses has been the subject of some controversy. Are they mostly affective, schizophreniform, or delirious? Glaser (245), in an early report, distinguished two types of psychosis: a primary affective disorder, either depressive or manic, and an organic reaction (toxic psychosis) with associated affective or paranoid-hallucinatory features, or both. A more recent review asserts that depression is the major form of mental disturbance induced by corticosteroids (244). About 15% of the reported reactions represented a hallucinatory-delusional psychosis (244). Some authors have pointed out that the majority of patients experience several types of psychotic symptoms, including confusion, in the course of a single psychotic episode; this makes classification of steroid-related mental disorders difficult (246). Clark et al. (247) maintained that the steroid psychoses lacked such features of delirium as confusion, memory impairment, and disorientation, instead exhibiting affective and schizophrenia-like symptomatology. This issue remains ambiguous, as does the incidence of delirium, if any, in patients treated with corticosteroids.

The EEG findings in steroid psychoses are also variable. In one series, about one-half of the records displayed some slowing of the background activity, but such changes could also occur in the absence of manifest psychopathology (245). The most frequently observed EEG changes in steroid psychoses include decreases in the amplitude and frequency of alpha activity, bursts of beta waves, and increased beta activity (248).

Several predisposing and facilitating factors have been claimed to increase the probability of steroid psychosis. They include high dosage, female sex, rapid increase in the dose or abrupt discontinuation of the drug, and coexistence of brain damage or disease of any etiology (244,248). Moreover, a mental disturbance is more likely to occur with cortisone or dexamethasone than with prednisone or prednisolone (248). It is noteworthy that withdrawal of corticosteroid drugs may precipitate a mental disturbance, which can take the form of delirium (249–251).

The pathophysiology of steroid psychoses has been the subject of much speculation, but no firm conclusions can be drawn (244). Relevant hypotheses have focused on electrolyte imbalance, increased excitability of the brain, and decreased cerebral serotonin level (12,244,252). Patients receiving corticosteroids frequently suffer from sleep-wake cycle disruption and sleep fragmentation (252). Prednisone has been found to reduce total REM sleep, to increase REM latency, and to induce intermittent awakening (12). These effects on the sleep-wake cycle have been ascribed to an increase in noradrenaline and alterations in central serotonergic activity (252). Such sleep disturbances can facilitate the development of delirium due to any organic factor. It must be concluded that we do not yet understand the pathogenesis of steroid psychoses.

Treatment of steroid psychosis involves gradual reduction of the dosage and either discontinuation of the drug or substitution of a different steroid. If the physician believes that continued steroid therapy is necessary, the dose should be reduced and the psychosis treated with haloperidol. Patients who become psychotic in the course of systemic lupus erythematosus treated with steroids sometimes present a diagnostic and therapeutic dilemma. Is the psychosis due to the drug or to the disease? Computed tomography and the EEG may aid the diagnosis of cerebral lupus. If it appears that the mental disturbance is caused by the lupus, steroids should be continued and the agitation and other psychotic symptoms should be treated with haloperidol.

Cytotoxic chemotherapeutic agents

After depression, delirium is the second most common psychiatric disorder encountered in cancer patients (253). In a substantial proportion of cases, delirium is a complication of cancer chemotherapy, since most of the more than 60 cytotoxic agents in current use have neurotoxic side effects (254–257). Limitations of space preclude a detailed discussion of the reported deliriogenic potential of all these drugs, and only the most important of them can be mentioned here. Readers are referred to appropriate reviews for more information (254–257).

L-Asparaginase may induce delirium accompanied by slowing of the EEG. In one series, 5 of 19 patients developed this complication (258). Delirium came on between days 2 and 19 after the initial injection, and the patients displayed a fluctuating level of consciousness and cognitive impairment. A change in mental status ranging from lethargy to coma was seen in 63% of patients treated with L-asparaginase who developed cerebrovascular complications, such as hemorrhage or thrombosis, during treatment (259). Such complications occur in 1% to 2% of patients and are some of the possible causes of delirium (259). Cerebral dysfunction or encephalopathy, including an acute confusional state, has been reported to occur in about 20% to 60% of patients treated with this agent (255). It may be due to toxic metabolic products, such as L-aspartate, L-glutamate, or ammonia, or to brain depletion of L-asparagine (255,258). Most patients are able to continue treatment despite persistent mild confusion or drowsiness, or both (255). The EEG returns to normal after the drug is stopped (255). In some cases, a delayed form of cerebral dysfunction and a subacute organic mental syndrome may follow treatment with L-asparaginase (255).

Cisplatin may precipitate delirium as a result of magnesium depletion (260). *Cytarabine* and related pyrimidine compounds may cause encephalopathy, notably when used in high doses (255,261). *Fluorouracil* and its analogue, *ftorufar,* may induce delirium, as well as an acute cerebellar sydrome (255,262). *Hexamethylenamine* has been reported to induce hallucinations, depression, and an acute encephalopathy (presumably delirium) in some patients (255). Similar psychotoxic effects have been reported with *isophosphamide* (257).

Immune reagents, such as interferon and interleukin-2, have recently been added to the treatment of cancer. They reportedly cause delirium and diffuse slowing of the EEG in some patients (263–266). Neuropsychiatric symptoms were displayed in one-half of the patients treated with *interleukin-2* and lymphokine-activated killer cells (263). These side effects usually developed toward the end of each treatment phase and appeared to be dose dependent. Treatment was the same as for delirium generally, and all patients recovered. The cause of the syndrome in these cases remains unknown (263). Delirium has also been observed during the treatment of cancer and viral hepatitis with *interferon* (264–266). Its development appears to be dose related, can disrupt therapy, and may be accompanied by suicidal tendencies (264). The pathogenesis of interferon-related delirium is unknown.

Methotrexate can cause both transient and permanent encephalopathy (255,267,268). As many as 60% of patients in some series developed meningeal irritation and arachnoiditis several hours after intrathecal methotrexate therapy (255). Stiff neck, headaches, fever, and lethargy characterize this side effect, which is probably a delirium. Dementia is a feature of methotrexate-induced leukoencephalopathy (255). Widespread depression of cerebral glucose metabolism was observed in a case of acute encephalopathy induced by high-dose methotrexate chemotherapy (267). There was associated EEG slowing. It appears that the drug can alter the blood-brain barrier and exert a direct neurotoxic effect, which may involve reduced glucose phosphorylation (267). PET scanning may help distinguish acute methotrexate encephalopathy from chronic leukoencephalopathy (267).

Procarbazine has been reported to cause somnolence and confusion in about 10% of patients given the drug orally (255). This side effect appears to represent delirium. The drug readily crosses the blood-brain barrier and inhibits the enzyme monoamine oxidase (269). Patients who are delirious from procarbazine should not be treated with phenothiazines, since it has a synergistic sedative effect with these drugs (269).

The *vinca alkaloids,* vincristine, vindesine, and vinblastine, may cause delirium (255,270). One of the effects of *vincristine* on the CNS is the excessive release of antidiuretic hormone, resulting in hyponatremia and delirium (270). Delirium may also occur in patients who have received accidental overdoses of the drug (270). Vincristine neurotoxicity is related to the dose and the frequency of administration. Patients older than 60 years are more susceptible to this effect than younger ones (270). *Vinblastine* is reported to cause depression or anxiety rather than delirium (256). Both this drug and *vindesine* have neurotoxic side effects similar to those of vincristine, but their neurotoxic potential is lower (255).

Disulfiram

Disulfiram (Antabuse), used in the treatment of alcoholism, induces delirium only on rare occasions (271). In the past, this drug was used in higher doses

(1–2 g/day), and a "reversible toxic encephalopathy" was reported to occur in 2% to 20% of patients treated with it (272). Delirium accounted for 75% of the psychotic reactions (273). More recently, much lower doses (250 mg) of disulfiram have been used, and the incidence of delirium caused by it has dropped drastically (271). Occasional reports of this complication do appear, however (274,275). An overdose of the drug may cause delirium (276).

The onset of disulfiram delirium may follow initiation of therapy by days to months. Prodromal symptoms, such as concentration difficulties, forgetfulness, anxiety, depression, and drowsiness, frequently precede the onset of the syndrome, which often features delusions; hallucinations are less common (277). Concurrent neurological signs may include ataxia, slurred speech, tremor, and Babinski reflexes (277). The EEG shows diffuse slowing. Seizures may occur. The delirium lifts a few days to weeks after discontinuation of disulfiram. Several mechanisms have been proposed to account for it: impaired oxygen consumption, accumulation of carbon disulfide, and increased cerebral dopamine concentration (277,278). The drug inhibits beta-hydroxylase and dopamine beta-hydroxylase (277). Treatment involves withdrawal of disulfiram and administration of haloperidol (277).

Histamine H_2-receptor antagonists

Following the introduction of *cimetidine* in 1976, a spate of letters to the editors of several journals reported delirium as a side effect of this drug (279,280). A worldwide survey of the adverse effects of this drug found, however, that this complication was uncommon, occurring in only 1.1 per 100,000 patients treated (281). Moreover, a review of over 800 documented cases of cimetidine overdosage concluded that it is not accociated with serious toxicity; delirium was not even mentioned (282). Cimetidine delirium is more likely to occur in the elderly and the very young, and in patients with hepatic or renal dysfunction, or both (283). Higher doses are also more likely to cause this adverse effect (283). Cimetidine is largely eliminated through the kidney; its elimination half-life is prolonged in the elderly and in those with renal insufficiency (284). In one study of severely ill patients treated with the drug, 17% developed delirium (285). These patients had both renal and hepatic dysfunction. A reduced dose is usually necessary in such patients. Delirium can occur 2 hours to 3 days after initiation of cimetidine therapy by either the oral or the intravenous route, and reverses within 2 days after discontinuation of the drug (286). The EEG may show diffuse slowing, with or without bursts of fast-wave activity (287). Some patients are lethargic and drowsy, while others are agitated, restless, hallucinating, and combative (286). Associated physical signs include slurred speech, dizziness, flushing, sweating, tachycardia, and dilated pupils (283,286).

The pathophysiology of cimetidine delirium is not fully understood. The syndrome may result from blockage of H_2 receptors in the CNS, notably in the mesencephalic reticular formation and posterior mamillary bodies (283,287). Histamine serves as a neurotransmitter and exerts a depressant action on the reticular activating system (283). Physostigmine has been used successfully in the treatment of cimetidine delirium (37). On the other hand, the syndrome may not respond to haloperidol (288). Discontinuation of the drug is usually sufficient.

Ranitidine is much less likely to cause delirium than cimetidine, but this side effect has occasionally been reported (40,289).

Lithium

Delirium is a common manifestation of lithium neurotoxicity that has been reported since the introduction of the drug to psychiatry in 1949 (290–293). A review of the over 200 published case reports of acute lithium toxicity occurring between 1948 and 1984 found that "impaired consciousness" (presumably delirium) was manifested by about 30% of the patients (291). Mild neurotoxicity features drowsiness, tremor, hypertonia, hyperreflexia, dysarthria, ataxia, muscle fasciculations, and nystagmus. More severe neurotoxicity is manifested by delirium and lethargy, and may progress to stupor, coma, and seizures (291). The EEG typically shows diffuse slowing (291). Delirium may occur at both therapeutic and toxic serum lithium levels. Levels above 2.0 mEq/l are usually toxic and hence more likely to precipitate the syndrome (294). Severe neurotoxicity often develops in the first week after initiation of treatment, unless an acute overdose has been ingested. Delirium tends to persist for up to 2 weeks after cessation of lithium therapy (294). In recent years, lower doses of the drug have been found to be therapeutically effective and its average 12-hour serum concentration is lower than in the past, i.e., about 0.7 mEq/L (295). As a result, side effects have become less frequent and less severe (295). Avoidance of acute intoxication is important, since in about 10% of patients persistent neurological sequelae, usually in the form of cerebellar dysfunction, may follow (296). A finding of generalized or paroxysmal EEG slowing in a patient receiving lithium, in the absence of other potential causes, should alert the clinician to the possibility of a current or impending neurotoxicity (297).

A number of factors have been postulated to promote lithium neurotoxicity: *Age* over 65 years is likely to be associated with more severe drug neurotoxicity (298). Changes in lithium pharmacokinetics have been observed in the elderly and indicate the need for lower doses in these patients (299). *Brain disease* is another putative factor, although the evidence is equivocal (292). *Sodium deficiency* leads to lithium retention and hence predisposes to neurotoxicity. The concurrent use of diuretics, with sodium depletion and dehydration, may have this effect (291). *Concomitant physical illness,* such as a febrile illness, renal insufficiency, and congestive heart failure, increases the risk of lithium neurotoxicity (292). *Drug interaction* is another important factor. Concurrent administration of phenothiazines, haloperidol, diuretics, nonsteroidal anti-inflammatory drugs, and methyldopa increases the susceptibility to lithium-induced delirium (291,292,300–302). *Psychiatric diagnosis* is also relevant. Schizophrenic and schizoaffective patients are more likely to develop neurotoxicity when treated with lithium than manic-depressives (292).

Several pathogenetic mechanisms have been proposed to account for the adverse neuropsychiatric effects of lithium. The ion blocks the release of noradrenaline and dopamine in the brain; it may alter the distribution of other ions, such as sodium, potassium, magnesium, and calcium; and it inhibits inositol phosphatase in cell membranes, and thus the formation of polyphosphoinositides that may mediate the action of acetylcholine and noradrenaline (124). None of these putative actions, however, can adequately account for lithium-induced delirium. The EEG changes indicate that the drug may have a direct toxic effect on the brain. It has been suggested that these changes may reflect thyroid dysfunction (297).

Treatment of lithium delirium involves reduction of the dose or discontinuation of the drug, correction of fluid and electrolyte imbalances, and symptomatic therapy. There are few contraindications to the use of haloperidol to control agitation. Careful monitoring of the symptoms of toxicity, of lithium serum levels, and of the EEG is indicated in patients known to be predisposed to the drug's neurotoxic potential. Concurrent use of the drugs that enhance that potential, notably diuretics, should be avoided.

Narcotic analgesics

Morphine rarely appears to cause delirium (109). *Meperidine,* on the other hand, was found to induce symptoms suggestive of the syndrome in 0.4% of 3,634 hospitalized medical patients (303). Very few reports explicitly referring to meperidine-induced delirium have been published, however (304,305). Some authors have suggested that the drug may induce the syndrome as a consequence of the anticholinergic activity of its active metabolite, normeperidine (304). Physostigmine has been used to reverse the delirium (304). Concurrent use of anticholinergic drugs can increase the risk of its development (304). Delirium may occur after only two or three injections of meperidine for pain relief; it features visual and auditory hallucinations, delusions, and agitation (304,305).

Pentazocine can induce delirium, but its incidence appears to be quite low.

Shortly after its introduction in 1967, reports of hallucinations and delirium began to appear (306–311). The incidence of neuropsychiatric side effects after therapeutic doses of the drug has been reported to range from 1% to 10% (308,309). The patients experience disorientation, hallucinations, "bizarre feelings," nightmares, and confusion (308,310). The poor quality of the published reports makes it difficult to decide whether the observed toxic symptoms represent delirium or some other organic mental syndrome such as hallucinosis. Unequivocal cases of pentazocine-induced delirium have been reported, however (307,311). The neurotoxic effects of the drug may be related to a rapid depletion of brain noradrenaline and dopamine (307). Pentazocine has been abused and a withdrawal syndrome can occur, but it does not feature delirium (307,310).

Propoxyphene rarely appears to cause delirium (312). The drug can lead to dependence, abuse, and withdrawal symptoms. An overdose can be fatal, as it causes CNS depression, which is manifested as coma and seizures rather than as delirium. *Methadone* also rarely causes the syndrome. I have not come across any reports of delirium due to *codeine.* Two new analgesics, *butorphanol,* and *nalbuphine,* are reported to induce "confusion" in about 1% of cases (312).

Nonnarcotic analgesics

Acetaminophen (paracetamol) in an overdose may cause acute hepatic necronecrosis and encephalopathy with delirium (313,314). Side effects with normal doses are rare, but a case of delirium following administration of therapeutic doses of a mixture of this drug and chlorzoxazone in a healthy young male has been reported (315).

Aspirin is among the most commonly used drugs. Salicylate poisoning is diagnosed in about 10% to 15% of patients admitted to poisoning centers (316). Intoxication with salicylates (salicylism) may be acute or chronic. Acute toxicity is usually either accidental or the result of an overdose taken in attempted suicide. In addition, intolerance to salicylates may result in a severe reaction following therapeutic doses (317). The elderly are more prone to develop salicylate intoxication, one manifestation of which may be delirium (318,319). Following a single large oral dose of salicylate, especially of the acid or its methyl ester, the patient may develop delirium with irritability, restlessness, and hallucinations (318,320,321). Delirium may also be a manifestation of chronic salicylism (322). Tinnitus, tremor, papilledema, hyperventilation, asterixis, convulsions, extensor plantar reflexes, and absent tendon reflexes have been observed among patients suffering from salicylism (318,321–323). Patients receiving high doses of aspirin may develop hepatitis and delirium (324,325). The syndrome can be facilitated by the concurrent administration of sedatives and by any disease, such as pulmonary insufficiency, accompanied by acidosis (323).

Delirium in salicylism appears to be mediated by metabolic changes, especially respiratory alkalosis that may be followed by metabolic acidosis, which exert adverse effects on brain function. There is a good correlation between the state of consciousness and the serum salicylate level (316). Salicylate may lower the brain glucose level (316). The EEG features a decrease in 8–9 Hz activity and an increase in 2–5 Hz activity (326). The clinical state in salicylism does not correlate reliably with the serum salicylate level, since one patient with a level of about 90 mg/100 ml may be comatose, while another may be awake and delirious (323). Treatment of salicylate intoxication consists of intravenous administration of fluids containing sodium bicarbonate (320).

Acute poisoning with both *phenacetin* and *acetanilid* may cause delirium. Patients who abuse phenacetin may develop renal papillary necrosis and uremia, and suffer delirium secondary to renal insufficiency (327).

Nonsteroidal anti-inflammatory agents, including ibuprofen, indomethacin, naproxen, sulindac, and tiaprofenic acid, have all been reported to cause delirium (328–334). The elderly are particularly prone to develop it (328,329,333,334). This adverse effect appears to occur more often with indomethacin than with the other agents (330,331).

Miscellaneous drugs

Practically every drug listed in the pharmacopeia may occasionally induce delirium in a susceptible, notably an elderly, individual. Many drugs can trigger it indirectly by virtue of their toxic effects on the liver or kidneys, for example, and the consequent functional failure of these organs. Other examples of such indirect induction of delirium include dilutional hyponatremia (333), precipitation of heat stroke (334), hypothyroidism (297), and hypoglycemia (335). By means of these and other intermediate mechanisms, many drugs that lack direct cerebrotoxic effects may bring about delirium. Clearly, to discuss all the drugs that have ever been reported to induce it would be both impossible and pointless. However, some agents outside of the groups already discussed may precipitate delirium and are important enough to be included in this section.

Aminophylline, theophylline, and *caffeine* have all been reported to induce delirium on occasion (336–340). The onset of delirium in a patient with chronic lung disease or pulmonary edema receiving aminophylline may herald the onset of a life-threatening status epilepticus (336). Iatrogenic or intentional theophylline overdosage can precipitate seizures and delirium (337).

Caffeine may occasionally induce delirium if used excessively in the form of diet pills or beverages (338–340).

Camphor poisoning is not uncommon in children and can induce delirium, seizures, and coma (341). Alexander and Purkinje are said to have ingested camphor in self-experiments and experienced the syndrome (109). Vincent van Gogh used strong doses of the drug for insomnia and may have suffered psychotic episodes as a result (342).

Clozapine has been reported to precipitate delirium (343). Patients who developed it were found to have raised levels of 5-hydroxy-indoleacetic acid in the CSF and reduced serotonin blood levels (343).

Colchicine overdose toxicity features delirium (344). *Cyclosporine* has been reported to cause severe CNS toxicity, including delirium, in patients undergoing liver or bone marrow transplantation (345,346). This effect has been found to be associated in some cases with hypomagnesemia (346) and in others with low total serum cholesterol (345). Computed tomography and magnetic resonance studies disclosed a severe, diffuse disorder of the white matter in patients who developed the syndrome after liver transplantation (345). *Ergot alkaloids* have been known for centuries to cause neurotoxicity, including delirium (347). Ergotism can feature diffuse cerebral vasoconstriction, which is probably responsible for the syndrome. *Gold* toxicity in the course of therapy for rheumatoid arthritis may include delirium (348). *Hypoglycemic agents* during oral therapy of adult-onset diabetes mellitus may cause severe encephalopathy, including delirium (349).

Ketamine, an intravenous anesthetic agent, produces a so-called dissociative anesthetic state (350–356). This drug can give rise to psychomimetic reactions that include hyperexcitability, depersonalization, body image disturbance, vivid dreams, hallucinations, and emergence delirium; these reactions occur in 5% to more than 30% of patients (350–352). The incidence of delirium proper is uncertain, since the published reports are not clear on this point. A study of 12,000 unselected administrations found the incidence to be 2.8% (351). Another study, however, found emergence delirium, defined as "confusion, with and without vocalization, excitement or irrational behavior," in over 30% of patients given ketamine in various doses (351). This discrepancy in the reported incidence of ketamine delirium apparently reflects differences in the definition of the syndrome. At least some of the psychomimetic reactions elicited by this agent seem to represent an organic hallucinosis or a dissociative state rather than delirium. A study of such reactions after low-dose ketamine infusion found that dreaming was the most frequent experience reported by the patients (353). A personal account of a "ketamine trip" offers a description of the unpleasant sensory disturbances and body image disturbances induced by this drug (354). The psychomimetic reactions are less likely to occur in children under 12 years of age and adults over 70 years (350). Animal experiments indicate that ketamine decreases the rate of glucose utilization in the hippocampus (356). EEG studies have demonstrated excitatory activity in both the thalamus and the limbic system without clinical evidence of seizure activity, indicating that the latter does not spread to the neocortex (352). Ketamine emergence reactions have been prevented by diazepam and lorazepam (352).

Local anesthetic agents readily cross the blood-brain barrier and hence may give rise to neurotoxic side effects, including delirium (357). *Nitrous oxide* has been used as both an inhalational anesthetic agent and a drug of abuse taken for its psychedelic effects. Delirium has been observed following prolonged exposure to this agent (358–360). Single doses are usually well tolerated. Nitrous oxide toxicity produces a clinical picture similar to that of vitamin B_{12} deficiency, including polyneuropathy and delirium (360,361).

Occasional cases of delirium have been observed with *phenelzine* (362), *podophyllin* (363,364), *sulfasalazine* (365), and *trazodone* (366).

Recreational (social, "street") drugs

A number of psychoactive substances have been used not for medicinal reasons but in order to alter mood or behavior (367). The current classification of mental disorders *(DSM-III-R)* lists 11 classes of such substances and indicates which of them may give rise to delirium (108). Some of these drugs are referred to in Chapter 12 (e.g., inhalants) or in previous sections of this Chapter (sedative-hypnotics, narcotics).

Alcohol is not included in *DSM-III-R* among the substances causing delirium. Only intoxication and alcohol idiosyncratic intoxication are defined. By contrast, Engel and Rosenbaum (368) have reported the induction of experimental delirium by oral administration of alcohol to healthy volunteers and chronic alcoholics, and asserted that it was an easy way of inducing "an acute delirium which is rapidly reversible." They observed clouding of consciousness that correlated with slowing of the EEG background activity. This issue remains unresolved.

Amphetamine and related sympathomimetic agents are included among the deliriogenic substances in *DSM-III-R*. Delirium is stated to occur within 1 hour of use and to disappear in about 6 hours. More rarely, it follows a period of intoxication (108). A review of the literature suggests that amphetamine typically induces an organic delusional disorder and only rarely a delirium (369). Intravenous use of amphetamine may cause cerebral vasculitis, which may give rise to delirium (370). *Phenylpropanolamine* may also cause vasculitis, as well as intracerebral hemorrhage and hypertensive encephalopathy (371). Cases of delirium due to this drug have been reported (371,372).

Other sympathomimetic agents used as *nasal sprays* or *diet pills* rarely cause the syndrome (373,374).

Cannabis is not listed in *DSM-III-R* among the substances of abuse causing delirium, but a number of published reports indicate strongly that high-potency preparations of the drug can in fact give rise to it (375,376). As one author asserts, symptoms of acute toxic psychosis precipitated by cannabis include excitement, confusion, disorientation, delusions, depersonalization, visual hallucinations, and "full-blown delirium" (376).

Cocaine delirium is included in *DSM-III-R* and has been reported in the literature (377–379). The syndrome develops within 24 hours of intake and ends in a matter of hours (108). An "excited delirium" in the course of cocaine intoxication may be a prelude to sudden death (379). The drug may induce a variety of serious and potentially lethal neurological complications, including seizures, stroke, subarachnoid hemorrhage, hyperthermia, and cerebral vasculitis (377,380). The acute psychiatric disturbances in cocaine toxicity have been ascribed to the drug's effects on various neurotransmitters, including noradrenaline, dopamine, and serotonin, or to kindling in limbic structures (377). Treatment is usually supportive and symptomatic; benzodiazepines given intravenously may help control agitation (379).

Hallucinogens are not listed as delirium-inducing substances in *DSM-III-R,* but one published report states that "confusion" was observed in 20% of patients admitted to a hospital as a result of ingestion of LSD (381). When LSD was administered intravenously to experimental subjects who were delirious after being given Ditran, an anticholinergic agent, they showed an increase in alertness, restlessness, perceptual distortions, and delusions (42). These behavioral changes were accompanied by a decrease in slow waves and an increase in fast activity in the EEG. In another study, Ditran delirium has been compared to and found to be different from LSD psychosis (382). One may tentatively conclude that the hallucinogens rarely, if ever, give rise to delirium.

Phencyclidine (PCP) is the last major drug of abuse with deliriogenic potential included in *DSM-III-R.* Delirium may occur within 24 hours after use or may arise up to a week following recovery from an overdose, and may last for up to a week (108). It is said to be less common than intoxication (108). PCP is structurally related to ketamine and was initially introduced as an anesthetic (Sernyl), but it was abandoned because of its frequent psychotomimetic side effects (383). It subsequently became a common and dangerous substance of abuse known under a variety of "street" names such as "angel dust," "crystal," "hog," "the pits," and "rocket fuel" (383). In one series of 1,000 cases of acute intoxication, an acute brain syndrome (presumably delirium) was noted in about 37% (384). Many of these patients were violent, agitated, hallucinating, and delusional; some were mute. Delirium is stated to be by far the most common psychiatric syndrome that brings the PCP user to medical attention (385). It appears to be dose related in duration and severity (385). The level of consciousness fluctuates, ranging from drowsiness to stupor and coma. The EEG features theta activity (385). Treatment involves the use of diazepam intravenously or haloperidol for agitation, and propranolol for tachycardia or hypertension (383,385). PCP has anticholinergic properties, and physostigmine has been used to counteract the delirium (38).

References

1. Lipowski, Z. J.: Delirum (acute confusional state), in Frederiks J. A. M. (ed): *Handbook of Clinical Neurology*. Vol 2 (No 46): *Neurobehavioural Disorders*. Amsterdam, Elsevier, pp 523-559.
2. Fraunfelder F. T., Meyer S. M.: Systemic reactions to ophthalmic drug preparations. *Med. Toxicol.* 1987;2:287–293.
3. Hamborg-Petersen B., Nielsen M. M., Thordal C.: Toxic effect of scopolamine eye drops in children. *Acta Ophthalmol.* 1984; 62:485–488.
4. Hollister L. E.: Drug-induced psychiatric disorders and their management. *Med. Toxicol.* 1986;1:428–448.
5. Danielson D. A., Porter J. B., Lawson D. H., et al: Drug-associated psychiatric disturbances in medical inpatients. *Psychopharmacology* 1981;74:105–108.
6. Crawshaw J. A., Mullen, P.E.: A study of benzhexol abuse. *Br. J. Psychiatry* 1984;145:300–303.
7. McIunis M., Petursson H.: Trixephenidyl dependence. *Acta Psychiatr. Scand.* 1984;69:538–542.
8. Pullen G. P., Best N. R., Maguire J.: Anticholinergic drug abuse: A common problem? *Br. Med. J.* 1984;289:612–613.
9. Blazer D. G., Federspiel C. F., Ray W. A., et al: The risk of anticholinergic toxicity in the elderly: A study of prescribing practices in two populations. *J. Gerontol.* 1983;38:31–35.
10. Sunderland T., Tariot P. N., Cohen R. M., et al: Anticholingergic sensitivity in patients with dementia of the Alzheimer type and age-matched controls. *Arch Gen Psychiatry* 1987;44:418–426.
11. Rouner B. W., David A., Lucal-Blaustein M. J., et al: Self-care capacity and anticholinergic drug levels in nursing home patients. *Am. J. Psychiatry* 1988;145:107–109.
12. Shader R. I. (ed): *Psychiatric Complications of Medical Drugs.* New York, Raven Pub, 1972.
13. Forbes T. R.: Why is it called "beautiful lady"? A note on belladonna. *Bull. N.Y. Acad. Med.* 1977;59:403–406.
14. Longo V. G.: Behavioral and electroencephalographic effects of atropine and related compounds. *Pharmacol. Rev.* 1966;18:965–996.
15. Ketchum J. S., Sidell F. R., Crowell E. B., et al: Atropine, scopolamine, and Ditran: Comparative pharmacology and antagonists in man. *Psychopharmacology (Berl.)* 1973;28:121–145.
16. Safer D. J., Allen R. P.: The central effects of scopolamine in man. *Biol. Psychiatry* 1971;3:347–355.

17. Forrer G. R.: Pharmacotoxic therapy with atropine sulfate. *J. Nerv. Ment. Dis.* 1953;117:226–233.
18. MacEwan G. W., Remick R. A., Noone J. A.: Psychosis due to transdermally administered scopolamine. *Can. Med. Assoc. J.* 1985;133:431–432.
19. Meck W. H., Church R. M.: Cholinergic modulation of temporal memory. *Behav. Neurosci.* 1987;101:457–464.
20. Warburton D. M., Wesnes K.: Drugs as research tools in psychology: Cholinergic drugs and information processing. *Neuropsychology* 1984;11:121–132.
21. Golinger R. C., Peet T., Tune L. E.: Association of elevated plasma anticholinergic activity in delirium in surgical patients. *Am. J. Psychiatry* 1987;144:1218–1220.
22. Summers W. K.: A clinical method of estimating risk of drug induced delirium. *Life Sci.* 1978;22:1511–1516.
23. Tune L. E., Holland A., Folstein M. F., et al: Association of postoperative delirium with raised serum levels of anticholinergic drugs. *Lancet* 1981;2:651–652.
24. Granacher R. P., Baldessarini R. J.: Physostigmine. *Arch. Gen. Psychiatry* 1975;32:375–380.
25. Granacher R. P., Baldessarini R. J.: The usefulness of physostigmine in neurology and psychiatry, in Klawans H.L. (ed): *Clinical Neuropharmacology,* Vol 1. New York, Raven Press, 1976, pp 63–79.
26. Johnson A. L., Hollister L. E., Berger P. A.: The anticholinergic intoxication syndrome: Diagnosis and treatment. *J. Clin. Psychiatry* 1981;42:313–317.
27. Kleinwächter I.: Beobachtung über die Wirkung des Calabar-Extracts gegen Atropin-vergiftung. *Berl. Klin. Wochenschr* 1864;1:369–371.
28. Crowell E. B., Ketchum J. S.: The treatment of scopolamine-induced delirium with physostigmine. *Clin. Pharmacol. Ther.* 1967;8:409–414.
29. Duvoisin R. C., Katz R. D.: Reversal of central anticholinergic syndrome in man by physostigmine. *J.A.M.A.* 1968;296:1963–1965.
30. Rumack B.: Anticholinergic poisoning: Treatment with physostigmine. *Pediatrics* 1973;52:449–451.
31. Berkowitz C. D.: Treatment of acute amantadine toxicity with physostigmine. *J. Pediatr.* 1979;95:144–145.
32. Daunderer M.: Akute Alkohol-Intoxikation: Physostigmin als Antidot gegen Äthanol. *Fortschr. Med.* 1978;96:1311–1312.
33. Artru A. A., Hui G. S.: Physostigmine reversal of general anesthesia for intraoperative neurological testing: Associated EEG changes. *Anesth. Analg.* 1986;65:1059–1062.
34. Avant G. R., Speeg K. V., Freemon F. R., et al: Physostigmine reversal of diazepam-induced hypnosis. *Ann. Intern. Med.* 1979;91:53–55.
35. Hoffman W. E., Albrecht R. F., Miletich D. J., et al: Cerebrovascular and cerebral effects of physostigmine, midazolam, and a benzodiazepine antagonist. *Anesth. Analg.* 1986;65:639–644.
36. Nilsson E.: Physostigmine treatment in various drug-induced intoxications. *Ann. Clin. Res.* 1982;14:165–172.
37. Mogilnicki S. R., Walker J. L., Finlayson D. C.: Physostigmine reversal of cimetidine-induced mental confusion. *J.A.M.A.* 1979;241:826–827.
38. Castellani S., Adams P. M., Giannini A. J.: Physostigmine treatment of acute phencyclidine intoxication. *J. Clin. Psychiatry* 1982;43:10–11.

39. Summers W. K., Allen R. E., Pitts F. N.: Does physostigmine reverse quinidine delirium? *West. J. Med.* 1981;135:411–414.
40. Goff D. C., Garber H. J., Jenike M. A.: Partial resolution of ranitidine-associated delirium with physostigmine: Case report. *J. Clin. Psychiatry* 1985;46:400–401.
41. Powers J. S., Decoskey D., Kahrilas P. J.: Physostigmine for treatment of delirium tremens. *J. Clin. Pharmacol.* 1981;21:57–60.
42. Itil T., Fink M.: EEG and behavioral aspects of the interactions of anticholinergic hallucinogens with centrally active compounds. *Prog. Brain Res.* 1968;28:149–168.
43. Bartus R. T., Dean R. L., Pontecorvo M. J., et al: The cholinergic hypothesis: A historical overview, current perspective, and future directions. *Ann. N.Y. Acad. Sci.* 1985;44:332–358.
44. Drachman D. A.: Central cholinergic system and memory, in Lipton M. A., DiMascio A., Killam K. F. (eds): *Psychopharmacology: A Generation of Progress.* New York, Raven Press, 1978, pp 651–662.
45. Warburton D. M., Wesnes K., Edwards J., et al: Scopolamine and the sensory conditioning of hallucinations. *Neuropsychobiology* 1985;14:198–202.
46. Petersen R. C.: Scopolamine-induced learning failures in man. *Psychopharmacology* 1977;52:283–289.
47. Nuotto E.: Psychomotor, physiological and cognitive effects of scopolamine and ephedrine in healthy man. *Eur. J. Clin. Pharmacol.* 1983;24:603–609.
48. Rupreht J., Dvoracek B.: Central anticholinergic syndrome in anesthetic practice. *Acta Anaesth. Belg.* 1976;27:45–60.
49. Risch S. C., Chohen R. M., Janowsky D. S., et al: Physostigmine induction of depressive symptomatology in normal human subjects. *Psychiatry Res.* 1981;4:89–94.
50. Blass J. P., Plum F.: Metabolic encephalopathies in older adults, in Katzman R., Terry R. D. (eds): *The Neurology of Aging.* Philadelphia, F. A. Davis, 1983; pp 189–220.
51. Mirakhur R. K., Clarke R. S. J., Dundee J. W., et al: Anticholinergic drugs in anesthesia. *Anaesthesia* 1978;33:133–138.
52. Anderson S., McGuire R., McKeown D.: Comparison of the cognitive effects of premedication with hyoscine and atropine. *Br. J. Anaesth.* 1985;57:169–173.
53. Smiler B. G., Bartholomew E. G., Sivak B. J., et al: Physostigmine reversal of scopolamine delirium in obstetric patients. *Am. J. Obstet. Gynecol.* 1973;116:326–349.
54. Kuhn J. A., Savage G. J.: Belladonna alkaloid psychosis. *Del. Med. J.* 1974;46:239–242.
55. Davies R. K., Tucker G. J., Harrow M., et al: Confusional episodes and antidepressant medications. *Am. J. Psychiatry* 1971;128:95–99.
56. Godwin C. D.: Case report of tricyclic-induced delirium at a therapeutic drug concentration. *Am. J. Psychiatry* 1983;140:1517–1518.
57. Heiser J. F., Wilbert D. E.: Reversal of delirium induced by tricyclic antidepressant drugs with physostigmine. *Am. J. Psychiatry* 1974;131:1275–1277.
58. Johnson P. B.: Physostigmine in tricyclic antidepressant overdose. *J.A.C.E.P.* 1976;5:443–445.
59. Kutcher S. P., Shulman K. I.: Desipramine-induced delirium at "subtherapeutic" concentrations: A case report. *Can. J. Psychiatry* 1985;30:368–369.

60. Livingston R. L., Zucker D. K., Isenberg K., et al: Tricyclic antidepressants and delirium. *J. Clin. Psychiatry* 1983;44:173–176.
61. Popkin M. K., Callies A. L., MacKenzie T. B.: The outcome of antidepressant use in the medically ill. *Arch. Gen. Psychiatry* 1985;42:1160–1163.
62. Preskorn S. H., Simpson S.: Tricyclic-antidepressant induced delirium and plasma drug concentration. *Am. J. Psychiatry* 1982;139:822–823.
63. Schmidt L. G., Grohmann R., Strauss A., et al: Epidemiology of toxic delirium due to psychotropic drugs in psychiatric hospitals. *Compr. Psychiatry* 1987;28:242–249.
64. Slovis T. L., Ott J. E., Teitelbaum D. T., et al: Physostigmine therapy in acute tricyclic antidepressant poisoning. *Clin. Toxicol.* 1971;4:451–459.
65. Tchen P., Weatherhead A. D., Richards N. G.: Acute intoxication with desipramine. *N. Engl. J. Med.* 1966;274:1197.
66. Helmchen H., Hippins H.; Die unerwunschten psychischen Wirkungen der Psychopharmaka. *Der Internist* 1967;9:336–344.
67. Cole J. O., Branconnier R., Salomon M., et al: Tricyclic use in the cognitively impaired elderly. *J. Clin. Psychiatry* 1983;44:14–19.
68. Chapin J. W., Wingard D. W.: Phsostigmine reversal of benzquinamide-induced delirium. *Anesthesiology* 1977;46:364–365.
69. Molloy D. W.: Memory loss, confusion, and disorientation in an elderly woman taking medicine. *J Am Geriatr. Soc* 1987;35:454–456.
70. Jones I. H., Stevenson J., Jordan A., et al: Pheniramine as hallucinogen. *Med. J. Aust.* 1973;1:382–386.
71. Malcolm R., Miller W. C.: Dimenhydrinate (dramamine) abuse: Hallucinogenic experiences with a proprietary antihistamine. *Am. J. Psychiatry* 1972;128:1012–1013.
72. Filloux F.: Toxic encephalopathy caused by topically applied diphenhydramine. *J. Pediatr.* 1986;108:1018–1020.
73. Jones J., Dougherty J., Cannon L.: Diphenhydramine-induced toxic psychosis. *Am. J. Emerg. Med.* 1986;4:369–371.
74. Köppel C., Ibe K., Tenczer J.: Clinical symptomatology of diphenhydramine overdose: An evaluation of 136 cases in 1982 to 1985. *Clin. Toxicol.* 1987;25:53–70.
75. Lee J. H., Turndorf H., Poppers P. J.: Physostigmine reversal of antihistamine-induced excitement and depression. *Anesthesiology* 1975;43:683–684.
76. Shawn D. H., McGuigan M. A.: Poisoning from dermal absorption of promethazine. *Can. Med. Assoc. J.* 1984;130:1460–1461.
77. Hays D. P., Johnson B. F., Perry R.: Prolonged hallucinations following a modest overdose of tripelennamine. *Clin. Toxicol.* 1980;16:331–333.
78. Bennett N. B., Kohn J.: Case report: Orphenadrine overdose. Cerebral manifestations treated with physostigmine. *Anesth. Intensive Care* 1976;4:157.
79. Ananth J. V., Jain R. C.: Benztropine psychosis. *Can. Psychiatr. Assoc. J.* 1973;18:409–414.
80. Bolin R. B.: Psychiatric manifestations of Artane toxicity. *J. Nerv. Ment. Dis.* 1960;131:256–259.
81. El-Yousef M. K., Janowsky D. S., Davis J. M., et al: Reversal of antiparkinsonian drug toxicity by physostigmine: A controlled study. *Am. J. Psychiatry* 1973;130:141–145.

82. Greenblatt D. J., Shader R. I.: Anticholinergics. *N. Engl. J. Med.* 1973;288:1215–1219.
83. Kulik A. V., Wilbur R.: Delirium and stereotypy from anticholinergic antiparkinsonian drugs. *Prog. Neuropsychopharmacol. Biol. Psychiatry* 1982;6:75–82.
84. McEvoy J. P., McCue M., Spring B., et al: Effects of amantadine and trihexyphenidyl on memory in elderly normal volunteers. *Am. J. Psychiatry* 1987;144:573–577.
85. Smith J. M.: Abuse of antiparkinson drugs: A review of the literature. *J. Clin. Psychiatry* 1980;41:351–354.
86. Stephens D. A.: Psychotoxic effects of benzhexol hydrochloride (Artane). *Br. J. Psychiatry* 1967;113:213–218.
87. Warnes H.: Toxic psychosis due to antiparkinsonian drugs. *Can. Psychiatr. Assoc. J.* 1967;12:323–326.
88. Woody G., O'Brien C. P.: Anticholinergic toxic psychosis in drug abusers treated with benztropine. *Compr. Psychiatry* 1974;15:439–442.
89. Angst J., Hicklin A.: Deliriöse Psychosen unter Neuroleptica und Antidepressiva. *Schweiz Med Wochenschr* 1967;97:546–549.
90. Beszterczey A., Pecknold J. C.: Toxic psychosis induced by high dosage of chlorpromazine therapy. *Can. Med. Assoc. J.* 1971;104;884–889.
91. Chaffin D. S.: Phenothiazine induced acute psychotic reaction: The psychotoxicity by a drug. *Am. J. Psychiatry* 1964;121:26–32.
92. Greenberg R. S., Joseph E. D.: A chlorpromazine organic psychotic reaction. *Mt. Sinai J. Med. N.Y.* 1962;29:165–171.
93. Helmchen H.: Delirante Abläufe unter psychiatrischen Pharmakotherapie. *Arch. Psychiatr. Nervenkr.* 1961;29:165–171.
94. Anielanczyk W.: Delirious syndrome after haloperidol administration. *Psychiatr. Pol.* 1973;7:219–221.
95. Sinaniotis C. A., Spyrides P., Vlachose P., et al: Acute haloperidol poisoning in children. *J. Pediatr.* 1978;93:1038–1039.
96. Veits H. R.: Haloperidol encephalopathy: Case report. *Milit. Med.* 1978;143:201–202.
97. Addonizio G., Susman V. L., Roth S. D.: Neuroleptic malignant syndrome: Review and analysis of 115 cases. *Biol. Psychiatry* 1987;22:1004–1020.
98. Levinson D. F., Simpson G. M.: Neuroleptic-induced extrapyramidal symptoms with fever. *Arch. Gen. Psychiatry* 1986;43:839–848.
99. Pearlman C. A.: Neuroleptic malignant syndrome: A review of the literature. *J. Clin. Psychopharmacol.* 1986;6:257–273.
100. Asher L. M., Cohen S.: The effect of banthine on the central nervous system. *Gastroenterology* 1951;17:178–183.
101. Ginsburg C. M., Angle C. R.: Diphenoxylate-atropine (Lomotil) poisoning. *Clin. Toxicol.* 1969;2:377–382.
102. Gowdy J. M.: Stramonium intoxication. *J.A.M.A.* 1972;221:585–587.
103. Jacobs K. W.: Asthmador: A legal hallucinogen. *Int. J. Addict.* 1974;9:503–512.
104. Shihab Z. M.: Psychotic reaction in an adult after topical cyclopentolate. *Ophthalmologica* 1980;181:228–230.
105. Allen M. D., Greenblatt D. J., Noel B. J.: Self-poisoning with over-the-counter hypnotics. *Clin. Toxicol.* 1979;15:151–158.

106. Hooper R. G., Conner C. S., Rumack B. H.: Acute poisoning from over-the-counter sleep preparations. *J.A.C.E.P.* 1979;8:98–100.
107. Brown J. K., Malone M. H.: "Legal highs"—constituents, activity, toxicology, and herbal folklore. *Clin. Toxicol.* 1978;12:1–31.
108. *Diagnostic and Statistical Manual of Mental Disorders,* ed 3 revised. Washington, DC, American Psychiatric Association, 1987.
109. DeBoor W.: *Pharmakopsychologie und Psychopathologie.* Berlin, Spring, 1956.
110. Isbell H., Altschul S., Kornetsky C. H., et al: Chronic barbiturate intoxication. *A.M.A. Arch. Neurol Psychiatry* 1950;64:1–28.
111. Gibson I. I.: Barbiturate delirium. *Practitioner* 1966;197:345–347.
112. Margetts E. L.: Chloral delirium. *Psychiatr. Q.* 1950;24:278–299.
113. Battin D. G. J., Varkey T. A.: Neuropsychiatric manifestations of bromide ingestion. *Postgrad. Med. J.* 1982;58:523–524.
114. De Keyser J., Maes V., Malfait R., et al: Bromism after prolonged use of carbromal. *Acta Neurol. Belg.* 1984;84:69–74.
115. Jinkins J. R., Chaleby K.: Acute toxic encephalopathy secondary to bromide sedative ingestion. *Neuroradiology* 1987;29:212.
116. Levin M.: Bromide delirium with unusual course. *Am. J. Psychiatry* 1953;110:130–132.
117. Levin M.: Eye disturbances in bromide intoxication. *Am. J. Ophthalmol.* 1960;50:478–483.
118. McDonald C. E., Owens D., Bolman W. M.: Bromide abuse: A continuing problem. *Am. J. Psychiatry* 1974;131:913–915.
119. Blaylock J. D.: Bromism: A persistent peril. *J. Arkansas Med. Soc.* 1973;70:130–135.
120. Carney M. W. P.: Five cases of bromism. *Lancet* 1971;2:523–524.
121. Berglund M., Nielsen S., Risberg J.: Regional cerebral blood flow in a case of bromide psychosis. *Arch. Psychiat. Nervenkr.* 1977;223:197–201.
122. Fried F. E., Malek-Ahmadi P.: Bromism: Recent perspectives. *South. Med. J.* 1975;68:220–222.
123. Tillim S. J.: Bromide intoxication and quantitative determination in serum. *Am. J. Psychiatry* 1957;114:232–236.
124. Baldessarini R. J.: *Chemotherapy in Psychiatry.* Cambridge, Mass, Harvard University Press, 1985.
125. Greenblatt D. J., Shader R. J., Abernethy D. R.: Current status of benzodiazepines. *N. Engl. J. Med.* 1983;309:354–358.
126. Tyrer P., Murphy S.: The place of benzodiazepines in psychiatric practice. *Br. J. Psychiatry* 1987;151:719–723.
127. Denson R.: Involuntary self-intoxication with triazolam. *Psychiatr. J. Univ. Ottawa* 1987;12:242–243.
128. Einarson T. R.: Hallucinations from triazolam. *Drug Intell. Clin. Pharm.* 1980;14:714–715.
129. France R. D., Krishnan R. R.: Behavioral toxicity with alprazolam. *J. Clin. Psychopharmacol* 1984;4:294.
130. Soldatos C. R., Sakkas P. N., Bergiannaki J. D., et al: Behavioral side effects of triazolam in psychiatric patients: Report of five cases. *Drug Intell. Clin. Pharm.* 1986;20:294–297.
131. Busto J., Kaplan H. L., Sellers E. M.: Benzodiazepine-associated emergencies in Toronto. *Am. J. Psychiatry* 1980;137:224–227.

132. Larson E. B., Kukull W. A., Buchner D., et al: Adverse drug reactions associated with global cognitive impairment in elderly persons. *Ann. Intern. Med.* 1987;107:169–173.
133. Salzman C.: Geriatric psychopharmacology. *Ann. Rev. Med.* 1985;36:217–228.
134. Everitt D. E., Avorn J.: Drug prescribing for the elderly. *Arch. Intern. Med.* 1986;146:2393–2396.
135. Essig C. F.: Newer sedative drugs that can cause states of intoxication and dependence of barbiturate type. *J.A.M.A.* 1966;196:714–717.
136. Zvin, I., Shalowitz M.: Acute toxic reaction to prolonged glutethimide administration. *N. Engl. J. Med.* 1962;266:496–498.
137. Haas D. C., Marasigan A.: Neurological effects of glutethimide. *J. Neurol. Neurosurg. Psychiatry* 1968;31:561–564.
138. Snavely S. R., Hodges G. R.: The neurotoxicity of antibacterial agents. *Ann. Intern. Med.* 1984;101:92–104.
139. Kline C. L., Highsmith L. S.: Toxic psychosis resulting from penicillin. *Ann. Intern. Med.* 1948;28:1057–1058.
140. Björnberg A., Selstam J.: Acute psychotic reaction after injection of procaine penicillin. *Acta Psychiatr. Scand.* 1960;35:129–139.
141. Conway N., Beck E., Somerville J.: Penicillin encephalopathy. *Postgrad. Med. J.* 1968;44:891–897.
142. Cummings J. L., Barritt C. F., Horan M.: Delusions induced by procaine penicillin: Case report and review of the syndrome. *Int. J. Psychiatry Med.* 1986–87;16:163–168.
143. Eggleston D. J.: Procaine penicillin psychosis. *Br. Dent. J.* 1980;148:73–74.
144. Silber T. J., D'Angelo L.: Psychosis and seizures following the injection of penicillin G procaine. *A.J.D.C.* 1985;139:335–337.
145. Trunet P., Bouvier A. M., Otterbein G., et al: Encephalopathies dues aux betalactamines. *Nouv. Press. Med.* 1982;11:1781–1784.
146. Levine P. H., Regelson W., Holland J. F.: Chloramphenicol-associated encephalopathy. *Clin. Pharmacol. Ther.* 1970;11:194–199.
147. Umstead G. S., Neumann K. H.: Erythromycin toxicity and acute psychotic reaction in cancer patients with hepatic dysfunction. *Arch. Intern. Med.* 1986;146:897–899.
148. Porot M., Destaing F.: Streptomycine et troubles mentaux. *Ann Med. Psychol.* 1950;108:47–53.
149. Byrd G. J.: Acute organic brain syndrome associated with gentamicin therapy. *J.A.M.A.* 1977;238:53–54.
150. Saker B. M., Musk A. W., Haywood E. F., et al: Reversible toxic psychosis after cephalexin. *Med. J. Aust.* 1973;1:497–498.
151. Lastnick G.: Psychotic symptoms with griseofulvin. *J.A.M.A.* 1974;229:1420–1421.
152. McCartney C. F., Hatley L. H., Kessler J. M.: Possible tobramycin delirium. *J.A.M.A.* 1982;247:1319.
153. Pratt T. H.: Rifampin-induced organic brain syndrome. *J.A.M.A.* 1979;241:2421–2422.
154. Kusumi R. K., Plouffe J. F., Wyatt R. H., et al: Central nervous system toxicity associated with metronidazole therapy. *Ann. Intern. Med.* 1980;93:59–60.
155. Jaeger A., Sauder P., Kopferschmitt J., et al: Clinical features and management of poisoning due to antimalarial drugs. *Med. Toxicol.* 1987;2:242–273.

156. Engel G. L., Romano J., Ferris E. B.: Effect of quinacrine (Atabrine) on the central nervous system. *Arch. Neurol. Psychiatry* 1947;58:337–350.
157. Evans R. L., Khalid S., Kinney J. L.: Antimalarial psychosis revisited. *Arch. Dermatol.* 1984;120:765–767.
158. Lindenmayer J. P., Vargas P.: Toxic psychosis following use of quinacrine. *J. Clin. Psychiatry* 1981;42:162–164.
159. Weisholtz S. J., McBride P. A., Murray H. W., et al: Quinacrine-induced psychiatric disturbances. *South. Med. J.* 1982;75:359–360.
160. Good M. J., Shader R. I.: Lethality and behavioral side effects of chloroquine. *J. Clin. Psychopharmacol.* 1982;2:40–47.
161. Girling D. J.: Adverse effects of antituberculosis drugs. *Drugs* 1982;23:56–74.
162. Pleasure H.: Psychiatric and neurological side effects of isoniazid and iproniazid. *Arch. Neurol. Psychiatry* 1954;72:313–320.
163. Yarbrough B. E., Wood J. P.: Isoniazid overdose treated with high-dose pyridoxine. *Ann. Emerg. Med.* 1983;12:303–305.
164. Bankier R. G.: Psychosis associated with cycloserine. *Can. Med. Assoc. J.* 1965;93:35–37.
165. Sharma G. S., Gupta P. K., Jain N. K., et al: Toxic psychosis due to isoniazid and ethionamide in a patient with pulmonary tuberculosis. *Tubercle* 1979;60:171–172.
166. Feldman S., Rodman J., Gregory B.: Excessive serum concentrations of acyclovir and neurotoxicity. *J. Infect. Dis.* 1988;157:385–388.
167. Burdge D. R., Chow A. W., Sacks S. L.: Neurotoxic effects during vidarabine therapy for herpes zoster. *Can. Med. Assoc. J.* 1985;132:392–395.
168. Cullis P. A., Cushing R.: Vidarabine encephalopathy. *J. Neurol. Neurosurg. Psychiatry* 1984;47:1351–1354.
169. Weddington W. W.: Delirium and depression associated with amphotericin B. *Psychosomatics* 1982;23:1076–1078.
170. Winn R. E., Bower J. H., Richards J. F.: Acute toxic delirium. *Arch. Intern. Med.* 1979;139:706–707.
171. Tollefson G.: Psychiatric implications of anticonvulsant drugs. *J. Clin. Psychiatry* 1980;41:295–302.
172. Trimble M. R., Reynolds E. H.: Anticonvulsant drugs and mental symptoms: A review. *Psychol. Med.* 1976;6:169–178.
173. Reynolds E. H.: Neurotoxicity of carbamazepine. *Adv. Neurol.* 1975;11:345–353.
174. Zaccara G., Paganini M., Campostrini R., et al: Hyperammonemia and valproate-induced alterations of the state of consciousness. *Eur. Neurol.* 1984;23:104–112.
175. Borison R. L.: Amantadine-induced psychosis in a geriatric patient with renal disease. *Am. J. Psychiatry* 1979;136:111–112.
176. Hausner R. S.: Amantadine-associated recurrence of psychosis. *Am. J. Psychiatry* 1980;137:240–242.
177. Postma J. U., Vantilburg W.: Visual hallucination and delirium during treatment with amantadine (Symmetrel). *J. Am. Geriatr. Soc.* 1975;23:212–215.
178. Einarson T. R., Turchet E. N.: Psychotic reaction to low-dose bromocriptine. *Clin. Pharmacol.* 1983;2:273–274.
179. Lieberman A. N., Kupersmith M., Gopinathan G., et al: Bromocriptine in Parkinson disease: Further studies. *Neurology* 1979;29:363–369.

180. Pearce I., Pearce J. M. S.: Bromocriptine in parkinsonism. *Br. Med. J.* 1978;1:1402–1404.
181. Serby M., Angrist B., Leiberman A.: Mental disturbances during bromocriptine and lergotrile treatment of Parkinson's disease. *Am. J. Psychiatry* 1978;135:1227–1229.
182. Shukla S., Turner W. J., Newman G.: Bromocriptine-related psychosis and treatment. *Biol. Psychiatry* 1985;20:326–328.
183. Smith R. C., Strong J. R., Hicks P. B., et al: Behavioral evidence for supersensitivity after chronic bromocriptine administration. *Psychopharmacology* 1979;60:241–246.
184. Celesia G. G., Barr A. N.: Psychosis and other psychiatric manifestations of levodopa therapy. *Arch. Neurol.* 1970;23:193–200.
185. Sroka H., Elizan T. S., Yahr M. D., et al: Organic mental syndrome and confusional states in Parkinson's disease. *Arch. Neurol.* 1981;38:339–342.
186. Nausieda P. A., Weiner W. J., Kaplan L. R., et al: Sleep disruption in the course of chronic levodopa therapy: An early feature of the levodopa psychosis. *Clin. Neuropharmacol.* 1982;5:183–194.
187. Beasley B. L., Nutt J. G., Davenport R. W., et al: Treatment with tryptophan of levodopa-associated psychiatric disturbances. *Arch. Neurol.* 1980;37:155–156.
188. Irwin M., Fuentenebro F., Marder S. R., et al: L-5-hydroxytryptophan-induced delirium. *Biol Psychiatry* 1986;21:673–676.
189. Billiard M., Besset A., Renaud B., et al: L'insomnie de l'encephalopathie bismutique. *Rev. EEG Neurophysiol.* 1977;7:147–152.
190. Burns R., Thomas D. W., Barron V. J.: Reversible encephalopathy possibly associated with bismuth subgallate ingestion. *Br. Med. J.* 1974;1:220–223.
191. Kruger G., Thomas D. J., Weinhardt F., et al: Disturbed oxidative metabolism in organic brain syndrome caused by bismuth in skin creams. *Lancet* 1976;2:485–487.
192. Supino-Viterbo V., Sicard C., Rivegliato M., et al: Toxic encephalopathy due to ingestion of bismuth salts: Clinical and EEG studies of 24 patients. *J. Neurol. Neurosurg. Psychiatry* 1977;40:748–752.
193. Weiss S.: Effect of the digitalis bodies on the nervous system. *Med. Clin. North Am.* 1932;15:963–982.
194. King J. T.: Digitalis delirium. *Ann. Intern. Med.* 1950; 1950;33:1360–1372.
195. Editorial: Digitalis: A neuroexcitatory drug. *Circulation* 52:739–742.
196. Sagel J., Matisonn R.: Neuropsychiatric disturbance as the initial manifestation of digitalis toxicity. *S. Afr. Med. J.* 1975;46:512–514.
197. Bigger J. T.: Digitalis toxicity. *J. Clin. Pharmacol.* 1985; 25:514–521.
198. Cuetter A. C., Ferrans V. J.: Neurological complications of cardiovascular therapy. *Curr. Probl. Cardiol.* 1987;12:159–211.
199. Eisendrath S. J., Sweeney M. A.: Toxic neuropsychiatric effects of digoxin at therapeutic serum concentrations. *Am. J. Psychiatry* 1987;144:506–507.
200. Gordon M., Goldberg L. M. C.: Clinical digoxin toxicity in the aged in association with co-administered verapamil. *J. Am. Geriatr. Soc.* 1986;34:659–662.
201. Portnoi V. A.: Digitalis delirium in elderly patients. *J. Clin. Pharmacol.* 1979;19:747–750.
202. Shear M. K., Sacks M. H.: Digitalis delirium: Report of two cases. *Am. J. Psychiatry* 1978;135:109–110.

203. Hansteen V., Jacobsen D., Knudsen K., et al: Acute, massive poisoning with digitoxin: Report of seven cases and discussion of treatment. *Clin. Toxicol.* 1981;18:679–692.
204. Closson R. G.: Visual hallucinations as the earliest symptom of digoxin intoxication. *Arch. Neurol.* 1983;40:386.
205. Wamboldt F. S., Jefferson J. W., Wamboldt M. Z.: Digitalis intoxication misdiagnosed as depression by primary care physicians. *Am. J. Psychiatry* 1986;143:219–221.
206. Kreeger R. W., Hammill S. C.: New antiarrhythmic drugs: Tocainide, mexiletine, flecainide, encainide, and amiodarone. *Mayo Clin. Proc.* 1987;62:1033–1050.
207. Alfano S. N., Leicht M. J., Skiendzielewski J. J.: Lidocaine toxicity following subcutaneous administration. *Ann. Emerg. Med.* 1984;13:465–467.
208. Saravay S. M., Marke J., Steinberg M. D., et al: "Doom anxiety" and delirium in lidocaine toxicity. *Am. J. Psychiatry* 1987; 144:159–163.
209. Vlay S. C., Mallis G. I.: Intravenous and oral lorcainide: Assessment of central nervous system toxicity and antiarrhythmic efficacy. *Am. Heart J.* 1986;111:452–455.
210. Crum I. D., Guidry J. R.: Procainamide-induced psychosis. *J.A.M.A.* 1978;240:1265–1266.
211. Gilbert G. J.: Quinidine dementia. *J.A.M.A.* 1977; 237:2093–2094.
212. Quintanilla J.: Psychosis due to quinidine intoxication. *Am. J. Psychiatry* 1957;113:1031–1032.
213. Bikadoroff S.: Mental changes associated with tocainide, a new antiarrhythmic. *Can. J. Psychiatry* 1987;32:219–221.
214. Husserl F. E., Messerli F. H.: Adverse effects of antihypertensive drugs. *Drugs* 1981;22:188–210.
215. Bartels D., Glasser M., Wang A., et al: Association between depression and propranolol use in ambulatory patients. *Clin. Pharm.* 1988;7:146–150.
216. Cummings J., Hebben N. A., Obler L., et al: Nonaphasic misnaming and other neurobehavioral features of an unusual toxic encephalopathy: Case study. *Cortex* 1980;16:315–323.
217. Kuhr B. M.: Prolonged delirium with propranolol. *J. Clin. Psychiatry* 1979;40:194–195.
218. McGahan D. J., Wojslaw A., Prasad V., et al: Propranolol-induced psychosis. *Drug Intell. Clin. Pharm.* 1984;18:601–603.
219. Miller F. A., Rampling D.: Adverse effects of combined propranolol and chlorpromazine therapy. *Am. J. Psychiatry* 1982;139:1198–1199.
220. Prakash R., Campbell T. W., Petrie W. M.: Psychoses with propranolol: A case report. *Can. J. Psychiatry* 1983;28:657–658.
221. Renick R. A., O'Kane J., Sparling T. G.: A case report of toxic psychosis with low-dose propranolol therapy. *Am. J. Psychiatry* 1981;138:850–851.
222. Orzack M. H. Branconnier R.: CNS effects of propranolol in man. *Psychopharmacology (Berl.)* 1973;29:299–306.
223. Fraunfelder F. T., Meyer S. M.: Systemic reactions to ophthalmic drug preparations. *Med. Toxicol.* 1987;2:287–293.
224. Shore J. H., Fraunfelder F. T., Meyer S. M.: Psychiatric side effects from topical ocular timolol, a beta-adrenergic blocker. *J. Clin. Psychopharmacol.* 1987;7:264–267.

225. Van Buskirk E. M.: Adverse reactions from timolol administration. *Ophthalmology* 1980;87:447–450.
226. Conner C. S., Watanabe A. S.: Clonidine overdose: A review. *Am. J. Hosp. Pharm.* 1979;36:906–911.
227. Hoffman W. F., Ladogana L.: Delirium secondary to clonidine therapy. *N.Y. State J. Med.* 1981;81:382–383.
228. Houston M. C.: Clonidine hydrochloride: Review of pharmacologic and clinical aspects. *Progr. Cardiovasc. Dis.* 1981;23:337–350.
229. Adler S.: Methyldopa-induced decrease in mental activity. *J.A.M.A.* 1974;230:1428–1429.
230. Hawkins D.J .: Acute organic brain syndrome psychosis with methyldopa therapy. *Mo. Med.* 1976;73:476–481.
231. Thornton W. E.: Dementia induced by methyldopa with haloperidol. *N. Engl. J. Med.* 1976;294:1222.
232. Kahn J. K.: Nifedipine-associated acute psychosis. *Am. J. Med.* 1986;81:705–706.
233. Da Silva O. A., De Melo R. A., Filho J. P. J.: Verapamil acute self-poisoning. *Clin. Toxicol.* 1979;14:361–367.
234. Jacobsen F. M., Sack D. A., James S. P.: Delirium induced by verapamil. *Am. J. Psychiatry* 1987;144:248.
235. Bertoni J. M., Schwartzman R. J., Van Horn G., et al: Asterixis and encephalopathy following metrizamide myelograph: Investigations into possible mechanisms and review of the literature. *Ann. Neurol.* 1981;9:366–370.
236. Cronqvist S. E., Holtas S. L., Laike T., et al: Psychic changes following myelography with metrizamide and iohexol. *Acta Radiol. (Diagn.)* 1984;25:369–373.
237. Davis R. J., Cummings J. L., Malin B. D., et al: Prolonged psychosis with first-rank symptoms following metrizamide myelography. *Psychosomatics* 1986;27:373–375.
238. France R. D., McCracken J.: Delirium following metrizamide myelography. *Psychosomatics* 1984;25:338–339.
239. Haley E. C.: Encephalopathy following arteriography: A possible toxic effect of contrast agents. *Ann. Neurol.* 1984;15:100–102.
240. Hauge O., Falkenberg H.: Neuropsychologic reactions and other side effects after metrizamide myelography. *A.J.N.R.* 1982;3:229–232.
241. Junck L., Marshall W. H.: Neurotoxicity of radiological contrast agents. *Ann. Neurol.* 1983;13:469–484.
242. Ratcliff G., Sandler S., Latchaw R.: Cognitive and affective changes after myelography: A comparison of metrizamide and iohexol. *A.J.N.R.* 1986;7:683–687.
243. Schmidt R. C.: Mental disorders after myelograph with metrizamide and other water-soluble contrast media. *Neuroradiology* 1980;19:153–157.
244. Ling M. H. M., Perry P. J., Tsuang M. T.: Side effects of corticosteroid therapy. *Arch. Gen. Psychiatry* 1981;38:471–477.
245. Glaser G. H.: Psychotic reactions induced by corticotrophin (ACTH) and cortisone. *Psychosom. Med.* 1953;15:280–291.
246. Hall R. C. W., Popkin M. K., Stickney S. K., et al: Presentation of the "steroid psychoses." *J. Nerv. Ment. Dis.* 1979;167:229–236.
247. Clark L. D., Bauer W., Cobb S.: Preliminary observations on mental disturbances occurring in patients under therapy with cortisone and ACTH. *N. Engl. J. Med.* 1952;246:205–216.
248. Von Zerssen D.: Mood and behavioral changes under corticosteroid therapy, in

Itil T. M., Laudahn G., Herrmann W. M. (eds): *Psychotropic Action of Hormones.* New York, Spectrum, 1976, pp 195–222.

249. Alpert E., Seigerman C.: Steroid withdrawal psychosis in a patient with closed head injury. *Arch. Phys. Med. Rehabil.* 1986;67:766–769.
250. Dixon R. B., Christy N. P.: On the various forms of corticosteroid withdrawal syndrome. *Am. J. Med.* 1980;68:224–230.
251. Yunus M. B., Morgan R. J., Barclay A. M., et al: Organic brain syndrome in rheumatoid arthritis after corticosteroid withdrawal. *J. Rheumatol.* 1985;12:636–637.
252. Nausieda P. A., Carvey P. M., Weiner W. J.: Modification of central serotonergic and dopaminergic behaviors in the course of chronic corticosteroid administration. *Eur. J. Pharmacol.* 1982;78:335–343.
253. Massie M. J., Holland J. C.: Consultation and liaison issues in cancer care. *Psychiatr. Med.* 1987;5:343–359.
254. Goldberg I. D., Bloomer W. D., Dawson D. M.: Nervous system toxic effects of cancer therapy. *J.A.M.A.* 1982;247:1437–1441.
255. Kaplan R. S., Wiernick P. H.: Neurotoxicity of antineoplastic drugs. *Semin. Oncol.* 1982;9:103–130.
256. Peterson L. G., Popkin M. K.: Neuropsychiatric effects of chemotherapeutic agents for cancer. *Psychosomatics* 1980;21:141–153.
257. Silberfarb P. M.: Chemotherapy and cognitive defects in cancer patients. *Ann. Rev. Med.* 1983;34:35–46.
258. Holland J., Fasaniello S., Ohnuma T.: Psychiatric symptoms associated with L-asparaginase administration. *J. Psychiatr. Res.* 1974;10:105–113.
259. Feinberg W. M., Swenson M. R.: Cerebrovascular complications of L-asparaginase therapy. *Neurology* 1988;38:127–133.
260. Matzen T. A., Martin R .L.: Magnesium deficiency psychosis induced by cancer chemotherapy. *Biol. Psychiatry* 1985;20:788–791.
261. Hwang T. L., Yung A., Estey E. H., Fields W. S.: Central nervous system toxicity with high-dose Ara-C. *Neurology* 1985;35:1475–1479.
262. Lynch H. T., Droszcz C. P., Albano W. A., et al: "Organic brain syndrome" secondary to 5-fluouracil toxicity. *Dis. Colon Rectum* 1981;24:130–131.
263. Denicoff K. D., Rubinow D. R., Papa M. Z., et al: The neuropsychiatric effects of treatment with interleukin-2 and lymphokine-activated killer cells. *Ann. Intern. Med.* 1987;107:293–300.
264. Renault P. F., Hoofnagle J. H., Park Y., et al: Psychiatric complications of long-term interferon alpha therapy. *Arch. Intern. Med.* 1987;147:1577–1580.
265. Smedley H., Katrak M., Sikora K., et al: Neurological effects of recombinant human interferon. *Br. Med. J.* 1983;286:262–264.
266. Suter C. C., Westmoreland B. F., Sharbrough F. W., et al: Electroencephalographic abnormalities in interferon encephalopathy: A preliminary report. *Mayo Clin. Proc.* 1984;59:847–850.
267. Phillips P. C., Dhawan V., Strother S. C., et al: Reduced cerebral glucose metabolism and increased brain capillary permeability following high-dose methotrexate chemotherapy: A positron emission tomographic study. *Ann. Neurol.* 1987;21:59–63.
268. Pochedly C.: Neurotoxicity due to CNS therapy for leukemia. *Med. Pediatr. Oncol.* 1977;3:101–115.
269. Weiss H. D., Walker M. D., Wiernik P. H.: Neurotoxicity of commonly used antineoplastic agents. *N. Engl. J. Med.* 1974;291:75–81.

270. Legha S. S.: Vincristine neurotoxicity. *Med. Toxicol.* 1986;1:421–427.
271. Branchey L., Davis W., Lee K. K., et al: Psychiatric complications of disulfiram treatment. *Am. J. Psychiatry* 1987;144:1310–1312.
272. Knee S. T., Razani J.: Acute organic brain syndrome: A complication of disulfiram therapy. *Am. J. Psychiatry* 1974;131:1281–1282.
273. Liddon S., Satran R.: Disulfiram (Antabuse) psychosis. *Am. J. Psychiatry* 1967;123:1284–1289.
274. Quail M., Karelse R. H.: Disulfiram psychosis. *S. Afr. Med. J.* 1980;57:551–552.
275. Weddington W. W., Marks R. C., Verghese J. P.: Disulfiram encephalopathy as a cause of the catatonia syndrome. *Am. J. Psychiatry* 1980;137:1217–1219.
276. Kirubakaran V., Liskow B., Mayfield D., et al: Case report of acute disulfiram overdose. *Am. J. Psychiatry* 1983;140:1513–1514.
277. Hotson J. R., Langston J. W.: Disulfiram-induced encephalopathy. *Arch. Neurol.* 1976;33:141–142.
278. Rainey J. M.: Disulfiram toxicity and carbon disulfide poisoning. *Am. J. Psychiatry* 1977;134:371–378.
279. Sonnenblick M., Rosin A. J., Weissberg N.: Neurological and psychiatric side effects of cimetidine—report of 3 cases with review of the literature. *Postgrad. Med. J.* 1982;58:415–418.
280. Strauss A.: Cimetidine and delirium: Assessment and management. *Psychosomatics* 1982;23:57–62.
281. Davis T. G., Pickett D. L., Schlosser J. H.: Evaluation of a worldwide spontaneous reporting system with cimetidine. *J.A.M.A.* 1980;243:1912–1914.
282. Krenzelok E. P., Litovitz T., Lippold K. P., et al: Cimetidine toxicity: An assessment of 881 cases. *Ann. Emerg. Med.* 1987;16:1217–1221.
283. McGuigan J. E.: A consideration of the adverse effects of cimetidine. *Gastroenterology* 1981;80:181–192.
284. Ritschel W. A.: Cimetidine dosage regimen for patients with renal failure and for geriatric patients. *Eur. J. Clin. Pharmacol.* 1982;23:501–504.
285. Schentag J. J., Calleri G., Rose J. Q., et al: Pharmacokinetic and clinical studies in patients with cimetidine-associated mental confusion. *Lancet* 1979;1:177–181.
286. Yudofsky S. C., Ahern G., Brockman R.: Agitation, disorientation, and hallucinations in patients on cimetidine. *Gen. Hosp. Psychiatry* 1980;3:233–236.
287. Van Sweden B., Kamphuisen H. A. C.: Cimetidine neurotoxicity. *Eur. Neurol.* 1984;23:300–305.
288. Miller A. A., Ambis D., Siegel J. H.: Cimetidine and mental confusion. *N. Engl. J. Med.* 1978;298:284–285.
289. Fennelly M. E.: Ranitidine-induced mental confusion. *Crit. Care Med.* 1987;15:1165–1166.
290. Agulnik P. L., Dimascio A., Moore P.: Acute brain syndrome associated with lithium therapy. *Am. J. Psychiatry* 1972;129:621–623.
291. El-Mallak L. R. S.: Acute lithium neurotoxicity. *Psychiatr. Dev.* 1986;4:311–328.
292. Johnson G. F. S.: Lithium neurotoxicity. *Aust. N.Z. J. Psychiatry* 1976;10:33–38.
293. Rifkin A., Quitkin F., Klein D. F.: Organic brain syndrome during lithium carbonate treatment. *Compr. Psychiatry* 1973;14:251–254.
294. De Paulo J. R., Folstein M. F., Correa E. I.: The course of delirium due to lithium intoxication. *J. Clin. Psychiatry* 1982;43:447–449.
295. Schou M.: Lithium treatment of manic-depressive illness. *J.A.M.A.* 1988;259:1834–1836.

296. Schou M.: Long-lasting neurological sequelae after lithium intoxication. *Acta Psychiatr. Scand.* 1984;70:594–602.
297. Struve F. A.: Lithium-specific pathological electroencephalographic changes: A successful replication of earlier investigative results. *Clin. Electroencephalogr.* 1987;18:46–53.
298. Smith R. E., Helms P. M.: Adverse effects of lithium therapy in the acutely ill elderly patient. *J. Clin. Psychiatry* 1982;43:94–99.
299. Hardy B. G., Shulman K. I., MacKenzie S. E., et al: Pharmacokinetics of lithium in the elderly. *J. Clin. Psychopharmacol.* 1987;7:153–158.
300. Keitner G. I., Rahman S.: Reversible neurotoxicity with combined lithium-haloperidol administration. *J. Clin. Psychopharmacol.* 1984;4:104–105.
301. Miller F., Menninger J.: Lithium-neuroleptic neurotoxicity is dose dependent. *J. Clin. Psychopharmacol.* 1987;7:89–91.
302. Yassa R.: Lithium-methyldopa interaction. *Can. Med. Assoc. J.* 1986;134:141–142.
303. Miller R. R., Jick H.: Clinical effects of meperidine in hospitalized medical patients. *J. Clin. Pharmacol.* 1978;18:180–189.
304. Eisendrath S. J., Goldman B., Douglas J., et al: Meperidine-induced delirium. *Am. J. Psychiatry* 1987;144:1062–1065.
305. MacVicar A. A.: Psychotic symptoms due to meperidine intoxication. *Can. Med. Assoc. J.* 1974;110:1237.
306. De Nosaquo N.: The hallucinatory effect of pentazocine (Talwin). *J.A.M.A.* 1969;210:502.
307. Kane F. J., Pokorny A.: Mental and emotional disturbance with pentazocine (Talwin) use. *South. Med. J.* 1975;68:808–811.
308. Miller R. R.: Clinical effects of pentazocine in hospitalized medical patients. *J. Clin. Pharmacol.* 1975;15:198–205.
309. Wood A. J. J., Moir D. C., Campbell C., et al: Medicines evaluation and monitoring group: Central nervous system effects of pentazocine. *Br. Med. J.* 1974;1:305–307.
310. Swanson D. W., Weddige R. L., Morse R. M.: Hospitalized pentazocine abusers. *Mayo Clin. Proc.* 1973;48:85–93.
311. Yost M. A., McKegney F. P.: Acute organic psychosis due to Talwin (pentazocine). *Conn. Med.* 1970;34:259–260.
312. Lewis J. R.: Evaluation of new analgesics. *J.A.M.A.* 1980;243:1465–1467.
313. Manoguerra A. S.: Acetoaminophen intoxication. *Clin. Toxicol.* 1979;14:151–155.
314. Sellers E. M., Freedman F.: Treatment of acetoaminophen poisoning. *Can. Med. Assoc. J.* 1981;125:827–829.
315. Liederman P. C., Boldus R. A.: Psychic side effects of a chlorzoxazone and acetoaminophen mixture. *J.A.M.A.* 1967;202:64–66.
316. Thisted B., Krantz T., Strom J., et al: Acute salicylate self-poisoning in 177 consecutive patients treated in ICU. *Acta Anesthesiol. Scand.* 1987;31:312–316.
317. Abrishami M. A., Thomas J.: Aspirin intolerance—a review. *Ann. Allergy* 1977;39:28–37.
318. Cupit G. C.: The use of non-prescription analgesics in an older population. *J. Am. Geriatr. Soc.* 1982;30 (Suppl):76–80.
319. Grigor R. R., Spitz P. W., Furst D. E.: Salicylate toxicity in elderly patients with rheumatoid arthritis. *J. Rheumatol.* 1987;14:60–66.

320. McGuigan M. A.: Death due to salicylate poisoning in Ontario. *Can. Med. Assoc. J.* 1986;135:891–894.
321. Steele T. E., Morton W. A.: Salicylate-induced delirium. *Psychosomatics* 1986;27:455–456.
322. Greer H. D., Ward H. P., Corbin K. B.: Chronic salicylate intoxication in adults. *J.A.M.A.* 1965;193:555–558.
323. Brown G. L., Wilson W. P.: Salicylate intoxication and the CNS. *Dis. Nerv. Syst.* 1971;32:135–140.
324. Petty B. G., Zahka K. G., Berstein M. T.: Aspirin hepatitis associated with encephalopathy. *J. Pediatr.* 1978;93:881–882.
325. Ulshen M. H., Grand R. J., Crain J. D., et al: Hepatotoxicty with encephalopathy associated with aspirin therapy in rheumatoid arthritis. *J. Pediatr.* 1978;93:1034–1047.
326. Fink M., Irwin P.: Central nervous system effects of aspirin. *Clin. Pharmacol. Ther.* 1982;32:362–365.
327. Murray R. M.: Personality factors in analgesic nephropathy. *Psychol. Med.* 1974;4:69–73.
328. Allison N., Shantz I.: Delirium due to tiaprofenic acid. *Can. Med. Assoc. J.* 1987;137:1022–1023.
329. Goodwin J. S., Regan M.: Cognitive dysfunction associated with naproxen and ibuprofen in the elderly. *Arthritis Rheum.* 1982;25:1013–1015.
330. Rhymer A. R., Gengos D. C.: Indomethacin. *Clin. Rheum. Dis.* 1979;5:541–552.
331. Schwartz J. I., Moura R. J.: Severe depersonalization and anxiety associated with indomethacin. *South. Med. J.* 1983;76:679–680.
332. Thornton T. L.: Delirium associated with sulindac. *J.A.M.A.* 1980;243:1630–1631.
333. Moses A. M., Miller M.: Drug-induced dilutional hyponatremia. *N. Engl. J. Med.* 1974;291:1234–1239.
334. Shibolet S., Lancaster M. C., Danon Y.: Heat stroke; A review. *Aviat. Space Environ. Med.* 1976;21:280–301.
335. Seltzer H. S.: Drug-induced hypoglycemia. *Diabetes* 1972;21:955–966.
336. Culberson C. G., Langston J. W., Herrick M.: Aminophylline encephalopathy: A clinical, electroencephalographic, and neuropathological analysis. *Trans. Am. Neurol. Assoc.* 1979;104:224–226.
337. Paloncek F. P., Rodrold K. A.: Evaluation of theophylline overdoses and toxicities. *Ann. Emerg. Med.* 1988; 17:135–144.
338. Shen W. W., D'Souza T. C. : Cola-induced organic brain syndrome. *Rocky Mt. Med. J.* 1979; 76:312–313.
339. Shaul P. W., Farrell M. K., Maloney M. J.: Caffeine toxicity as a cause of acute psychosis in anorexia nervosa. *J. Pediatr.* 1984; 105: 493–495.
340. Stillner V., Popkin M. K., Pierce C. M.: Caffeine-induced delirium during prolonged competitive stress. *Am. J. Psychiatry* 1978; 135:855–856.
341. Aronow R., Spigiel R. W.: Implications of camphor poisoning. *Drug Intell. Clin. Pharm.* 1976; 10:631–634.
342. Monroe R. R.: The episodic psychoses of Vincent van Gogh. *J. Nerv. Ment. Dis.* 1978; 166:480–488.
343. Banki C. M., Vojnik M.: Comparative simultaneous measurement of cerebrospinal fluid 5-hydroxyindoleacetic acid and blood serotonin levels in delirium tremens and clorazapine-induced delirious reaction. *J. Neurol. Neurosurg. Psychiatry* 1978; 41:420–424.

344. Stapczynski J. S., Rothstein R. J., Gaye W. A., Niemann JT: Colchicine overdose: Report of two cases and review of the literature. *Ann. Emerg. Med.* 1981; 10:364–369.
345. De Groen P. C., Aksamit A. J., Rakela J., et al.: Central nervous system toxicity after liver transplantation. *N. Engl. J. Med.* 1987; 317:861–866.
346. Thompson C. B., Sullivan K. M., June C. H., Thomas E. D.: Association between cyclosporin neurotoxicity and hypomagnesemia. *Lancet* 1984;2:116–1120.
347. Senter H. J., Lieberman A. N., Pinto R.: Cerebral manifestations of ergotism. *Stroke* 1976;7:88–92.
348. Perry R. P., Jacobsen E. S.: Gold induced encephalopathy: Case report. *J. Rheumatol.* 1984;11:233–234.
349. Turkington R. W.: Encephalopathy induced by oral hypoglycemic agents. *Arch. Intern. Med.* 1977;137:1082–1083.
350. Seibert C. P.: Recognition, management, and prevention of neuropsychological dysfunction after operation. *Int. Anesthesiol. Clin.* 1986;24:39–59.
351. Knox J. W. D., Bovill J. G., Clarke R. S. J., et al: Clinical studies of induction agents. XXXVI: Ketamine. *Br. J. Anaesth.* 1970;42:875–888.
352. Reich DL, Silvay G: Ketamine: An update on the first twenty-five years of clinical experience. *Can. J. Anaesth.* 1989;36:186–197.
353. Klausen N. O., Wiberg-Jorgensen F., Chraemmer-Jorgensen B.: Psychomimetic reactions after low-dose ketamine infusion. *Br. J. Anaesth.* 1983;55:297–301.
354. Johnstone R. E.: A ketamine trip. *Anesthesiology* 1973;39:460–461.
355. Schwedler M., Miletich D. J., Albrecht R. F.: Cerebral blood flow and metabolism following ketamine administration. *Can. Anaesth. Soc. J.* 1982;29:222–226.
356. Oguchi K., Arakawa K., Nelson S. R., et al: The influence of loperidol, diazepam, and physostigmine on ketamine-induced behavior and brain regional glucose utilization in rat. *Anesthesiology* 1982;57:353–358.
357. Mather L. E., Tucker G. T., Murphy T. M., et al: Cardiovascular and subjective central nervous system effects of long-acting local anesthetics in man. *Anaesth. Intens. Care* 1979;2:215–221.
358. Brodsky L., Zuniga J.: Nitrous oxide: A psychotogenic agent. *Compr. Psychiatry* 1975;16:185–188.
359. Jastak J. T., Malamed S. F.: Nitrous oxide sedation and sexual phenomena. J.A.D.A. 1980;101:38–40.
360. Sterman A. B., Coyle P. K.: Subacute toxic delirium following nitrous oxide abuse. *Arch. Neurol.* 1983;40:446–447.
361. Heyer E. J., Simpson D. M., Bodis-Wollner I., et al: Nitrous oxide: Clinical and electrophysiologic investigation of neurologic complications. *Neurology* 1986;36:1618–1622.
362. White P. D.: Myoclonus and episodic delirium associated with phenelzine: A case report. *J. Clin. Psychiatry* 1987;48:340–341.
363. Filley C. M., Graff-Radford N. R., Lacy J. R., et al: Neurologic manifestations of podophyllin toxicity. *Neurology* 1982;32:308–311.
364. Stoudemire A., Baker N., Thompson T. L.: Delirium induced by topical application of podophyllin: A case report. *Am. J. Psychiatry* 1981;138:1505–1506.
365. Smith M. D., Gibson G. E., Rowland R.: Combined hepatotoxicity and neurotoxicity following sulphasalazine administration. *Aust. N.Z. J. Med.* 1982;12:76–80.
366. Damlouji N. F., Ferguson J. M.: Trazodone-induced delirium in bulimic patients. *Am. J. Psychiatry* 1984;141:434–435.

367. Pickens R. W., Heston L. L. (eds): *Psychiatric Factors in Drug Abuse.* New York, Grune & Stratton, 1979.
368. Engel G. L., Rosenbaum M.: Delirium. III. Electroencelphalographic changes associated with acute alcoholic intoxication. *Arch. Neurol. Psychiatry* 1945;53:44–50.
369. Ellinwood E. H.: Amphetamine psychosis: A multidimensional process. *Semin. Psychiatry* 1969;1:208–226.
370. Bostwick D. G.: Amphetamine induced cerebral vasculitis. *Hum. Pathol.* 1981;12:1031–1033.
371. Glick R., Hoying J., Cerullo L., et al: Phenylpropanolamine: An over-the-counter drug causing central nervous system vasculitis and intracerebral hemorrhage. *Neurosurgery* 1987;20:969–974.
372. Bernstein E., Diskant B. M.: Phenylpropanolamine: A potentially hazardous drug. *Ann. Emerg. Med.* 1982;11:311–315.
373. Khan S. A., Spiegel D. A., Jobe P. C.: Psychotomimetic effects of anorectic drugs. *A.F.P.* 1987;36:107–111.
374. Snow S. S., Logan T. P., Hollender M. H.: Nasal spray "addiction" and psychosis: A case report. *Br. J. Psychiatry* 1980;136:297–299.
375. Ghodse A. H.: Cannabis psychosis. *Br. J. Addict.* 1986;81:473–478.
376. Schwartz R. H.: Marijuana: An overview. *Pediatr. Clin. North Am.* 1987;34:305–317.
377. Lowenstein D. H., Massa S. M., Rowbotham M. C., et al: Acute neurologic and psychiatric complications associated with cocaine abuse. *Am. J. Med.* 1987;83:841–846.
378. Murray J. B.: An overview of cocaine use and abuse. *Psychol. Rep.* 1986;59:243–264.
379. Wetli C. V., Fishbain D. A.: Cocaine-induced psychosis and sudden death in recreational cocaine users. *J. Forensic Sci.* 1985;30:873–880.
380. Kaye B. R., Fainstat M.: Cerebral vasculitis associated with cocaine abuse. *J.A.M.A.* 1987;258:2104–2106.
381. Ungerleider J. T., Fisher D. D., Fuller M.: The dangers of LSD. *J.A.M.A.* 1966;197:389–392.
382. Wilson R. E., Shagass C.: Comparison of two drugs with psychotomimetic effects (LSD and Ditran). *J. Nerv. Ment. Dis.* 1964;138:277–286.
383. Rappolt R. T., Gay G. R., Farris R. D.: Phencyclidine (PCP) intoxication: Diagnosis in stages and algorithms of treatment. *Clin. Toxicol.* 1980;16:509–529.
384. McCarron M. M., Schulze B. W., Thompson G. A., et al: Acute phencyclidine intoxication: Incidence of clinical findings in 1,000 cases. *Ann. Emerg. Med.* 1981;10;237–242.
385. Pearlson G. D.: Psychiatric and medical syndromes associated with phencyclidine (PCP) abuse. *Johns Hopkins Med. J.* 1981;148:25–33.

12

Poisons

Many exogenous substances can give rise to delirium. Those currently used as medical drugs are discussed in Chapter 11. In this chapter, industrial toxic agents, inhalants abused for their psychoactive effects, and poisons of animal, mushroom, and plant origin are reviewed. They may cause delirium as a result of accidental exposure, mostly at work, or of intentional intake for suicidal, homicidal, or recreational purposes. The literature on the psychotoxic effects of these substances is generally inadequate. Psychiatrists have shown little interest in this aspect of psychopathology (1). The purpose of behavioral toxicology is to fill the gap (1,2). Psychiatric effects of poisons are generally poorly described in the literature, and writers use inconsistent and undefined terms in this regard. Terms such as "behavioral changes," "mental effects," "psychosis," and "confusion" are commonly used and mean little, as no attempt is usually made to define them and to specify operational or diagnostic criteria for their application. As a result, it is often impossible to know what mental disorder the author has observed and is discussing.

Books on toxicology are quite inconsistent in their treatment of the psychopathological effects of chemical agents. Speaking specifically of delirium, some textbook writers fail to mention it at all (3), while others list toxic substances that have been reported to induce it (4). One writer lists over 60 potentially deliriogenic agents, including drugs, industrial chemicals, poisonous plants and mushrooms, and venoms (4). Another textbook writer asserts that delirium is one of the most common effects of a toxic substance on the

CNS, notably on the reticular formation (5). This statement is probably correct, but more evidence is needed to support it. The incidence of delirium due to industrial poisons is unknown. It appears that simple intoxication and reversible dementia are the most common organic mental syndromes due to industrial poisons. Intoxication, as currently defined, features maladaptive behavior and relatively mild disturbances of cognition, attention, wakefulness, judgment, emotional control, and psychomotor behavior (6). Delirium is likely to occur in a person who is acutely and relatively severely poisoned, or who is chronically intoxicated but suffers acute cognitive decompensation as a result of either an increased concentration of the toxic agent in the body or concurrent exposure to some other potentially deliriogenic factor. Psychological stress may also play a contributory role in such decompensation. Regardless of the toxic agent involved, prodromal symptoms, such as disturbance of the sleep-wake cycle, nightmares, lethargy, irritability, anxiety, depression, and fleeting hallucinations, often herald the onset of a full-blown delirium. This may be the first event that leads to a psychiatric and medical evaluation of a person suffering from chronic intoxication in an industrial setting.

Only those toxic agents whose deliriogenic potential has been reasonably well documented and that are practically important because of their prevalence will be reviewed. In many cases, I have interpreted reports that a given substance has been observed to cause confusion or disorientation as presumptive evidence that delirium was actually involved. In some instances, this interpretation may have been incorrect. We must tolerate uncertainty in this area.

Alcohols

Ethyl alcohol is discussed in Chapter 11. Two other alcohols deserve mention as possibly deliriogenic: ethylene glycol and methanol.

Ethylene glycol has low toxicity but, when ingested accidentally or intentionally in a large dose, it may give rise to serious intoxication that can involve the brain and is often fatal (7–9). A wide variety of neurological abnormalities, as well as delirium, stupor, and coma, are common. Severe metabolic acidosis is usually present.

Methanol poisoning shares many clinical and biochemical characteristics with ethylene glycol intoxication (10). Both of these substances are metabolized to toxic metabolites that are responsible for metabolic acidosis. The onset of symptoms is typically delayed by as much as 72 hours following ingestion of methanol; symptoms include visual disturbances, lethargy, confusion, stupor, and coma. Treatment involves the administration of alkali and ethanol and hemodialysis (10).

Aliphatic Hydrocarbons

The aliphatic hydrocarbons include saturated and unsatured series. The saturated series consists of methane, ethane, propane, and butane gases, as well as liquids and solids. Methane is biologically inert and exerts a toxic effect only by replacing oxygen. Saturated hydrocarbons, from propane through the octanes, have increasingly strong narcotic properties; confusion is one of their many effects on the central nervous system (11). Vertigo, headache, convulsions, and coma may follow exposure to the vapors of these compounds.

Aromatic hydrocarbons

The aromatic hydrocarbons are based on benzene and molecules that incorporate one or more benzene rings. Their chief sources are coal and petroleum. They are used mostly as solvents and synthetic substrates, and some of them have been abused for their psychoactive effects.

Benzene acute intoxication may feature euphoria, dizziness, headache, staggering gait, delirium, and loss of consciousness (12,13). Shortness of breath, irritability, and unsteadiness on walking may persist for several weeks. Acute benzene intoxication has been called "benzol jag" by industrial workers because of its symptoms resembling drunken behavior with confusion (11).

Toluene, xylene, and *styrene* are less toxic than benzene. Acute toxicity involves CNS depression and encephalopathy. The latter may feature all the manifestations of narcosis, including euphoria, fatigue, reduced psychomotor activity, delirium, and coma. Much of the literature on the neurotoxicity of industrial solvents has focused on chronic exposure to these substances in the workplace (13–18). Evidence shows that long-term exposure to these chemicals can result in cognitive impairment and other psychological abnormalities that may or may not be reversible. Thus, simple intoxication and dementia appear to be the most common organic mental syndromes induced by chronic exposure to industrial solvents. Acute intoxication, notably with toluene, has been reported mostly in the context of solvent abuse and will be discussed in a later section.

Halogenated hydrocarbons

These compounds are widely used in industry as solvents and for chlorine use in the manufacture of plastics, pesticides, and other goods. Several of them have been reported to induce delirium (19).

Carbon tetrachloride is one of the most toxic common solvents and can affect the CNS. The neurological symptoms and signs tend to appear early in cases of acute poisoning and may dominate the clinical picture. Headache, vertigo, weakness, blurring of vision, tremor, paresthesias, and drowsiness are the initial manifestations, followed in some cases by delirium and coma (19,20).

Ethylene dichloride intoxication may feature "mental confusion" (3).

Methyl bromide is used as a fumigant and insecticide. Intoxication is uncommon and often includes neurotoxic effects, which fall into three stages: 1. a premonitory stage with headache, vertigo, and gait disturbance; 2. a cerebral irritation stage with delirium, twitching, and seizures; and 3. a recovery stage, which may last for several years and may be marked by hallucinations, memory impairment, aphasia, and incoordination (21). Methyl bromide poisoning may present as delirium and may be misdiagnosed as a functional psychosis (22). In a child, it may resemble Reye's syndrome (21).

Methyl chloride is a gas used mainly as a chemical intermediate and as a foaming agent in the production of foamed plastics. Its toxic symptoms include drowsiness, blurred vision, dizziness, ataxia, nightmares, restlessness, and delirium (23).

Methylene chloride, a solvent, can cause acute intoxication, which may include neuropsychological symptoms such as headache, dizziness, and a sensation of drunkenness (24). It is not clear whether delirium can occur.

Trichloroethylene, a solvent, can cause encephalopathy characterized by impaired short memory, irritability, a sense of drunkenness, and a "spacey" feeling (25). In some cases, euphoria, excitement, dizziness, drowsiness, and delirium may be present (2,11).

Carbon disulfide (CS_2)

This colorless, transparent fluid is used mostly in the manufacture of viscose rayon and in cold vulcanization of rubber. Reports of severe mental symptoms in workers poisoned by it appeared in the nineteenth century and were labelled "carbon disulfide neurosis" (26). One early report referred to it as "acute mania"; it was, in fact, delirium (11). Following months or even years of exposure, some workers suddenly became delirious and displayed excitement and hallucinations. A variety of symptoms of chronic CS_2 intoxication have been reported: irritability, depression, impaired psychomotor function and concentration, somatization, insomnia, bad dreams, temper outbursts, and memory loss (2,11,26–28). Acute CS_2 poisoning may feature delirium, which can occur in a setting of chronic intoxication and the related cognitive impairment, depression, and an organic personality syndrome (2). The pathophysiology of the behavioral toxicity of CS_2 is not well understood. The agent is believed to interfere with certain respiratory enzymes in the brain and thus with cerebral oxidative metabolism. Inhibition of brain monoamine oxidase has been reported. In some cases of poisoning, a decrease in the number of cerebral cortical ganglion cells has been observed (27,28).

Carbon monoxide (CO)

CO poisoning is an important cause of illness and death as a result of accidental or deliberate exposure. Over 3,000 deaths per year from such poisoning occur in the United States (29). CO inhalation is a common means of suicide, especially with the use of automobile exhaust fumes. Accidental exposure may result from leaking gas mains, black smoke inhalation during a fire, and inadequate venting of furnaces. Symptoms of acute CO intoxication are protean and include neuropsychiatric manifestations (29–33). The incidence of delirium in this context has been reported to be between 17% and 25% (31). The syndrome may be a presenting feature of acute CO poisoning or can follow emergence from coma. It may last for only hours or for up to 4 weeks (32). Moreover, it may be a manifestation of delayed postanoxic encephalopathy, which comes on, after a lucid interval, as long as 3 weeks after the initial exposure. Suddenly, delirium and/or other symptoms of cerebral dysfunction appear, and the patient may become comatose and die.

CO combines with hemoglobin to form carboxyhemoglobin (COHb). The resulting hypoxia is believed to be the main basis of CO toxicity. Confusion occurs with COHb levels of 40% to 50% (29) and is accompanied by headache, palpitations, nausea, dizziness, and excitement (29–33). COHb levels of 50% to 60% result in coma (3). CO gives rise to parenchymal necrosis in vulnerable areas of cerebral gray matter, including the globus pallidus, cerebral cortex, hippocampus, cerebellum, and substantia nigra (30). Permanent neuropsychiatric sequelae include dementia, amnestic syndrome, and organic personality syndrome (29–32). Treatment includes the monitoring and management of cardiac arrhythmias and oxygenation (20).

Esters

Dimethyl sulfate, an important alkylating agent, is primarily an irritant producing inflammation of the eyes, upper airway, and skin, but it has also been reported to cause delirium (3).

Glyceryl trinitrate can induce hypotension, tachycardia, vomiting, and headache ("powder head"). More intense exposure can given rise to delirium, especially in conjunction with alcohol (11).

Nitrites have been abused to enhance sexual pleasure. Amyl, butyl, and isobutyl nitrites can cause hypotension. Toxic effects of amyl nitrite inhalation include rapid flushing of the face, vertigo, weakness, headache, restlessness, and delirium (34). Syncope and death from cardiovascular collapse may follow inhalation of volatile nitrites ("poppers," "locker room") during sexual intercourse (34).

Fluorohydrocarbons

These compounds have narcotic properties in high concentrations. A syndrome called "polymer-fume fever" has been described in persons exposed to decomposition products of fluoroplastics (11). Fluorohydrocarbons of the Freon type are used as propellants for deodorant sprays. Inhalation of the latter can result in confusion, hallucinations, excitement, cognitive impairment, and muscular incoordination (35). These reported symptoms of intoxication probably represent delirium.

Hydrogen Sulfide

This highly poisonous gas is formed by the decay of organic matter containing sulfur, such as sewage and industrial waste water in tanneries, abattoirs, and glue factories. The gas acts rapidly and causes severe histotoxic anoxia by inhibition of cytochrome oxidase (36). In lower concentrations (50 to 500 ppm) it causes hyperpnea. Exposure to 1,000 ppm results in rapid loss of consciousness. Removal from the poisoned environment can result in equally rapid arousal and eventually complete recovery. If apnea occurs, it is often followed by convulsions, collapse, and death (36). Exposure to concentrations insufficient to result in loss of consciousness may induce delirium. Treatment involves injection of an intravenous solution of sodium nitrite (36).

Metals and metalloids

Toxic metals, such as arsenic, cadmium, lead, and mercury, are ubiquitous in the modern industrial environment (37). Intoxication with some of them, or their compounds, may give rise to delerium.

Arsenic is widely used in herbicides, insecticides, and rodenticides. Highly poisonous, it has been used for centuries for homidical purposes. Acute encephalopathy may result from intoxication with this metal and feature delirium (38–40). Symptoms develop 30 minutes to several hours following ingestion, either accidental or intentional. Cardiac arrhythmia may occur and cause death. It is worth noting that arsenic poisoning can follow ingestion of moonshine, i.e., illicit whiskey (41). Treatment involves the use of a chelating agent (38). Delirium can be a feature of acute *arsine* poisoning (42).

Lead seldom causes acute encephalopathy today (43). In the nineteenth century, the cerebral form of plumbism was called "encephalopathia saturnina" and featured delirium, convulsions, and coma. This form of lead poisoning rarely occurs in adults today but may be seen in association with other symptoms of poisoning in children (43). In adults, it is most likely to follow ingestion of illicit whiskey (43). Chronic lead poisoning may produce neurotoxic effects such as fatigue, irritability, insomnia, nervousness, headache, and cognitive impairment (37,43).

Tetraethyl lead may cause acute encephalopathy, which in its more severe form can feature delirium with hallucinations, paranoid delusions, and excitement (44). The incidence of this encephalopathy in industrial settings appears to be low today due to the precautions used by industry. On the other hand, tetraethyl poisoning may follow gasoline sniffing by children and adolescents (45). Blood levels of lead are elevated, and levels of erythrocytic delta-aminolevulinic acid are markedly decreased. The EEG is diffusely slowed. Treatment of acute lead poisoning involves the use of chelating agents.

Manganese appears to give rise mostly to chronic intoxication, which can involve behavioral toxicity in the form of "manganese madness" that resembles schizophrenia (46). It is not clear whether delirium ever occurs.

Mercury can cause poisoning in its elemental form, used in industry, and in the form of its organic compounds, notably methylmercury (37). Mercurialism is one of the oldest forms of industrial intoxication (47). Elemental mercury vaporizes readily at room temperature and may be inhaled. Inorganic mercury can give rise to both acute and chronic poisoning, but its toxic effects on the CNS are less severe than those of its organic compounds (48). Elemental mercury is most likely to cause acute intoxication by inhalation of the vapor. It has a high degree of fat solubility and may alter the permeability of cerebral blood vessels. Intoxicated patients tend to have poor concentration and recent memory deficits but do not seem to develop delirium (49).

Intoxication with organic compounds of mercury, notably *methylmercury,* used as a pesticide, is largely confined to the CNS (48,50,51). Early symptoms include paresthesias and other signs of peripheral neuropathy (38). Moderately intoxicated individuals display clouding of the sensorium, which may progress to akinetic mutism and coma (50). Delirium seems to be a relatively uncommon manifestation of mercurialism.

Nickel can give rise to acute poisoning as a result of inhalation of nickel carbonyl. "Mental confusion," as well as convulsions, have been observed (11).

Thallium is an extremely toxic metal. It is used at times as a homicidal or suicidal agent and is found in the pharmaceutical, glass, and dye industries (52). Its clinical manifestations are often initially neuropsychiatric and may include delirium (53).

Zinc can cause acute intoxication, which may feature lethargy and confusion (54).

Solvent-inhalant abuse

Solvent-inhalant abuse is the deliberate inhalation of volatile organic substances other than conventional anesthetic gases (55). The substances involved fall into three groups: organic solvents, hydrocarbon mixtures such as gasoline and lighter fuel, and aerosol propellants.

Prior to the current epidemic of solvent-inhalant abuse, there had been episodes of illicit inhalation of anesthetic gases, such as nitrous oxide and ether. Over the past 25 years, a dramatic increase in the abuse of volatile solvent-inhalants has occurred (56). A wide range of products have been abused: various cements, nail polish remover, ink, lacquer thinners, glue, lighter fluid, cleaning fluid, tyepwriter correction fluid, gasoline, antifreeze, virtually all products packaged in aerosol cans, and pure solvents (toluene, acetone, ethyl ether) (55,57). The chemical constituents of the abused products include a variety of aliphatic, aromatic, and halogenated hydrocarbons; ketones; esters, such as amyl acetate; alcohols, such as butyl and propyl alcohols; glycols; and ethers (55). Some of the most frequently implicated chemicals, such as toluene, carbon tetrachloride, and trichloroethylene, have already been discussed as potentially deliriogenic substances. Their combinations encountered in the various abused products may induce delirium when they are inhaled in high concentrations to achieve a euphoric, hallucinatory, or delirious state. Acute intoxication from inhalation of organic solvents has been referred to as "inhalation psychosis," which appears to be toxic delirium (58). Populations at risk include adults whose work brings them into contact with solvent-inhalants, as well as children and adolescents (56).

Toxic effects of the solvent-inhalants include those on kidney and liver functions, blood, and the CNS (55). Sudden death may occur as a result of asphyxiation, cardiac arrhythmia, respiratory arrest, and liver failure (56). Lead encephalopathy may result from gasoline sniffing (45,59). In acute intoxication with at least some of these agents, the EEG shows slowing of the background activity (58,60). The pathophysiology of solvent inhalation is incompletely understood. The inhaled vapors enter the blood rapidly and pass the blood-brain barrier to exert their neurotoxic effects. Hydrocarbons in general are CNS depressants, but excitement tends to precede narcosis and loss of consciousness. Initially, the sniffer tends to experience a feeling of euphoria and excitement, followed by hallucinations and delusions. As the concentration of the inhaled vapor increases, drowsiness and progressive loss of alertness and awareness develop; finally, loss of consciousness occurs. The hallucinations are visual or auditory, or both. They are typically pleasant and often grandiose, with the inhaler figuring as a hero. On occasion, however, the hallucinations may be frightening, with visions of fierce animals or threatening, ghost-like figures, for example. Illusions and hallucinations of floating or spinning are not uncommon. Distortions of space and visual perception may occur. In *gasoline* intoxication, some disorientation, memory impairment, and other cognitive deficits are found, depending on the degree of CNS toxicity. Repeated intoxication may lead to progressive dementia and cerebellar ataxia (61).

Withdrawal symptoms associated with chronic, heavy use of solvent-inhalants include delirium and seizures (56). They begin within hours or a few days after cessation of abuse and respond to diazepam (56).

Synthetic organic insecticides

The two major classes of insecticides in current use are the *organophosphates* and the *carbamates.* The latter, by contrast to the former, do not cause neurotoxicity (62). Poisoning with organophosphates is usually the consequence of a suicidal attempt, an accident, or, rarely, usage for homicidal purposes (62). In mild to moderate intoxication, the patient tends to be alert and oriented, and complains of such symptoms as headache, dizziness, blurred vision, tremor, incoordination, weakness, and abdominal cramps. Acute poisoning may feature "depressed level of consciousness," confusion, and toxic psychosis (62–64). The description of these mental effects in the literature is so inadequate that it is impossible to be sure if they represent delirium. Decreased vigilance, slowing of information processing, psychomotor retardation, memory impairment, anxiety, and depression are the reported psychopathological effects of organophosphate toxicity in humans (65,66). EEG abnormalities, especially frontocentral slowing, have been observed in men exposed to these insecticides (67,68). Whether these effects represent delirium is not clear, but this is possible.

Organophosphate insecticides act as irreversible cholinesterase inhibitors (62). As a result of their action, acetylcholine accumulates at synapses, causing overstimulation and consequent disruption of transmission in both the central and the peripheral nervous systems. Treatment of poisoning involves atropinization (62).

Poisonous animals, mushrooms, and plants

Delirium may be induced by ingestion of certain *fishes,* such as ciguatera (69), or by envenomation by certain *snakes,* such as the Eastern coral snake (70), or by spiders, such as the brown recluse spider (71).

Ingestion of poisonous *mushrooms,* notably those of the *Amanita* genus, may also cause delirium (72–74).

A number of *plants* contain deliriogenic substances (75,76). Most notable among them in North America are those of the Solanaceae family which contain belladonna alkaloids. Deadly nightshade *(Atropa belladonna),* Jimson weed *(Datura stramonium),* devil's trumpet *(Datura metel),* dunal *(Datura metaloides),* angel's trumpet *(Datura suavolens),* and black henbane *Hyoscyamus niger)* are the North American plants that contain belladonna alkaloids and cause poisoning. These plants yield a mixture of the alkaloids atropine and scopolamine and are a common cause of anticholinergic delirium (75–78). Ingestion of Solanaceae plants may be accidental, especially in children, or deliberate for the purpose of inducing a hallucinatory state. Jimson weed poisoning due to deliberate abuse by adolescents and young adults is not uncommon, especially in the autumn, when seeds are readily available (78). Similarly, delirium due to ingestion of angel's trumpet appears to be on the rise because of the popularity of this plant as a hallucinogen (77). Treatment of poisoning with these plants is the same as for anticholinergic delirium generally and is discussed in Chapter 11.

One other deliriogenic plant should be mentioned because of its historical interest: *wormweed (Arthemisia absinthium).* Essential oils derived from this and from certain other plants, such as mugwort *(Artemisia vulgaris),* sage *(Salvia officinalis),* and tansy *(Tanacetum vulgare),* contains thujone, a psychoactive substance (79,80). Its effects have been known since antiquity (79). Thujone-containing plants were formerly used in certain alcoholic beverages, notably absinthe, which was well known to poets and artists of the nineteenth century such as Baudelaire, Van Gogh, and others (80). Thujone can induce delirium.

References

1. Weiss B.: Intersections of psychiatry and toxicology. *Int. J. Ment. Health* 1985;14:7–25.
2. Feldman R. G., Ricks N. L., Baker E. L.: Neuropsychological effects of industrial toxins: A review. *Am. J. Industr. Med.* 1980;1:211–227.
3. Patty F. A.: *Industrial Hygiene and Toxicology.* New York, Wiley Interscience, 1962.
4. Von Oettingen W. F.: Poisoning. *A Guide to Clinical Diagnosis* and Treatment, ed 2. Philadelphia, WB Saunders, 1958, pp 89–90.
5. Casarett L. J., Doull J. (eds): *Toxicology. The Basic Science of Poisons.* New York, Macmillan, 1975.
6. *Diagnostic and Statistical Manual of Mental Disorders,* ed 3 revised. Washington, DC, American Psychiatric Association, 1987.
7. Berger J. R., Ayyar D. R.: Neurological complications of ethylene glycol intoxication. *Arch. Neurol.* 1981;38:724–726.
8. Binder L. S., Postma R.: Ethylene glycol intoxication. *Tex. Med.* 1986;82:33–35.
9. Jacobsen D., Ostby N., Bredesen J. E.: Studies on ethylene glycol poisoning. *Acta Med. Scand.* 1982;212:11–15.
10. Jacobsen D., McMartin K. E.: Methanol and ethylene glycol poisonings. *Med. Toxicol.* 1986;1:309–334.

11. Hamilton A., Hardy H. L.: *Industrial Toxicology,* ed 3. Acton, Mass, Publishing Sciences Group, 1974.
12. Haley T. J.: Evaluation of the health effects of benzene inhalation. *Clin. Toxicol.* 1977;11:531–548.
13. Bruckner J. V., Peterson R. G.: Toxicology of aliphatic and aromatic hydrocarbons, in Sharp C. W., Brehm M. L. (eds): *Review of Inhalants: Euphoria to Dysfunction.* Washington, DC, National Institute on Drug Abuse, 1977, pp 124–163.
14. Baker E. L., Smith T. J., Landrigan P. J.: The neurotoxicity of industrial solvents: A review of the literature. *Am. J. Industr. Med.* 1985;8:207–217.
15. Eskelinen L., Luisto M., Tenkanen L., et al: Neuropsychological methods in the differentiation of organic solvent intoxication from certain neurological conditions. *J. Clin. Exp. Neuropsychol.* 1986;8:239–256.
16. Flodin U., Edling C., Axelsen O.: Clinical studies of psycho-organic syndromes among workers with exposure to solvents. *Am. J. Industr. Med.* 1984;5:287–295.
17. Gregersen P., Klausen H., Elsnal C. U.: Chronic toxic encephalopathy in solvent-exposed painters in Denmark 1976–1980: Clinical cases and social consequences after a 5-year follow-up. *Am. J. Industr. Med.* 1987;11:399–417.
18. Linz D. H., de Garmo P. L., Morton W. E., et al: Organic solvent-induced encephalopathy in industrial painters. *J. Occup. Med.* 1986;28:119–125.
19. Haddad L. M., Winchester J. F. (eds): *Poisoning and Drug Overdosage.* Philadelphia, WB Saunders, 1983, pp 780–783.
20. Ruprah M., Mant T. G. K., Flanagan R. J.: Acute carbon tetrachloride poisoning in 19 patients. Implications for diagnosis and treatment. *Lancet* 1985;1:1027–1029.
21. Shield L. K., Coleman T. L., Markesbery W. R.: Methylbromide intoxication: Neurologic features, including simulation of Reye syndrome. *Neurology* 1977;27:959–962.
22. Zatuchni J., Hong K.: Methyl bromide poisoning seen initially as psychosis. *Arch. Neurol.* 1981;38:529–530.
23. Scharnweber H. C., Spears G. N., Cowles S. R.: Chronic methyl chloride intoxication in six industrial workers. *J. Occup. Med.* 1974;16:112–113.
24. Rasmussen K., Sabroe S.: Neuropsychological symptoms among metal workers exposed to halogenated hydrocarbons. *Scand. J. Soc. Med.* 1986;14:161–168.
25. McCunney R. J.: Diverse manifestations of trichloroethylene. *Br. J. Industr. Med.* 1988;45:122–126.
26. Davidson M., Feinleib M.: Carbon disulfide poisoning: A review. *Am. Heart J.* 1972;83:100–114.
27. Hanwinen H.: Psychological picture of manifest and latent carbon disulphide poisoning. *Br. J. Industr. Med.* 1971;28:374–381.
28. Mancuso T. F., Locke B. Z.: Carbon disulphide as a cause of suicide. *J. Occup. Med.* 1972;14:595–606.
29. Dolan M. C.: Carbon monoxide poisoning. *Can. Med. Assoc. J.* 1985;133:392–398.
30. Ginsberg M. D.: Carbon monoxide intoxication: Clinical features, neuropathology and mechanisms of injury. *Clin. Toxicol.* 1985;23:281–288.
31. Smith J. S., Brandon S.: Acute carbon monoxide poisoning—3 years of experience in a defined population. *Postgrad. Med. J.* 1970;46:65–70.
32. Smith J. S., Brandon S.: Morbidity from carbon monoxide poisoning at three-year follow-up. *Br. Med. J.* 1973;1:318–321.
33. Zimmerman S. S., Truxal B.: Carbon monoxide poisoning. *Pediatrics* 1981;68:215–224.

34. Haley T. J.: Review of the physiological effects of amyl, butyl, and isobutyl nitrites. *Clin. Toxicol.* 1980;16:317–329.
35. Kramer R. A., Pierpaoli P.: Hallucinogenic effect of propellant components of deodorant sprays. *Pediatrics* 1971;48:322–323.
36. Smith R. P., Gosselin R. E.: Hydrogen sulfide poisoning. *J. Occup. Med.* 1979;21:93–97.
37. Landrigan P. J.: Occupational and community exposures to toxic metals: Lead, cadmium, mercury and arsenic. *West. J. Med.* 1982;137:531–539.
38. Fuortes L.: Arsenic poisoning. *Postgrad. Med.* 1988;83:233–244.
39. Schoolmeester W. L., White D. R.: Arsenic poisoning. *South. Med. J.* 1980;73:198–208.
40. Zaloga G. P., Deal J., Spurling T., et al: Case report: Unusual manifestations of arsenic intoxication. *Am. J. Med. Sci.* 1985;289:210–214.
41. Gerhardt R. E., Crecelius E. A., Hudson J. B.: Trace element contents of moonshine. *Arch. Environ. Health* 1980;35:332–334.
42. Parish G. G., Glass R., Kimbrough R.: Acute arsine poisoning in two workers cleaning a clogged drain. *Arch. Environ. Health* 1979;34:224–227.
43. Cullen M. R., Robins J. M., Eskenazi B.: Adult inorganic lead intoxication: Presentation of 31 new cases and a review of recent advances in literature. *Medicine* 1983;62:221–247.
44. Beattie A. D., Moore M. R.: Tetraethyl-lead poisoning. Lancet 1972;2:12–15.
45. Boecky R. L., Postl B., Coodin F. J.: Gasoline sniffing and tetraethyl lead poisoning. *Pediatrics* 1977;60:140–145.
46. Banta R. G., Markesberry W. R.: Elevated manganese levels associated with dementia and extrapyramidal signs. *Neurology* 1977;27:213–216.
47. Maurissen J. P. J.: History of mercury and mercurialism. *N.Y. State J. Med.* 1981;81:1902–1909.
48. Williamson A. M., Teo R. K. C., Sanderson J.: Occupational mercury exposure and its consequences for behavior. *Int. Arch. Occup. Environ. Health.* 1982;50:273–286.
49. Vroom F. Q., Greer M.: Mercury vapour intoxication. *Brain* 1972;95:305–318.
50. Bakir F., Rustam H., Tikriti S., et al: Clinical and epidemiological aspects of methylmercury poisoning. *Postgrad. Med. J.* 1980;56:1–10.
51. Gerstner H. B., Huff J. E.: Selected case histories and epidemiologic examples of human mercury poisoning. *Clin. Toxicol.* 1977;11:131–150.
52. Thompson D. F.: Management of thallium poisoning. *Clin. Toxicol.* 1981;18:979–990.
53. Bank W. J., Pleasure D. E., Suzuki K., et al: Thallium poisoning. *Arch. Neurol.* 1972;26:456–464.
54. Chobanian S. J.: Accidental ingestion of liquid zinc chloride: Local and systemic effects. *Ann. Emerg. Med.* 1981;10:91–93.
55. Hayden J. W., Comstock E. G.: The clinical toxicology of solvent abuse. *Clin. Toxicol.* 1976;9:169–184.
56. Westermeyer J.: The psychiatrist and solvent-inhalant abuse: Recognition, assessment, and treatment. *Am. J. Psychiatry* 1987;144:903–907.
57. Barnes G. E., Vulcano B. A.: Bibliography of the solvent abuse literature. *Int. J. Addict.* 1979;14:401–421.
58. Glaser F. B.: Inhalation psychosis and related states. *Arch. Gen. Psychiatry* 1966;14:315–322.

59. Goldings A. S., Stewart R. M.: Organic lead encephalopathy: Behavioral change and movement disorder following gasoline inhalation. *J. Clin. Psychiatry* 1982;43:70–72.
60. Seshia S. S., Rajani K. R., Boeckx R. L., et al: The neurological manifestations of chronic inhalation of leaded gasoline. *Dev. Med. Child Neurol.* 1978;20:323–334.
61. Valepy R., Sumi S. M., Copass M. K., et al: Acute and chronic progressive encephalopathy due to gasoline sniffing. *Neurology* 1978;28:507–508.
62. Tafuri J., Roberts J.: Organophosphate poisoning. *Ann. Emerg. Med.* 1987;16:193–202.
63. Minton N. A., Murray V. S. G.: A review of organophosphate poisoning. *Med. Toxicol.* 1988;3:350–375.
64. Perold J. G., Bezuidenhout D. J. J.: Chronic organophosphate poisoning. *S. Afr. Med. J.* 1980;57:7–9.
65. Levin H. S., Rodnitsky R. L.: Behavioral effects of organophosphate pesticides in man. *Clin. Toxicol.* 1976;9:391–405.
66. Namba T., Nolte C. T., Jackrel J., et al: Poisoning due to organophosphate insecticides. *Am. J. Med.* 1971;50:475–492.
67. Dille J. R., Smith P. W.: Central nervous system effects of chronic exposure to organophosphate insecticides. *Aerospace Med.* 1964;35:475–480.
68. Metcalf D. R., Holmes H. H.: EEG, psychological, and neurological alterations in humans with organophosphorus exposure. *Ann. N.Y. Acad. Sci.* 1969;160:357–365.
69. Lawrence D. N., Enriquez M. B., Lumish R. M., et al: Ciguatera fish poisoning in Miami. *J.A.M.A.* 1980;244:254–258.
70. Kitchens C. S., Van Mierop L. H. S.: Envenomation by the Eastern coral snake *(Micrurus fulvius fulvius). J.A.M.A.* 1987;258:1615–1618.
71. Wong R. C., Hughes S. E., Voorhees J. J.: Spider bites. *Arch. Dermatol.* 1987;123:98–104.
72. Lampe K. F., McCann M. A.: Differential diagnosis of poisoning by North American mushrooms, with particular emphasis on *Amanita phalloides*-like intoxication. *Ann. Emerg. Med.* 1987;16:956–962.
73. McCormick D. J., Avbel A. J., Gibbons R. B.: Nonlethal mushroom poisoning. *Ann. Intern. Med.* 1979;90:332–335.
74. Hanrahan J. P., Gordon M. A.: Mushroom poisoning. *J.A.M.A.* 1984;251:1057–1061.
75. Brown J. K., Malone M. H.: "Legal highs"—constituents, activity, toxicology, and herbal folklore. *Clin. Toxicol.* 1978;12:1–31.
76. Hardin J. W., Arena J. M.: *Human Poisoning from Native and Cultivated Plants.* Durham, NC, Duke University Press, 1974.
77. Hall R. C. W., Popkin M. K., McHenry L. E.: Angel's trumpet psychosis: A central nervous system anticholinergic syndrome. *Am. J. Psychiatry* 1977;134:312–314.
78. Klein-Schwartz W., Oderda G. M.: Jimson weed intoxication in adolescents and young adults. *A.J.D.C.* 1984;138:737–739.
79. Albert-Puleo M.: Mythobotany, pharmacology, and chemistry of thujone-containing plants and derivatives. *Econ. Botany* 1978;32:65–74.
80. Vogt D. D., Montagne M.: Absinthe: Behind the emerald mask. *Intern. J. Addict.* 1982;17:1015–1029.

13

Alcohol and Drug Withdrawal

A censensus has recently been reached regarding the definition of terms in the area of substance abuse (1). "Withdrawal" has been defined as "cessation of drug or alcohol use by an individual in whom dependence is established" (1, p 557). "Withdrawal syndrome" refers to "the onset of a predictable constellation of signs and symptoms involving altered activity of the central nervous system after the abrupt discontinuation of, or rapid decrease in, dosage of a drug" (1, p 557). In this chapter, delirium due to withdrawal of alcohol and drugs will be discussed.

Alcohol withdrawal delirium (delirium tremens)

Definition

DSM-III-R (2) contains two forms of alcohol withdrawal syndrome: *uncomplicated alcohol withdrawal* and *alcohol withdrawal delirium.* The essential feature of the latter is stated to be a delirium that occurs within a week after withdrawal (as defined above) of alcohol. This disorder has also been called "delirium tremens." Its diagnostic criteria include marked autonomic hyperactivity (2). The associated features are vivid hallucinations, either visual, auditory, or tactile; delusions; agitation; and a coarse, irregular tremor (2). If seizures, "rum fits," also follow withdrawal, they always precede the development of delirium. The latter usually occurs after 5 to 15 years of heavy drinking and lasts for several days (2).

DSM-III-R makes a welcome attempt to standardize the terminology of and the diagnostic criteria for the alcohol withdrawal syndrome, a condition whose clinical features and boundaries have been a subject of controversy for decades (3–5). The term "delirium tremens" was introduced by Sutton (6) in 1813 and is still widely, if imprecisely, used by clinicians (7). Actually the whole area of mental disorders related to alcohol abuse has been plagued by terminological chaos (8). This makes it difficult to draw conclusions from the published studies regarding the incidence, pathophysiology, and treatment of alcohol withdrawal delirium. It is hoped that once the new classification and terminology become widely followed, a more consistent use of the terms and diagnostic criteria will result, facilitating advances in knowledge about the management of alcohol-related mental disorders. Meanwhile, it is impossible to review the literature in this field without using the term "delirium tremens."

Clinical features

The incidence of alcohol withdrawal delirium is unknown but is considered to be low. Some writers have estimated that fewer than 1% of alcoholics develop delirium tremens (4). In one large study, the syndrome was diagnosed in about 40% of 1,026 alcoholics hospitalized for acute mental and physical disturbances associated with drinking—hardly a representative population (9).

The age of patients varies from study to study and averages 40 to 50 years (4). Men develop alcohol withdrawal delirium four to five times as often as women. Delirium tremens usually occurs in alcoholics with a history of drinking for 5 to 15 years, mostly for more than 10 years (4). Symptoms of withdrawal generally develop 7 to 24 hours after cessation of drinking and include coarse tremors of the hands or tongue; nausea or vomiting; malaise; autonomic nervous system hyperactivity manifested by tachycardia, sweating, and elevated blood pressure; anxiety; irritability; insomnia; nightmares; and transient illusions and hallucinations (2). This stage may be followed by convulsive seizures, which usually occur within 3 days after cessation of drinking (10,11). Delirium, considered to be the most severe form or stage of the alcohol withdrawal syndrome, develops 72 to 96 hours after cessation of drinking (5). This sequence of events is not invariable: seizures may not develop at all, and delirium may occur without preceding seizures (10,11). If it does develop, it becomes manifest after 3 to 4 days of the tremulous-hallucinatory stage and follows that stage, according to different reports, in 5% to 45% of cases.

Clinical features of the alcohol withdrawal delirium are typically those of the hyperalert-hyperactive variant of delirium, described in Chapters 4 and 5. The emotional tone varies and may range from amusement to panic or rage. An early personal account of delirium tremens, published in 1844, speaks of the "horror" that a patient may experience (12). A large Swedish study has provided a wealth of information on the frequency of the various symptoms in patients with the syndrome (9). Severe disorientation was noted in one-half of the patients; no patient was fully oriented, although about one in five displayed only a mild degree of disorientation. Visual hallucinations were noted in 97%, auditory hallucinations in 79%, and gustatory or olfactory ones, or both, in 6% of 552 patients with delirium tremens. Delusions of persecution were observed in 35% of the patients. Anxiety occurred in 65%, euphoria in 41%, depression in 13%, irritability in 48%, and aggressivity in 32%. Coarse tremor was noted in 92% of the patients on admission. General psychomotor hyperactivity was exhibited by 92%, picking movements with fingers by 78%, and episodes of clonic muscle jerks by 23%. One-third of the patients sweated profusely, and one in five had vomiting or diarrhea, or both. Fever was found in 57% and tachycardia (more than 90 bpm) in 94%. Both systolic and diastolic blood pressures were elevated in about two-thirds of the patients in this series. The duration of delirium averaged 3 days, and the syndrome seldom lasted for more than one week. The mortality rate was 3%. Other authors assert that in recent years the mortality rate in delirium tremens has dropped to less than 1% (4).

Large-scale studies (3–5,9), like the one just quoted, have helped to clarify the clinical features and natural history of delirium tremens but provide relatively little information about the finer aspects of the patients' psychiatric symptoms and the quality of the subjective experience. Clinical studies of individual patients offer interesting data on these aspects of the syndrome.

De Boor (13) has summarized the more important German studies in this area, notably those of Bonhoeffer, Kraepelin, and Naecke. Some of these earlier investigators pointed out that not all patients with delirium tremens experience frightening hallucinations, as is often assumed. Many of these hallucinations are marked by occupational and otherwise nonthreatening content. Hallucinations of animals were reported by only one-third of one series of patients, by contrast to 70% in another study. The hallucinated animals may be small, but in the majority of cases they seem to be life-sized. Large, mythological animals may fill the vision of some patients. Not all of them hallucinate rats and mice, as is popularly believed: in one study, quoted by de Boor, not a single patient reported such hallucinatory contents. Patients tend to hallucinate many objects or animals simultaneously. Whole scenes, as well as inanimate objects, people, and plants, may form the main content of the visual hallucinations. On the whole, the patients tend to accept their misperceptions as real. Auditory hallucinations consist mostly of threatening and abusive voices, but some patients hallucinate music, for example. Pressure on the eyeball may elicit visual hallucinations. Patients tend to be suggestible and can be readily talked into hallucinating various objects or figures. Illusions are very common. Contents of dreams that the patient had experienced in the past may appear as hallucinations in delirium tremens.

A recent study compared the hallucinations of alcoholics and "functional psychotics" (14). Human content predominated in both groups, but the alcoholics reported more animal content than the psychotics (mostly schizophrenics). Human voices predominated in the auditory hallucinations of both groups, but alcoholics heard relatively more animal sounds. The species involved in their animal-content hallucinations were mostly insects, reptiles, rodents, and predatory mammals. These patients also tended to experience tactile hallucinations of insects on the skin (formication). The investigators concluded that the most frequent hallucinations of alcoholics involve an emotionally negative animal content.

Another study has focused on auditory elementary hallucinations in delirium tremens (15). They were found in 50% of the patients and included simple phasic noises, such as clicks, reports, fluttering, and fading sounds. Tinnitus was reported by 40% of the patients. Moreover, about one-half of the patients experienced unstructured visual hallucinations in the form of shadows, spots, and flashes of light. The investigators hypothesize that the noises experienced in delirium tremens do not represent hallucinations but rather real noises produced by excessive contractions of the stapedius, tensor tympani, and tensor veli palatini muscles.

Other investigators have explored the relationship between hallucinations and *sleep disturbances* in alcohol withdrawal delirium (16). An alcoholic typically suffers from insomnia, which may lead to a heavy drinking bout. Gradually, nightmares develop and begin to interrupt whatever sleep the patient may secure, but additional intake of alcohol may initially suppress them. After a while the nightmares return, and the patient becomes increasingly uncertain about whether he or she is asleep and dreaming or awake and hallucinating. A predominantly waking state with hallucinations follows. Initially, the hallucinations tend to come on when the patient is alone, at night, or in the dark, and closes the eyes. This development may be arrested if the patient succeeds in obtaining sound sleep. An intimate relationship appears to exist between dreams and hallucinations in these patients (see also Chapter 6).

Other investigators have compared the subjective experience of delirium tremens with that of a state of altered awareness induced by LSD (16). Both states were characterized by misperceptions, increased alertness, and a subjectively increased train of thought. They differed, however, in that the delirium tremens was marked by the belief that the experienced hallucinations represented real perceptions, by paranoid delusions, and by anxiety or depression. In another experiment, it was observed that subjects given both an anticholinergic agent (Ditran) and LSD showed a clinical picture resembling that of delirium tremens more closely than when either drug alone was administered (17).

The clinical picture of delirium tremens helps to establish the diagnosis (4). Patients are usually communicative and relate their experiences freely. They tend to be absorbed by their hallucinations, vigilant, hyperactive, agitated, restless, and tremulous. As in all types of delirium, both the cognitive-attentional deficits and the hallucinatory experiences tend to fluctuate in severity during the daytime and are most conspicuous at night.

Etiology

From the time delirium tremens was first described and identified at the turn of the nineteenth century up to recently, a controversy had persisted regarding its etiology. While some medical writers considered it to be the consequence of alcohol withdrawal in heavy drinkers, others regarded it as a direct result of excessive drinking (4). Studies carried out in the 1950s confirmed the relationship between ethanol and the withdrawal syndrome, whose severity appeared to depend on the amount and duration of alcohol consumption (18). Isbell et al. (19), in their classic experimental study, demonstrated that abrupt withdrawal of alcohol from chronically intoxicated subjects induces an abstinence syndrome that may feature convulsions or delirium, or both. Not only abrupt cessation, but also a reduction in ethanol intake, may precipitate a withdrawal syndrome. A similar conclusion was reached by Victor and Wolfe (5) on the basis of their own studies and those of others. Tremulousness, hallucinations, seizures, and delirium characterize the syndrome. Delirium tremens requires heavy drinking for many weeks or months by a person who has, in most cases, abused alcohol for 5 or more years (3,5). In one study, the patients had a mean daily consumption of 1 liter of whiskey or 2 liters of wine for a mean period of about 17 years (3). Severe withdrawal syndrome may also occur in patients who do not consume large quantities of ethanol but who take sedative-hypnotic drugs that have cross tolerance with ethanol at the same time (18). Other hypotheses about the etiology of delirium tremens include such factors as hypomagnesemia, cirrhosis of the liver, deficiency of thiamine, and fat embolism (19). However, there is now a broad consensus that the withdrawal hypothesis of delirium tremens has the strongest empirical support (18,19). Some authors assert that withdrawal is a necessary, but not a sufficient condition to elicit it (18).

Delirium tremens does not develop in all alcoholics—its incidence is estimated to range from less than 1% to 15% (4)—and this raises the question of whether individual *predisposing factors* exist. Genetic, psychological, nutritional, and socioeconomic factors have been proposed to predispose an alcoholic to the development of delirium tremens (4,20).

Precipitating factors have been postulated to include the drinking pattern, dietary intake, gastrointestinal symptoms, infection, inflammation, trauma, and hepatic insufficiency (4,5). Free-choice drinking pattern, decreased food intake, gastritis, acute infection, and trauma due to accident or surgery have all been observed to increase both the probability and the severity of alcohol withdrawal delirium.

Pathophysiology and pathogenesis

The pathophysiology and pathogenesis of the alcohol withdrawal delirium are still poorly understood. Ethanol is a CNS depressant whose prolonged, excessive intake results in the development of physical dependence and tolerance (4). The withdrawal of alcohol in a dependent individual is characterized by a relatively rapid transition from CNS depression to *hyperexcitability* (18,21). Explanatory hypotheses about the alcohol withdrawal syndrome and delirium involve the concepts of cellular adaptation to alcohol, denervation or disuse, supersensitivity, and rebound (4). Cells are believed to adapt to alcohol, and thus homeostasis is achieved. When alcohol is withdrawn, compensatory mechanisms are activated and some functions that had been suppressed by it become transiently exaggerated; rebound hyperexcitability of the CNS results. More specifically, it appears that alcohol may act primarily on the reticular activating system of the midbrain. During withdrawal, disuse supersensitivity of this structure is accompanied by increased cortical excitability. Repeated episodes of the alcohol withdrawal syndrome have been hypothesized to activate a *kindling* process by producing hyperexcitability of the limbic system and resulting in progressively severe withdrawal symptoms such as seizures and delirium (22,23).

Several other pathophysiological mechanisms have been proposed to account for the clinical manifestations of alcohol withdrawal delirium and related withdrawal symptoms. They include metabolic disturbances, alterations in metabolism and release of neurotransmitters, disordered sleep-wake cycle, and the characteristics of neuronal receptors. None of these mechanisms fully explains all the signs and symptoms (18).

The metabolic derangements that have been postulated to underlie at least some of the features of the alcohol withdrawal syndrome include *respiratory alkalosis* and *hypomagnesemia* (4,5,18,19,24–26). Early in alcohol withdrawal, patients begin to hyperventilate, and this leads to a respiratory alkalosis (18). Serum magnesium levels drop during this stage (18,24–26), but tend to return to normal prior to the development of delirium; hence, the role of hypomagnesemia in the alcohol withdrawal syndrome has been questioned (5,18). Hyperventilation-induced respiratory alkalosis may result in seizures. Lowered CO_2 tension may cause cerebral vasoconstriction, reduced CBF, and thus hypoxia. rCBF has been found to be reduced during the first 2 days of withdrawal and to be particularly marked in patients with clouded sensorium (27). It has been suggested that the latter may reflect brain stem dysfunction, while hallucinations could be related to cortical dysfunction (27). More recently, deficiencies of fatty acids, prostaglandins, and zinc have been implicated in the withdrawal syndrome (18).

All the known *neurotransmitters* appear to be affected during the alcohol withdrawal period (28). Particular attention has been paid to *noradrenaline* (29,30). CSF levels of noradrenaline are elevated in the alcohol withdrawal syndrome (29), as are those of its major metabolite, 3-methoxy-4-hydroxyphenylglycol (MHPG) (30). Repeated withdrawals may lead to kindling and successively enhanced noradrenergic overactivity (30). Pituitary responsiveness to corticotropin-releasing hormone, which increases the firing rate of cerebral noradrenergic neurons, is blunted (30). It is possible that enhanced central noradrenergic activity, possibly coupled with reduced central cholinergic activity, may underlie some of the core characteristics of the alcohol withdrawal delirium, such as hyperalertness, hyperactivity, and overactivity of the sympathetic nervous system. The EEG findings in this syndrome seem to support this hypothesis.

During alcohol withdrawal, the EEG usually shows low-voltage fast activity and a paucity or absence of alpha rhythm (31–34). The main activity may be below the alpha range (33). These EEG changes differ from those found in alcohol intoxication, as well as in many other deliria, in which reduction of alertness and wakefulness is accompanied by general slowing of the background activity (see Chapter 7). This suggests that different biochemical mechanisms, such as increased noradrenergic activity, distinguish alcohol withdrawal delirium.

Sleep disturbances in alcohol withdrawal delirium are discussed in Chapter 5. Their relationship to the phenomenology of the syndrome remains intriguing but unresolved.

Finally, some investigators have proposed that changes in the physical properties of *neuronal membranes* could be related to the alcohol withdrawal syndrome (28). This hypothesis is still a subject of investigation.

Treatment

A variety of therapeutic regimens have been claimed to be effective in the alcohol withdrawal syndrome (4,5,18,35–40), but no single approach to treatment has gained universal acceptance. One author asserts that the most effective therapy for alcohol withdrawal delirium is to try to prevent its occurrence (3). It is important to distinguish between the proposed treatments for the alcohol withdrawal syndrome with and without delirium. A comprehensive review of the voluminous literature on this subject is beyond the scope of this book. The following account will focus on the prevention and management of delirium.

The *objectives* of the treatment of alcohol withdrawal include 1. prevention of serious complications, such as delirium, seizures, and arrhythmias; 2. relief of subjective symptoms; 3. management of delirium once it has developed; and 4. preparation for long-term rehabilitation (18,38).

The first decision to be made in a case of alcohol withdrawal is whether to hospitalize the patient. Mild withdrawal does not require hospitalization, but a major episode does. A *supportive environment* offering reassurance, frequent monitoring of signs and symptoms, and reality orientation has been reported to be effective in over two-thirds of patients with a mild alcohol withdrawal syndrome (38,40,41). Such an environment can be provided in a detoxification center or a hospital. When alcohol withdrawal is marked by delirium or seizures, or is associated with medical illness, injury, or physical dependence on other drugs, hospitalization is mandatory. It appears that even though supportive treatment reduces the general symptoms of withdrawal, it does not prevent delirium, seizures, or arrhythmias; hence, patients in moderate to severe withdrawal should have the benefit of pharmacotherapy (38).

Pharmacotherapy is the cornerstone of management of the more severe alcohol withdrawal syndrome, including the withdrawal delirium. *Benzodiazepines* are currently the drugs of choice (18,36–39). Several studies have indicated that early treatment with these drugs reduces the incidence of delirium from 6% to about 4% (18). Practically all the currently available benzodiazepines have been studied and found effective (38). Chlordiazepoxide, diazepam, oxazepam, and lorazepam are most often used (37,38). The choice of the drug appears to be less important than the adjustment of its dosage to calm the patient (39). It follows that no suggested dosage schedule should be followed rigidly. The objective is to achieve sedation but to avoid oversedation. The usual strategy is to give larger doses on the first day and to lower them progressively on subsequent days (38). A typical regimen on the first day involves multiple doses of diazepam (20–40 mg) or chlordiazepoxide (100–400 mg) (38). Alternatively, lorazepam (1–2 mg orally or sublingually three times a day) or oxazepam (15–30 mg orally three times a day) may be administered. Some writers recommend an oral loading dose of diazepam (20 mg) every 1–2 hours until clinical improvement occurs (38). All hospitalized patients in moderate to severe withdrawal should be loaded with at least 60 mg of diazepam (38). A patient with hepatic disease should be given three daily doses of oxazepam (15–30 mg) or lorazepam (1–2 mg). In the case of severe agitation, rapid sedation is needed and hence parenteral administration is preferable. Diazepam, 10–20 mg/hr, may be administered intravenously until the patient is calm. In the case of delirium, the oral diazepam may have to be supplemented with intramuscular haloperidol, 2.5–5 mg/hr.

Many other drugs have been used in the treatment of the alcohol withdrawal syndrome, including delirium. Phenothiazines, barbiturates, paraldehyde, and antihistamines are not recommended because of their undesirable side effects (42). Clonidine has been recommended as an alternative to benzodiazepines (35). A beta blocker, atenolol, has been used recently, along with benzodiazepines, to help control a hyperadrenergic state, but it appears to be of little value in preventing the onset of delirium (36). Another beta blocker, propranolol, may reduce the severity of the tremor and has been used to treat cardiac arrhythmias, but it tends to induce hallucinations and delirium (43). Anticonvulsant drugs have been claimed to prevent seizures and, in some cases, to sedate the patient, but the evidence of their efficacy is inconclusive, except in patients with epilepsy or a history of recurrent withdrawal seizures (36,38). Physostigmine has been reported to be effective in a few cases of delirium tremens (44). In Europe, chlormethiazole appears to be the preferred drug for the treatment of the syndrome (45).

In summary, for the treatment of the alcohol withdrawal delirium, a combination of a benzodiazepine and haloperidol is recommended.

General management of uncomplicated alcohol withdrawal, as well as one with an alcohol withdrawal delirium, involves a thorough examination, correction of electrolyte and fluid imbalances, and treatment of any concurrent medical disease or complications.

When first seen, every patient should be carefully examined for evidence of injury, especially head trauma; infection; subdural hematoma; pneumonia; and hepatic failure. X-rays of the chest and skull and lumbar puncture may be indicated (5,39). Serum levels of electrolytes, including magnesium, and other routine blood tests should be carried out.

Any medical complications that may be present require immediate appropriate treatment. Constant observation and repeated examination of the patient are essential. Precautions against self-injury or injury to others by a severely agitated and delusional delirious patient are mandatory. Such a patient may have to be restrained in a lateral or prone position until sedation occurs in response to pharamcotherapy. A special attendant or a member of the family should stay with the patient if circumstances allow it. The importance of supportive nursing care has already been mentioned.

Dehydration, electrolyte imbalance, and vitamin deficiency must be corrected. Hypomagnesemia and hypokalemia may be present in a patient with alcohol withdrawal delirium, may cause cardiac arrhythmias, and should be corrected. Magnesium sulfate, 2 g every 6 hours intravenously during the first day, has been recommended for patients with hypomagnesemia, cardiac arrhythmia, and intact renal function (36,39). A patient who is malnourished or dehydrated should be given intravenous fluids (dextrose and saline solution) (39). Thiamine deficiency is common among alcoholics; hence, it is advisable to administer 100 mg of thiamine parenterally at least once, followed daily by oral vitamin supplements.

ECT therapy has been used occasionally to treat delirium tremens (46), but its value in this condition is questionable and it is seldom applied.

Sedative-hypnotic withdrawal

Abrupt reduction in dosage or cessation of any sedative-hypnotic drug may result in a withdrawal syndrome, with delirium as one of its severe manifestations. These drug withdrawal deliria are clinically similar to the alcohol withdrawal delirium. They are typically characterized by global cognitive impairment, attention disturbances, restlessness, agitation, irritability, insomnia, visual and auditory hallucinations, delusions, and anxiety. In addition, somatic symptoms are regularly present and may include seizures, tremor, sweating, fever, tachycardia, reduced or elevated blood pressure, weakness, anorexia, nausea, vomiting, and rapid weight loss (47–52). In the past, barbiturates were the most often abused sedative-hypnotics, and withdrawal of them commonly induced delirium or seizures, or both. More recently, benzodiazepines have become the most commonly used and abused drugs in this category; withdrawal of them is much less likely to precipitate delirium. Thus, even though the general features of the drug withdrawal delirium are similar, regardless of which sedative-hypnotic is involved, the readiness with which its withdrawal produces delirium varies widely from one drug, or class of drugs, to another. For this reason, they are discussed in separate sections.

Barbiturates

Classic experimental studies by Isbell et al. (52) demonstrated conclusively that abrupt reduction of the dosage or withdrawal of a barbiturate drug in a person who is chronically intoxicated and dependent produces an abstinence syndrome that often features delirium. The subjects received secobarbital sodium, pentobarbital sodium, or amobarbital sodium in doses that were gradually increased to a maximum of 1.3–3 g daily. The total period of intoxication ranged from 92 to 144 days. Twelve hours after abrupt withdrawal of the barbiturate, the subjects began to complain of anxiety and weakness, and displayed anorexia, insomnia, and a coarse tremor of the hands and face. From 24 to 30 hours after the last dose, these symptoms worsened; in addition, the subjects developed muscle twitching, vomiting, and increased startle responses. After 30 to 60 hours following withdrawal, most subjects developed convulsions. Delirium came on 36 hours to 13 days following the last dose. All patients recovered. The EEG during withdrawal showed paroxysmal bursts of high-amplitude, slow waves (four to six cycles per second). These changes preceded grand mal seizures. Increased percentages of 6–7 c/sec waves persisted for about 2 weeks.

Wikler (53) has summarized earlier studies on barbiturate withdrawal. He points out that delirium usually develops in about 60% of the cases between the fourth and seventh days of abstinence, and may or may not be preceded by convulsions. The symptoms are worse at night. The delirium lasts for a period ranging from a few days to about 2 weeks. Sudden recovery may follow prolonged, spontaneous sleep. In some patients, however, recovery progresses gradually. Administration of barbiturates does not abolish the delirium. Intake of as little as 1.0 g of a barbiturate daily for a month or more may be sufficient to result in delirium after rapid withdrawal of the drug. The EEG changes during the withdrawal syndrome include diffuse slowing of the background activity and high-voltage, bilaterally synchronous bursts of spikes, sharp waves, irregularly shaped delta waves, or 2–4 c/sec "spike and dome" complexes. These changes generally subside by the fourth or fifth day, but mild slowing of the background activity may persist longer. EEG changes druing the phase of delirium are difficult to assess because of muscle artifacts.

Considerable attention has been devoted to the role of sleep disturbances in the barbiturate withdrawal delirium. It has been hypothesized that REM sleep rebound may be responsible for its occurrence (54). Barbiturates suppress REM sleep initially, but then tolerance develops and REM levels return to baseline. On rapid withdrawal of the drug, there is an immediate rebound of REM sleep that persists for several weeks. Mental activity concomitant with REM sleep intrudes into wakefulness and constitutes delirium. This attractive hypothesis was challenged by investigators who failed to confirm that REM rebound occurs regularly after a period of barbiturate-induced REM suppression (55). Other researchers studied sleep patterns in patients suffering from delirium due to alcohol and meprobamate withdrawal, conditions believed to have the same underlying mechanisms as the barbiturate withdrawal delirium (56). No rebound increases in REM sleep were observed. This issue remains unresolved (see also Chapter 6 and 7).

Other studies have concluded that withdrawal symptoms are most likely to occur in patients abusing short-acting barbiturates, which are rapidly excreted, as determined by their blood levels (57).

Two major hypotheses have been advanced to account for barbiturate dependence and withdrawal (58): 1. chronic disuse hyperexcitability and 2.

neurotransmitter surfeit and supersensitivity of receptors. The first hypothesis asserts that chronic barbiturate intoxication suppresses the CNS and that, upon rapid withdrawal of the drug, a hyperexcitability resembling that following denervation or chronic disuse of tissue results. The same explanation has been offered to account for the withdrawal phenomena in alcohol and other CNS depressant dependence. These drugs display cross-tolerance, i.e., one of them can substitute for another in suppressing specific abstinence symptoms. The second hypothesis asserts that CNS depressants bring about accumulation of a neurotransmitter in the presynaptic terminals and in the axons of presynaptic neurons. After withdrawal of the depressant drug, there is release of excess neurotransmitter, resulting in exaggerated responses to stimuli. A related hypothesis proposes that the observed hyperexcitability in withdrawal states results from an increase in the number of receptors in the postsynaptic areas. These issues remain unresolved.

TREATMENT

Phenobarbital has been most widely used in the treatment of the barbiturate withdrawal syndrome (38,48–50,59). This drug has a slow elimination rate, a wider margin of safety between intoxication and CNS depression, and anticonvulsant properties (59). A 30-mg dose of phenobarbital can be used for each 100 mg of pentobarbital or its equivalent (49). Stabilization doses should be maintained for 2 days and then decreased by 30 mg each day (49). A loading-dose approach using this drug has been recommended by some writers (38,59). It involves giving phenobarbital orally at a rate of 120 mg/hr until a predetermined end point of its effect is reached, i.e., nystagmus, ataxia, dysarthria, or emotional lability (59). Haloperidol may be used to relieve agitation (60).

Nonbarbiturate sedative-hypnotics

Both the older drugs, such as chloral hydrate and paraldehyde, and the newer ones, introduced since 1950, are capable of inducing intoxication, dependence, and withdrawal delirium that are practically indistinguishable from those due to barbiturates (47,48,51,61). These drugs are listed in Table 13–1, and relevant references are given in parentheses. Benzodiazepines, being by far the most commonly used sedative-hypnotics today, are discussed separately in the next section.

Benzodiazepines

Long-term therapeutic use as well as abuse of benzodiazepines leads to physical dependence manifested by an abstinence syndrome on withdrawal (74–79). Most patients experience relatively mild symptoms including anxiety,

TABLE 13–1 Nonbarbiturate Sedative-Hypnotics

Benzodiazepines (see next section)
Chloral hydrate (62)
Chlormethiazole (63)
Ethchlorvynol (64,65)
Ethinamate (66)
Glutethimide (67,68)
Meprobamate (69)
Methaqualone (70,71)
Methyprylon (72)
Paraldehyde (73)

tremor, paresthesias, muscle twitching, hypersensitivity to visual and auditory stimuli, insomnia, tinnitus, and depersonalization (75,76,79). In a minority of cases, seizures or delirium, or both, may occur (76,79). The incidence of benzodiazepine withdrawal delirium is uknown, but the syndrome appears to be uncommon and is much more likely to occur following withdrawal from high doses, especially when other drugs, notably alcohol, are taken concurrently (79). Only a few scattered reports of delirium due to withdrawal of various benzodiazepine drugs can be found in the literature. Table 13-2 lists the studies reported to date.

The EEG in patients experiencing benzodiazepine withdrawal shows prominent fast activity, but confusion, if present, tends to be associated with diffuse slow-wave activity (51,89). It has been hypothesized that delirium due to hypnotic-sedative (including benzodiazepine) withdrawal could result from an acute reduction in the neurotransmitter gamma-aminobutyric acid (GABA), the major inhibiting transmitter in the CNS (90). This reduction could disrupt sleep and lead to increased REM sleep. Another hypothesis asserts that the appearance of a withdrawal syndrome in a proportion of benzodiazepine users could result from a rebound reaction and from hypersensitivity of benzodiazepine receptors in the brain (79).

Management of the benzodiazepine withdrawal syndrome involves prevention of severe symptoms, including delirium and seizures, which are most

TABLE 13–2 Benzodiazepines and Reported Withdrawal Delirium

Alprazolam (80–82)
Bromazepam (83)
Chlordiazepoxide (47, 84)
Clorazepate (85)
Diazepam (47,86)
Lorazepam (87)
Triazolam (88)

likely to develop if a benzodiazepine drug has been rapidly withdrawn. It follows that the cardinal rule is to reduce the dosage *gradually* (38,75,76,79). For patients with acute withdrawal symptoms diazepam loading (20 mg/hr orally) can be used until the symptoms subside (38). A beta-receptor blocker, such as propranolol, may help relieve some of the unpleasant symptoms of autonomic nervous system arousal (76,79). If delirium occurs, haloperidol may be used to control agitation (86).

Miscellaneous drugs

Delirium has occasionally been reported following withdrawal of drugs other than sedative-hypnotics.

Baclofen is a muscle relaxant used for muscle spasms and spasticity in multiple sclerosis and spinal cord injury. Its abrupt discontinuation may produce delirium (91,92).

Amphetamine withdrawal delirium has been reported, but the evidence for it is open to question (93,94).

Opiate withdrawal very seldom, if ever, features delirium (13,53). One case of the syndrome has been reported recently, but the patient had advanced cancer and severe pain, and was given very high doses of morphine (95).

Propoxyphene dependence and withdrawal have been observed. Delirium may occasionally be a feature of the withdrawal (47,96).

Thiothixene withdrawal delirium has been reported after abrupt withdrawal of the drug from a schizophrenic patient (97). Neuroleptics do not generally have this effect.

Tricyclic antidepressants, when withdrawn, may given rise to a variety of symptoms, very occasionally accompanied by delirium, but the evidence for it is weak (98,99).

References

1. Rinaldi R. C., Steindler E. M. Wilford B. B., et al: Clarification and standardization of substance abuse terminology. *J.A.M.A.* 1988;259:555–557.
2. *Diagnostic and Statistical Manual of Mental Disorders,* ed 3 revised. Washington, DC, American Psychiatric Association, 1987.
3. Cutshall B. J.: The Saunders-Sutton syndrome: An analysis of delirium tremens. *Q. J. Stud. Alcohol* 1965;26:423–448.
4. Gross M. M., Lewis E., Hastey J.: Acute alcohol withdrawal syndrome, in Kissin H., Begleiter H. (eds): *The Biology of Alcoholism,* Vol 3. New York, Plenum Press, 1973, pp 191–263.
5. Victor M., Wolfe S. M.: Causation and treatment of the alcohol withdrawal syndrome, in Bourne P., Fox R. (eds): *Alcoholism: Progress in Research and Treatment.* New York, Academic Press, 1973, pp 137–169.

6. Sutton T.: *Tracts on Delirium Tremens, on Peritonitis and on Some Other Inflammatory Affections.* London, Underwood, 1813.
7. Kramp P., Hemmingsen R.: Delirium tremens. Some clinical features. Part 1. *Acta Psychiatr. Scand.* 1979;60:393–404.
8. Cutting J.: A reappraisal of alcohol psychoses. *Psychol. Med.* 1978;8:285–295.
9. Salum I. (ed): Delirium tremens and certain other acute sequels of alcohol abuse. *Acta Psychiatr. Scand.,* Suppl. 235, 1972.
10. Hillbom M. E.: Occurrence of cerebral seizures provoked by alcohol abuse. *Epilepsia* 1980;21:459–466.
11. Newsom J. A.: Withdrawal seizures in an in-patient alcoholism program, in Galanter M. (ed): *Currents in Alcoholisms,* Vol 6. New York, Grune & Stratton, 1979, pp 11–14.
12. Root J.: *The Horrors of Delirium Tremens.* New York, J Adams, 1844.
13. De Boor W.: *Pharmakopsychologie und Psychopathologie.* Berlin, Springer Verlag, 1956.
14. Deiker T., Chambers H. E.: Structure and content of hallucinations in alcohol withdrawal and functional psychosis. *J. Stud. Alcohol* 1978;39:1831–1840.
15. Saravay S. M., Pardes H.: Auditory elementary hallucinations in alcohol withdrawal psychosis. *Arch. Gen. Psychiatry* 1967;16:652–658.
16. Ditman K. S., Whittlesey J. R. B.: Comparison of the LSD-25 experience and delirium tremens. *Arch. Gen. Psychiatry* 1959;1:47–57.
17. Itil T., Fink M.: Anticholinergic drug-induced delirium: Experimental modification, quantitative EEG and behavioral correlations. *J. Nerv. Ment. Dis.* 1966;143:492–507.
18. Hemmingsen R., Kramp P.: Delirium tremens and related clinical states. *Acta Psychiatr. Scand.* 1988, Suppl. 345, 78:94–107.
19. Isbell H., Fraser H. F., Wikler A., et al: An experimental study of the etiology of "rum fits" and delirium tremens. *Quart. J. Stud. Alc.* 1955;16:1–33.
20. Whitwell F. D.: A study into the aetiology of delirium tremens. *Br. J. Addict.* 1975;70:156–161.
21. Majchrowicz E.: Biologic properties of ethanol and the biphasic nature of ethanol withdrawal syndrome, in Tarter R. E., Van Thiel D. H. (eds): *Alcohol and the Brain. Chronic Effects.* New York, Plenum, 1985.
22. Ballenger J. C., Post R. M.: Kindling as a model for alcohol withdrawal syndromes. *Br. J. Psychiatry* 1978;133:1–14.
23. Brown M. E., Anton R. F., Malcolm R., et al: Alcohol detoxification and withdrawal seizures: Clinical support for a kindling hypothesis. *Biol. Psychiatry* 1988;23:507–514.
24. Hoes M. J.: The significance of the serum levels of vitamin B-1 and magnesium in delirium tremens and alcholism. *J. Clin. Psychiatry* 1979;40:476–479.
25. Meyer J. G., Urban K.: Electrolyte changes and acid base balance after alcohol withdrawal. *J. Neurol.* 1977;215:135–140.
26. Stendig-Lindberg G.: Hypomagnesemia in alcohol encephalopathies. *Acta Psychiatr. Scand.* 1974;50:465–480.
27. Berglund M., Risberg J.: Regional cerebral blood flow during alcohol withdrawal. *Arch. Gen. Psychiatry* 1981;38:351–355.
28. Goldstein D. B.: The alcohol withdrawal syndrome. A view from the laboratory, in Galanter M. (ed): *Recent Development in Alcoholism,* Vol 4. New York, Plenum, 1986, pp 231–240.

29. Hawley R. J., Major L. F., Schulman E. A., et al: CSF levels of norepinephrine during alcohol withdrawal. *Arch. Neurol.* 1981;38:289–292.
30. Linnoila M.: Alcohol withdrawal and noradrenergic function. *Ann. Intern. Med.* 1987;107:875–889.
31. Allahyari H., Deisenhammer E., Weiser E.: EEG examination during delirium tremens. *Psychiatr. Clin.* 1976;9:21–31.
32. Schear H. E.: The EEG pattern in delirium tremens. *Clin. Electroencephalogr.* 1985;16:30–32.
33. Van Sweden B.: The EEG in chronic alcoholism. Part 1. The EEG in alcohol addicts presenting with psychosis. *Clin. Neurol. Neurosurg.* 1983;85:3–11.
34. Wikler A., Pescor F. T., Fraser H. F., et al: Electroencephalographic changes associated with chronic alcoholic intoxication and the alcohol abstinence syndrome. *Am. J. Psychiatry* 1956;113:106–114.
35. Baumgartner G. R., Rowen R. C.: Clonidine vs chlordiazepoxide in the management of acute alcohol withdrawal syndrome. *Arch. Intern. Med.* 1987;147:1223–1226.
36. Liskow B. I., Goodwin D. W.: Pharmacological treatment of alcohol intoxication, withdrawal and dependence: A critical review. *J. Stud. Alcohol* 1987;48:356–370.
37. Rosenbloom A. J.: Optimizing drug treatment of alcohol withdrawal. *Am. J. Med.* 1986;81:901–904.
38. Sellers E. M.: Alcohol, barbiturate and benzodiazepine withdrawal syndromes: Clinical management. *Can. Med. Assoc. J.* 1988;139:113–118.
39. Thompson W. L.: Management of alcohol withdrawal syndrome. *Arch. Intern. Med.* 1978;138:278–283.
40. Whitfield, E. L., Thompson, G., Lamb A., et al: Detoxification of 1,024 alcoholic patients without psychoactive drugs. *J.A.M.A.* 1978;293:1409–1410.
41. Shaw J. M., Kolesar G. S., Sellers E. M., et al: Development of optimal treatment tactics for alcohol withdrawal. 1. Assessment and effectiveness of supportive care. *J. Clin. Psychopharmacol.* 1981;1:382–387.
42. Sellers E. M., Kalant H.: Drug therapy: Alcohol intoxication and withdrawal. *N. Engl. J. Med.* 1976;294:757–762.
43. Jacob M. S., Zilm D. H., MacLeod S. M., et al: Propranolol-associated confused states during alcohol withdrawal. *J. Clin. Psychopharmacol.* 1983;3:185–187.
44. Powers J. S., Decoskey D., Kahrilas P. J.: Physostigmine for treatment of delirium tremens. *J. Clin. Pharmacol.* 1981;21:57–60.
45. Schied H. W., Braunschweiger M., Schupamann A.: Treatment of delirium tremens in German psychiatric hospitals: Results of a recent survey. *Acta Psychiatr. Scand.* 1986;73 (Suppl 329):153–156.
46. Dudley W. H. C., Williams J. G.: Electroconvulsive therapy in delirium tremens. *Compr. Psychiatry* 1972;13:257–260.
47. Fruensgaard K.: Withdrawal psychosis: A study of 30 consecutive cases. *Acta Psychiatr. Scand.* 1976;53:105–118, 1976.
48. Khantzian E. J., McKenna G. J.: Acute toxic and withdrawal reactions associated with drug use and abuse. *Ann. Intern. Med.* 1979;90:361–372.
49. Liappas I. A., Jenner F. A., Vicente B.: Withdrawal syndromes. *J. R. Coll. Physicians Lond.* 1987;21:214–218.
50. Perry P. J., Alexander B.: Sedative/hypnotic dependence: Patient stabilization, tolerance testing, and withdrawal. *Drug Intell. Clin. Pharm.* 1986;20:532–537.

51. Duncan J.: Neuropsychiatric aspects of sedative drug withdrawal. *Hum. Psychopharmacol* 1988;3:171–180.
52. Isbell H., Altschul S., Dornetsky C. H., et al: Chronic barbiturate intoxication. *Arch. Neurol. Psychiatry* 1950;64:1–28.
53. Wikler A.: Neurophysiological aspects of the opiate and barbiturate abstinence syndrome. *Proc. Assoc. Res. Nerv. Ment. Dis.* 1953;32:269–286.
54. Evans J. I., Lewis S. A.: Drug withdrawal state. *Arch. Gen. Psychiatry* 1968;19:631–634.
55. Feinberg I., Hibi S., Caveness C., et al: Absence of REM rebound after barbiturate withdrawal. *Science* 1974;185:534–535.
56. Tachibana M., Tanaka K., Hishikawa Y., et al: A sleep study of acute psychotic states due to alcohol and meprobamate addiction. *Adv. Sleep Res.* 1975;2:177–205.
57. Wulff M. H.: *The Barbiturate Withdrawal Syndrome.* Copenhagen, Munksgaard, 1959.
58. Gault F. P.: A review of recent literature on barbiturate addiction and withdrawal. *Bol. Estud. Med. Biol.* 1976;29:75–83.
59. Robinson G. M., Sellers, E. M., Janecek E.: Barbiturate and hypnosedative withdrawal by a multiple oral phenobarbital loading dose technique. *Clin. Pharmacol. Ther.* 1981;30:71–76.
60. Snyder R.: Haloperidol in barbiturate detoxification. *Milit. Med.* 1977;142:885–886.
61. Allgulander C.: Dependence on sedative and hypnotic drugs. *Acta Psychiatr. Scand.* 1978; Suppl 270.
62. Margetts E. L.: Chloral delirium. *Psychiatr. Q.* 1950;24:278–299.
63. Hession M. A., Verma S., Bhakta K. G. M.: Dependence on chlormethiazole and effects of its withdrawal. *Lancet* 1979;1:953–954.
64. Flemenbaum H., Gunby B.: Ethchlorvynol (Placidyl) abuse and withdrawal. *Dis. Nerv. Syst.* 1971;32:188–192.
65. Wood H. P., Flippin H. F.: Delirium tremens following withdrawal of ethchlorvynol. *Am. J. Psychiatry* 1965;121:1127–1129.
66. Ellinwood E. H., Ewing J. A., Hoaken P. C. S.: Habituation to ethinamate. *N. Engl. J. Med.* 1962;266:185–186.
67. Johnson F. A., Van Buren H. C.: Abstinence syndrome following glutethimide intoxication. *J.A.M.A.* 1962;180:1024–1027.
68. Lloyd E. A., Clark L. D.: Convulsions and delirium incident to glutethimide (Doriden) withdrawal. *Dis. Nerv. Syst.* 1959;20:524–526.
69. Haizlip T. M., Ewing J. A.: Meprobamate habituation: A controlled clinical study. *N. Engl. J. Med.* 1961;258:1181–1186.
70. Kato M.: An epidemiological analysis of drug dependence in Japan. *Int. J. Addict.* 1969;4:591–621.
71. Ewart R. B. S., Priest R. G.: Methaqualone addiction and delirium tremens. *Br. Med. J.* 1967;3:92–93.
72. Jensen G. R.: Addiction to Noludar: A report of two cases. *N.Z. Med. J.* 1960;59:431–432.
73. Kehrer F.: Uber Abstinenzpsychosen bei chronischen Vergiftungen. *Z. Neur.* 1910;3:485–502.
74. Ashton H.: Benzodiazepine withdrawal: Outcome in 50 patients. *Br. J. Addict.* 1987;82:665–671.

75. Busto U., Sellers E. M., Naranjo C. A., et al: Withdrawal reaction after long-term therapeutic use of benzodiazepines. *N. Engl. J. Med.* 1986;315:854–859.
76. Editorial: Treatment of benzodiazepine dependence. *Lancet* 1987;1:78–79.
77. Greenblatt D. J., Shader R. I., Abernethy D. R.: Current status of benzodiazepines (Second of two parts). *N. Engl. J. Med.* 1983;309:410–426.
78. Higgitt A. C., Lader M. H., Fonagy P.: Clinical management of benzodiazepine dependence. *Br. Med. J.* 1985;291:688–690.
79. Owen R. T., Tyrer P.: Benzodiazepine dependence: A review of the evidence. *Drugs* 1983;25:385–398.
80. Browne J. L., Hauge K. J.: A review of alprazolam withdrawal. *Drug Intell. Clin. Pharm.* 1986;20:837–841.
81. Levy A. B.: Delirium and seizures due to abrupt alprazolam withdrawal: Case report. *J. Clin. Psychiatry* 1984;38–39.
82. Zipursky R. B., Baker R. W., Zimmer B.: Alprazolam withdrawal delirium unresponsive to diazepam: Case report. *J. Clin. Psychiatry* 1985;46:344–345.
83. Bowing J.: Entzugsdelirien unter Bromazepam (Lexotamil). *Nervenarzt* 1981;52:293–297.
84. Hollister L. E., Motzembecker F. P., Degan R. O.: Withdrawal reactions from chlordiazepoxide (Librium). *Psychopharmacologia* 1961;2:63–68.
85. Allgulander C., Borg S.: A case report: A delirious abstinence syndrome associated with clorazepate (Tranxilene). *Br. J. Addict.* 1978;73:175–177.
86. Leung F. W., Guze P. A.: Diazepam withdrawal. *West. J. Med.* 1983;138:255–257.
87. Stewart R. B., Salem R. B., Steinberg C.: A case report of lorazepam withdrawal. *Am. J. Psychiatry* 1980;137:1113–1114.
88. Heritch A. J., Capwell R., Roy-Byrne P. R.: A case of psychosis and delirium following withdrawal from triazolam. *J. Clin. Psychiatry* 1987;48:168–169.
89. VanSweden B.: The EEG in hypnosedative drug withdrawal and dependence. *Eur. Arch. Psychiatr. Neurol. Sci.* 1984;234:268–274.
90. Cowen P. J., Nutt D. J.: Abstinence symptoms after withdrawal of tranquilizing drugs: Is there a common neurochemical mechanism? *Lancet* 1982;2:360–362.
91. Harrison S. A., Wood C. A.: Hallucinations after preoperative baclofen discontinuation in spinal cord injury patients. *Drug Intell. Clin. Pharm.* 1985;19:747–749.
92. Terrence C. F., Fromm G. H.: Complications of baclofen withdrawal. *Arch. Neurol.* 1981;38:588–589.
93. Askevold F.: The occurrence of paranoid incidents and abstinence delirium in abusers of amphetamine. *Acta Psychiatr. Scand.* 1959;4:145–164.
94. Streltzer J., Leigh H.: Amphetamine abstinence psychosis—does it exist? *Psychiatr. Opinion* 1977;13:47–51.
95. Kumor K. M., Grochow L. B., Hausheer F.: Unusual opioid withdrawal syndrome. A case-report. *Lancet* 1987;1:720–721.
96. Strode S. W.: Propoxyphene dependence withdrawal. *A.F.P.* 1985;32:105–108.
97. Ferholt J. B., Stone W. N.: Severe delirium after abrupt withdrawal of thiothixene in a chronic schizophrenic patient. *J. Nerv. Ment. Dis.* 1970;150:400–403.
98. Lawrence J. M.: Reactions to withdrawal of antidepressants, antiparkinsonian drugs, and lithium. *Psychosomatics* 1985;26:869–877.
99. Santos A. B., McCurdy L.: Delirium after abrupt withdrawal from doxepin: Case report. *Am. J. Psychiatry* 1980;137:239–240.

14

Metabolic Disorders (Encephalopathies)

This important class of etiological factors in delirium comprises systemic disorders of metabolism, due to organ failure for example, that have deleterious secondary effects on brain metabolism. The term "encephalopathy" is often used in this context (1–4), but its definition is anything but consistent in the medical literature. A recently published medical dictionary (5) defines it as 1. any disease or degenerative condition of the brain; and 2. an acute reaction of the brain to a variety of toxic or infective agents, without any actual inflammation such as occurs in encephalitis (5, p 937). Posner (4) proposes that the term "metabolic encephalopathy" be used to refer to the behavioral changes resulting from diffuse or widespread multifocal failure of cerebral metabolism (4, p 645). Delirium, according to him, denotes the wakeful stage of metabolic encephalopathy, which may be primary or secondary to extra-cerebral disease. For Lockwood (2), metabolic encephalopathies constitute a group of disorders due to failure of organs other than the brain that results in cerebral dysfunction caused by three pathogenic mechanisms: 1. the presence of a toxin or the accumulation of a metabolic waste product, as in liver failure; 2. deficiency of an essential metabolic substrate, as in hypoxia or hypoglycemia; and 3. disturbance of the internal milieu of the brain, as in water intoxication.

As the above discussion illustrates, the term "encephalopathy" is variously defined, and its boundaries differ from author to author. It is not identical to "delirium." Disorders that some writers would include under the term "encephalopathy" are discussed in other chapters of this book. This chapter describes those *systemic* disorders that are usually considered "metabolic," and result from failure or dysfunction of organs other than the brain, or from disturbances of the internal milieu, or both. They are listed in Table 14–1.

TABLE 14–1 Systemic Metabolic Disorders Causing Delirium

- A. Deficiency of oxygen or substrate for cerebral metabolism
  - 1 Hypoxia
  - 2. Hypoglycemia
- B. Organ failure or dysfunction
  - 1. Hepatic encephalopathy
  - 2. Uremic and dialysis encephalopathies
  - 3. Hypercapnic encephalopathy
  - 4. Pancreatic encephalopathy
  - 5. Endocrinopathies
    - a. Panhypopituitarism
    - b. Hypothyroidism
    - c. Hyperthyroidism
    - d. Hypoparathyroidism
    - e. Hyperparathyroidism
    - f. Hypoadrenalism
    - g. Hyperadrenalism
    - h. Diabetes mellitus
- C. Other systemic diseases
  - 1. Cancer
  - 2. Carcinoid syndrome
  - 3. Porphyria
  - 4. Wilson's disease
- D. Disorders of fluid, electrolyte, and acid-base balance
  - 1. Hyponatremia
  - 2. Hypernatremia
  - 3. Hypokalemia
  - 4. Hyperkalemia
  - 5. Hypocalcemia
  - 6. Hypercalcemia
  - 7. Hypomagnesemia
  - 8. Hypermagnesemia
  - 9. Hypophosphatemia
  - 10. Acidosis
  - 11. Alkalosis
- E. Vitamin deficiency or excess
- F. Disorders of temperature regulation
  - 1. Hypothermia
  - 2. Hyperthermia (heat stroke)
- G. Miscellaneous disorders

Deficiency of oxygen or substrate

Hypoxia

Hypoxia is a reduction of the oxygen concentration or tension in the body. The importance of an adequate oxygen supply for cerebral function and the major consequences of hypoxia for the latter are discussed in Chapter 7. The normal brain in a conscious human accounts for about 20% of the total body basal oxygen consumption. The level of awareness is quite closely correlated with the CMR. The metabolic basis of consciousness or awareness is twofold: 1. appropriate transmembrane ion gradients must be maintained to protect communication between cells; 2. appropriate neurotransmitters must be synthesized, released, and inactivated to enable such communication (6). Moreover, the postsynaptic membranes must be in an excitable state. Hypoxia alters cerebral blood flow and oxygen uptake in conscious persons (7). Blood flow increases, which helps to maintain a normal or near-normal brain energy state (7). The CMR for oxygen generally increases and then decreases as hypoxia rises (7). Reduced oxygen availability inhibits acetylcholine metabolism, an effect that has been proposed to account for the mental changes induced by hypoxia (7). The metabolism of catecholamine is depressed, and the GABA brain concentration increases (7). When oxygen or substrate, or both, are lacking, cerebral function fails before there is evidence of depletion of brain energy reserves. Psychological symptoms and EEG changes tend to precede any detectable failure in brain energy metabolism and may reflect changes in neurotransmitter metabolism. Thus, pathways subserving communication between cells are especially vulnerable to metabolic failure and hence to hypoxia (6).

The supply of oxygen to the brain depends on the CBF and the oxygen content of the blood. CBF depends on the cerebral perfusion pressure, i.e., the difference between the mean systemic arterial pressure and the cerebral venous blood pressure. The level of the mean systemic arterial blood pressure at which brain damage is produced in humans is about 50 mm Hg (8). The lower limit of oxygen saturation of arterial blood for normal mental function is 85%. The limit for consciousness is 55% to 60% saturation (9). Oxygen deprivation for 1 or 2 minutes, especially in a person with cerebrovascular disease, is liable to be followed by delirium and stupor. Hypoxic damage to the brain may occur in a variety of clinical conditions characterized by an inadequate supply of oxygen or glucose to the neurons. Areas of the brain that are selectively vulnerable to hypoxia include the arterial boundary zones, Ammon's horns, the thalamus, and the cerebellum (8).

Graham (8) distinguishes six categories of cerebral hypoxia: 1. stagnant, which may be ischemic and due to local or generalized arrest of the blood supply, or oligemic, which is due to local or generalized reduction of the blood supply; 2. anoxia and hypoxia due to absence of oxygen in the lungs or to reduced pulmonary oxygen tension; 3. anemic, which results from an abnormally low hemoglobin concentration or from unavailability of hemoglobin for oxygen transport, as in CO poisoning; 4. histotoxic, due to poisoning of respiratory enzymes in the neurons; 5. hypoglycemic; and 6. febrile convulsions and status epilepticus. Other authors speak of hypoxic, hypobaric, anemic, and histotoxic hypoxia (7). Hypoxic hypoxia features decreased oxygen content of the inspired air; hypobaric hypoxia occurs with decrased atmospheric pressure; anemic hypoxia is characterized by reduced oxygen-carrying capacity of the blood; and histotoxic hypoxia involves reduced ability of the tissues to utilize oxygen, even though an adequate amount is available. Most of the pathological conditions that give rise to cerebral ischemia-hypoxia are discussed in other chapters of this book. They include cardiac arrest and arrhythmias, myocardial infarction, acute pulmonary embolism, congestive heart failure, vasculitides, cerebral embolism or thrombosis, multi-infarct dementia, CO poisoning, and cerebral malaria. In this section, the focus is on some of the remaining conditions resulting in cerebral hypoxia and thus capable of inducing delirium.

Acute mountain sickness may include delirium. The mental effects of acute exposure to high altitude are related to the degree of oxygen unsaturation of the arterial blood (9). There is no general agreement regarding the degree of acute hypoxia necessary to cause the earliest signs of decrement in cognitive performance. Some investigators have found no evidence of impairment on a free-recall memory test and on a scanning task in subjects acutely exposed to simulated altitudes of 12,000 feet (10). The critical altitude for psychological changes seems to fall between 4,000 and 5,000 m (11). At 5,000 m, a marked deterioration in cognitive ability has been observed (11). Some writers assert that memory and intelligence begin to show disturbance at 12,000 to 18,000 feet, depending on the rapidity of ascent, duration of exposure, and individual susceptibility (9). The accepted limit for normal mental function is 85% oxygen saturation of the arterial blood, which corresponds to an altitude of 10,000 feet for people breathing air and 33,000 feet for those breathing oxygen (9). Hillary is said to have spent 10 minutes on the summit of Mount Everest, i.e., at about 27,700 feet, before he began to notice confusion (9). Ambulatory EEG recordings obtained from mountaineers at heights ranging from 4,115 m to 6,220 m found only a marked reduction in stage 4 sleep (12). Psychopathological features of acute mountain sickness include psychomotor, mood, memory, judgment, and orientation disturbances (13). Moreover, complications, such as pulmonary edema, can also affect consciousness.

Delirium has been observed in a few subjects at altitudes of about 6,000 m (13). Acetazolamide counteracts cognitive impairment due to acute mountain sickness (14).

Near-drowning can result in "blunted consciousness" characterized by a combination of lethargy, disorientation, confusion, agitation, and combativeness (15). Most patients who show these features survive and make an uneventful recovery (15).

Decompression sickness results from liberation of gases into body fluids and tissues during or after decompression at too fast a rate. Cerebral ischemia and raised intracranial pressure follow, and delirium may occur (16). Under hyperbaric conditions to which divers may be exposed the EEG shows increased slow activity (17). Similar EEG changes have been reported in *hypobaric hypoxia* (18).

Nitrogen narcosis can occur in divers using compressed air. The mental symptoms include initial mild impairment of cognitive functions, followed by confusion and hallucinations (19).

Anemia may result in delirium when the oxygen-carrying capacity of the blood falls by more than one-half. Acute confusional state has been reported in elderly patients suffering from severe anemia. The condition cleared up after blood transfusion (20).

Hypoglycemia

Delirium is one of the four manifestations of hypoglycemic encephalopathy, the other three being coma, a stroke-like form, and an epileptic attack with single or multiple general convulsions (21). The signs and symptoms of hypoglycemia can be divided into two groups: adrenergic and neuroglucopenic (22). The former include hunger, tremulousness, anxiety, sweating, tachycardia, and palpitations. The latter include headache, weakness, confusion, abnormal behavior, seizures, and coma. Some authors distinguish between acute and chronic neuroglucopenia; delirium can occur as a feature of either condition (23). Recurrent severe hypoglycemic episodes, as well as a single prolonged coma, may result in dementia or, less often, in an organic amnestic syndrome. A study of 850 cases of islet-cell tumors found an incidence of psychiatric disorders of 12% (24). About one-half of these patients failed to show improvement in mental status after surgery, underscoring the importance of early diagnosis and proper treatment of hypoglycemia.

The causes of fasting hypoglycemia can be classified into four major groups (25): 1. organic hypoglycemia, in which a recognizable anatomic lesion exists (e.g., hyperinsulinism due to pancreatic islet beta-cell disease, nonpancreatic tumors, and pituitary and adrenocortical hypofunction); 2. deficiency of a specific hepatic enzyme (in infancy and childhood); 3. functional hypoglycemia, in which there is no demonstrable anatomical lesion (e.g., severe inanition); and 4. hypoglycemia due to exogenous agents, such as alcohol, insulin, and oral hypoglycemic and other drugs (26,27). Postprandial, or reactive, hypoglycemia, such as that after gastrectomy, may occasionally feature delirium (28).

In hospitalized patients, hypoglycemia is most often seen in association with diabetes, renal insufficiency, liver disease, infections, shock, pregnancy, neoplasia, and burns (29). Administered insulin is by far the most common direct cause of hypoglycemia in diabetic patients, who represent the largest single group of those with hypoglycemic episodes (29). A study of 125 patient visits to a hospital emergency room for symptomatic hypoglycemia found that diabetes, alcohol, and sepsis, alone or in combination, accounted for 90% of the visits (30). Confusion was a presenting symptom in about 20% of the cases. Some patients present with factitious hypoglycemia due to surreptitious insulin use (31).

Insulinoma is a rare tumor occurring more often in women and in older persons (32). Hypoglycemic symptoms may occur for several or more years before the diagnosis is made, appear irregularly, and vary in duration. Their onset is typically in the late afternoon or in the early morning before breakfast. Confusion or abnormal behavior has been observed in about 80% of these patients (32). Mental confusion alone has been noted in 30% of patients in one series (33). In most cases, hypoglycemic episodes occur spasmodically at first and are separated by symptom-free intervals of weeks or months. These may be fewer than six episodes per year (33). Gradually, the frequency, duration, and severity of hypoglycemia increase. Delirium may be misdiagnosed as a functional psychiatric illness, and the patient's underlying organic disease may remain unrecognized for years (34).

Hypoglycemic symptoms are the same, regardless of their underlying cause. Neuroglucopenia and delirium depend for their development on the rate and degree of decrease in blood glucose concentration, as well as on individual susceptibility, which is variable. The arterial blood glucose concentration at which neuropsychiatric symptoms appear varies considerably but is seldom above 40 mg/100 ml. In one study, confusion was associated with blood glucose levels averaging 32 mg/100 ml (30). Blood glucose levels as low as 20 mg/100 ml, or even less, have been recorded in symptom-free subjects. In most cases of spontaneous hypoglycemia giving rise to symptoms, the glucose concentration is 30 mg/100 ml or less (23). In healthy men subjected to a 24-hour fast, plasma glucose levels do not fall below 60 mg/100 ml, but in healthy premenopausal women, such levels are generally lower and may fall to 58 mg/100 ml (25).

Apart from delirium, neuropsychiatric symptoms of hypoglycemia, or rather neuroglucopenia, may include outbursts of anger and violent behavior, paranoid delusions, catalepsy, and perceptual disturbances such as macropsia, micropsia, and visual hallucinations (24). Hypoglycemic symptoms have been misdiagnosed as hysteria, schizophrenia, mania, and endogenous depression (35). In one series of 91 patients with hyperinsulinism, a psychiatric diagnosis was initially made in 16 (36). It is likely that failure to diagnose delirium in these patients resulted in the misdiagnosis.

The EEG in hypoglycemia shows diffuse slowing, epileptiform activity, or foci of slow activity (24). A shift to lower frequencies has been observed with experimentally induced mild hypoglycemia when blood glucose levels were reduced to 35 to 49 mg/100 ml (37). In general, there is a direct correlation between the blood glucose level and the EEG changes (3).

The importance of glucose as the only (except in extreme starvation) substrate for cerebral energy metabolism is discussed in Chapter 7. Coupled with the small reserves of glucose and glycogen within the CNS, the dependence on this source of energy renders the brain uniquely vulnerable to large decreases in systemic glucose supply (3,38). Acute hypoglycemia usually results from excessive insulin administration or secretion. Function may be restored if the hypoglycemia is corrected by intravenous glucose, but pronounced residual deficits may remain (38). Patients with unexplained delirium, seizures, or coma should immediately receive glucose and thiamine (30).

Organ failure or dysfunction

Hepatic encephalopathy

Hepatic encephalopathy (HE) is a disturbance of brain function that can complicate any form of liver disease and in which consciousness is particularly affected (39). It can also be viewed as a neuropsychiatric syndrome whose clinical manifestations range from slight changes in mental status to delirium and coma (39,40). Abnormal behavior and disorders of consciousness have been noted in patients with liver disease since antiquity. Accounts of delirium occurring in this context were first published in the nineteenth century (39).

Three clinical forms of HE have been distinguished (39): chronic portal-systemic encephalopathy (PSE), cirrhosis with a precipitant, and acute liver failure. Cirrhosis with a precipitant is the most common form. Delirium can occur in all three types of HE. It can appear in cirrhosis when encephalopathy is precipitated by excessive diuresis, gastrointestinal hemorrhage, infection, alcohol ingestion, surgery, and drugs such as opiates, barbiturates, neuroleptics, and antihistamines. Chronic PSE may feature intermittent episodes of delirium related to such precipitants as increased dietary intake of protein or infection. Acute liver failure is usually due to viral hepatitis, acetaminophen self-poisoning, alcoholic hepatitis, drugs such as halothane and methyldopa, and poisoning with carbon tetrachloride or mushrooms. Delirium in acute liver failure may be preceded by euphoria or depression, posturing, antisocial behavior, nightmares, headache, dizziness, and drowsiness. It tends to be of the hyperactive type, with psychomotor overactivity, noisy and belligerent behavior, and seizures (39,41). The prognosis is poor.

Clinical features of delirium due to chronic liver disease are variable. The early stages of encephalopathy feature irritability, restlessness, confusion, and asterixis (40). Somnolence during the day and insomnia at night are also common initial features. Patients tend to be slow in speech and movement and apathetic. They may show memory impairment, inability to concentrate, constructional apraxia, spatial disorientation, a tendency to wander aimlessly, unformed visual hallucinations, and macropsia. These symptoms tend to fluctuate from day to day and precede the onset of delirium, stupor, or coma by days or weeks. Psychometric tests show intellectual, psychomotor, and attentional deficits in these patients (42–45). Delirium may be difficult to distinguish from the more chronic cognitive and attentional deficits that accompany chronic liver disease and subclinical HE (45). It is typically hypoactive, but with intermittent agitation and restlessness. The patient may be apathetic, depressed, or euphoric. Speech is usually slurred and monotonous, and may feature perseveration and dysphasia. Visual hallucinations are commonly present and usually simple, i.e., colored (usually green or red) stars or flashing lights. An occasional patient may experience complex visual hallucinations of whole scenes. Catatonic posturing may occur (46). In an alcoholic patient, symptoms of HE may be mixed with those of delirium tremens (47). Flapping tremor (asterixis) and other neuromuscular abnormalities accompany the delirium (39,40,44). The patient may at any time progress to stupor and coma and may display delirium again after emerging from the coma.

The EEG in HE shows changes during both wakefulness and sleep (39,48–52). There is a fairly good correlation between the EEG abnormality and the clinical stage of HE (50). The mean frequency of the background activity slows down to the delta range. Initially, there is an increase in amplitude and a slight slowing. As the patient becomes stuporous, further slowing and an increase in wave amplitude appear. Triphasic waves occur in hepatic coma and carry a poor prognosis. The EEG changes may initially be more severe than the mental state of the patient indicates and can persist after the mental disorder has lifted. EEG recordings should be part of the routine assessment of patients with liver disease, as they are diagnostically useful even though the changes are nonspecific and occur in other encephalopathies (50). These changes can be found before the overt clinical features of HE appear (50).

Sleep is profoundly disturbed (49). There is reduction in slow-wave sleep, absence of stage 4 sleep, increase in the percentage of REM sleep, and gradual breakdown of the sleep-wake cycle as the encephalopathy progresses. Correlations have been found between the severity of clinical features, waking EEG changes, and arterial ammonia levels on the one hand, and EEG characteristics and the duration and organization of sleep on the other (49).

The diagnosis of delirium due to HE depends on the history, clinical features, and laboratory tests. A history of chronic liver disease or alcohol abuse, or both, is suggestive but not conclusive. The patient may be delirious due to alcohol or drug withdrawal, intoxication with drugs, or other factors. A history of changes in personality, hypersomnia, reversal of the sleep pattern, and impaired performance at work should be looked for (50). Clinical features are helpful. General psychomotor hypoactivity; slow, monotonous, and slurred speech; mask-like face; perseveration; asterixis and other neurological signs elicited on physical examination are all suggestive of HE. Patients with acute liver failure are usually, but not invariably (53), jaundiced, but in those with chronic cirrhosis jaundice may not be conspicuous (40). Laboratory tests include the EEG, examination of the CSF, blood chemistries, and neuropsychological testing. The EEG changes have already been described. Visual evoked potential recordings have been reported to be helpful in differentiating the stages of encephalopathy (54). The CSF is usually clear and colorless but shows an elevated level of glutamine, a finding claimed to distinguish between hepatic and other forms of encephalopathy (40). CSF lactate levels are elevated and reportedly correlate well with the clinical stage (55). Blood and CSF ammonia levels are usually, but not invariably, elevated. Measurement of blood ammonia can be useful in following the clinical condition of a patient (40). HE is virtually always present when the blood ammonia concentration exceeds 3 mg/ml, but about 10% of patients with severe encephalopathy have levels within the normal range. Hypoglycemia, alkalosis, and hypokalemia are common in liver failure and can aggravate the encephalopathy (39). Various diagnostic psychometric tests have been recommended (45,50). The number connection and trailmaking tests are particularly useful (50,56,57). A study of patients being assessed for liver transplantation showed that 30% of them were delirious (57). The mini-mental state and Trailmaking Tests A and B enabled a reliable differentiation between delirious and nondelirious patients.

Pathogenesis of HE has been the subject of much research, speculation, and controversy (2,3,38,40,58–61). A number of mechanisms have been proposed that can only be listed here:

1. Hyperammonemia. Blood and CSF ammonia levels are raised in most patients with HE but do not correlate with the level of awareness. Hyperammonemia induced experimentally in humans was accompanied by lowered altertness, decreased interaction with other people, and tremor (62).
2. False neurotransmitters, such as octopamine, formed by bacterial action in the colon and replacing noradrenaline and dopamine. This hypothesis

remains controversial despite the arousal effect of levodopa in acute liver failure and of bromocriptine in some patients with chronic HE (63).

3. Elevated levels of GABA acting as an inhibiting neurotransmitter and causing impairment of brain function. It is hypothesized that an endogenous substance with benzodiazepine agonist-like properties contributes to HE by potentiating GABA-ergic neurotransmission (61).
4. Elevated levels of tryptophan and serotonin—a controversial hypothesis (63).
5. Elevated short-chain fatty acids and mercaptans exerting a neurotoxic effect. The role of these substances in the production of mental symptoms in HE remains open to question.

Treatment of delirium due to hepatic disease involves treatment of the underlying condition, as well as the symptoms. A discussion of the former is beyond the scope of this book. In general, medical treatment aims at recognizing and treating precipitating factors, facilitating removal of toxic products, and avoiding iatrogenic complications (64). Sedative and analgesic drugs should, if possible, be avoided. If the patient is sufficiently agitated to need sedation, oxazepam or lorazepam can be used (65). Phenothiazines and haloperidol are contraindicated. Levodopa and bromocriptine have been reported to improve mental status in some patients but are not recommended for routine treatment (64).

Uremic and dialysis encephalopathies

UREMIC ENCEPHALOPATHY

Uremic encephalopathy is an acute or subacute organic mental syndrome occurring in patients with acute or chronic renal failure when renal function falls below 10% of normal (66). In 1868, Addison (67) wrote *On The Disorders of the Brain Connected with Diseased Kidneys* and noted "psychotic manifestations." Baker and Knutson (68) have distinguished six psychiatric syndromes complicating uremia: 1. an asthenic form, characterized by malaise, fatigue, poor memory and concentration, and gradual progression to stupor, coma, and death; 2. acute delirium, by far the most common syndrome; 3. a schizophrenic form, featuring catatonic symptoms; 4. a depressed form; 5. a manic form; and 6. a paranoid form. The asthenic form appears to represent what would be called "dementia" today. This classification reflects the wide variety of mental changes observed in uremic encephalopathy and noted by more recent authors (66,69–71). Delirium is a common feature of both acute and chronic uremic encephalopathy.

Stenback and Haapanen (72) studied delirium in patients with acute renal failure, as well as in those suffering from chronic kidney disease. The criterion of inclusion in the study was azotemia, defined as a blood urea level of 50 mg/100 ml or higher. The patients were divided into two groups: those with a serum urea concentration of 50 to 199 mg/100 ml and over ("low urea" group) and those with a concentration of 250 mg/100 ml and over ("high urea" group). Delirium was observed in about 35% of the patients with acute renal failure and in about 45% of those with chronic renal failure. The syndrome was more likely to accompany serum urea concentrations higher than 250 mg/100 ml; about 80% of all cases of delirium fell into the high urea group. Convulsions often accompanied delirium in chronic renal failure. Multiple metabolic disturbances were found to accompany delirium in such failure and were thought to have contributed to the occurrence of the syndrome. They included increased blood urea levels, hyponatremia, hypochloremia, hypokalemia, hyperkalemia, hypocalcemia, hypermagnesemia, and metabolic acidosis. Autopsy findings in patients dying from renal failure showed neuronal degeneration, mostly in the cerebral cortex, reticular formation, and sensory nuclei of the brain stem (72).

Acute uremic encephalopathy can complicate acute renal failure or supervene in the course of chronic kidney disease with chronic encephalopathy. Patients suffering from the latter disease show various combinations of cognitive-attentional deficits, poor concentration, depression, apathy, fatigue, insomnia, drowsiness, personality changes, irritability, restlessness, slurred speech, reduced libido, and social withdrawal (66,68–77). Studies have consistently found lower performance IQ scores compared to verbal IQ scores in patients with chronic renal failure (76). Poor performance on tests of choice-reaction time, auditory short-term memory, serial 7s, number recall, mental arithmetic, and time perception has been reported (73–75). In a stable phase of chronic encephalopathy, the patients are oriented. Evidence of cognitive deficits is usually present when the blood urea nitrogen level is only moderately raised (less than 200 mg/100 ml), but it may not be apparent on bedside clinical testing unless the level of 200 mg/100 ml is exceeded (75). The neuropsychiatric disorders in uremia show no regular correlation with either blood urea nitrogen level or the multiple metabolic and biochemical disturbances. One patient may be delirious with a blood urea nitrogen level of 50 mg/100 ml or less, while another patient may be nondelirious with a level over 200 mg/100 ml. On the whole, however, delirium does occur more often when the blood urea nitrogen level exceeds 250 mg/100 ml, especially when such a change develops rapidly (72). It may come on whenever the chronic kidney disease progresses rapidly, or a sudden change in electrolyte concentration develops, or both. Other precipitating factors include water intoxication, hypertensive encephalopathy, systemic and urinary infections, congestive heart failure, intravascular coagulation, and Wernicke's encephalopathy (75).

Clinical features of delirium in uremia have been referred to as the "hyper-excitable syndrome" because of the symptoms of irritability, hallucinations, aggressive behavior, and CNS and neuromuscular hyperexcitability (75). The patient is often anxious and restless, but may be depressed or euphoric. Psychomotor activity may shift suddenly from lethargy to excitement and vice versa. Baker and Knutson (68) describe these features vividly: "The entire course of the illness may shift rapidly from states of overactivity with aggressiveness, crying, laughing, singing, dancing, and swearing to states of lethargy with incoherent muttering, self-condemnatory delusions, mutism, or even catatonia" (p 685). Hallucinations, both visual and auditory, are common, fleeting, and frightening. Delusions, usually persecutory, may be present. Neuromuscular dysfunction in the form of asterixis, akinesia, rigidity, choreoathetosis, trismus, myoclonus, catatonia, and oculogyria may be present. Convulsions may occur.

The EEG in uremic encephalopathy is usually abnormal during both wakefulness and sleep (66,69,70,75,78–80). There is slowing of background activity, with frequencies of 5 to 6 c/sec. Bursts of paroxysmal slow waves and spike discharges may occur. The blood urea nitrogen level tends to correlate best with the EEG (78). The sleep EEG in uremia features reduced slow-wave (stages 3 and 4) and REM stages and an increased number of awakenings. The changes are similar to those found in hepatic encephalopathy. A correlation has been observed between increased blood urea nitrogen levels and the disturbance of sleep (79).

Pathogenesis of uremic encephalopathy is still poorly understood (66,69,81). Uremia is associated with decreased brain oxygen consumption (81). A disturbance of cerebral neurotransmitters and an accumulation of a false neurotransmitter, octopamine, have been found in patients with uremic encephalopathy (82). A pathophysiological role in the brain dysfunction of uremia has been established only for parathyroid hormone (PTH), a putative neurotoxin (69). Such dysfunction may possibly result from a PTH-mediated increase in brain calcium (66). These changes may underlie the mental symptoms.

Treatment of delirium in patients with uremic encephalopathy involves, as always, identification and treatment of the underlying cause or causes. Otherwise, the general measures discussed in Chapter 10 apply.

DIALYSIS ENCEPHALOPATHY

Encephalopathy with delirium may complicate not only acute and chronic renal failure but also the treatment of these conditions. The dialytic treatment of end-stage renal disease can be complicated by two distinct CNS disorders: *dialysis dysequilibrium (DDS)* and *dialysis dementia* (69,83,84). The former features headache, muscular twitching and cramps, tremors, blurring of vision, seizures, restlessness, dizziness, and confusion (69,83,84). The patient may display depression or euphoria, irritability, agitation or lethargy, hallucinations, paranoid delusions, and disordered behavior (84). The syndrome may appear during or up to 24 hours after hemodialysis, and recovery can take several days. The EEG may be abnormal but is not diagnostic (66,69). It has been suggested that DDS is due to brain edema resulting from CNS acidosis (66,69). DDS is particularly likely to occur in rapid hemodialysis, and has become less frequent and milder since the introduction of modern techniques (69,75). Mahoney and Arieff (69) assert that the diagnosis of DDS has become a wastebasket for a variety of disorders that can complicate renal failure and should be one of exclusion. Disorders that may mimic it include subdural hematoma, nonketotic hyperosmolar coma with hyperglycemia, dialysis dementia, hypoglycemia, hyponatremia, hypercalcemia, malignant hypertension, Wernicke's encephalopathy, and drugs (69). Flurazepam and diazepam have been implicated in some cases (85). All these factors may bring about delirium in a hemodialyzed patient. In some cases, its etiology cannot be established (86,87). Psychological stress caused by dialysis is believed to precipitate delirium, but this hypothesis remains untested (86,87).

Dialysis dementia (DD) (also referred to as "dialysis encephalopathy") is a progressive and often fatal neuropsychiatric complication in patients on chronic hemodialysis (66,69,83,88). It features speech disorders, multifocal myoclonus, dementia, and EEG abnormalities. Delirium and seizures may occur (83,89,90). Some writers claim that the symptoms of DD may fluctuate in severity and thus suggest a reversible organic mental syndrome (91). The differential diagnosis between DDS, DD, and a subacute or chronic encephalopathy with a reversible dementia is difficult yet important, since the prognosis in these three disorders is vastly different: DDS is a transient disorder, subacute and chronic encephalopathies are potentially reversible, and DD is progressive and frequently fatal. DD may develop suddenly or insidiously after many months or a few years of dialysis. Symptoms may initially be intermittent and often are worse during dialysis. The first symptom is usually a speech disorder featuring stammering, hesistancy, and even speech arrest (83). As DD progresses, the speech disturbance worsens and includes dysarthria, dyspraxia, and dysphasia. There is progressive dementia and personality change, and episodes of delirium may develop (83,89,90). Seizures, asterixis, twitching, motor apraxia, and myoclonic jerks often occur. The patients gradually lose their ability to communicate and ambulate. Death follows as a result of sepsis, suicide, or removal from dialysis (83). EEG abnormalities are essential for the diagnosis of DD (83). They may precede the onset of overt clinical symptoms by 6 months and feature multifocal bursts of high-amplitude delta activity with spikes and sharp waves (69,83,91). As DD progresses, the EEG background activity slows (69,91). The EEG abnormalities suggest involvement of the reticular formation and the cerebral cortex (92). Psychological studies have confirmed the presence of dementia in these patients (93,94). An inverse correlation has been reported between prescribed oral aluminum and cognitive function, but there is no correlation with cumulative exposure to aluminum in water used to manufacture dialysate (94).

Pathogenesis of DD remains controversial. Most of its outbreaks have been associated with high levels of aluminum in the dialysate (69,88,95). It has been hypothesized that excessive aluminum in the brain plays a causal role in the pathophysiology of DD by inhibiting cerebral metabolism (96). Dialysis with deionized water and very low aluminum levels in the dialysate resulted in no new cases of DD in a dialysis unit where the incidence of DD had been unusually high (97). Some authors, however, maintain that DD most likely represents a final common pathway for a variety of etiological factors (69).

The differential diagnosis of DD is important. The clinical similarity between reversible and progressive dialysis encephalopathy makes diagnostic errors difficult to avoid. A combination of speech disorders, progressive dementia, language disorders, episodes of delirium, and marked EEG abnormalities noted earlier, developing in a patient who has been on dialysis for more than 1 year, point to the diagnosis of DD. Yet a patient showing such symptoms has improved on clonazepam (98). Other similar patients have reportedly recovered after renal transplantation (99) and subtotal parathyroidectomy (100). Every effort should be made to rule out the treatable causes of delirium and dementia listed earlier before concluding that the patient suffers from DD (69). The treatment of DD will not be discussed here.

Renal transplantation is another treatment of chronic renal failure that may be complicated by delirium (101). A study of renal homograft recipients revealed significant psychopathology in 32% of 292 patients studied (102). Psychiatric symptoms had been present in 38% of these patients prior to transplantation. Preoperative organic mental disorders were usually relieved by successful transplantation. About 10% of the patients developed delirium or some other organic mental syndrome postoperatively. Administration of steroids, defective renal function, sepsis, and hypertension were the most frequent etiological factors. Depression was common both in the patients who became delirious and in those who did not. Seven patients attempted suicide.

Following renal transplantation, delirium may develop in the immediate postoperative period, probably in reaction to anesthetics, analgesics, and sedative-hypnotics (101). At a later stage, other factors may be implicated. Old infections may be reactivated as a result of increased susceptibility to them in patients treated with immunosuppressive drugs. A high incidence of CNS infections has been reported in renal transplant recipients (75). Bacterial and fungal infections of the meninges, brain abscess, toxoplasmosis, and viral encephalitis have all been observed in these patients and may cause delirium. Malignant neoplasms, especially involving the brain, have been reported in renal transplant recipients (75). Progressive multifocal leukoencephalopathy is a rare complication after renal transplantation and results in dementia, which may be initially mistaken for delirium. Permanent brain damage may occur during uremic or dialysis encephalopathy and cannot be reversed by renal transplantation. In one study, about 50% of transplant patients showed cognitive deficits suggestive of dementia (103). Such patients are likely to have a history of medical complications in the course of dialysis.

Hypercapnic encephalopathy

Delirium may occur as a manifestation of hypercapnic (pulmonary, respiratory) encephalopathy (21,104–110). Respiratory failure, defined as inadequate or impaired gas exchange, can be due to pulmonary or extrapulmonary diseases. The resulting encephalopathy is a consequence of the cerebral effects of hypoxia or hypercarbia, or both, and may feature delirium (110). Chronic respiratory insufficiency in a patient with chronic obstructive pulmonary disease (COPD), its most common cause, may be interspersed with episodes of acute pulmonary decompensation, hypoxia-hypercapnia, encephalopathy, and delirium. These episodes can be precipitated by such factors as bronchopulmonary infection, surgical procedures, and sedatives or inappropriate oxygen therapy (106). Respiratory failure can also occur in a patient with normal lungs as a consequence of decreased total ventilation caused by such conditions as obstruction of the upper airways, trauma to the chest, or myasthenia gravis. Cor pulmonale, hypotension, and electrolyte imbalance may contribute to the onset of delirium in the course of COPD (107). The highest incidence of the syndrome is associated with PCO_2 levels below 70–80 mm Hg (109). However, no consistent correlation has been found between the degree of mental disturbance and the degree of deviation from normal in the concentration of any chemical in the blood (107). Patients usually show both hypoxia and hypercapnia, but the mental changes are attributable mainly to the latter and not to the associated hypoxemia (109). Hypercapnia can give rise to CO_2 narcosis, which features confusion as well as drowsiness, headache, hypertension, tachycardia, sweating, multifocal myoclonus, and asterixis (109,110). Coma and death may follow. Hallucinations, delusions, and "mania" were observed in 14% of 50 patients suffering from acute pulmonary decompensation (107). These symptoms were likely those of delirium.

The EEG in patients with pulmonary encephalopathy show slowing of the background activity, theta and delta waves, and increased voltage (105). Night sleep in this disorder is often disturbed, with reduced total sleep time, frequent awakenings, and consequent excessive daytime somnolence (111–

113). It is conceivable that relative sleep deprivation in COPD could contribute to the onset of delirium.

Patients with severe COPD and both hypoxemia and hypercapnia may develop delirium, stupor, or coma after administration of oxygen, which removes the stimulus of hypoxia needed to maintain respiration in the presence of hypercapnia. As a result, the latter increases and consciousness becomes further reduced (21). Oxygen should be administered in low doses. This therapy results in improved cognition in patients with COPD (114).

Pathogenesis of pulmonary encephalopathy and the related delirium seems to involve a combination of hypercapnia, hypoxemia, and congestive heart failure (21). Rapid changes in the arterial blood carbon dioxide tension ($PaCO_2$) level are more likely to result in mental confusion than chronic hypercapnia. Experimentally induced acute hypercapnia produces mental confusion when the $PaCO_2$ reaches about 70 mm Hg; by contrast, patients with COPD may be mentally clear with $PaCO_2$ levels of 60 to 70 mm Hg and are said to tolerate levels of up to 90 mm Hg (107). In one reported series of patients with COPD, obvious mental changes were observed at $PaCO_2$ levels ranging from 48 to 148 mm Hg (107). Moderate hypercapnia ($PaCO_2$ of 50 to 60 mm Hg) in humans approximately doubles the CBF and concurrently results in a reduction of brain glucose metabolism (115). Thus, hypercapnia appears to resemble barbiturate anesthesia and hypoglycemia in that the brain becomes partially depleted of carbohydrate substrate and has to oxidize endogenous substrate to sustain energy production (115). It has been hypothesized that most of the clinical effects of hypercapnia are due, at least partly, to intracellular acidosis in the brain (21,109). A decrease in cerebral glucose metabolism due to hypercapnia could lead to decreased synthesis of acetylcholine, which might result in cognitive impairment and delirium (109).

Treatment of delirium in patients with respiratory failure involves, first of all, correction of the underlying hypoxemia, hypercapnia, electrolyte imbalance, and other relevant organic disturbances. Sedation should be avoided as far as possible to avoid further compromise of respiration. If the patient is severely agitated, haloperidol can be used (see Chapter 10). To correct the insomnia that is commonly present, I have used oral hydroxyzine without ill effects.

Pancreatic encephalopathy

Delirium may complicate pancreatic disease, especially acute pancreatitis (116–122). Benos (117,118) claims that at least 168 such cases had been reported in the medical literature by 1973, and the reported incidence of the encephalopathy ranges from 4% to 53%. Delirium comes on 48 to 72 hours after the onset of acute pancreatitis and lasts for several days (116). It is often mistaken for delirium tremens, which it markedly resembles (116,118). Schuster and Iber (121) studied 30 patients with pancreatitis and compared them with 30 alcoholic patients admitted with the diagnosis of pneumonia. Sixteen (53%) of the patients with pancreatitis displayed an "acute hallucinatory psychosis." Hallucinations were visual, auditory, or both. In the comparison group of alcoholics with pneumonia, 13% developed delirium. Most of the patients with pancreatitis had an "impressive alcoholic background." The authors concluded that pancreatitis is more likely to precipitate delirium in alcoholic patients than pneumonia. Alcohol withdrawal did not seem to be the cause of delirium in the patients with pancreatic disease. Estrada et al. (119) found encephalopathy in 35% of patients with acute pancreatitis and observed a direct relationship between the encephalopathy and an increase in the CSF lipase level. The EEG shows diffuse or multifocal slow activity (21).

Pathogenesis of pancreatic encephalopathy is not known. Various putative pathogenic factors have been proposed, among them cerebral and pulmonary fat embolism, hypoxia, hypoglycemia, disseminated intravascular coagulation, toxic effects of pancreatic enzymes on the brain, hypocalcemia, and hyperosmolality (21,117,120,122). The pathology involves mostly widespread demyelinization and diffuse petechial hemorrhages in the brain (122). Diagnosis is based on the evidence of acute pancreatitis, multifocal neurological signs, delirium, and diffuse slowing of the EEG. Treatment with antienzymes is claimed to improve the prognosis (122).

Endocrinopathies

PANHYPOPITUITARISM

Delirium can occur as a complication of panhypopituitarism (PHP), but its frequency in this disorder is unknown (123). In a series of 100 patients with verified PHP, 64% had presented with psychiatric symptoms (124). Early literature on Simmond's disease contains reports of associated delirium (125). Sheehan and Summers (126), in their classic paper on PHP, refer to mental symptoms, including delusions, hallucinations, and depression. The more recent literature contains only scattered references to delirium in the course of pituitary deficiency (127–130). Delirium may precede or follow coma in PHP or may be the only disorder of consciousness in a given patient (128,129). Hypoglycemia, electrolyte disturbances, hypothermia, and hypotension may be jointly responsible for both delirium and coma.

HYPOTHYROIDISM

Beaumont (123) asserts that mental symptoms are nearly always present in hypothyroidism. The description of such symptoms in the published reports is usually so poor that it is impossible to be sure what kind of mental disorder was present. Frequently used terms such as "myxedema psychosis" or "myxedema madness" are of no diagnostic value. Browning et al. (131) assert that the psychosis of myxedema is actually delirium, which is probably due to a disturbance of cerebral metabolism, as indicated by the slowing and lowering of the EEG voltage. However, in five of the seven patients studied by those authors, the "sensorial impairment" could only be detected by formal testing and seemed to be quite stable and prolonged—hardly a clinical picture of delirium. A review of the literature suggests that delirium is quite uncommon in hypothyroidism, and is most likely to occur in thyroidectomized patients and in those who have undergone a rapid change in thyroid status as a result of medical treatment; however, organic affective and delusional syndromes appear to be much more common (132–134). Easson (135) quotes Kraepelin, who asserted that, in myxedematous patients, "in rare cases there may appear conditions of confusion with hallucinations and delusions." Easson himself could find only 19 patients among those admitted to the Mayo Clinic between 1947 and 1958 who displayed psychosis, mostly paranoid or depressive, or both. He postulated that psychosis in these patients is related to the stress occasioned by internal and external bodily changes. Royce (136), in his review of severe impairment of consciousness (mostly coma) in myxedema, notes that about 100 such cases were reported between 1953 and 1963. Hypoxia, hypercarbia, hyponatremia, and hypopituitarism were the main factors believed to be responsible. Hypothermia and administration of drugs, such as barbiturates and phenothiazines, could also have this effect. It is conceivable that the same factors could be responsible for the occasional delirium.

Memory impairment, mental and psychomotor slowness, and some degree of intellectual deterioration are very common manifestations of hypothyroidism. They are of slow onset and usually long duration, and thus represent *dementia* of varying severity that is reversible with thyroid therapy (123,124,137–139). Psychoses, mostly paranoid or depressive, with visual or auditory hallucinations, may be superimposed on the dementia or occur independently, but they seem to be uncommon.

The EEG in hypothyroidism is usually abnormal, with mild slowing of the alpha rhythm and a poor or absent response to eye opening and closing (140). About 25% of patients have low-voltage, diffusely slowed records. These changes tend to improve in parallel with the clinical improvement. A decrease in sleep stages 3 and 4, as well as sleep apnea, have been noted in some patients (140,141). CBF and the metabolic rate are reduced. All these factors may contribute to the delirium occasionally seen in hypothyroidism and to dementia.

HYPERTHYROIDISM

Delirium is a rare complication of hyperthyroidism today. As mentioned earlier, however, one must keep in mind that the issue of psychiatric diagnosis is often quite muddled in published reports. For example, a recent article on the relationship between thyroid disease and mental illness (142) states that "reversible confusional states occur rarely but delirium or clouding of consciousness is usually present" (p 103). It is difficult to draw any conclusion from this confusing and contradictory statement. The incidence of delirium in hyperthyroidism is said to be about 3% or 4% (143), and was apparently higher in the past when thyroid crisis or storm was a relatively common event (144). An occasional hyperthyroid patient may present with lethargy and delirium. This condition is most common in the elderly ("apathetic thyrotoxicosis"), and may be followed by coma and death unless it is diagnosed and treated (145,146). Untreated hyperthyroid patients display relatively mild attentional-cognitive deficits on psychological testing (147,148). Generalized anxiety disorder and major depression appear to be the most common psychiatric disorders (147).

The EEG is often abnormal. Hyperthyroid patients show reduced alpha activity and increased beta activity (148). In more severe hyperthyroidism, slow background activity may appear. CBF is usually increased (21).

Delirium may occur episodically in the course of *Hashimoto's thyroiditis* (148,149).

HYPOPARATHYROIDISM

This endocrinopathy may be idiopathic or follow thyroidectomy. Delirium has been reported in hypoparathyroidism and, in one small series of patients, represented the most common form of psychosis (150,151). "Mental changes" have been found in about 17% of 71 patients of hypoparathyroidism in a recent report from China; confusion with hallucinations was observed in two of them (152). Other mental symptoms in that series included anxiety and depression. Reversible dementia has also been reported and has responded to treatment with alfacalcidol (153). Both delirium and dementia in hypoparathyroidism result from hypocalcemia. Delirium may also occur after parathyroidectomy (154).

HYPERPARATHYROIDISM

Organic mental syndromes, notably delirium and dementia, are relatively common in hyperparathyroidism, especially in the elderly (155–161). Delirium usually occurs with plasma calcium levels at or about 16 mg/100 ml but may also develop with lower concentrations. It tends to come on abruptly and is a presenting feature of hyperparathyroid crisis (162). Depression, memory impairment, fatigue, lethargy, and drowsiness are common features. Hypercalcemia, hypomagnesemia, and increased PTH levels are believed to be responsible for the psychiatric symptoms in this disorder (161). They tend to recede, completely or partially, in response to surgical and medical treatment.

HYPOADRENALISM (ADDISON'S DISEASE)

"Mental changes" are said to occur in 60% to 90% of patients with Addison's disease (124, 138). The reported "changes" or abnormalities include delirium, dementia, depression, apathy, and paranoid psychosis. Stoll (163), in his monograph based on a study of 33 patients with Addison's disease, states that delirium occurs most often in acute and terminal failure of the adrenal cortex, and urges that this cause be systematically ruled out in all cases of delirium. He notes that a diffuse organic psychosyndrome (presumably dementia) of relatively mild degree is surprisingly common. Plum and Posner (21) assert that a large proportion of untreated or inadequately treated patients with Addison's disease are "mildly delirious." Elderly patients with adrenal insufficiency often display intermittent confusion (164). The pathogenesis of delirium in this encephalopathy probably involves a combination of factors, including removal of the cortisone effect on the brain, hyponatremia, hyperkalemia, hypoglycemia, and hypotension (21).

HYPERADRENALISM (CUSHING'S SYNDROME)

Psychiatric disturbances are a very common feature of Cushing's syndrome (CS) (165–167). Estimates of their frequency vary but, with systematic assessment of mental status, are about 80% (165–167). Affective, mostly depressive, disorders are by far the most common (165–167). Cognitive impairment, notably memory, attention, and concentration deficits, have been observed in the majority of patients with CS (166,168). Delirium has been reported but appears to be uncommon (166,169–172). It is said to be associated with advanced disease and with particularly high cortisol and ACTH levels (166). On occasion, delirium may be a presenting feature of occult CS (172). Regestein et al. (171) observed delirium in five of seven patients with CS; all five were over 65 years of age, indicating that any metabolic disorder is more likely to cause delirium in an elderly rather than a younger patient. The EEG in CS is usually either normal or shows mild slowing of background acitvity, excessive fast activity, and minor paroxysmal discharges (173).

Pathogenesis of delirium in CS appears to be related to hypercortisolemia and its direct effects on the brain (21). Excessive ACTH may be at least partly responsible in some cases (166). Cortisol hypersecretion may contribute to the cognitive dysfunction in depression (174), and ACTH has been found to impair selective attention (175). Given these findings, it is surprising that delirium does not occur more often in CS. The psychiatric aspects of exogenous steroids are discussed in Chapter 11.

DIABETES MELLITUS

Delirium, as well as stupor and coma, may result from a number of complications of diabetes mellitus (DM) (21). DM was found to account for nearly

15% of the etiological factors in delirium in elderly patients screened during a prevalence study of the syndrome in a general hospital (176). Acute diabetic complications are common in the elderly (177). Elderly diabetics are especially vulnerable to hypoglycemic reactions in response to insulin, sulfonylurea drugs, or neoplasm. Moreover, one complication is particularly important with geriatric patients: hyperosmolar nonketotic diabetic coma (177).

Diabetic ketoacidosis most often follows infection, insulin deficiency, cardiovascular accidents, and trauma (178). About 70% of patients display clouding of consciousness, and about 10% present in coma (178). The state of consciousness in these patients does not correlate with blood glucose levels, hydrogen ions, electrolytes, or ketone bodies, but it does correlate with plasma osmolality (178). Experimentally induced acute and chronic hyperglycemia in rats is associated with reduced rCBF (179).

Hyperosmolar nonketotic diabetic coma typically occurs in the elderly (177,180–183). Clouding of consciousness, sometimes with visual hallucinations and other features of delirium, is often present and may be the presenting feature (177,180–183). As many as one-half of the patients have either untreated or undiagnosed DM (177). A variety of precipitating factors may be involved, including drugs that decrease insulin secretion, interfere with its action, or promote dehydration (177). Hypothermia and other factors may have the same effect (177). The patient is typically sleepy, lethargic, and confused, and progresses to stupor and coma. Focal neurological signs and generalized convulsions may be present. Prolonged mental confusion follows treatment on occasion (181). Plasma glucose concentrations usually exceed 600 to 800 mg/100 ml (177).

Hypoglycemia is discussed in an earlier section of this chapter.

Diabetic lactic acidosis can follow ketoacidosis or administration of oral hypoglycemic agents (21). Symptoms are similar to those of any other severe metabolic acidosis and may include confusion.

Other systemic diseases

Cancer

Delirium is a recognized complication of cancer, but its incidence and prevalence are variously estimated and actually unknown (184). After depression, the syndrome is claimed to represent the second most common psychiatric disorder among cancer patients (185). In one series of 546 such patients, it was diagnosed in 15% (184). Delirium appears to be particularly common in terminal cancer patients, 50% to 85% of whom were observed to display it in two small series (186,187). Organic mental syndrome was diagnosed in 40% of 100 consecutive patients with cancer referred for psychiatric consultation

(188), and delirium was found in 10% of such referred patients in a cancer hospital (189). In general, the prevalence of organic mental disorders among cancer patients is reported to be 8% (190).

Delirium in cancer patients may be due to a number of factors, occurring singly or in various combinations. These factors fall into two major groups: first, intracranial, including primary and secondary neoplasms of the brain and meningeal carcinomatosis; and second, indirect cerebral effects of systemic cancer or its treatment (21,184,185,188). Delirium due to brain neoplasm is discussed in Chapter 17, and that caused by chemotherapeutic agents is reviewed in Chapter 11. In this section, only the indirect cerebral effects of systemic cancer are discussed and are listed in Table 14–2.

Metabolic encephalopathy is one of the most common, if not the most common, causes of delirium in cancer patients (21,184,185,188,191,192). It may be misdiagnosed as brain metastases, as exemplified by a study of patients who died of bronchogenic carcinoma (193). Brain metastases had been diagnosed clinically in 44% of those patients but were histologically proven in only 20%. Delirium ("disturbances of consciousness") was present in about 80% of all patients suspected of having brain metastases and was almost equally distributed among those who proved to have a brain tumor and those who did not. It follows that at least as many patients without cerebral metastases displayed delirium. The most frequent causes of delirium included respiratory failure and hypercalcemia. In a group of 100 cancer patients referred for psychiatric consultation, 40% had an organic mental syndrome (OMS)

TABLE 14–2 Nonmetastatic Causes of Delirium

A. Disordered metabolic or endocrine function
   1. Hepatic encephalopathy
   2. Uremic encephalopathy
   3. Respiratory encephalopathy
   4. Hypercalcemia
   5. Hypoglycemia
   6. Hyponatremia or water intoxication
   7. Hyperserotonemia
   8. Hyperadrenalism
   9. Hyperthyroidism
B. Vascular and hematopoietic disorders
   1. Anemia
   2. Erythrocytemia
   3. Thrombocytopenia
   4. Hyperviscosity and increased coagulability of the blood
   5. Cerebral infarction
C. Malnutrition
D. Infection
E. Paraneoplastic encephalopathy
F. Encephalopathy secondary to therapy

and less then one-fifth of those with an OMS had documented evidence of cerebral metastases (188). A study of cancer patients with encephalopathy referred for a neurological consultation found that about 40% suffered from metabolic brain disease, notably hepatic or uremic encephalopathy and hypercalcemia (21). In many patients several factors, metabolic or otherwise, may contribute to the onset of delirium; all these potential causes need to be looked for and corrected, if possible, if the syndrome is to subside. In an occasional patient, delirium may be a presenting feature of cancer in the absence of cerebral metastases (194).

The causes of metabolic encephalopathy among cancer patients are listed in Table 14–2. All of them are discussed in other sections of this chapter.

Vascular and hematopoietic disorders are less common causes of encephalopathy and delirium than metabolic disordrs. *Hyperviscosity* is usually associated with dysproteinemias, such as excessive macroglobulinemia in multiple myeloma. The patient typically presents with delirium, lethargy, and somnolence (195). The EEG is diffusely slowed. Delirium in this condition is believed to be at least partly due to concurrent hypercalcemia. *Disseminated intravascular coagulation* was the most common vascular disease responsible for encephalopathy in one study (21), and delirium may be one of its manifestations (196). *Thrombocytopenia* associated with cancer may give rise to delirium as a result of bleeding into the brain. *Anemia,* due to malnutrition, depression of bone marrow, blood loss, chronic infection, radiotherapy, or chemotherapy, is common, and while it is unlikely to cause delirium unless very severe, it may contribute to it as a result of cerebral hypoxia.

Malnutrition is common in advanced cancer, especially that involving the gastrointestinal tract. Avitaminosis may be associated with it and may cause delirium.

Infection, such as diffuse sepsis, may cause encephalopathy and delirium (21).

Paraneoplastic encephalopathy (PE) or "remote effects" of cancer on the nervous system tends to occur in patients with systemic malignancy and is caused by neither metastases to the brain nor any of the identifiable nonmetastatic effects of cancer on the nervous system (191). This condition is uncommon and may precede the diagnosis of cancer, and its etiology is unknown (191). Hallucinations, paranoid ideation, and bizarre behavior have been reported in 24% of a small series of patients with PE (197). Paraneoplastic syndromes that may give rise to delirium include *limbic encephalitis, progressive multifocal leukoencephalopathy,* and *diffuse polioencephalopathy* (191,192,198,199). Limbic encephalitis is an uncommon complication of cancer, particularly of oat cell carcinoma of the lung. Mental symptoms are common and include confusion and dementia (200). Progressive multifocal leukoencephalopathy may complicate especially Hodgkin's disease and leukemia, and occasionally features delirium (201). Diffuse polioencephalopathy may present with delirium or dementia (198).

There are other potential metabolic and vascular mechanisms whereby cancer may give rise to delirium. It follows that if the latter develops in a patient known to have a neoplasm, a search for the various treatable and potentially reversible etiological factors must be undertaken. On the other hand, delirium may on occasion be the presenting feature of occult neoplasm; this possible cause should always be considered, especially in an older patient.

Treatment of delirium in a cancer patient should follow the general guidelines discussed in Chapter 10. Some authors have recommended intravenous administration of large doses of haloperidol (as much as 350 mg in 24 hours), combined with up to 240 mg daily of lorazepam, to control agitation in delirious, critically ill cancer patients (202). Other writers point out, however, that some of these patients respond readily to relatively small doses of antipsychotic drugs, such as haloperidol. Hence, the initial response must be assessed and the dosage of the drug adjusted according to the patient's response, rather than following a fixed schedule (203). I agree with this more conservative approach.

Carcinoid syndrome

This syndrome is of some interest for the student of delirium because of its association with disorders of indole metabolism. Major et al. (204) found episodes of confusion or altered consciousness in 35% of 22 patients with carcinoid tumor. These episodes, presumably delirium, are said to have overlapped with depressive and anxiety disorders. The investigators hypothesized that decreased levels of brain serotonin were responsible for both the confusion and depression in their patients. In another study, only 6 of 219 patients with a carcinoid tumor had encephalopathy believed to be due to liver failure (205). Lehmann (206) claimed that "confusion" is the most common abnormality in patients with carcinoid syndrome, occurring in about 25%. He reported on his own patient, who displayed florid delirium followed by catatonic stupor. Slowing of the EEG accompanied the delirium.

Serotonin does not penetrate the blood-brain barrier; hence, a functional deficiency of this neurotransmitter in the brain may coexist with its high blood levels. Production of serotonin by a carcinoid tumor accounts for about 60% of dietary tryptophan, and an insufficient quantity of this compound is available for the synthesis of serotonin in the brain. Administration of L-tryptophan may decrease the delirium in a patient with carcinoid syndrome (207). Delirium was reported in a patient with hyperserotonemia in the absence of a carcinoid tumor (207). Some, but not all, patients with carcinoidosis treated with parachlorphenylalanine (PCPA) developed delirium and slowing of the

EEG (208). The drug does not cause mental symptoms in normal subjects (204). It has been proposed that tryptophan deficiency and lowered brain serotonin levels may be responsible for delirium and depression in patients with carcinoid tumors, as well as in patients with pellagra and those treated with PCPA and levodopa (204,209). This issue remains unresolved.

Porphyria

In its acute intermittent form, porphyria is notorious for the frequency and diversity of its associated mental symptoms. Delirium appears to be the most common mental disorder complicating acute porphyria (210). Its frequency in three large series of patients ranged from 18% to 52% (211). Delirium in this disease may vary from mild to severe and may progress to coma. An acute attack typically involves exposure to a precipitating event, such as intake of barbiturates, sulfonamides, anticonvulsants, and certain non-steroidal anti-inflammatory agents (212); alcohol excess; infection; or menstruation (213). The resulting symptoms usually include severe abdominal pain, pains and paresthesias in the extremities, nausea, vomiting, tachycardia, fever, and delirium (214). CNS involvement has been reported in the majority of patients (213,214). The EEG shows diffuse slowing in about 80% of cases (214). Some patients display schizophrenia-like features and may be misdiagnosed as suffering from a functional psychosis (211,213).

The pathogenesis of acute intermittent porphyria is still obscure. It has been hypothesized that delta-aminolevulinic acid or porphobilinogen, or both, may produce all the mental symptoms of the acute attack by modifying synaptic transmission in the CNS (213).

Wilson's disease

A variety of psychiatric symptoms and disorders have been reported to occur in Wilson's disease (WD) (hepatolenticular degeneration), an inborn error of metabolism involving deposition of copper in various organs, notably the liver and brain (215). In a recent series of 31 patients with WD, 34.5% presented first with psychiatric symptoms; delirium was not mentioned (216). More patients are referred initially to psychiatrists than to other specialists (217). Neuropsychological deficits, mostly in the areas of memory and motor functioning, have been found in neurologically impaired patients with WD (218). Delirium has been reported only infrequently and probably occurs only as a manifestation of hepatic encephalopathy. It has been suggested that psychiatric patients under 30 years of age should be screened with a ceruloplasmin determination to rule out WD (217). Treatment of delirium in this disease should be the same as in HE and involve administration of benzodiazepines rather than of neuroleptics, which could affect liver function and increase the dystonia that is usually present (217).

Disorders of fluid, electrolyte, and acid-base balance

Brain function may be affected by disturbance of the electrolyte concentration for two major reasons: first, there may be a deficiency or excess of blood or whole-body electrolytes affecting the brain secondarily; and second, a primary disorder of the brain may result in a disturbance of the salt–water balance, which in turn affects cerebral function. The blood-brain barrier is freely permeable to water; hence, changes in the osmolality of the serum are readily transmitted to the CSF and the extracellular fluid of the brain. By contrast, penetration of inorganic cations and anions from blood into the brain is slow. Disturbances of the concentrations of potassium, calcium, and magnesium in the blood do not have a marked effect on the CNS functions because of the mechanisms that tend to keep the ionic composition of the CSF and the extracellular fluid of the brain relatively stable (219). By contrast, the brain is highly vulnerable to rapid changes in serum osmolality. Serum osmolalities below about 260 mEq/l or above 350 mEq/l are likely to produce cerebral changes and related symptoms (21). An increase in osmolality leads to increased cellular water content and tissue swelling, while a decrease results in shrinkage of the brain (21).

Delirium is a prominent, if not the most common, psychiatric manifestation of acute electrolyte, fluid, and acid-base disorders. Many clinical conditions bring about delirium as a consequence of such disorders. Burns, major surgery, renal failure, and infections are common examples of conditions that are often associated with delirium and are partly mediated by fluid and electrolyte imbalance. Japanese workers reportedly found such imbalance in about 70% of patients with delirium due to various organic diseases (220). In some of these cases, the duration of the delirium was significantly shorted when the imbalance was corrected. Hyponatremia or hypokalemia, or both, with or without hypochloremia, were the most frequently observed electrolyte abnormalities. A wide variety of drugs have been implicated in a whole range of electrolyte disorders (221).

Hyponatremia

Dilution or depletion, or both, of body sodium stores results in hyponatremia (222). The possible etiological factors include drugs such as diuretics, antidepressants, lithium, and neuroleptics (221,223,224); excessive parenteral fluids (225); renal disease (222); inappropriate secretion of antidiuretic hormone (SIADH) (222,223); and excessive water drinking (226). Self-induced hyponatremia and water intoxication as a result of polydipsia in psychiatric, notably schizophrenic, patients has attracted much attention in recent years (226–232). The reported prevalence of polydipsia in chronically ill psychiatric patients ranges from 6% to 17%, and it is estimated that up to one-half of these patients with polydipsia develop symptoms of water intoxication (226).

Mental symptoms of hyponatremia are related to the serum sodium level and the rapidity of its fall, as well as to the etiology (222). Insidious development of hyponatremia may be tolerated until the serum sodium level falls to about 100 mEq/l. Early symptoms include impaired sensation of taste, anorexia, fatigue, headache, muscle cramps, thirst, and mild confusion. With more severe hyponatremia, delirium and convulsions may appear. Confusion tends to occur with serum sodium levels of about 115 mEq/l. Coma, irreversible brain damage, and death may follow (222,225,233). The EEG changes in hyponatremia involve loss of alpha activity and irregular discharges of high-amplitude theta waves (222).

Treatment involves fluid restriction and administration of demeclocycline (226). In patients with severe hyponatremia, serum sodium levels should not be normalized too rapidly so that neurological complications may be avoided (233,234).

Hypernatremia

Hypernatremia is a common problem in elderly hospitalized patients (235). It can be acute or chronic, and its manifestations reflect high osmolality of body fluids. The causes of hypernatremia are varied and often multifactorial, including febrile illness with increased water loss and hyperventilation; CNS lesions; diarrhea; nonketotic hyperosmolar coma; dehydration; nasogastric hyperalimentation; and severe burns.

The rapidity with which hypernatremia develops influences its effects on mental function. Gradual onset may allow consciousness to be undisturbed despite serum sodium levels of 170 mEq/l or higher. Depression of consciousness otherwise tends to occur with sodium levels of 160 mEq/l or higher (21,235) and correlates with the severity of the hypernatremia (235). Delirium, lethargy, stupor, and coma are the usual manifestations of hypernatremic encephalopathy (21,222,235). The EEG shows varying degrees of slow-wave activity but may be normal (222). Permanent brain damage may follow hypernatremia, especially in children and the elderly (222,235).

Hypokalemia

Delirium may be caused by hypokalemia but appears to be relatively uncommon. Profound hypokalemia can occur in familiar periodic paralysis, for example, without any mental symptoms (236). Hypokalemia may result from vomiting, diarrhea, diabetic ketoacidosis, laxative addiction, renal tubular acidosis, and other conditions. Diuretics are a particularly important cause of this disorder, as they are among the drugs most often prescribed for the elderly (237). Common symptoms of hypokalemia include muscular weakness and cramps, lethargy, apathy, drowsiness, and irritability. Delirium has been reported (220,236).

Hyperkalemia

It is claimed that an organic mental syndrome is the most frequent manifestation of hyperkalemia (238). This disorder can be precipitated or exaggerated by a variety of drugs, including non-steroidal anti-inflammatory agents and potassium-sparing diuretics. Delirium may be caused indirectly as a result of cardiac arrhythmias induced by elevated serum potassium levels.

Hypocalcemia

Delirium, irritability, fatigue, weakness, and depression are common features of hypocalcemia, which is most often due to hypoparathyroidism, sepsis, renal failure, malabsorption syndrome, and certain drugs such as phenytoin (238). Acute hypocalcemia is often seen in critically ill patients in the intensive care unit and necessitates intravenous calcium therapy (239).

Some patients develop symptoms when serum calcium levels fall rapidly below 8.5 mg/100 ml; others, with chronic hypocalcemia, may remain symptom free with calcium levels as low as 5–6 mg/100 ml. Delirium is most likely to develop when hypocalcemia develops acutely. Muscle weakness and cramps, paresthesias, tetany, and seizures may precede or accompany delirium. The EEG shows progressive slowing of background activity with falling calcium levels, as well as low-voltage, fast activity and sharp waves and spikes (240).

Hypercalcemia

Hypercalcemia is a serious and potentially lethal complication of many diseases, notably the malignant ones (241,242). It may be acute or chronic. Delirium may not only be caused by hypercalcemia but is also its presenting feature (243). Neuropsychiatric symptoms may develop when calcium levels are only 12 mg/100 ml, yet they may be absent with levels as high as 16 mg/l. Such symptoms may include, in addition to delirium, lassitude, drowsiness, anxiety, depression, stupor, and coma. Anorexia, nausea, vomiting, headache, and difficulty in walking are among common early symptoms (243).

Confusion tends to correlate with serum calcium levels (244). Since hypercalcemia presents a life-threatening medical emergency, it is important to keep in mind that delirium may be its presenting manifestation. Hypercalcemia should be suspected in a delirious patient with cancer (242).

The EEG in hypercalcemic patients shows diffuse slowing of background activity interrupted by high-voltage bursts of delta waves (240,245). These abnormalities tend to subside within 2 months of the start of therapy. In some patients the EEG is normal. This has prompted the suggestion that factors other than hypercalcemia must be present in order for the EEG changes to appear (246).

Hypomagnesemia

Delirium is a recognized feature of hypomagnesemia (238,247). The latter usually occurs in association with other electrolyte abnormalities, such as hypocalcemia and hypokalemia, and it may be difficult to determine its specific clinical effects and psychiatric features (219). Hypomagnesemia may be a result of starvation, malabsorption syndrome, chronic alcoholism, diuretics, severe diarrhea, aldosteronism, and other conditions (247). Levels of about 1 mEq/l may precipitate delirium and seizures at times, while levels as low as 0.3 mEq/l may produce no symptoms. Depression, apathy, anxiety, weakness, tremor, muscle fasciculations, irritability, tetany, and occasionally seizures may accompany mental changes (247). Manifestations of hypomagnesemia are believed to stem from the role of magnesium in activating and generating adenosine triphosphate (ATP) and cyclic adenosine monophosphate and in regulating neuromuscular transmission (247).

Hypermagnesemia

Hypermagnesemia is much less common than hypomagnesemia but, like the latter, may be potentially life-threatening (245). Its most common causes are severe renal failure and treatment with magnesium-containing antacids. Many elderly patients are at increased risk of hypermagnesemia as a result of the increased load and reduced excretion. The initial presenting features include drowsiness, lethargy, and weakness. Some patients may remain alert, however, even at plasma concentrations greater than 5 mEq/l (248). Narcosis and coma may occur. It is not clear whether and how often delirium develops.

Hypophosphatemia

This condition has many causes, such as diabetic ketoacidosis, acute and chronic alcoholism, severe burns, respiratory alkalosis, and intravenous hyperalimentation (249,250). Two biochemical abnormalities appear to be responsible for the clinical manifestations of hypophosphatemia: depletion of intracellular ATP and tissue hypoxia (250). These abnormalities are believed to be responsible for CNS and neuromuscular symptoms. A report on a small group of patients with a history of caloric deprivation who were treated with an oral diet or intravenous hyperalimentation notes that the majority of them developed confusion, with or without hallucinations, during the treatment (249). All these patients, however, had evidence of liver disease and were alcoholics. It is not clear if the observed delirium was etiologically related to hypophosphatemia or is ever a feature of it.

Acidosis

Acidosis is an arterial blood pH below 7.40. Primary respiratory acidosis occurs with increased PCO_2, while primary metabolic acidosis involves compensatory hyperventilation and decreased PCO_2. A patient with metabolic alkalosis may hyperventilate and develop compensatory respiratory acidosis which is discussed in the section on hypercapnic encephalopathy.

Metabolic acidosis occurs in a variety of conditions, such as renal failure; diabetic ketoacidosis; lactic acidosis; and methanol, ammonium chloride, and salicylate intoxication (251). Acidosis interferes with brain energy metabolism (21). All the metabolic acidoses give rise to hyperpnea, followed by confusion and, at times, stupor, coma, and convulsions (21). D-Lactate acidosis, for example, has been reported to precipitate confusion in 63% of patients who had jejunoileal bypass (252). Other conditions associated with acidosis are discussed in this and other chapters.

Alkalosis

Metabolic alkalosis is the acid-base disturbance most often encountered in the hospital setting (251). It may result from loss of acid through vomiting, chloride depletion, excessive intake of alkalis, hypercapnia, or hypersecretion of mineralocorticoids. Respiratory alkalosis occurs when CO_2 removal by the lungs exceeds its production in the body, with resulting hypocapnia. It may follow hyperventilation, mechanical overventilation, pneumonia, or hepatic failure. Lethargy and mental confusion are more likely to result from alkalosis than stupor or coma (21). These effects are unlikely to develop unless the systemic pH exceeds 7.55 (251). Coexisting hypocalcemia or cerebrovascular disease appears to predispose to disturbances of consciousness during alkalosis (251). Hypoventilation secondary to metabolic alkalosis can augment hypoxia and thus contribute to the mental symptoms (21).

Acute respiratory alkalosis results in constriction of cerebral arterioles with a consequent reduction of CBF and brain hypoxia. Mild confusion and EEG slowing follow. These changes seem to occur more readily in younger individuals (35 years of age or less), probably due to their greater cerebral vascular reactivity. Excessive hyperventilation results in a reduction of cerebral oxidative metabolism. Voluntary hyperventilation for about 3 minutes tends to induce symptoms such as lightheadedness, faintness, a feeling of unreality, blurring of vision, chest pain, paresthesias, and occasionally syncope (253). In an occasional case, hallucinations may appear (254). The EEG shows generalized slowing. These effects amount to a mild acute confusional state (255,256).

Vitamin deficiency or excess

Deficiency of several vitamins can result in cognitive disorders, including delirium and dementia. The conditions most often associated with vitamin deficiencies in North America include old age, especially if combined with dementia or depression, or both; alcoholism; gastrointestinal disease; poverty; food faddism; anorexia nervosa; and iatrogenic factors such as renal hemodialysis, intravenous hyperalimentation, certain drugs, gastrectomy, gastric partition, and jejunoileal bypass. Delirium due to vitamin deficiencies in the elderly occurs even in the developed countries (257). Malnutrition is not uncommon among hospitalized patients (258) and is in many cases iatrogenic (259). Deficiencies of cyanocobalamine (vitamine B_{12}), folic acid, niacin, and thiamine are reasonably well established as potential causes of delirium. The status of vitamin C, riboflavin, and pyridoxine deficiencies in this respect is unclear.

Vitamin B_{12} deficiency is known to give rise to organic mental syndromes (260–267). The precise nature of these conditions is not clear, since many writers refer to "organic psychosis," "dementia," "organic change," or "organic states," i.e., mostly meaningless diagnostic labels. Some authors are more specific and speak of delirium or acute confusional state. Clearly, delirium does occur in vitamin B_{12} deficiency, as explicitly stated in some published repotts or inferred from clinical descriptions of the patients' symptoms (260,261,263,266,267). The true incidence of delirium is impossible to determine because of the semantic problems referred to above. It appears that the majority of the reported patients suffered from a more or less reversible dementia rather than delirium. Samson et al. (263), however, found delirium in 13 of 14 patients with pernicious anemia, and MacDonald Holmes (261) observed "confusion and memory defect" in all 14 of his patients. If the organic mental syndrome is not treated properly, an irreversible dementia of some severity is liable to develop (261,263). It is therefore important to rule out vitamin B_{12} deficiency in a patient presenting with unexplained delirium or dementia. Moreover, one should keep in mind that psychiatric manifestations of vitamin B_{12} deficiency may precede any abnormality of the peripheral blood or bone marrow or any signs of subacute combined degeneration of the spinal cord (268).

Vitamin B_{12} deficiency occurs most often in pernicious anemia. Other causes include nutritional deficiency, intestinal malabsorption, gastrectomy, and drugs, notably anticonvulsants.

The EEG in patients with vitamin B_{12} deficiency and an associated organic mental syndrome shows diffuse slowing of the background activity, which correlates well with the clinical findings (263). Improvement in both the EEG and the mental state follows administration of vitamin B_{12} and coincides with the maximum reticulocyte response (263). CBF is increased and CMR is decreased in patients with pernicious anemia.

Folate deficiency is not well established as a cause of delirium. Published reports on psychiatric manifestations speak only of reversible dementia and do not mention delirium (269–271). It is thus unclear whether folate deficiency ever gives rise to this syndrome.

Nicotinic acid (niacin) deficiency is manifested clinically as pellagra, a disease characterized by dermatitis, diarrhea, and dementia (272). Gregory (273), in his thorough review of psychiatric syndromes associated with pellagra, asserts that they constitute another triad of three D's: depression, delirium, and dementia. Early reports on mental symptoms in pellagra make a clear reference to delirium in this condition. Spies et al. (274), for example, state that the most common type of psychosis in pellagra features loss of memory, disorientation, confusion, and confabulation. These authors further state that delirium may also occur. Jolliffe et al. (275) coined the term "nicotinic acid deficiency encephalopathy," characterized by clouding of consciousness, cogwheel rigidity, and grasp and sucking reflexes. One-half of their 150 patients showed no other signs of pellagra. These articles appeared at a time when endemic pellagra was still prevalent in the United States; it has since been eradicated, and only sporadic cases continue to appear (276). Two small series of cases published in the past decade or so give discrepant data: one found temporal disorientation and impairment of recent memory in 5 of 18 patients (276), while the other noted confusion in the history of all of 20 patients who came to necropsy (272). These latter patients had all been chronic alcoholics and had been diagnosed as suffering from delirium tremens. Pellagra was not suspected clinically, since the classical cutaneous signs were absent; these patients had "pellagra sine pelle agra" (272). The authors concluded that it is important to recognize pellagra in chronic alcoholic patients if brain damage is to be avoided.

The importance of niacin and nicotinamide for brain function stems from their role as precursors of the pyridine nucleotide cofactors (3). Deficiency of the vitamin results in profound functional and structural changes in the CNS.

The most consistenct neuropathological abnormality in pellagra is central chromatolysis of the neurons in various areas of the brain, including Betz cells (272).

Confirmation of the diagnosis of pellagra involves either a trial of niacin therapy or the urinary excretion of 2-pyridone. Determination of the plasma tryptophan level may help the diagnosis if the level is found to be low (276).

Thiamine deficiency is regarded by some writers as a classical example of a metabolic encephalopathy (277). Malnutrition of any cause may result in thiamine deficiency. It is most often encountered in association with chronic alcoholism but is by no means confined to alcoholics. Severe thiamine deficiency has been reported in gastrointestinal disease, hyperemesis gravidarum, starvation, and in patients on renal hemodialysis and in those treated with intravenous fluids or hyperalimentation (278–282).

Thiamine deficiency gives rise to Wernicke's encephalopathy, a syndrome first described by Wernicke (283) in 1881. He drew attention to the diagnostic triad in this condition, i.e., confusion, nystagmus, and ataxia. Other features include ophthalmoplegia and a severe memory deficit, with or without confabulation. In one large study, 56% of the patients displayed a "global confusional state" on admission (284). This statement suggests that they were delirious. A medical editorial states explicitly that spatiotemporal disorientation in patients with Wernicke's encephalopathy may lead to delirium and coma (285). The encephalopathy is relatively common, and its diagnosis is often missed (280). The delirium in this condition is typically of the hypoalert-hypoactive variety, with apathy, severe disorientation, and marked memory impairment. Hallucinations are uncommon unless delirium tremens coexists. The delirium may persist for up to 2 months after institution of treatment, but symptoms usually begin to subside within several days (283). As delirium clears up, a chronic amnestic (Korsakoff) syndrome emerges and may or may not be reversible (283).

Gibson et al. (277) have proposed that acetylcholine synthesis, as well as synaptic transmission, are decreased in severe thiamine deficiency. Acetylcholine is an important neurotransmitter in the reticular activating system and plays a crucial role in attention, memory, learning, and consciousness, aspects of brain function impaired not only in Wernicke's encephalopathy but also in other metabolic encephalopathies, as well as in delirium. The role of the cholinergic system in the latter is discussed in Chapter 7.

Early diagnosis and treatment of Wernicke's encephalopathy are essential if a chronic and possibly irreversible organic amnestic syndrome is to be prevented (286). Treatment with parenteral thiamine is mandatory.

Hypervitaminosis due to excessive intake of vitamins A and D may occasionally lead to delirium. Hypervitaminosis due to excessive vitamin A can result in hypercalcemia, increased intracranial pressure, pseudotumor cerebri, and delirium (287–289). Affected patients have taken high doses (at least 150,000 units daily) of vitamin A for prolonged periods.

Hypervitaminosis D has been reported most often during the treatment of surgical hypoparathyroidism, rheumatoid arthritis, osteoarthritis, and osteomalacia (290,291). Hypercalcemia develops in vitamin D intoxication. Confusion has been noted in this condition (290).

Disorders of temperature regulation

Hypothermia

Hypothermia is a drop in the body's core temperature to 35°C or less. "Accidental hypothermia" refers to an unintended decrease in core body temperature in the absence of a primary CNS disease involving the thermoregulatory center (292–295). The elderly are especially vulnerable to this common disorder as a result of a variety of predisposing factors, such as CNS, cardiovascular, infectious, endocrine, or renal disease; use of drugs such as ethanol, phenothiazines, and antidepressants; poor living conditions; and malnutrition (292). Many victims of hypothermia are intoxicated with alcohol. With core temperatures between 33° and 35°C (mild hypothermia), consciousness is usually unimpaired but retrograde amnesia has been reported (294). In moderate hypothermia (core temperature between 30° and 33°C), consciousness is impaired, and in severe hypothermia (core temperature below 30°C) the patient is usually comatose (294). Infection is a major associated disorder in hypothermia, and impaired mental status is significantly more common among infected patients (296).

Cooling causes a progressive slowing of the EEG and increased latency of evoked potentials (297,298). Hypothermia results in depression of synaptic transmission due to impaired transmitter release, as well as slowing of axonal conduction (297). The former disorder is probably largely responsible for confusion in hypothermia.

Hyperthermia (heat stroke)

Heat stroke is usually associated with a core temperature of more than 40.6°C and anhidrosis; it can be either exertional or nonexertional (299–302). Malignant hyperthermia is a hypermetabolic state with core temperatures higher than 41°C caused by anesthetic gases and muscle relaxants (303). Heat stroke is particularly prevalent in hot climates, during heat waves in urban areas, and in hot industrial environments. Psychiatric patients are at risk for heat stroke, notably schizophrenics taking antipsychotic or other drugs with anticholinergic effects (304). Exertional heat stroke among distance runners, including joggers, has attracted attention with the growing popularity of recreational running (305,306).

Delirium is a common feature of heat stroke. The onset of the stroke is usually sudden and manifested clinically either by delirium, with agitated and aggressive behavior and vivid hallucinations, or by coma (299–302). Seizures, hyperirritability, rigidity, muscle cramps, coarse tremor, dystonic movements, ataxia, and opisthotonus may occur. Delirium usually precedes the onset of coma. After regaining consciousness, many patients report vivid, frightening dreams (301). Delirium may also come on after recovery from coma and may last for several days. Irreversible brain damage and associated mental symptoms may occur. Hyperthermia causes an increase in CBF and CMR. Edema or congestion of the brain is usually present. At or just above 42°C, brain energy failure develops (115).

Miscellaneous disorders

It is neither possible nor useful to list every disorder that may give rise to delirium on occasion. However, several disorders, not referred to elsewhere in this book, are clinically of some importance and hence deserve brief mention.

Allergy, notably to certain foods, is claimed by some authors to cause confusional states (307). The validity of this claim is open to question, however. *Angioedema* and *urticaria* may be associated with a mild encephalopathy and "alteration of consciousness" (308).

Systemic mastocytosis has been reported to be associated with delirium in some patients (309).

Electrical injury may give rise to confusion (310,311). In one series it was observed in 50% of the patients (311). Restlessness and "disoriented behavior," presumably delirium, have been observed in persons struck by lightning (312). Delirium may occur following ECT (314–314). Some authors have reported an acute mental syndrome after ECT but state that it did not meet the criteria for delirium; however, these criteria comprise items not considered essential for the diagnosis of delirium, according to *DSM-III* (315). The syndrome can develop after ECT on occasion, but its incidence is unknown (314).

Radiation injury, a complication of radiotherapy of the CNS, has been reported to cause confusion in some patients (316).

References

1. Braunwald E., Isselbacher K. J., Petersdorf R. G., et al (eds): *Harrison's Principles of Internal Medicine.* ed 11. New York, McGraw-Hill, 1987.
2. Lockwood A. H.: Metabolic encephalopathies: Opportunities and challenges. *J. Cereb. Blood Flow Metab.* 1987;7:523–526.
3. McCandless D. W. (ed): *Cerebral Energy Metabolism and Metabolic Encephalopathy.* New York, Plenum Press, 1985.
4. Posner J. B.: Delirium and exogenous metabolic brain disease, in Beeson P. B., McDermott W., Wyngaarden J. B. (eds): *Cecil Textbook of Medicine.* ed 15. Vol 1. Philadelphia, WB. Saunders, 1979, pp 644–651.
5. Becker E. L., Landau S. I. (eds): *International Dictionary of Medicine and Biology.* Vol 1. New York, Wiley, 1986.
6. Siesjö B. K.: Metabolic basis of consciousness. *The 11th World Congress of Neurology.* Amsterdam, Excerpta Medica, 1977, p 671.
7. Gibson G. E.: Hypoxia, in McCandless D. W. (ed): *Cerebral Energy Metabolism and Metabolic Encephalopathy.* New York, Plenum Press, 1985, pp 43–78.
8. Graham D. I.: Pathology of hypoxic brain damage in man. *J. Clin. Pathol.* 1978; 30 Suppl 11:170–180.
9. Pugh L. G. C. E.: The effect of acute and chronic exposure to low-oxygen supply on consciousness, in Schaefer K. E. (ed): *Environmental Effects on Consciousness.* New York, Macmillan, 1962, pp 106–116.
10. Crow T. J., Kelman G. R.: Psychological effects of mild acute hypoxia. *Br. J. Anaesth.* 1973;45:335–337.
11. Nelson M.: Psychological testing at high altitudes. *Aviat. Space Environ. Med.* 1982;53:122–126.
12. Finnegan T. P., Abraham P., Docherty T. B.: Ambulatory monitoring of the electroencephalogram in high altitude mountaineers. *Electroencephalogr. Clin. Neurophysiol.* 1985;60:220–224.
13. Ryn Z.: Nervous system and altitude syndrome of high altitude asthenia. *Acta Med. Pol.* 1979;20:155–169.
14. White A. J.: Cognitive impairment of acute mountain sickness and acetazolamine. *Aviat. Space Environ. Med.* 1984;55:598–603.
15. Modell J. H., Graves S. A., Kuck E. J.: Near-drowning: Correlation of level of consciousness and survival. *Can. Anaesth. Soc. J.* 1980;27:211–215.
16. Peters B. H., Levine H. S., Kelly P. J.: Neurologic and psychologic manifestations of decompression illness in divers. *Neurology* 1977;27:125–127.
17. Dolmierski R., Maslowski J., Matousek M., et al: EEG changes under hyperbaric conditions: Spectral analysis during simulated diving. *Acta Neurol. Scand.* 1988;77:437–439.
18. Kraaier V., Van Huffelen A. C., Wieneke G. H.: Quantitative EEG changes due to hypobaric hypoxia in normal subjects. *Electroencephalogr. Clin. Neurophysiol.* 1988;69:303–312.
19. Edmonds C., Thomas R. L.: Medical aspects of diving—part 3. *Med. J. Aust.* 1972;2:1300–1304.
20. Cassaigne J. Y., Duflo B., Pequignot H.: Confusion mentale et anemie chez le sujet age. *Concours Medi.* 1973;29:80–83.
21. Plum F., Posner J. B.: *The Diagnosis of Stupor and Coma,* ed 3. Philadelphia, FA Davis, 1980.

22. Field J. B.: Hypoglycemia. *Endocrinol. Metab. Clin. North Am.* 1989;18:27–43.
23. Marks V., Rose C. F.: *Hypoglycemia,* ed 2. Raven Press, New York, 1987.
24. Laurent J., Debry G., Floquet J.: *Hypoglycemic Tumors.* Amsterdam, Excerpta Medica, 1971.
25. Fajans S. S., Floyd J. C.: Fasting hypoglycemia in adults. *N. Engl. J. Med.* 1976;294:766–772.
26. Seltzer H. S.: Drug-induced hypoglycemia. *Diabetes* 1972;21:955–966.
27. Turkington R. W.: Encephalopathy induced by oral hypoglycemic drugs. *Arch. Intern. Med.* 1977;137:1082–1083.
28. Hafken L., Leichter S., Reich T.: Organic brain dysfunction as a possible consequence of postgastrectomy hypoglycemia. *Am. J. Psychiatry* 1975;132:1321–1324.
29. Fischer K. F., Lees J. A., Newman J. H.: Hypoglycemia in hospitalized patients. *N. Engl. J. Med.* 1986;315:1245–1250.
30. Malouf R., Brust J. C. M.: Hypoglycemia: Causes, neurological manifestations, and outcome. *Ann. Neurol.* 1985;17:421–430.
31. Grunberg G., Weiner J. L., Silverman R., et al: Factitious hypoglycemia due to surreptitious administration of insulin. *Ann. Intern. Med.* 1988;108:252–257.
32. Service J. F., Dale A. J. D., Elveback L. R., et al: Insulinoma. Clinical and diagnostic features of 60 consecutive cases. *Mayo Clin. Proc.* 1976;51:417–429.
33. Frerichs H., Creutzfeldt W.: Hypoglycemia. 1. Insulin secreting tumors. *Clin. Endocrinol. Metab.* 1976;5:747–767.
34. Boyd I. H., Cleveland S. E.: Psychiatric symptoms masking an insulinoma. *Dis. Nerv. Syst.* 1967;28:457–458.
35. Todd J., Martin F. R. R., Dewhurst K. E.: Mental symptoms due to insulinomata. *Br. Med. J.* 1962;2:828–831.
36. Breidahl H. D., Priestley J. T., Rynearson E. H.: Clinical aspects of hyperinsulinism. *J.A.M.A.* 1956;160:198–201.
37. Engel G. L., Webb J. P., Ferris E. B.: Quantitative electroencephalographic studies of anoxia in humans; comparison with acute alcoholic intoxication and hypoglycemia. *J. Clin. Invest.* 1945;24:691–697.
38. Editorial: Hypoglycaemia and the nervous system. *Lancet* 1985;2:759–760.
39. Sherlock S.: *Diseases of the Liver and Biliary System.* ed 6. Oxford, Blackwell, 1981.
40. Fraser C. L., Arieff A. I.: Hepatic encephalopathy. *N. Engl. J. Med.* 1985;313:865–873.
41. Zacharski L. R., Litin E. M., Mulder D. W., et al: Acute fatal hepatic failure presenting with psychiatric symptoms. *Am. J. Psychiatry* 1970;127:382–386.
42. Gilberstadt S. J., Gilberstadt H., Zieve L., et al: Psychomotor performance defects in cirrhotic patients without overt encephalopathy. *Arch. Intern. Med.* 1980;140:519–521.
43. Rehnstrom S., Simert G., Hansson J. A., et al: Chronic hepatic encephalopathy. A psychometrical study. *Scand. J. Gastroenterol.* 1977;12:305–311.
44. Steigman F., Clowdus B. F.: *Hepatic Encephalopathy.* Springfield, Ill, Charles C Thomas, 1971.
45. Tarter R. E., Hegedus A. M., Van Theil D. H.: Neuropsychiatric sequelae of portal-systemic encephalopathy: A review. *Int. J. Neurosci.* 1984;24:203–216.
46. Jaffe N.: Catatonia and hepatic dysfunction. *Dis. Nerv. Syst.* 1967;28:606–608.

47. Davidson E. A., Solomon P.: The differentiation of delirium tremens from impending hepatic coma. *J. Ment. Sci.* 1958;104:326–333.
48. Hawkes C. H., Brunt P. W.: The current status of the EEG in liver disease. *Dig. Dis.* 1974;19:75–80.
49. Kurtz D., Zenglein J. P., Girardel M., et al: Etude du sommeil nocturne au cours de l'encephalopathie porto-cave. *Electroencephalogr. Clin. Neurophysiol.* 1972;33:167–178.
50. Pappas S. C., Jones E. A.: Methods for assessing hepatic encephalopathy. *Semin. Liver Dis.* 1983;3:298–307.
51. Trewby P. N., Casemore C., Williams R.: Continuous bipolar recording of the EEG in patients with fulminant hepatic failure. *Electroencephalogr. Clin. Neurophysiol.* 1978;45:107–110.
52. Van der Rijt C. C. D., Schalm S. W., De Groot G. H., et al: Objective measurement of hepatic encephalopathy by means of automated EEG analysis. *Electroencephalogr. Clin. Neurophysiol.* 1984;57:423–426.
53. Jasson L., Goldin H.: Acute anicteric hepatitis manifested by coma and delirium. *N.Y. State J. Med.* 1961;61:1587–1588.
54. Zeneroli M. L., Pinelli G., Gollini G., et al: Visual evoked potential: A diagnostic tool for the assessment of hepatic encephalopathy. *Gut* 1984;25:291–299.
55. Yao H., Sadoshima S., Fujii K., et al: Cerebrospinal fluid lactate in patients with hepatic encephalopathy. *Eur. Neurol.* 1987;27:182–187.
56. Conn H. O.: Trailmaking and number-connection tests in the assessment of mental state in portal systemic encephalopathy. *Am. J. Dig. Dis.* 1977;22:541–550.
57. Trzepacz P. T., Maue F. R., Coffman G.: Neuropsychiatric assessment of liver transplantation candidates: Delirium and other psychiatric disorders. *Int. J. Psychiatry Med.* 1986–87;16:101–111.
58. Bade J. C., Schafer K.: Psychophysiology of chronic hepatic encephalopathy. *Hepatogastroenterology* 1985;32:259–266.
59. Fischer J. E., Baldessarini R. J.: False neurotransmitters and hepatic failure. *Lancet* 1971;2:75–80.
60. Jones E. A., Schafer D. F., Ferenci P., et al: The neurobiology of hepatic encephalopathy. *Hepatology* 1984;4:1235–1242.
61. Mullen K. D., Martin J. V., Mendelson W. B., et al: Could an endogenous benzodiazepine ligand contribute to hepatic encephalopathy? *Lancet* 1988;1:457–459.
62. Eichler M.: Psychological changes associated with induced hyperammonemia. *Science* 1964;144:886–888.
63. Editorial: Hepatic encephalopathy today. *Lancet*1984;1:489–491.
64. Jensen D. M.: Portal-systemic encephalopathy and hepatic coma. *Med. Clin. North Am.* 1986;70:1081–1091.
65. Misra P.: Hepatic encephalopathy. *Med. Clin. North Am.* 1981;65:209–226.
66. Teschan P. E., Arieff A. I.: Uremic and dialysis encephalopathies, in McCandless D. W. (ed): *Cerebral Energy Metabolism and Metabolic Encephalopathy.* New York, Plenum Press, 1985, pp 263–285.
67. Addison T.: *On the Disorders of the Brain Connected with Diseased Kidneys.* London, Sydenham Society, 1868.
68. Baker A. B., Knutson J.: Psychiatric aspects of uremia. *Am. J. Psychiatry* 1946;102:683–687.

69. Mahoney C. A., Arieff A. I.: Uremic encephalopathies: Clinical, biochemical, and experimental features. *Am. J. Kidney Dis.* 1982;2:324–336.
70. Marshall J. R.: Neuropsychiatric aspects of renal failure. *J. Clin. Psychiatry* 1979;40:81–85.
71. Stewart R. S., Stewart R. M.: Neuropsychiatric aspects of chronic renal disease. *Psychosomatics* 1979;20:524–531.
72. Stenback A., Haapanen E.: *Azotemia and Psychosis.* Copenhagen, Munksgaard, 1967.
73. Ginn H. E.: Neurobehavioral dysfunction in uremia. *Kidney Int.* 1975; (Suppl 2) 7:217–221.
74. McDaniel J. W.: Metabolic and CNS correlates of cognitive dysfunction with renal failure. *Psychophysiology* 1971;8:704–713.
75. Nissenson A. R., Levin M. L., Klawans H. L., et al: Neurological sequelae of end stage renal disease (ESRD). *J. Chronic Dis.*1977;30:705–733.
76. Osberg J. W., Meares G. J., McKee D. C., et al: Intellectual functioning in renal failure and chronic dialysis. *J. Chronic Dis.* 1982;35:445–457.
77. Ryan J. J., Souheaver G. T., De Wolfe A. S.: Intellectual deficit in chronic renal failure. *J. Nerv. Ment. Dis.* 1980;168:763–767.
78. Hughes R. J.: Correlations between EEG and chemical changes in uremia. *Electroencephalogr. Clin. Neurophysiol.* 1980;48:583–594.
79. Passouant P., Cadilhac J., Baldy-Moulinser M., et al: Etude du sommeil nocturne chez des uremiques chroniques soumis a une epuration extrarenale. *Electroencephalogr. Clin. Neurophysiol.* 1970;29:441–449.
80. Teschan P. E.: Electroencephalographic and other neurophysiological abnormalities in uremia. *Kidney Int.* (Suppl 2)1975;7:210–216.
81. Mahoney C. A., Sarnacki P., Arieff A. I.: Uremic encephalopathy: Role of brain energy metabolism. *Am. J. Physiol.* 1984;247:527–532.
82. Jeppson B., Freund H. R., Gimmon Z., et al: Blood-brain barrier derangement in uremic encephalopathy. *Surgery* 1982;92:30–35.
83. Alfrey A. C.: Dialysis encephalopathy syndrome. *Ann. Rev. Med.* 1978;29:93–98.
84. Jack R., Rabin P. L., McKinney T. D.: Dialysis encephalopathy: A review. *Int. J. Psychiatry Med.* 1983–84;13:309–326.
85. Taclob L., Needle M.: Drug-induced encephalopathy in patients on maintenance hemodialysis. *Lancet* 1976;2:704–705.
86. Glick I. D., Goldfield M. D., Kounat P. J.: Recognition and management of psychosis associated with hemodialysis. *Calif. Med.* 1973;119:56–59.
87. Merrill R. H., Collins J. L.: Acute psychosis in chronic renal failure: Case reports. *Milit. Med.* 1974;139:622–624.
88. Arieff A. I.: Aluminum and the pathogenesis of dialysis encephalopathy. *Am. J. Kidney Dis.* 1985;6:317–321.
89. Burks J. S., Alfrey A. C., Huddlestone J., et al: A fatal encephalopathy in chronic hemodialysis patients. *Lancet* 1976;1:764–768.
90. Chokroverty S., Buretman M. E., Berger V., et al: Progressive dialytic encephalopathy. *J. Neurol. Neurosurg. Psychiatry*1976;39:411–419.
91. Hughes J. R., Schreeder M. T.: EEG in dialysis encephalopathy. *Neurology* 1980;30:1148–1154.
92. Mahurkar S. D., Meyers L., Cohen J., et al: Electroencephalographic and radionuclide studies in dialysis dementia. *Kidney Int.* 1978;13:306–315.

93. Madison D. L., Baehr E. T., Bazell M., et al: Communicative and cognitive deterioration in dialysis dementia: Two case studies. *J. Speech Hear. Dis.* 1977;42:238–246.
94. Jackson M., Warrington E. K., Roe L. J., et al: Cognitive function in hemodialysis patients. *Clin. Nephrol.* 1987;27:26–30.
95. Van De Vyver F. L., Silva F. J. E., D'Haese P. C. D., et al: Aluminum toxicity in dialysis patients. *Contrib. Nephrol.* 1987;55:198–220.
96. Lai J. C. K., Blass J. P.: Inhibition of brain glycolysis by aluminum. *J. Neurochem.* 1984;42:438–446.
97. Rozas V. V., Port F. K., Rute W. M.: Progressive dialysis encephalopathy from dialysate aluminum. *Arch. Intern. Med.* 1978;138:1375–1377.
98. Trauner D. A., Clayman M.: Dialysis encephalopathy treated with clonazepam. *Ann. Neurol.* 1979;6:555–556.
99. Sullivan P. A., Murnaghan D. J., Callaghan N.: Dialysis dementia: Recovery after transplantation. *Br. Med. J.* 1977;2:740–741.
100. Ball J. H., Butkus D. E., Madison D. S.: Effect of subtotal parathyroidectomy on dialysis dementia. *Nephron* 1977;18:151–155.
101. Procci W. R.: Psychiatric aspects of renal transplantation, in Chattarjee S. N. (ed): *Renal Transplantation.* New York, Raven Press, 1980, pp 163–188.
102. Penn I., Bunch D., Olenik D., et al: Psychiatric experience with patients receiving renal and hepatic transplants, in Castelnuovo Tedesco P. (ed): *Psychiatric Aspects of Organ Transplantation.* New York, Grune & Stratton, 1971, pp 133–144.
103. Waniek W., Pach J., Hartmann H. G., et al: Hirnleistungsstörungen bei Patienten eines Dialyse-Transplantations-Programms. *Schweiz. Med. Wochenschr.* 1977:107–832–835.
104. Arieff A. J., Buckingham W. B.: Fluctuating "acute dementia" due to emphysema with pulmonary insufficiency. *Trans. Am. Neurol. Assoc.* 1970;95:203–205.
105. Austen F. K., Carmichael M. W., Adams R. D.: Neurologic manifestations of chronic pulmonary insufficiency. *N. Engl. J. Med.* 1957;257:579–590.
106. Chitkara R. K., Khan F. A.: Neurologic manifestations of lung disease. *Semin. Respir. Dis.* 1988;9:395–402.
107. Dulfano M. J., Ishikawa S.: Hypercapnia: Mental changes and extrapulmonary complications. *Ann. Intern. Med.* 1965;63:829–841.
108. Grant I., Heaton R. K., McSweeny A. J., et al: Neuropsychologic findings in hypoxemic chronic obstructive pulmonary disease. *Arch. Intern. Med.* 1982;142:1470–1476.
109. Miller A. L.: Carbon dioxide narcosis, in McCandless D. W. (ed): *Cerebral Energy Metabolism and Metabolic Encephalopathy.* New York, Plenum Press, 1985, pp 143–162.
110. Rogers R. M. (ed): *Respiratory Intensive Care.* Springfield, Ill, Charles C Thomas, 1977.
111. Fleetham J., West P., Mezon B., et al: Sleep, arousals, and oxygen desaturation in chronic obstructive pulmonary disease. *Am. Rev. Respir. Dis.* 1982;126:429–433.
112. Guilleminault C., Cummiskey J., Motta J.: Chronic obstructive airflow disease and sleep studies. *Am. Rev. Respir. Dis.* 1980;122:397–406.
113. Phillips B. A., Cooper K. R., Burke T. V.: The effect of sleep loss on breathing in chronic obstructive pulmonary disease. *Chest* 1987;91:29–32.

114. Anthonisen N. R.: Long-term oxygen therapy. *Ann. Intern. Med.* 1983;99:519–527.
115. Siesjö B. K.: *Brain Energy Metabolism.* New York, Wiley, 1978.
116. Benos J.: Encephalopathia pancreatica. *Munch. Med. Wochenschr.* 1973;115:1842–1844.
117. Benos J.: Funktionpsychosen und neurologische Ausfälle bei Pankreatitis. *Med. Clin.* 1974;69:1185–1192.
118. Benos J.: Zur Differentialdiagnose der deliranten Psychose bei akuter Pankreatitis vom Alkoholdelir. *A. Allgemeinmed.* 1973;49:1172–1173.
119. Estrada R. V., Moreno J., Martinez E., et al: Pancreatic encephalopathy. *Acta Neurol. Scand.* 1979;59:135–139.
120. Johnson D. A., Tong N. T.: Pancreatic encephalopathy. *South. Med. J.* 1977;70:165–167.
121. Schuster M. M., Iber F. L.: Psychosis with pancreatitis. *Arch. Intern. Med.* 1965;116:228–233.
122. Sharf B., Bental E.: Pancreatic encephalopathy. *J. Neurol. Neurosurg. Psychiatry* 1971;34:357–361.
123. Beaumont P. J. V.: Endocrines and psychiatry. *Br. J. Hosp. Med.* 1972;17:485–497.
124. Smith C. K., Barish J., Carrea J., et al: Psychiatric disturbances in endocrinologic disease. *Psychosom. Med.* 1972;34:69–86.
125. Wadsworth R. C., McKeon C.: Pathologic and mental alterations in a case of Simmond's disease. *Arch. Neurol. Psychiatry* 1941;46:272–296.
126. Sheehan H. L., Summers V. K.: The syndrome of hypopituitarism. *Q. J. Med.* 1949;18:319–362.
127. Court J., Diaz F.: Disturbances of consciousness in Sheehan's Syndrome. *Rev. Med. Chile* 1973;101:780–783.
128. Khanna S., Ammini A., Saxena S., et al: Hypopituitarism presenting as delirium. *Int. J. Psychiatry Med.* 1988;18:89–92.
129. Parker R. R., Isaacs A. D., McKerron C. G.: Recoverable organic psychosis after hypopituitary coma. *Br. Med. J.* 1976;1:132–133.
130. Leiberman D. M.: Pituitary deficiency and paranoid psychosis. *Psychiatr. J. Univ. Ottawa* 1980;5:113–117.
131. Browning T. B., Atkins R. W., Weiner H.: Cerebral metabolic disturbances in hypothyroidism. *Arch. Intern. Med.* 1954;93:938–950.
132. Berrios G. E., Leysen A., Samuel C., et al: Psychiatric morbidity following total and partial thyroidectomy. *Acta Psychiatr. Scand.* 1985;72:369–373.
133. Josepheon A. M., MacKenzie T. B.: Thyroid-induced mania in hypothyroid patients. *Br. J. Psychiatry* 1980;137:222–228.
134. Schofield A., Bracken P.: Thyroid-induced psychosis in myxoedema. *Irish Med. J.* 1983;76:495–496.
135. Easson W. M.: Myxedema with psychosis. Arch. Gen. Psychiatry 1966;14:277–283.
136. Royce P. C.: Severely impaired consciosness in myxedema—a review. *Am. J. Med. Sci.* 1971;261:46–50.
137. Asher R.: Myxoedematous madness. *Br. Med. J.* 1949;2:255–262.
138. Hall R. C. W., Stickney S., Beresford T. P.: Endocrine disease and behavior. *Integr. Psychiatry* 1986;4:122–135.

139. Olivarius B. D., Roder E.: Reversible psychosis and dementia in myxedema. *Acta Psychiatr. Scand.* 1970;46:1–13.
140. Hooshmand H., Sarhaddi S.: Hypothyroidism in adults and children. EEG findings. *Clin. Electroencephalogr.* 1975;6:61–67.
141. Orr W. C., Males J. L., Imes N. K.: Myxedema and obstructive sleep apnea. *Am. J. Med.* 1981;7:1061–1066.
142. White A. J., Barraclough B.: Thyroid disease and mental illness: A study of thyroid disease in psychiatric admissions. *J. Psychosom. Res.* 1988;32:99–106.
143. Burch E. A., Messervy T. W.: Psychiatric symptoms in medical illness: Hyperthyroidism revisited. *Psychosomatics* 1978;19:34–40.
144. Jamieson G. R., Wall J. H.: Psychoses associated with hyperthyroidism. *Psychiatr. Q.* 1936;10:464–480.
145. Gambert S. R., Escher J. E.: Atypical presentation of endocrine disorders in the elderly. *Geriatrics* 1988;43:69–78.
146. Griffin M. A., Solomon D. H.: Hyperthyroidism in the elderly. *J. Am. Geriatr. Soc.* 1986;34:887–892.
147. Trzepacz P. T., McCue M., Klein I., et al: A psychiatric and neuropsychological study of patients with untreated Graves' disease. *Gen. Hosp. Psychiatry* 1988;10:49–55.
148. Hall R. C. W., Popkin M. K., De Vaul R., et al: Psychiatric manifestations of Hashimoto's thyroiditis. *Psychosomatics* 1982;23:337–342.
149. Thrush D. C., Boddie H. G.: Episodic encephalopathy associated with thyroid disorders. *J. Neurol. Neurosurg. Psychiatry* 1974;37:696–700.
150. Greene J. A., Swanson L. W.: Psychosis in hypoparathyroidism. *Ann. Intern. Med.* 1941;14:1233–1236.
151. Sugar O.: Central neurological complications of hypoparathyroidism. *Arch. Neurol. Psychiatry* 1953;70:86–107.
152. Shu-lian Y., Chang-Lua W, Ying-kun F: Neurologic and psychiatric manifestations in hypoparathyroidism. *Chinese Med. J.* 1984;97:267–272.
153. Mateo D., Gimenez-Roldan S.: Dementia in idiopathic hypoparathyroidism. *Arch. Neurol.* 1982;39:424–425.
154. Mikkelsen E. J., Reider A. A.: Post-parathyroidectomy psychosis: Clinical and research implications. *J. Clin. Psychiatry* 1979;40:352–358.
155. Alarcon R. D., Franceschini J. A.: Hyperparathyroidism and paranoid psychosis. Case report and review of the literature. *Br. J. Psychiatry* 1984;145:477–486.
156. Borer M. S., Bhanot V. K.: Hyperparathyroidism: Neuropsychiatric manifestations. *Psychosomatics* 1985;26:597–601.
157. Joborn C., Hetta J., Frisk P., et al: Primary hyperparathyroidism in patients with organic brain syndrome. *Acta Med. Scand.* 1986;219:91–98.
158. Kleinfeld M., Peter S., Gilbert G. M.: Delirium as the predominant manifestation of hyperparathyroidism: Reversal after parathyroidectomy. *J. Am. Geriatr. Soc.* 1984;32:689–690.
159. Lafferty F. W.: Primary hyperparathyroidism. *Arch. Intern. Med.* 1981;141:1761–1766.
160. Petersen P.: Psychiatric disorders in primary hyperparathyroidism. *J. Clin. Endocrinol. Metab.* 1968;28:1491–1495.
161. Sier H. C., Hartnell J., Morley J. E., et al: Primary hyperparathyroidism and delirium in the elderly. *J. Am. Geriatr. Soc.* 1988;36:157–170.

162. Wang C. A., Guyton S. W.: Hyperparathyroid crisis. *Ann. Surg.* 1979;190:782–790.

163. Stoll W. A.: *Die Psychiatrie des Morbus Addison.* Stuttgart, Thieme, 1953.

164. Moss C. N., England M. L., Kowal J.: Adrenal insufficiency (Addison's disease) in the elderly. *J. Am. Geriatr. Soc.* 1985;33:63–68.

165. Haskett R. F.: Diagnostic categorization of psychiatric disturbance in Cushing's syndrome. *Am. J. Psychiatry* 1985;142:911–916.

166. Starkman M. N., Schteingart D. E.: Neuropsychiatric manifestations of patients with Cushing's syndrome. *Arch. Intern. Med.* 1981;141:215–219.

167. Cohen S. I.: Cushing's syndrome: A psychiatric study of 29 patients. *Br. J. Psychiatry* 1980;136:120–124.

168. Starkman M. N., Schteingart D. E., Schork M. A.: Correlation of bedside cognitive and neuropsychological tests in patients with Cushing's syndrome. *Psychosomatics* 1986;27:508–511.

169. Gerson S. N., Miclat R.: Cushing disease presenting as atypical psychosis followed by sudden death. *Can. J. Psychiatry* 1985;30:223–224.

170. Kramlinger K. G., Peterson G. C., Watson P. K., et al: Metyrapone for depression and delirium secondary to Cushing's syndrome. *Psychosomatics* 1985;26:67–71.

171. Regestein Q. R., Rose L. I., Williams G. H.: Psychopathology in Cushing's syndrome. *Arch. Intern. Med.* 1971;130:114–117.

172. Saad M. F., Adams F., Mackay B., et al: Occult Cushing's disease presenting with acute psychosis. *Am. J. Med.* 1984;76:759–766.

173. Tucker R. P., Weinstein H. E., Schteingart D. E., et al: EEG changes and serum cortisol levels in Cushing's syndrome. *Clin. Electroencephalogr.* 1978;9:32–37.

174. Rubinow D. R., Post R. M., Savard R., et al: Cortisol hypersecretion and cognitive impairment in depression. *Arch. Gen. Psychiatry* 1984;41:279–283.

175. Born J., Brauninger W., Fehm-Wolfsdorf G., et al: Dose-dependent influences on electrophysiological signs of attention in humans after neuropeptide ACTH 4–10. *Exp. Brain Res.* 1987;67:85–92.

176. Freedman D. K., Troll L., Mills A. B., et al: *Acute Organic Disorder Accompanied by Mental Symptoms.* Sacramento, California Department of Mental Hygiene, 1965.

177. Lipson L. G. (ed): Diabetes mellitus in the elderly. *Am. J. Med.* 1986;80 (Suppl 5A): 1–56.

178. Alberti K. G. M. M., Nattrass M.: Severe diabetic ketoacidosis. *Med. Clin. North Am.* 1978;62:799–814.

179. Duckrow R. B., Beard D. C., Brennan R. W.: Regional cerebral blood flow decreases during chronic and acute hyperglycemia. *Stroke* 1987;18:52–58.

180. Arieff A. I., Carroll H. J.: Cerebral edema and depression of sensorium in nonketotic hyperosmolar coma. *Diabetes* 1974;23:525–531.

181. Braaten J. T.: Hyperosmolar nonketotic diabetic coma: Diagnosis and management. *Geriatrics* 1987;42:83–92.

182. Khardori R., Soler N. G.: Hyperosmolar hyperglycemic nonketotic syndrome. *Am. J. Med.* 1984;77:899–904.

183. Maccario M.: Neurological dysfunction associated with nonketotic hyperglycemia. *Arch. Neurol.* 1968;19:525–534.

184. Fleishman S., Lesko L.: Delirium and dementia, in Holland J. C., Rowland J. H. (eds): *Psycho-oncology: The Psychological Care of the Patient with Cancer.* New York, Oxford University Press, in press.
185. Massie M. J., Holland J. C.: Psychiatry and oncology, in Grinspoon L. (ed): *Psychiatric Update,* Vol 111. Washington, DC, American Psychiatric Press, 1984, pp 239–256.
186. Bruera E., Chadwick S., Weinlick A., et al: Delirium and severe sedation in patients with terminal cancer. *Cancer Treat. Rep.* 1987;71:787–788.
187. Massie M. J., Holland J., Glass E.: Delirium in terminally ill cancer patients. *Am. J. Psychiatry* 1983;140:1048–1050.
188. Levine P. M., Silberfarb P. M., Lipowski Z. J.: Mental disorders in cancer patients. A study of 100 psychiatric referrals. *Cancer* 1978;42:1385–1391.
189. Davis B. D., Fernandez F., Adams F., et al: Diagnosis of dementia in cancer patients. *Psychosomatics* 1987;28:175–179.
190. Derogatis L. R., Morrow G. R., Fetting J., et al: The prevalence of psychiatric disorders among cancer patients. *J.A.M.A.* 1983;249:751–757.
191. Posner J. B.: Neurological complications of cancer. *Med. Clin. North Am.* 1979;63:783–800.
192. Shapiro W. R.: Remote effects on the central nervous system: encephalopathy. *Adv. Neurol.* 1976;15:101–117.
193. Schmid-Wermser I., Nagel G. A., Schmid A. H.: Zur klinischen Diagnose von Hirnmetastasen beim Bronchuskarzinom. *Schweiz. Med. Wochenschr.* 1974;104:464–468.
194. Hughes G. S., Turner R. C.: Hypernephroma presenting as acute delirium. *J. Urol.* 1983;130:539–540.
195. Alkan M. L., Mayersdorf A., Dvilansky A.: Electroencephalographic and encephalopathic findings in multiple myeloma: Hyperviscosity versus hypercalcemia. *Clin. Electroencephalogr.* 1975;6:16–22.
196. Reagan T. J., Okazaki H.: The thrombotic syndrome associated with carcinoma. *Arch. Neurol.* 1974;31:390–395.
197. Cornelius J. R., Soloff P. H., Miewald B. K.: Behavioral manifestations of paraneoplastic encephalopathy. *Biol. Psychiatry* 1986;21:686–690.
198. Brain (Lord), Norris F. H.: *The Remote Effects of Cancer on the Nervous System.* New York, Grune & Stratton, 1965.
199. Henson R. A., Urich H.: *Cancer and the Nervous System. The Neurological Manifestations of Systemic Malignant Disease.* Oxford, Blackwell, 1982.
200. Kaplan A. M., Itabashi H. H.: Encephalitis associated with carcinoma. *J. Neurol. Neurosurg. Psychiatry* 1974;37:116–117.
201. Canning B., Kobayashi R. M., Kaplan C. G., et al: Progressive multifocal leukoencephalopathy. *West. J. Med.* 1976;125:364–369.
202. Adams F., Anderson B. S., Fernandez F.: Emergency pharmacotherapy of delirium in the critically ill cancer patient. *Psychosomatics* 1986;27:33–37.
203. Peterson L. G., Leipman M., Bongar B.: Psychotropic medications in patients with cancer. *Gen. Hosp. Psychiatry* 1987;9:313–323.
204. Major L. F., Brown L., Wilson W. P.: Carcinoid and psychiatric symptoms. *South. Med. J.* 1973;66:787–790.
205. Patchell R. A., Posner J. B.: Neurologic complications of carcinoid. *Neurology* 1986;36:745–749.

206. Lehmann J.: Mental disturbances followed by stupor in a patient with carcinoidosis. *Acta Psychiatr. Scand.* 1966;42:153–161.
207. Southren A. L., Warner R. R. P., Christoff N. I., et al: An unusual neurologic syndrome associated with hyperserotonemia. *N. Engl. J. Med.* 1959;260:1265–1268.
208. Engelman K., Lovenberg W., Sjoerdsma A.: Inhibition of serotonin synthesis by para-chlorophylalanine in patients with carcinoid syndrome. *N. Eng. J. Med.* 1967;277:1103–1108.
209. Lehmann J.: Tryptophan deficiency stupor: A new psychiatric syndrome. *Acta Psychiatr. Scand.* 1982;300 (Suppl) 1–57.
210. Roth N.: The psychiatric syndromes of porphyria. *J. Neuropsychiatry* 1968;4:32–44.
211. Rowland L. P.: Acute intermittent porphyria: Search for an enzymatic defect with implications for neurology and psychiatry. *Dis. Nerv. Syst.* 1961;22:1–12.
212. Magnus I. A.: Drugs and porphyria. *Br. Med. J.* 1984;288:1474–1475.
213. Becker D. M., Kramer S.: The neurological manifestations of porphyria: A review. *Medicine* 1977;56:411–423.
214. Stein J. A., Tschudy D. P.: Acute intermittent porphyria. *Medicine* 1970;49:1–16.
215. Dening T. R.: Psychiatric aspects of Wilson's disease. *Br. J. Psychiatry* 1985;147:677–682.
216. Starosta-Rubinstein S., Young A. B., Kluin K., et al: Clinical assessment of 31 patients with Wilson's disease. *Arch. Neurol.* 1987;44:365–370.
217. Cartwright G. E.: Diagnosis of treatable Wilson's disease. *N. Engl. J. Med.* 1978;298:1347–1350.
218. Medalia A., Isaacs-Glaberman K., Scheinberg I. H.: Neuropsychological impairment in Wilson's disease. *Arch. Neurol.* 1988;45:502–504.
219. Maxwell M. H., Kleeman C. R. (eds): *Clinical Disorders of Fluid and Electrolyte Metabolism.* New York, McGraw-Hill, 1972.
220. Koizumi J., Shiraishi H., Ofuku K., et al: Duration of delirium shortened by the correction of electrolyte imbalance. *Jpn. J. Psychiatr. Neurol.* 1988;42:81–88.
221. Nanji A. A.: Drug-induced electrolyte disorders. *Drug Intell. Clin. Pharm.* 1983; 17:175–185.
222. Arieff A. I., Guisado R.: Effects on the central nervous system of hypernatremic and hyponatremic states. *Kidney Int.* 1976;10:104–116.
223. Parker W. A.: Imipramine-induced syndrome of inappropriate antidiuretic hormone secretion. *Drug Intell. Clin. Pharm.* 1984;18:890–894.
224. Sandifer M. G.: Hyponatremia due to psychotropic drugs. *J. Clin. Psychiatry* 1983;44:301–303.
225. Arieff A. I.: Hyponatremia, convulsions, respiratory arrest, and permanent brain damage after elective surgery in healthy women. *N. Engl. J. Med.* 1986;314:1529–1535.
226. Illowsky B. P., Kirch D. G.: Polydipsia and hyponatremia in psychiatric patients. *Am. J. Psychiatry* 1988;145:675–683.
227. Cronin R. E.: Psychogenic polydipsia with hyponatremia: Report of eleven cases. *Am. J. Kidney Dis.* 1987;9:410–416.
228. Delva N. J., Crammer J. L.: Polydipsia in chronic psychiatric patients. *Br. J. Psychiatry* 1988;152:242–245.

229. Ferrier I. N.: Water intoxication in patients with psychiatric illness. *Br. Med. J.* 1985;291:1594–1596.
230. Jos C. J., Evenson R. C., Mallya A. R.: Self-induced water intoxication. A comparison of 34 cases with matched controls. *J. Clin. Psychiatry* 1986;47:368–370.
231. Hariprasad M. K., Eisinger R. P., Nadler I. M., et al: Hyponatremia in psychogenic polydipsia. *Arch. Intern. Med.* 1980;140:1639–1642.
232. Singh S., Padi M. H., Bullard H., et al: Water intoxication in psychiatric patients. *Br. J. Psychiatry* 1985;146:127–131.
233. Sterns R. H.: Severe symptomatic hyponatremia: Treatment and outcome. *Ann. Intern. Med.* 1987;107:656–664.
234. Ayus J. C., Krothapalli R. K., Arieff A. I.: Treatment of symptomatic hyponatremia and its relation to brain damage. *N. Engl. J. Med.* 1987;317:1190–1195.
235. Snyder N. A., Feigal D. W., Arieff A. I.: Hypernatremia in elderly patients. *Ann. Intern. Med.* 1987;107:309–319.
236. Mitchell W., Feldman F.: Neuropsychiatric aspects of hypokalemia. *Can. Med. Assoc. J.* 1968;92:49–51.
237. Bayer A. J., Farag R., Browne S., et al: Plasma electrolytes in elderly patients taking fixed combination diuretics. *Postgrad. Med. J.* 1986;62:159–162.
238. Webb W. L., Gehi M.: Electrolyte and fluid imbalance: Neuropsychiatric manifestations. *Psychosomatics* 1981;22:199–203.
239. Zaloga G. P., Chernow B.: Hypocalcemia in critical illness. *J.A.M.A.* 1986;256:1924–1929.
240. Swash M., Rowan A. J.: Electroencephalographic criteria of hypocalcemia and hypercalcemia. *Arch. Neurol.* 1972;26:218–228.
241. Lee D. B. N., Zawada E. T., Kleeman C. R.: The pathophysiology and clinical aspects of hypercalcemic disorders. *West J. Med.* 1978;129:278–320.
242. Mundy G. R., Ibbotson K. J., D'Souza S. M., et al: The hypercalcemia of cancer. *N. Engl. J. Med.* 1984;310:1718–1727.
243. Lehrer G. M.: Neuropsychiatric presentation of hypercalcemia. *Mt. Sinai J. Med. N.Y.* 1960;27:10–18.
244. Byrne E. J., Hosking D. J., Jameson C.: Serial assessment of serum calcium correlates with mental state. *Int. J. Geriatr. Psychiatry* 1987;2:163–168.
245. Cornette M., Grisar T.: A study of clinical signs and EEG profiles in hypercalcemic encephalopathy. *Acta Neurol. Belg.* 1977;77:129–143.
246. Etheridge J. E., Grabow J. D.: Hypercalcemia without EEG abnormalities. *Dis. Nerv. Syst.* 1971;32:479–482.
247. Berkelhammer C., Bear R. A.: A clinical approach to common electrolyte problems: Hypomagnesemia. *Can. Med. Assoc. J.* 1985;132:360–368.
248. Ratzan R. M., Chapron D. J., Mumford D., et al: Uncovering magnesium toxicity. *Geriatrics* 1980;35:75–86.
249. Silvis S. E., DiBartolomeo A. G., Aaker H. M.: Hypophosphatemia and neurological changes secondary to oral caloric intake. *Am. J. Gastroenterol.* 1980;73:215–222.
250. Stoff J. S.: Phosphate homeostasis and hypophosphatemia. *Am. J. Med.* 1982;72:489–495.
251. Riley L. J., Ilson B. E., Narins R. G.: Acute metabolic acid-base disorders. *Crit. Care Clin.* 1987;5:699–724.
252. Thurn J. R., Pierpont G. L., Ludvigsen C. W., et al: D-Lactate encephalopathy. *Am. J. Med.* 1985;79:717–721.

253. Engel G. L., Ferris E. B., Logan M.: Hyperventilation: Analysis of clinical symptomatology. *Ann. Intern. Med.* 1947;27:683–704.
254. Allen T. E., Angus B.: Hyperventilation leading to hallucinations. *Am. J. Psychiatry* 1968;125:632–637.
255. Keskimaki I., Sainio K., Sovijarvi A. R. A., et al: EEG and end-tidal carbon dioxide concentration in the hyperventilation syndrome. *Electroencephalogr. Clin. Neurophysiol.* 1980;50:496–501.
256. Magarian G. J., Olney R. K.: Absence spells. Hyperventilation as a previously unrecognized cause. *Am. J. Med.* 1984;76:905–909.
257. Mitra M. L.: Confusional states in relation to vitamin deficiencies in the elderly. *J. Am. Geriatr. Soc.* 1971;19:536–545.
258. Weinsier R. L., Hunker E. M., Krumdieck C. L., et al: Hospital malnutrition. A prospective evaluation of general medical patients during the course of hospitalization. *Am. J. Clin. Nutr.* 1979;32:418–426.
259. Young R. C., Blass J. P.: Iatrogenic nutritional deficiences. *Ann. Rev. Nutr.* 1982;2:201–207.
260. Evans D. L., Edelsohn G. A., Golden R. N.: Organic psychosis without anemia or spinal cord symptoms in patients with vitamin B_{12} deficiency. *Am. J. Psychiatry* 1983;140:218–221.
261. MacDonald Holmes J.: Cerebral manifestations of vitamin B_{12} deficiency. *Br. Med. J.* 1956;2:1394–1398.
262. Reynolds E. H.: Neurological aspects of folate and vitamin B_{12} metabolism. *Clin. Haematol.* 1976;5:661–696.
263. Samson D. C., Swisher S. N., Christian R. M., et al: Cerebral metabolic disturbance and delirium in pernicious anemia. *Arch. Int. Med.* 1952;90:4–14.
264. Shorvon S. D., Carney M. W. P., Chanarin I., et al: The neuropsychiatry of megaloblastic anaemia. *Br. Med. J.* 1980;281:1036–1043.
265. Shulman R.: The present status of vitamin B_{12} and folic acid deficiency in psychiatric illness. *Can. Psychiatr. Assoc. J.* 1972;17:205–216.
266. Webb M. G. T., Weir D. G., Moore J. N. P.: Diagnosis of vitamin B_{12} deficiency in psychiatric patients. *J. Irish Med. Assoc.* 1971;64:403–408.
267. Zucker D. K., Livingston R. L., Nakra R., et al: B_{12} deficiency and psychiatric disorders: Case report and literature review. *Biol. Psychiatry* 1981;16:197–205.
268. Lindenbaum J., Healton E. B., Savage D. G., et al: Neuropsychiatric disorders caused by cobalamin deficiency in the absence of anemia or macrocytosis. *N. Eng. J. Med.* 1988;318:1720–1728.
269. Sapira J. D., Tullis S., Mullaly R.: Reversible dementia due to folate deficiency. *South. Med. J.* 1975;68:776–778.
270. Shulman R.: An overview of folic acid deficiency and psychiatric illness, in Botez M. I., Reynolds E. H. (eds): *Folic Acid in Neurology, Psychiatry, and Internal Medicine.* New York, Raven Press, 1979, pp 463–474.
271. Strachan R. W., Henderson J. G.: Dementia and folate deficiency. *Q. J. Med.* 1967;36:189–204.
272. Ishii N., Nishihara Y.: Pellagra among chronic alcoholics: Clinical and pathological study of 20 necropsy cases. *J. Neurol. Neurosurg. Psychiatry* 1981;44:209–215.
273. Gregory I.: The role of nicotinic acid (niacin) in mental health and disease. *J. Ment. Sci.* 1955;101:85–109.

274. Spies T. D., Aring C. D., Gelperin J., et al: The mental symptoms of pellagra. *Am. J. Med. Sci.* 1938;196:461–475.
275. Jolliffe N., Bowman K. M., Rosenblum L. A., et al: Nicotinic acid deficiency encephalopathy. *J.A.M.A.* 1941;114:307–312.
276. Spivak J. L., Jackson D. L.: Pellagra: An analysis of 18 patients and a review of the literature. *Johns Hopkins Med. J.* 1977; 140:295–309.
277. Gibson G., Barclay L., Blass J.: The role of the cholinergic system in thiamin deficiency. *Ann. N.Y. Acad. Sci.* 1982;378:382–403.
278. Anderson S. H., Charles T. J., Nicol A. D.: Thiamine deficiency at a district general hospital: Report of five cases. *Q. J. Med.* 1985;55:15–32.
279. Hartman E. E., Sweet J. J., Elvart A. C.: Neuropsychological effects of Wernicke's encephalopathy as a consequence of hyperemesis gravidarum. *Int. J. Clin. Neuropsychol.* 1985;7:204–207.
280. Harper C. G.: Wernicke's encephalopathy: A more common disease than realized. *J. Neurol. Neurosurg. Psychiatry* 1979;42:226–231.
281. Jagadha V., Deck J. H. N., Halliday W. C., et al: Wernicke's encephalopathy in patients on peritoneal dialysis or hemodialysis. *Ann. Neurol.* 1987;21:78–84.
282. Velez R. J., Myers B., Guber M. S.: Severe acute metabolic acidosis (acute beriberi): An avoidable complication of total parenteral nutrition. *J. Parenter. Enter. Nutr.* 1985;9:216–219.
283. Wernicke C.: *Lehrbuch der Gehirnkrankheiten fur Ärzte und Studierende.* Vol 2. Kassel, Fischer, 1881.
284. Victor M., Adams R. D., Collins G. H.: *The Wernicke-Korsakoff Syndrome.* Philadelphia, FA Davis, 1971.
285. Editorial: Wernicke's encephalopathy. *Br. Med. J.* 1979;2:291–292.
286. Editorial: Wernicke's preventable encephalopathy.*Lancet* 1979;1:1122–1123.
287. Lippe B., Hensen L., Mendoza G., et al: Chronic vitamin A intoxication. *Am. J. Dis. Child.* 1981;135:634–636.
288. Ragavan V. V., Smith J. E., Bilezikian J. P.: Case report: Vitamin A toxicity and hypercalcemia. *Am. J. Med. Sci.* 1982;283:161–164.
289. Restak R. M.: Pseudotumor cerebri, psychosis, and hypervitaminosis. *Am. J. Nerv. Ment. Dis.* 1972;155:72–75.
290. Paterson C. R.: Vitamin-D poisoning: Survey of causes in 21 patients with hypercalcemia. *Lancet* 1980;1:1164–1165.
291. Schwartzman M. S., Franck W. A.: Vitamin D toxicity complicating the treatment of senile, postmenopausal, and glucocorticoid-induced osteoporosis. *Am. J. Med.* 1987;82:224–230.
292. Celestino F. S., Van Noord G. R., Miraglia C. P.: Accidental hypothermia in the elderly. *J. Fam. Pract.* 1988;26:259–267.
293. Danzl D. F., Pozos R. S.: Multicenter hypothermia survey. *Ann. Emerg. Med.* 1987;16:1042–1055.
294. Lonning P. E., Skulberg A., Abyholm F.: Accidental hypothermia. *Acta Anaesthesiol. Scand.* 1986;30:601–613.
295. Martyn J. W.: Diagnosing and treating hypothermia. *Can. Med. Assoc. J.* 1981;125:1089–1097.
296. Lewin S., Brettman L. R., Holzman R. S.: Infections in hypothermic patients. *Arch. Intern. Med.* 1981;141:920–925.

297. Fitzgibbon T., Hayward J. S., Walker D.: EEG and visual evoked potentials of conscious man during moderate hypothermia. *Electroencephalogr. Clin. Neurophysiol.* 1984;58:48–54.
298. Markand O. N., Lee B. I., Warren C., et al: Effects of hypothermia on brainstem auditory evoked potentials in humans. *Ann. Neurol.* 1987;22:507–513.
299. Carter B. J., Cammermeyer M.: A phenomenology of heat injury: The predominance of confusion. *Milit. Med.* 1988;153:118–126.
300. Graham B. S., Lichtenstein M. J., Hinson J. M., et al: Nonexertional heatstroke. *Arch. Intern. Med.* 1986;146:87–90.
301. Shibolet S., Lancaster M. C., Danon Y.: Heat stroke: A review. *Aviat. Space Environ. Med.* 1976;47:280–301.
302. Tucker L. E., Stanford J., Graves B., et al: Clinical heatstroke: Clinical and laboratory assessment. *South. Med. J.* 1985;78:20–25.
303. Rosenberg H.: Clinical presentation of malignant hyperthermia. *Br. J. Anaesth.* 1988;60:268–273.
304. Bark N. M.: Heatstroke in psychiatric patients: Two cases and a review. *J. Clin. Psychiatry* 1982;43:377–380.
305. Hart L. E., Egier B. P., Shimizu A. G., et al: Exertional heat stroke: The runner's nemesis. *Can. Med. Assoc. J.* 1980;122:1144–1150.
306. Young M., Sciurba F., Rinaldo J.: Delirium and pulmonary edema after completing a marathon. *Am. Rev. Respir. Dis.* 1987;136:737–739.
307. Campbell M. B.: Neurological allergy. *Rev. Allergy* 1968;22:80–89.
308. Sunder T. R., Balsam M. J., Vengrow M. I.: Neurological manifestations of angioedema. *J.A.M.A.* 1982;247:2005–2007.
309. Rogers M. P., Bloomingdale K., Murawski B. J., et al: Mixed organic brain syndrome as a manifestation of systemic mastocytosis. *Psychosom. Med.* 1986;48:437–447.
310. Kobernick M.: Electrical injuries: Pathophysiology and emergency management. *Ann. Emerg. Med.* 1982;11:633–638.
311. Silversides J.: The neurological sequelae of electrical injury. *Can. Med. Assoc. J.* 1964;91:195–204.
312. Peters W. J.: Lightning injury. *Can. Med. Assoc. J.* 1983;128:148–150.
313. Daniel W. F., Weiner R. D., Grovitz H. F., et al: ECT-induced delirium and further ECT: A case report. *Am. J. Psychiatry* 1983;140:922–924.
314. Leechuy I., Abrams R., Kohlhaas J.: ECT-induced postictal delirium and electrode placement. *Am. J. Psychiatry* 1988;145:880–881.
315. Summers W. K., Robins E., Reich T.: The natural history of acute organic mental syndrome after bilateral electroconvulsive therapy. *Biol. Psychiatry* 1979;14:905–912.
316. McMahon T., Vahora S.: Radiation damage to the brain: Neuropsychiatric aspects. *Gen. Hosp. Psychiatry* 1986;8:437–441.

15

Infections

For centuries, delirium was inextricably linked with fever by medical writers (see Chapter 1). In his influential book *Five Dissertations on Fever,* published at the turn of the nineteenth century, Fordyce (1) devoted a good deal of attention to this link. He observed that delirium arises frequently in the course of a febrile illness and results from loss of sleep. This hypothesis prevailed for about three centuries and continues to challenge researchers. Fordyce maintained that two types of delirium occur in fever: one without any "material affection" of the brain and the other with "fullness of the vessels of the brain."

"Fever delirium" was formerly regarded as a prototype of delirium generally, and acute infectious diseases were believed to be its most common causes (2). Typhoid fever, pneumonia, and septicemia were the infections most often implicated. Delirium due to infection was thought to result from a combination of pathogenetic factors such as anemia or hyperemia of the brain, toxemia, and high fever (3). It was classified according to the timing of its onset in relation to fever: it could precede the latter, occur at its height, come on at the stage of effervescence, or arise during convalescence ("delirium of collapse"). Delirium at the height of fever was regarded as the most common form (4,5). Delirium of collapse was believed to be due to anemia of the brain, impaired nutrition and sleep deprivation (4).

In recent years, less attention has been paid to infectious diseases as a cause of delirium. As a journal editorial puts it, "The current preoccupation with non-infective causes of organic psychosis and the successful control of infection have diverted attention away from infective causes, yet these are relatively common causes in Britain and very common in other parts of the world" (6, p 214). A book on fever (7) emphasizes that delirium is one of the most frequently encountered complications of infectious diseases, especially of meningitis, encephalitis, typhoid fever, typhus, pneumonia, malaria, influenza, rheumatic fever, and puerperal fever. Moreover, a growing clinical and public health problem is presented by the infections in the *elderly,* in whom any infectious disease may feature delirium and present in an atypical fashion (8–11). Fever, for example, may be absent, yet delirium be present. It is generally recognized that the syndrome often arises in the course of an infection in a *child,* but the literature on this topic is scarce and epidemiological studies are lacking (12,13). Delirium can complicate any infection in childhood and is claimed to occur in children as young as 16 months (13). Infectious diseases are highly prevalent in the *tropical countries.* Meningitis, encephalitis, typhoid fever, brucellosis, malaria, pneumonia, and trypanosomiasis are all common in the tropics and often feature delirium (14–16).

One may conclude that, despite medical advances, infectious diseases remain common and constitute an important class of organic causes of delirium among the elderly, children, the poor, and the inhabitants of tropical and developing countries.

Pathogenesis of infectious delirium

Little is known about this subject, and the old hypotheses referred to earlier still stand. Pyrexia and toxemia still need to be considered as possible factors. One author (17) has proposed that the putative pathogenetic factors in infectious delirium fall into three groups: 1. infections within the CNS giving rise to direct toxic effects, such as necrosis, inflammation and edema of the brain, and inhibition of cerebral enzyme systems; 2. systemic infections causing cerebral ischemia-hypoxia, an abnormal ionic and acid-base environment in the brain, or both; and 3. reactions to drugs used to treat the infection.

More recently, attention has been directed to CNS *neurotransmitters* (18–20). Several authors have proposed that encephalopathy associated with sepsis, for example, could involve disturbances in cerebral synaptic transmission and energy production due to a toxic mechanism (18–20). False neurotransmitters, increased brain concentrations of serotonergic and reduced levels of catecholaminergic neurotransmitters, and formation of disseminated microabscesses in the brain may all be involved in the pathogenesis of septic encephalopathy (18–20).

Other investigators have focused on the pathogenesis of *fever,* whose role in precipitating delirium in the course of an infectious disease has been postulated for centuries. Fever is a conspicuous sign of the acute-phase response to a microbial invasion and is considered to be an effect of a polypeptide, interleukin-1, which appears to be identical with the endogenous pyrogen, the mediator of fever (21,22). Interleukin-1 has also been found to induce slow-wave sleep and may be responsible for the increased sleeping that accompanies many infectious diseases (21). How this finding can be reconciled with the old notion that sleep loss may account, at least in part, for delirium in a febrile illness is by no means clear. In the elderly, the febrile response may be impaired or absent in the course of an infection, and delirium is very common (22,23).

Certain effects of fever appear to be relevant to delirium (7). Hyperthermia induced in animals has been shown to result in an increase in CMR for oxygen by about 5% per 1°C increase in body temperature (24). At constant $PaCO_2$, there is a corresponding increase in CBF. It appears that 42°C is a critical temperature, one above which enzyme inactivation occurs (24). Fever, by increasing brain energy demansds, may be potentially harmful in the presence of cerebral ischemia-hypoxia, hypoglycemia, or both. Blood pyruvate and lactate levels are abnormally elevated in human febrile infections (25). This finding has been tentatively explained as being secondary to increased breakdown of glucose and glycogen. Various factors have been suggested to account for these metabolic changes. Increased turnover of cellular constitutents, enhanced ionic permeability of excitable membranes, thiamine deficiency, release of adrenaline, and alkalosis have all been implicated (24,25).

Fever has been shown to affect sleep and dreams, as well as the EEG (26–29). Artificially induced fever was accompanied by sleep changes; there were more awakenings, as well as a reduction of stage 4 sleep and stage 1-REM (28). These findings differ from those of the action of interleukin-1 (21). The investigators speculated that the observed changes reflected the effect of fever on the arousal mechanism in the brain. This hypothesis was subsequently challenged by other researchers, who concluded, on the basis of animal experiments, that no direct relationship could be found between fever and sleep disturbance; the latter was most likely due to an action of bacterial products, such as a mucopeptide, independent of fever (27). Thus, it appears that either fever alone, or bacterial toxins, or both can produce abnormalities in the sleep cycle. Patients with fever may experience nightmares and either insomnia or daytime sleepiness (29). EEGs recorded in adult patients during fever secondary to focal, extracranial infection showed a high frequency of abnormal tracings (29). The abnormalities consisted mostly of paroxysmal slow waves (29). This study, however, involved only a small number of patients and must be replicated before any conclusions can be drawn about the effects of fever on the EEG.

Some investigators have focused on the effects on performance of *experimentally induced infections* (30,31). In one study, tularemia and sandfly fever were induced in volunteers (30). The subjects displayed decrements in performance that were greatest, but did not correlate, with fever and showed marked individual variation. This interesting work brings out the fact that some persons become delirious with slight fever, while others remain lucid even when the body temperature is considerably elevated in the course of an infection. Indeed, in the experiments just cited, some volunteers performed well in spite of fever. Decrements in performance were generally most marked on active tasks such as arithmetic computation. Volunteers with experimentally induced influenza showed attentional deficits, which the investigators hypothesized to be mediated by interferon or some other related mediator (31). These studies documented that even relatively minor infections might adversely influence certain cognitive functions or attention, or both.

In summary, our understanding of the pathogenesis and pathophysiology of infectious delirium is negligible. A few suggestive clues have emerged from the limited research carried out to date and cited above. It appears that the pathogenesis of delirium due to infection is multifactorial and may involve different mechanisms, depending on the nature of the infection, its location, and the presence and degree of fever. Future studies, such as those on septic encephalopathy cited above, may help to clarify the pathophysiological processes whereby delirium is induced by the various infections.

Infections associated with delirium

Both intracranial and systemic infections can give rise to delirium. To discuss all of them here would be pointless; only those that are either common or more often associated with the syndrome will be considered and are listed in Table 15–1. It should be emphasized once again that any infection is much more likely to cause delirium in an elderly patient than in a younger one (8,9,32).

Intracranial infections

These infections are often accompanied by delirium (33). They should be considered in the differential diagnosis, especially when its etiology is not readily established. Neurological signs are usually present but may be absent, and the infection can present clinically with delirium as its most conspicuous feature. This is particularly liable to occur in the case of encephalitis.

TABLE 15–1 INFECTIOUS DISEASES CAUSING DELIRIUM

A. Intracranial Infections
   1. Viral encephalitis (herpes simplex, herpes zoster, etc.)
   2. Acquired immune deficiency syndrome
   3. Reye's syndrome
   4. Postinfectious encephalomyelitis
      a. Syndenham's chorea
      b. Cat scratch disease
      c. Lyme disease
      d. Pertussis
   5. Bacterial meningitis, including the tuberculosis form
   6. Aseptic (viral) meningitis
   7. Acute poliomyelitis
   8. Brain abscess
   9. Spirochetal infections: neurosyphilis, Lyme disease
   10. Fungal infections: actinomycosis, candidiasis, coccidioidomycosis, cryptococcosis, histoplasmosis, mucormycosis
   11. Protozoal infections: amebiasis, malaria, toxoplasmosis, trypanosomiasis
   12. Helminthic infections: cysticercosis, schistosomiasis, trichinosis

B. Systemic Infections
   1. Bacteremia, septic shock
   2. Infective endocarditis
   3. Intra-abdominal infections
   4. Pneumonia
      a. Mycoplasma infections
      b. Plague
      c. Psittacosis
   5. Toxic shock syndrome
   6. Typhoid fever
   7. Typhus and other rickettsioses
   8. Viral infections
      a. Influenza
      b. Acute viral hepatitis

VIRAL ENCEPHALITIS

This disease is commonly associated with delirium of some severity. Acute viral encephalitis may be epidemic or endemic. The former is most often caused by members of the arbovirus group. The sporadic cases are most often due to herpes simplex virus (34,35). Less common causes include mumps, influenza, herpes zoster, coxsackie, cytomegalovirus, rubella, rubeola, rabies, enteroviruses, and Epstein-Barr virus. Acute encephalitis of any etiology may be associated with delirium, which can be the presenting feature. In one series of 191 adult patients with acute encephalitis, "psychic disorders" were noted in about 40% (35). The authors do not specify the exact nature of these "disorders," and one can only assume that they represent delirium. This assumption may or may not be correct, since encephalitis can on occasion give rise to an organic delusional or affective disorder rather than frank delirium, the most common psychiatric manifestation (36–39). Some patients display symptoms giving the impression of schizophrenia or mania (39). Catatonia, marked disinhibition manifested verbally and behaviorally, free expression of normally unconscious wishes and impulses, florid hallucinations, paranoid delusions, depersonalization, and other symptoms have resulted in the erroneous diagnosis of a functional psychosis (39). Yet, careful examination of the patient's mental status generally elicits evidence of fluctuating cognitive and attentional deficits indicating the presence of delirium; this should lead to investigations to establish its etiology. In case of doubt, an amobarbital interview may be used for a diagnosis, since it tends to accentuate the cognitive impairment and hence increases the probability that the patient is suffering from an organic rather than a functional psychosis (39). Moreover, this technique may allow examination of the mental status in an extremely agitated or mute patient. Amobarbital may at times precipitate severe hypotension in an encephalitic individual and should be injected slowly. The EEG is usually abnormal in encephalitis and shows diffuse bilateral slowing (34). In herpes simplex encephalitis it may feature periodic complexes of sharp and slow waves, but these changes tend to appear relatively late in the course of the disease (38). Nevertheless, the EEG is claimed to be the most useful diagnostic aid, even in comparison with computed tomography scanning (34,38).

Several forms of encephalitis deserve special mention because of their clinical importance. *Acquired immune deficiency syndrome (AIDS)* is frequently complicated by disorders of the CNS, including delirium (40,48). AIDS-related dementia (ARD), a subacute encephalitis caused by human immunodeficiency virus (HIV) infection, is the most frequent and important neuropsychiatric complication (40–47). Moreover, some patients who are neither clinically demented nor show gross neurological abnormalities display evidence of cerebral involvement on comprehensive neuropsychological testing and magnetic resonance imaging (43). It has been estimated that up to two-thirds of AIDS patients who do not develop some other CNS disease may develop dementia (46). The early features of this disorder include impairment of cognitive and motor functions and of behavior. The most frequent early symptoms are forgetfulness and reduced ability to concentrate (46). Confusion was observed at an early stage in about 25% of the patients in one series (46). Apathy and withdrawal are also common early symptoms. An occasional patient presents with psychosis. Delirium can be the initial symptom of ARD and has been reported to occur in about 40% of cases of late dementia (45). Patients with ARD are predisposed to the development of delirium in response to psychoactive drugs, infection, and metabolic disorders (45). Several studies have indicated that the incidence of the syndrome in AIDS patients is about 30% (44,47). Its etiology includes a variety of CNS infections, notably cytomegalovirus (48) and herpes simplex/zoster encephalitis, cryptococcosis, and *Toxoplasma gondii* CNS infection (44). Additional potential causes of delirium include CNS lymphoma, systemic lymphoma, and Kaposi's sarcoma with CNS involvement, metabolic encephalopathy, and therapeutic agents such as psychotropic drugs and those used for the treatment of the underlying disease azidothymidine (AZT) and g-(1,3-dihydroxy-2-propoxymethyl) guanine (DHPG) (44,45). Clearly, delirium is a common disorder in AIDS patients that can be due to a variety of possible causes occurring singly or in combination. Its management should follow the guidelines discussed in Chapter 9.

Infectious mononucleosis is relatively common and hence deserves special attention. On occasion, it may give rise to encephalitis or meningoencephalitis and present with delirium (49,50). Estimates of the frequency of acute neurological presentations in this infection range from 1% to 5%; the incidence of delirium is unknown (50).

Encephalitis lethargica is mostly of historical importance (51,52), but it still occurs in endemic form (53,54). A pandemic of encephalitis in the years 1916–1919 gave rise to a large literature that contains a wealth of clinical observations relevant to organic psychiatry (51,52). Three types of early manifestations were discussed: lethargic, hyperkinetic, and amyostatic. In the course of the disease, one form may predominate or all three may occur in various combinations and sequences. Delirium was a common feature of all three types, thus demonstrating that the syndrome may be associated with hypoactivity, hyperactivity, or shifts from one form of psychomotor activity to its opposite. Bizarre behavior, restlessness, and excitement were the features of the hyperkinetic type and often resulted in the erroneous diagnosis of catatonic schizophrenia. Sleep disturbances were common, and ranged from marked somnolence in the lethargic form to total insomnia at night and inversion of the sleep-wake cycle in the hyperkinetic type (51). Of special interest is the fact that a disease of the brain may give rise to such a wide range of psychopathological manifestations, many of which had been traditionally viewed as "functional" rather than of organic origin (52). Observations of patients with this infection have helped to expand the concept of organic mental syndromes, reflected in the current classification of mental disorders, and to blur the distinction between the organic and the functional ones.

Reye's syndrome, an encephalopathy with fatty degeneration of the viscera, notably the liver, is usually associated with delirium (55–57). Typically, a viral infection, most often influenza or varicella, is followed in 3 to 5 days by the onset of severe vomiting. The patients are initially irritable and lethargic but remain oriented (56). Some of them remain lethargic throughout, while others progress to an agitated delirium and may ultimately develop coma, decerebrate and decorticate posturing, hyperventilation, and hyperpyrexia. Death occurs in about 25% to 40% of cases (56). The encephalopathy usually persists for 1 to 4 days and may be followed by permanent neurological impairment. Reye's syndrome is particularly common in children but may also occur in adults (55). Its pathogenesis is still incompletely understood, but it appears to involve multiple metabolic disturbances manifested by hyperammonemia, free fatty acidemia, and lactic acidosis (56). Salicylate ingestion during the antecedent illness and prior to the onset of Reye's syndrome appears to be casually related to the latter condition (55–57). Treatment involves lowering the raised intracranial pressure (55).

POSTINFECTIOUS ENCEPHALOMYELITIS

This group of syndromes includes focal or diffuse involvement of the CNS that follows an infectious illness or immunization. Cell-mediated immunity is believed to be the predominant pathogenic mechanism (58). Postinfectious encephalomyelitis is most often associated with viral infections, such as measles (59), but it may also occur after bacterial infections, mycoplasma pneumonia, vaccination, and immunization (58). The onset is typically sudden, several days to weeks after the preceding illness, with high fever, meningism, seizures, focal neurological signs, and delirium (58,59). Sudden onset of confusion has been observed in about one-half of the patients with measles encephalomyelitis (59).

Other postinfectious neurological syndromes can follow bacterial infections, including *Sydenham's chorea* (59,60), *cat scratch disease* (61), *Lyme disease* (62,63), and *pertussis* (64). Delirium can occur in all of them.

Bacterial meningitis

In a series of 875 patients with bacterial meningitis, confusion was observed in about 20% of the cases and was highest (40%) in pneumococcal meningitis (65). In the elderly, bacterial meningitis has been reported to feature delirium in 57% of one series of patients and was highest (92%) in those with pneumococcal infection (66).

Tuberculous meningitis is most often encountered in children and young adults, but it can also occur in the elderly (67,68). Delirium typically sets in about 2 weeks after the onset of other symptoms of the infection and is accompanied by a disproportionately severe impairment of memory resembling Wernicke's encephalopathy (67).

ASEPTIC MENINGITIS

This disease is usually due to a viral infection. Delirium is common but tends to be relatively mild (69,70).

Acute poliomyelitis

This viral infection may be complicated by delirium in about 15% of cases, as was observed during the Boston epidemic of 1955 (71). All of the delirious patients were in the acute febrile phase of the disease, and all had signs of bulbar or bulbospinal involvement. Most of them were treated in a respirator. The delirium lasted for 5 days to 6 weeks, the average duration being about 2 weeks. A striking feature was the pleasurable, nonfrightening nature of the hallucinations. Kinesthetic illusions and hallucinations were unusually common and seemed to be suggested by the sounds and motions produced by the respirator. The investigators speculated that lesions in the midbrain and the diencephalon might be responsible for the delirium. Perceptual deprivation associated with treatment in a respirator may have been a contributing factor (72).

Brain abscess

Typically, brain abscess presents with headache, focal neurological signs, and reduced awareness. Delirium may be a manifestation of a rapidly expanding abscess or may be accompanied by intracranial hypertension (73). The presence of a pericranial infection (ear, mastoid, sinuses) or of an infection in another part of the body, such as infective endocarditis, provides a suggestive diagnostic clue.

SPIROCHETAL INFECTIONS

Neurosyphilis is still encountered with some frequency. Acute meningoencephalitis is currently one of its most common symptomatic forms and often features confusion (74,75). An acute confusional state has also been observed in some patients with general paresis (76).

Lyme disease has already been referred to.

Fungal infections

Invasion of the CNS by fungi can give rise to the syndromes of meningitis or encephalitis, or a combination of both (77). Delirium is a common feature of these diseases, which include *actinomycosis, candidiasis, coccidioidomycosis, cryptococcosis, histoplasmosis,* and *mucormycosis* (77). Fungal infections of the CNS are most often encountered in compromised hosts such as patients with AIDS or those treated with corticosteroids or immunosuppressive agents. Symptoms indicative of delirium have been reported to occur in 50% of patients with cryptococcosis (78), and also appear to be common in coccidioidomycosis (79) and mucormycosis (77).

PROTOZOAL INFECTIONS

Amebic meningoencephalitis often features confusion (80). *Cerebral malaria,* a potentially fatal complication of *Plasmodium falciparum* infection, involves a diffuse encephalopathy with hyperpyrexia and delirium (81–83). Stupor, convulsions, and coma may follow. In one report, the patients displayed vivid hallucinations, paranoid delusions, and agitation (83). On occasion, a diagnostic problem may arise when a patient with cerebral malaria presents with what appears to be a functional psychosis (81,82). Multifocal cerebral ischemia and hypoxia appear to underly the delirium in these cases, but hyperpyrexia may also play a part in its development. *Toxoplasmosis,* an infection caused by *Toxoplasma gondii,* may result in diffuse encephalopathy, meningoencephalitis, and single or multiple mass lesions in the brain (84). Delirium can be a feature of this infection, as was noted in the section on AIDS (44,85,86).

Trypanosomiasis, or sleeping sickness, transmitted by the bite of the tsetse fly, can cause meningoencephalitis and is often accompanied by delirium as well as a disordered sleep-wake cycle, usually consisting of diurnal somnolence and nocturnal insomnia (87).

HELMINTHIC INFECTIONS

Infections by this group of parasites can involve the CNS and give rise to delirium. *Cysticercosis,* an infection caused by *Taenia solium,* can cause dementia as well as confusion (88,89). A review of patients studied in the United States reports that "altered mental status" was observed in 9% to 26% in several series of cases of neurocysticercosis (88). *Schistosomiasis* can also involve the brain. Treatment of this disease with oxamniquine has been reported to precipitate "distortion of reality" and hallucinations, suggestive of delirium, in the majority of a small series of patients (90). *Trichinosis* with CNS involvement may be accompanied by delirium in 70% of cases (91,92). The syndrome usually occurs in the second week of the infection as a manifestation of meningoencephalitis caused by the larvae of *Trichinella spiralis.* The EEG shows diffuse slowing of background activity (91).

Systemic infections

Systemic infections are among the most important causes of delirium in children and the elderly, who are liable to develop it in the course of any infectious disease. The elderly are more likely to become delirious during an infection than are younger adults. Even a urinary tract infection may precipitate confusion in an older patient. Infections to which the elderly are particularly prone include pneumonia, influenza, tuberculosis, urinary tract infection, gram-negative bacteremia, intra-abdominal sepsis, infective endocarditis, and herpes zoster virus (8,9,32). The more common and important systemic infections that can give rise to delirium will be briefly reviewed.

Bacteremia in the elderly commonly results from urinary tract infection with gram-negative organisms and may be manifested only by delirium and agitation (93). Older patients are more likely to present with afebrile bacteremia, which has a high mortality; confusion may be its presenting feature. In one series of patients with pneumococcal bacteremia, 50% presented with an altered mental status (presumably delirium) (94). In a study of elderly patients, 87% displayed "depressed consciousness" (95). Bacteremia in the elderly may be associated with septic shock and delirium (96).

Infective endocarditis is currently more common in the elderly than in young adults (97). Atypically, an older patient may present with delirium without fever (97–99). The mental symptoms may range from mild confusion to a full-blown delirium with hallucinations and delusions. Delirium has been reported to occur in 38% to 50% of patients and is especially common in the elderly (98,99). In some cases, patients were initially admitted to a psychiatric service because of their psychotic symptoms, which were thought to represent a functional psychosis (100).

Intra-abdominal infections, such as cholecystitis, appendicitis, and diverticulitis, in the elderly can be associated with delirium (101).

Pneumonia is a common infection in the elderly; mental confusion can be its presenting feature (102,103). In *Legionnaire's disease,* pneumonia may be associated with cerebral involvement and delirium (104,105). Infection by *Mycoplasma pneumoniae* is said to account for up to 20% of all pneumonia cases in the general population, and can cause meningoencephalitis and other neurological complications (106,107). Delirium has been reported (106–108). *Psittacosis* typically presents with pneumonitis and severe headache; delirium has been reported in 12% of cases (109). *Plague* may take the form of a pneumonia and commonly features delirium. Defoe (110), in his account of the Great Plague in England, in 1665, wrote, "when the distemper was at its height it generally made them raving and delirious . . . and many who were not tied threw themselves out of windows" (110, p 177).

Toxic shock syndrome (TSS), a multisystemic disease, occurs most often in menstruating women but has also been known to affect men and nonmenstruating women (111,112). It follows *Staphylococcus aureus* infections of the respiratory tract that can complicate influenza and influenza-like illness (111). Infections by *S. aureus* in other clinical settings, such as surgical wound infections and in postpartum women, can also be complicated by TSS (112). Immunological response and competence appear to be implicated in its pathogenesis. Toxins produced by *S. aureus* may be the cause of TSS, an illness characterized by fever, hypotension, erythroderma, and multisystem involvement. Delirium occurs in most patients (112).

Typhoid fever has long been recognized as a cause of delirium (113). The term "typhoid state" has been used by many writers to refer to a muttering delirium in the course of typhoid fever and other acute infections (113). In tropical countries, this state occurs in about one-half of the patients with typhoid fever (114), but it appears to be less common in Western countries (113,115). A report from India states that fever or neuropsychiatric manifestations were the most common presenting features in a series of 246 patients (116). In about 30% of these patients the onset of the disease was acute, with delirium and convulsions. Delirium is usually severe and may last for up to 3 weeks after the fever has subsided (114,116); it is not a bad prognostic sign. Its severity is not related to the height of the temperature (116). The pathogenesis of the syndrome in typhoid fever is unclear. Circulating bacteria and endotoxins do not seem to play a major role (117).

Typhus and other rickettsial infections, such as Rocky Mountain spotted fever, have been notorious for their association with delirium (118,119). Until the 1830s no distinction had been made between typhus and typhoid (120). Delirium was observed as a relatively common complication of the former during its epidemic in New York City in 1847 (121). Guttman (119) published a remarkable account of his observations on psychiatric complications of typhus, personally observed and experienced during World War II. Delirium of varying severity was commonly seen at all stages of the disease: the prodromal, the height, and the decrudescence. In some cases, including his own, the syndrome featured rich, vivid hallucinatory and dream-like experiences.

Viral infections may give rise to delirium without apparently invading the CNS (122). Among the earliest symptoms of many such acute infections are impairment of attention and reduction of the speed of mental activity (30,31). These disturbances may be regarded as prodromal symptoms of delirium, which may or may not become fully manifest. Loss of interest in reading, difficulty in marshaling one's thoughts, mild depression, and hypersensitivity to bright light and noise are additional features of the early phase of an acute viral infection, such as influenza. Gould (122) regards these symptoms as indicative of a mild delirium. The syndrome may become clearly manifest if the illness becomes severe, or if the patient has a pronounced susceptibility to the syndrome or is elderly.

Published reports often make it impossible to establish if the delirium observed in patients suffering from a viral infection was due to a direct invasion of the CNS and the development of encephalitis, meningitis, or meningoencephalitis, or if it represented an encephalopathy with no evidence of direct CNS involvement by the pathogen. *Influenza,* for example, appears to give rise to such an encephalopathy at times (123). Reye's syndrome, referred to earlier, may account for at least some of these cases (124). *Acute viral hep-*

atitis may possibly give rise to the same type of encephalopathy (125–127). Neuropsychiatric manifestations of this infection can precede the onset of jaundice and cause a diagnostic problem in an occasional case (126).

In summary, both intracranial and systemic infections are important organic causes of delirium notably in children and the elderly. The pathogenesis and pathophysiology of the syndrome are poorly understood and appear to be multifactorial. In the elderly, delirium may be the presenting feature of an infectious disease in the absence of fever. Such a disease must always be considered in the differential diagnosis if death is to be avoided as a result of failure to treat the underlying infection.

References

1. Fordyce G.: *Five Dissertations on Fever.* 2nd American ed. Boston, Bedlington and Ewer, 1823.
2. Swift H. M.: Delirium and delirious states. *Bost. Med. Surg. J.* 1907; 157:687–692.
3. Verco: Delirium. *St. Bart Hosp. Rep. (Lond.)* 1877; 13:332–342.
4. Weber H.: On delirium or acute insanity during the decline of acute diseases, especially the delirium of collapse. *Med. Chir. Trans. (Lond.)* 1865;30:135–159.
5. Hirsch W.: A study of delirium. *N.Y. Med. J.* 1899;70:109–115.
6. Editorial: Organic psychosis. *Br. Med. J.* 1974;2:214–215.
7. Villaverde M. M., MacMillan C. W.: Fever. *From Symptoms to Treatment.* New York, Van Nostrand Reinhold, 1978.
8. Schneider E. L.: Infectious diseases in the elderly. *Ann. Intern. Med.* 1983;98:395–400.
9. Yoshikawa T. T.: Geriatric infectious diseases: An emerging problem. *J. Am. Geriatr. Soc.* 1983;31:34–39.
10. Berman P., Hogan D. B., Fox R. A.: The atypical presentation of infection in old age. *Age Ageing* 1987;16:201–207.
11. Freedman D. K., Troll L., Mills A. B., et al: *Acute Organic Disorder Accompanied by Mental Symptoms.* Sacramento, Calif, Dept of Mental Hygiene, 1965.
12. Bollea G.: Acute organic psychoses in childhood, in Howells J. G. (ed): *Modern Perspectives in International Child Psychiatry.* New York, Brunner Mazel, 1971, pp 706–732.
13. Kanner L.: *Child Psychiatry* 4th ed. Springfield, Ill., Charles C Thomas, 1972, pp 329–337.
14. Black R. H.: Tropical diseases of psychiatric importance. *Papua New Guinea Med. J.* 1976;19:19–23.
15. Buchan T.: Organic confusional states. *S. Afr. Med. J.* 1972;46:1340–1343.
16. Editorial: Temporary mental confusion in a medical ward. *Cent. Afr. J. Med.* 1974;20:127–129.
17. Wallace J. F.: Infectious delirium. *Southwest. Med.* 1969;50:181–183.
18. Hasselgren P. O., Fischer J. E.: Septic encephalopathy. *Intensive Care Med.* 1986;12:13–16.
19. Jackson A. C., Gilbert J. J., Young G. B., et al: The encephalopathy of sepsis. *Can. J. Neurol. Sci.* 1985;12:303–307.

20. Winder T. R., Minuk G. Y., Sargeant E. J., et al: Gamma-aminobutyric acid (GABA) and sepsis-related encephalopathy. *Can. J. Neurol. Sci.* 1988;15:23–25.
21. Dinarello C. A.: Interleukin-1 and the pathogenesis of the acute-phase response. *N. Engl. J. Med.* 1984;311:1413–1418.
22. Norman D. C., Grahn D., Yoshikawa T. T.: Fever and aging. *J. Am. Geriatr. Soc.* 1985;33:859–863.
23. Berman P., Fox R. A.: Fever in the elderly. *Age Ageing* 1985;14:327–332.
24. Siesjö B. K., Carlsson C., Hagerdal M., et al: Brain metabolism in the critically ill. *Crit. Care Med.* 1976;4:283–294.
25. Bilbert V. E.: Blood pyruvate and lactate during febrile human infections. *Metabolism* 1968;17:943–951.
26. Dubois M., Sato S., Leese E., et al: Electroencephalographic changes during whole body hyperthermia in humans. *Electroencephalogr. Clin. Neurophysiol.* 1980;50:486–495.
27. Kadlecova O., Masek K., Rotta J., et al: Fever and sleep cycle changes induced by bacterial products. *J. Hyg. Epidemiol. Microbiol. Immunol.* 1974;18:472–475.
28. Karacan I., Wolff S. M., Williams R. L., et al: The effects of fever on sleep and dreams. *Psychosomatics* 1968;9:331–339.
29. Lifshitz A., Lopez M., Fiorelli S., et al: The electroencephalogram in adult patients with fever. *Clin. Electroencephalogr.* 1987;18:85–88.
30. Alluisi E. A., Beisel W. R., Bartelloni P. J., et al: Behavioral effects of tularemia and sandfly fever in man. *J. Infect. Dis.* 1973;128:710–717.
31. Smith A. P., Tyrrell D. A. J., Al-Nakib W., et al: The effects of experimentally induced respiratory virus infections on performance. *Psychol. Med.* 1988;18:65–71.
32. Yoshikawa T. T.: Important infections in elderly persons. *West. J. Med.* 1981;135:441–445.
33. Oill P. A., Yoshikawa T. T., Yamauchi T.: Infectious disease emergencies. Part I: Patients presenting with an altered state of consciousness. *West. J. Med* 1976;125:36–46.
34. Kennard C., Swash M.: Acute viral encephalitis. Its diagnosis and outcome. *Brain* 1981;104:129–148.
35. Koshiniemi M., Manninen V., Vaheri A., et al: Acute encephalitis. *Acta Med. Scand.* 1981;209:115–120.
36. Oommen K. J., Johnson P. C., Ray C. G.: Herpes simplex type 2 virus encephalitis presenting as psychosis. *Am. J. Med.* 1982;73:445–448.
37. Schlitt M., Lakeman F. D., Whitley R. J.: Psychosis and herpes simplex encephalitis. *South. Med. J.* 1985;78:1347–1350.
38. Tenser R. B.: Herpes simplex and herpes zoster. *Neurol. Clin.* 1984;2:215–240.
39. Wilson L. G.: Psychiatric aspects of acute viral encephalitis, in Kurstak E., Lipowski Z. J., Morozov P. V. (eds): *Viruses, Immunity, and Mental Disorders.* New York, Plenum Medical Book, 1987, pp 413–422.
40. Elder G. A., Sever J. L.: Neurologic disorders associated with AIDS retroviral infection. *Rev. Infect. Dis.* 1988;10:286–302.
41. Faulstich M. E.: Psychiatric aspects of AIDS. *Am. J. Psychiatry* 1987;144:551–556.
42. Gabuzda D. H., Hirsch M. S.: Neurologic manifestations of infection with human immunodeficiency virus. *Ann. Intern. Med.* 1987;107:383–391.

43. Grant I., Atkinson J. H., Hesselink J. R., et al: Evidence for early central nervous system involvement in the acquired immunodeficiency syndrome (AIDS) and other human immunodeficiency virus (HIV) infections. *Ann. Intern. Med.* 1987;107:828–836.
44. Loewenstein R. J., Rubinow D. R.: Psychiatric aspects of AIDS. The organic mental syndromes, in Kurstak E., Lipowski Z. J., Morozov P. V. (eds): *Viruses, Immunity, and Mental Disorders.* New York, Plenum Medical Book Co, 1987, pp 95–107.
45. McArthur J. C.: Neurologic manifestations of AIDS. *Medicine* 1987;66:407–437.
46. Navia B. A., Jordan B. D., Price R. W.: The AIDS dementia complex: 1. Clinical features. *Ann. Neurol.* 1986;19:517–524.
47. Perry S. W., Tross S.: Psychiatric problems of AIDS inpatients at the New York Hospital: Preliminary report. *Public Health Rep.* 1984;99:200–206.
48. Post M. J. D., Hensley G. T., Moskowitz L. B., et al: Cytomegalic inclusion virus encephalitis in patients with AIDS: CT, clinical, and pathologic correlation. *A.J.N.R.* 1986;7:275–280.
49. Hendler N.: Infectious mononucleosis and psychiatric disorders, in Kurstak E., Lipowski Z. J., Morozov P. V. (eds): *Viruses, Immunity, and Mental Disorders.* New York, Plenum Medical Book Co, 1987, pp 81–94.
50. Leavell R., Ray C. G., Ferry P. C., et al: Unusual acute neurologic presentations with Epstein-Barr virus infection. *Arch. Neurol.* 1986;43:186–188.
51. Hoenig J., Abbey S.: Von Economo's disease (encephalitis lethargica). Lessons for psychiatry, in Kurstak E., Lipowski Z. J., Morozov P. V.: *Viruses, Immunity, and Mental Disorders.* New York, Plenum Medical Book Co, 1987, pp 423–439.
52. Ward C. D.: Encephalitis lethargica and the development of neuropsychiatry. *Psychiatr. Clin. North Am.* 1986;9:215–224.
53. Editorial: Encephalitis lethargica. *Lancet* 1981;2:1386–1397.
54. Johnson J.: Encephalitis lethargica, a contemporary cause of catatonic stupor. *Br. J. Psychiatry* 1987;151:550–552.
55. Ede R. J., Williams R.: Reye's syndrome in adults. *Br. Med. J.* 1988,296:517–518.
56. Heubi J. E., Partin J. C., Partin J. S., et al: Reye's syndrome: Current concepts. *Hepatology* 1987;7:155–164.
57. Hurwitz E. S., Barrett M. J., Bregman D., et al: Public Health Service study of Reye's syndrome and medications. *J.A.M.A.* 1987;257:1905–1911.
58. Evans O. B.: Parainfections neurologic diseases. *Semin. Neurol.* 1985;5:288–297.
59. Johnson R. T., Griffin D. E., Hirsch R. L., et al: Measles encephalomyelitis—clinical and immunologic studies. *N. Engl. J. Med.* 1984;310:137–141.
60. Chien L. T., Economides A. N., Lemmi H.: Syndenham's chorea and seizures. *Arch. Neurol.* 1978;35:382–385.
61. Lewis D. W., Tucker S. H.: Central nervous system involvement in cat scratch disease. *Pediatrics* 1986;77:714–721.
62. Parke A.: From New to old England: The progress of Lyme disease. *Br. Med. J.* 1987;294:525–526.
63. Steere A. C., Bartenhagen N. H., Craft J. E., et al: The early clinical manifestations of Lyme disease. *Ann. Intern. Med.* 1983;99:76–82.
64. Davis L. E., Burstyn D. G., Manclark C. R.: Pertussis encephalopathy with a normal brain biopsy and elevated lymphocytosis-promotion factor antibodies. *Pediatr. Infect. Dis.* 1984;3:448–451.

65. Bohr V., Hansen B., Jessen O., et al: Eight hundred and seventy-five cases of bacterial meningitis. *J. Infection* 1983;7:21–30.
66. Gorse G. J., Thrupp L. D., Nudleman K. L., et al: Bacterial meningitis in the elderly. *Arch. Intern. Med.* 1984;144:1603–1607.
67. Cybulska E., Rucinski J.: Tuberculous meningitis. *Br. J. Hosp. Med.* 1988;33:63–66.
68. Dixon P. E., Hoey C., Cayley A. C. D.: Tuberculous meningitis in the elderly. *Postgrad. Med. J.* 1984;60:586–588.
69. Butler I. J., Johnson R. T.: Central nervous system infections. *Pediatr. Clin. North Am.* 1974;21:649–668.
70. Rosenthal M. S.: Viral infections of the central nervous system. *Med. Clin. North Am.* 1974;58:593–603.
71. Holland J. C. B., Coles M. R.: Neuropsychiatric aspects of acute poliomyelitis. *Am. J. Psychiatry* 1957;114:54–63.
72. Mendelson J., Solomon P., Lindemann E.: Hallucinations of poliomyelitis patients during treatment in a respirator. *J. Nerv. Ment. Dis.* 1958;126:421–428.
73. Beller A. J., Sahar A., Praiss I.: Brain abscess. *J. Neurol. Neurosurg. Psychiatry* 1973;36:757–768.
74. Hotson J. R.: Modern neurosyphilis: A partially treated chronic meningitis. *West. J. Med.* 1981;135:191–200.
75. Simon R. P.: Neurosyphilis. *Arch. Neurol.* 1985;42:606–613.
76. Bockner S., Coltart N.: New cases of G.P.I. *Br. Med. J.* 1961;1:18–20.
77. Salaki J. S., Louria D. B., Chmel H.: Fungal and yeast infections of the central nervous system. *Medicine* 1984;63:108–132.
78. Sobel R. A., Ellis W. G., Nielsen S. L., et al: Central nervous system coccidioidomycosis. *Hum. Pathol.* 1984;15:980–995.
79. Yoshikawa T. T., Fujita N., Grinnell V., et al: Management of central nervous system cryptococcosis. *West. J. Med.* 1980;132:123–133.
80. Butt C. G.: Primary amebic meningoencephalitis. *N. Engl. J. Med.* 1966;274:1473–1476.
81. Blocker W. W., Kastl A. J., Daroff R. B.: The psychiatric manifestations of cerebral malaria. *Am. J. Psychiatry* 1968;125:88–92.
82. Kean B. H., Reilly P. C.: Malaria—The mime. *Am. J. Med.* 1976;61:159–164.
83. Wintrob R. M.: Malaria and the acute psychotic episode. *J. Nerv. Ment. Dis.* 1973;156:306–317.
84. Cowley F. K., Jenkins K. A., Remington J. S.: *Toxoplasma gondii* infection of the central nervous system. *Hum. Pathol.* 1981;12:690–698.
85. Bach M. C., Armstrong R. M.: Acute toxoplasmic encephalitis in a normal adult. *Arch. Neurol.* 1983;40:596–597.
86. Minto A., Roberts F. J.: The psychiatric complications of toxoplasmosis. *Lancet* 1959;1:1180–1182.
87. Antoine P.: Etude neurologique et psychologique des malades trypanosomes et leur evolution. *Ann. Soc. Belg. Med. Trop.* 1977;57:227–247.
88. Earnest M. P., Reller L. B., Filley C. M., et al: Neuocysticercosis in the United States: 35 cases and a review. *Rev. Infect. Dis.* 1987;9:961–979.
89. Grisolia J. S.: CNS cysticercosis. *Arch. Neurol.* 1982;39:540–544.
90. Istre G. R., Fontaine R. E., Tarr J., et al: Acute schistosomiasis among Americans rafting the Omo river, Ethiopia. *J.A.M.A.* 1984;251:508–510.
91. Barr R.: Human trichinosis. *Can. Med. Assoc. J.* 1966;95:912–916.

92. Dalessio D. J., Wolff H. G.: *Trichinella spiralis* infection of the central nervous system. *Arch. Neurol.* 1961;4:407–417.
93. Polly S. M., Sanders W. E.: Surgical infections in the elderly: Prevention, diagnosis, and treatment. *Geriatrics* 1977;32:88–97.
94. Chang J. I., Mylotte J. M.: Pneumococcal bacteremia. *J. Am. Geriatr. Soc.* 1987;35:747–754.
95. Van Dijk J. M., Rosin A. J., Rudenski B.: Septicaemia in the elderly. *Practitioner* 1982;226:1439–1143.
96. Holloway W. A., Reinhardt J.: Septic shock in the elderly. *Geriatrics* 1984;39:48–54.
97. Cantrell M., Yoshikawa T. T.: Aging and infective endocarditis. *J. Am. Geriatr. Soc.* 1983;31:216–222.
98. Bademosi O., Falase A. O., Jaiyesimi F., et al: Neuropsychiatric manifestations of infective endocarditis: A study of 95 patients at Ibadan, Nigeria. *J. Neurol. Neurosurg. Psychiatry* 1976;39:325–329.
99. Greenlee J. E., Mandell G. L.: Neurological manifestations of infective endocarditis: A review. *Stroke* 1973;4:958–963.
100. Hermans P. E.: The clinical manifestations of infective endocarditis. *Mayo Clin. Proc.* 1982;57:15–21.
101. Normal D. C., Yoshikawa T. T.: Intraabdominal infections in the elderly. *J. Am. Geriatr. Soc.* 1983;31:677–684.
102. Niederman M. S., Fein A. M.: Pneumonia in the elderly. *Geriatr. Clin. North Am.* 1986;2:241–268.
103. Verghese A., Berk S. L.: Bacterial pneumonia in the elderly. *Medicine* 1983;62:271–285.
104. Cheung M. T.: Eight cases of Legionnaires' disease. *Can. Med. Assoc. J.* 1980;123:639–644.
105. Lees A. W., Tyrrell W. F.: Severe cerebral disturbance in Legionnaires' disease. *Lancet* 1978;2:1335–1338.
106. Cassell G. H., Cole B. C.: Mycoplasmas as agents of human disease. *N. Engl. J. Med.* 1981;304:80–89.
107. Decaux G., Szyper M., Ectors M., et al: Central nervous system complications of *Mycoplasma pneumoniae. J. Neurol. Neurosurg. Psychiatry* 1980;43:883–887.
108. Moskal M. J., Kaylarian V. H., Doro J. M.: Psychosis complicating *Mycoplasma pneumoniae* infection. *Pediatr. Infect. Dis.* 1984;3:63–66.
109. Yung A. P., Grayson M. L.: Psittacosis—A review of 135 cases. *Med. J. Aust.* 1988;148:228–233.
110. Defoe D.: *A Journal of the Plague Year.* New York, Penguin Books, 1966.
111. MacDonald K. L., Osterholm M. T., Hedberg C. W., et al: Toxic shock syndrome. *J.A.M.A.* 1987;257:1053–1058.
112. Wright S. W., Trott A. T.: Toxic shock syndrome: A review. *Ann. Emerg. Med.* 1988;17:268–273.
113. Verghese A.: The "typhoid state" revisited. *Am. J. Med.* 1985;79:370–372.
114. Osuntokun B. O., Bademosi O., Ogunremi K., et al: Neuro-psychiatric manifestations of typhoid fever in 959 patients. *Arch. Neurol.* 1972;27:7–13.
115. Klotz S. A., Jorgensen J. H., Buckwold F. J., et al: Typhoid fever. *Arch. Intern. Med.* 1984;144:533–537.
116. Khosla S. N., Srivastava S. C., Gupta S.: Neuropsychiatric manifestations of typhoid. *J. Trop. Med. Hyg.* 1977;80:95–98.

117. Butler T., Bell W. R., Levin J., et al: Typhoid fever. *Arch. Intern. Med.* 1978;138:407–410.
118. Gorman R. J., Saxon S., Snead O. C.: Neurologic sequelae of Rocky Mountain spotted fever. *Pediatrics* 1981;67:354–357.
119. Guttman O.: Psychic disturbances in typhus fever. *Psychiatr. Q.* 1952;26:478–491.
120. Smith D. C.: Gerhard's distinction between typhoid and typhus and its reception in America, 1833–1860. *Bull. Hist. Med.* 1980;54:368–385.
121. Gelston A. L., Jones T. C.: Typhus fever: Report of an epidemic in New York City in 1847. *J. Infect. Dis.* 1977;136:813–821.
122. Gould J.: Virus disease and psychiatric ill-health. *Br. J. Clin. Pract.* 1975;11:1-5.
123. Hochberg F. H., Nelson K., Janzen W.: Influenza type B-related encephalopathy. *J.A.M.A.* 1975;231:817–821.
124. Kennedy C. R., Robinson R. O., Valman H. B., et al: A major role for viruses in acute childhood encephalopathy. *Lancet* 1986;1:989–991.
125. Apstein M. D., Koff E., Koff R. S.: Neuropsychological dysfunction in acute viral hepatitis. *Digestion* 1979;19:349–358.
126. Friedlander W. J.: Neurologic signs and symptoms as a prodrome to viral hepatitis. *Neurology* 1956;6:574–579.
127. Liebowitz S., Gorman W. F.: Neuropsychiatric complications of viral hepatitis. *N. Engl. J. Med.* 1952;246:932–937.

16

Vascular Diseases

Cerebrovascular diseases (CVD)

Vascular diseases of the brain constitute an important class of organic causes of delirium, which is, in turn, one of the most common psychiatric manifestations of CVD. In one study, CVD was found to be the second most frequent cause of delirium in 562 patients diagnosed in a neuropsychiatric hospital (1). In a more recent study of 35 delirious elderly patients, stroke was the most common cause of delirium (2). Whether these findings have general validity is open to question, however. It is generally accepted that systemic diseases are a more common cause of delirium than intracranial diseases in patients of any age. Moreover, medical drugs are likely to be the primary cause of the syndrome in the elderly. In the following discussion, both the acute and the chronic vascular diseases of the brain are considered in relation to delirium and are listed in Table 16–1.

CVD has three major components (3): 1. decreased perfusion pressure due to a pathological process such as atherosclerosis, embolism, thrombosis, or vasculitis, and consequently an inadequate supply of the metabolic substrates necessary to sustain normal brain function; 2. pathophysiological change in the metabolism of the brain, which may be transient or persistent; and 3. focal or general cerebral dysfunction, or both. Focal cerebral dysfunction includes transient ischemic attacks (TIAs), progressing stroke, and completed stroke. "General cerebral dysfunction" refers to general ischemia of the brain result-

TABLE 16–1 Cerebrovascular Diseases Causing Delirium

Transient ischemic attacks
Cerebral thrombosis, embolism
Subarachnoid hemorrhage
Multi-infarct dementia
Subdural hematoma
Hypertensive encephalopathy
Migraine
Cerebral vasculitis
Multifocal cerebral ischemia

ing from a reduction in its blood supply due to conditions such as cardiac arrest. Delirium may be a manifestation of any pathological process or event resulting in cerebral ischemia. The latter may involve the carotid or the vertebrobasilar arterial system, or both.

Transient ischemic attacks (TIAs)

These are episodes of focal cerebral dysfunction of vascular origin, rapid onset, and brief duration (less than 24 hours) (4). An attack may involve either the carotid or the vertebrobasilar arterial system. Visual hallucinations and "mental changes" are reported to occur in less than 3% of carotid artery TIA's (5); whether delirium occurs is unclear. Vertebrobasilar TIAs are reported to feature "mental changes" in about 5% of cases (5). Delirium does not seem to be common.

Cerebral infarction and embolism

CEREBRAL INFARCTION

A study of 661 patients with stroke, confirmed by computed tomography scan or at autopsy, demonstrated disorientation or confusion in 33% of those with cerebral infarction (6). Only six patients presented with "acute delirium." In another study, only 13 of 302 patients with a stroke confirmed by autopsy presented with confusional state (7). In 1967, Horenstein et al. (8) reported on nine patients with sudden agitated delirium resulting from unilateral or bilateral infarction of the fusiform or lingual gyri. A similar case was reported by Medina et al. (9) in 1974. The patient, a 78-year-old man, was blind in addition to being delirious. Since then, a number of reports have appeared on delirum following infarction of the right thalamus (10), posterior cerebral artery (11–13), and right middle cerebral artery (14–16). It appears that infarction in the territory of the left posterior cerebral artery is sufficient to produce delirium, but not all patients with such infarctions become delirious (11). Patients with infarctions in the territory of the right middle cerebral artery (RMCA) may present with an agitated confusional state (14–16). In one series of cases with RMCA infarction, only 2 of 46 patients presented with this state (16), and in another study, 36 of 60 patients with an acute confusional state had lesions in the right hemisphere (15). A recent report from Japan claims that 61% of 41 patients with infarction with RMCA distribution displayed an acute confusional state ACS (what I refer to as "hypoalert-hypoactive delirium"), and 15% manifested acute agitated delirium (AAD) ("hyperalert-hyperactive delirium" in this book) (14). The authors conclude that acute confusional state is one of the most common features of infarction in the RMCA territory and is linked to damage to the right frontostriatal region—which, they assert, is important in the regulation of global attention. The right hemisphere is claimed to be dominant for directed attention (14). The causative lesion in AAD is said to involve the right middle temporal gyrus and to occur with infarction in the territory of the inferior division of the RMCA (14). In AAD, emotional aspects rather than attention are claimed to be involved (14). These speculations suggest a distinct pathogenesis and an anatomical localization for the two types of delirium. Their validity must be tested by future studies. It is not clear at this time what, if any, significance these hypotheses may have for delirium generally. One must beware of reductionistic localizationism in this area, considering that the vast majority of cases both hyperactive and hypoactive delirium do not involve focal lesions but rather *widespread* reduction of cerebral oxidative metabolism and disturbance of neurotransmission. Moreover, as noted above, agitated delirium can be caused by infarctions of the *left* posterior cerebral artery territory and is thus not confined to those in the territory of the RMCA. The issue of focal versus diffuse cerebral involvement in the pathogenesis of delirium awaits the results of future research with tools such as PET.

Internal carotid artery occlusion may have a sudden onset, with delirium among the presenting features (17–19).

Symptoms of obstruction within the *vertebrobasilar* arterial system depend on the site of occlusion or stenosis, the degree, and the availability of collateral flow. Complete occlusion of the main trunk of the basilar artery usually leads to death. Incomplete obstruction is more common, and may result in various transient and fluctuating or permanent disorders and deficits, such as deafness, vertigo, or drop attacks, which reflect dysfunction of the brain stem. Visual disturbances are usually present and may include fortification spectra, blurring of vision, hemianopic field defects, and visual hallucinations (20,21). Occipital headaches, ataxia, bilateral paresthesias over the body, akinetic mutism, hemiplegia, and other manifestations may occur in various combinations. Delirium of some severity may accompany these symptoms. Infarction of the *posterior cerebral artery* has already been referred to.

CEREBRAL EMBOLISM

Cerebral embolism may originate in the heart or lungs, or in one of the arteries to the brain, notably the carotid. Embolism due to a cardiac source commonly results from a cardiac arrhythmia, valvular heart disease, myocardial infarction, or subacute bacterial endocarditis. Fat and air embolism can also occur, the former following trauma to the musculoskeletal system, particularly in multiple fractures. The onset of symptoms is typically rapid, and the patient usually becomes confused rather than unconscious. A convulsion may occur initially. In one series of patients with the *fat embolism syndrome,* "changes in sensorium" were observed in 41 of 54 patients (22). The full syndrome develops 12 hours to 3 days after injury and may feature "agitated confusion" (23). The EEG abnormalities in fat embolism consist of diffuse delta and theta waves. *Air embolism* may result from mediastinal emphysema or pneumothorax and may lead to delirium, loss of consciousness, or both.

Subarachnoid hemorrhage

In subarachnoid hemorrhage of the primary type, initial bleeding occurs directly into the subarachnoid space and is often due to a ruptured intracranial aneurysm or an angioma. Symptoms develop suddenly, and severe headache is typically the first to appear. Disturbance of consciousness ranging from confusion to coma follows. Confusion has been reported in up to 50% of cases (24–26). It may accompany the headache initially and may be followed by coma, or loss of consciousness may be transient and succeeded by confusion. Some of the reported patients suddenly developed severe head pain and confusion as long as 10 days before lapsing into coma. Other patients were admitted to the hospital with confusion and a history of transient unconsciousness within hours or a few days. Meningeal irritation, with or without other neurological signs and symptoms, accompanies the delirium. Warning signs of an impending rupture of an intracranial aneurysm may include lethargy and visual hallucinations (27). Delirium usually clears up within a week, but may occasionally persist for several weeks and gradually merge with a more chronic dementia, which may be partly reversible. Neuropsychological testing of 48 patients who had undergone surgery for subarachnoid hemorrhage due to an aneurysm found that the majority had a good outcome, i.e., no more than a mild deficit (28).

In about 5% of cases, subarachnoid hemorrhage is caused by an intracranial *arteriovenous malformation.* Intellectual deterioration or "mental changes" have been reported in 15% to 50% of these patients, but some investigators found none (29). The reason for this discrepancy is obscure. In a few reported cases, "mental confusion" caused the patient to seek help (30).

Trauma due to *cardiac catherization* or *angiography* may occasionally result in thromboembolism and delirium (31,32). A toxic reaction to contrast agents (see Chapter 11) should be ruled out.

Multi-infarct dementia (MID)

This type of dementia results from multiple small or large infarcts, and is most often associated with hypertension or extracerebral vascular disease, or both (33–35). Most such infarcts are currently believed to be secondary to disease of extracranial arteries and the heart, and only in a minority of cases are due to atherosclerosis of cerebral vessels (35). Thromboembolism from extracranial sources is thought to be the chief cause of cerebral infarcts. Dementia results from repeated, accumulated small and larger strokes. The validity of MID as a distinct clinical entity has recently been questioned (36), but the concept has persisted. Some authors assert that the specificity, sensitivity, and reliability of the *DSM-III* criteria for MID are not justified on either clinical or pathological grounds (37). Be that as it may, the concept of MID continues to be widely used. Two types have been distinguished: cortical and subcortical (38). Nocturnal confusion has been observed in 40% of the cases of the former type but in only 14% of the latter type (38). MID is claimed to account for about 12% to 20% of the cases of dementia (36). Its course is characterized by an abrupt onset, a stepwise progression, and a fluctuating course (35). Its course is punctuated by episodes of delirium, which clears up and leaves in its wake increased cognitive deficits. Focal neurological signs, such as weakness, dysphagia, dysarthria, and brisk reflexes, accompany the delirium. Fluctuations in cognitive deficits in MID appear to be related to those in CBF (39). Diagnosis of MID is based on the history, physical examination, EEG, computed tomography scanning, and magnetic resonance imaging (34).

Subcortical arteriosclerotic encephalopathy (Binswanger's disease) may give rise to slowly progressive dementia as a result of bilateral white matter disease (40). Episodes of stroke and delirium may occur in the initial phase of the disease (41).

Subdural hematoma (SH)

Delirium is among the most common features of this condition (42–48). In one study of 79 patients with subacute or chronic SH, 52.2% had delirium (42). Mental changes, usually referred to in the published reports as "confusion," "memory loss," "somnolence," "stupor," or "lethargy," are among the most important and most readily missed presenting manifestations of SH. Disorientation and confusion, symptoms usually indicating the presence of delirium, are the most common mental status abnormalities (42–48). These clinical features are especially prominent in elderly patients, who may not display the typical manifestations of increased intracranial pressure, such as headache and papilledema (44,45). The patients may be misdiagnosed as having stroke, senile dementia, or an unspecified psychiatric disorder. At times, the diagnosis has been delayed until an autopsy was carried out. The patient will usually die or suffer irreversible brain damage and dementia unless an early diagnosis is made and proper operative treatment is instituted. In one early study, 60% of patients over 65 years of age died before SH was diagnosed (45). Computed tomography is an accurate and safe diagnostic aid (47).

The peak incidence of SH is during the sixth and seventh decades of life (44). About one-half of all cases occur in persons 60 years of age or older. A history of head trauma is absent in about 35% to 50% of patients (44). The trauma may be minor, such as a tumble out of bed. Symptoms tend to develop insidiously and usually include those of increased intracranial pressure and focal neurological signs (47). Delirium or dementia may develop subacutely or in a stepwise manner. Somnolence, confusion, disorientation, and memory impairment may dominate the clinical picture in elderly patients with chronic SH. It is important to maintain a high level of suspicion of SH in any patient with or without a history of head trauma who develops unexplained acute confusional state or focal neurological signs, or both (47).

Hypertensive encephalopathy

This syndrome consists of a sudden rise in blood pressure, usually preceded by severe headache and followed by generalized seizures, delirium or coma, or cortical blindness, without focal abnormalities (48). The symptoms may last for minutes, hours, or days and usually, but not always, have no sequelae. In a few cases, dementia may follow (48). The encephalopathy may complicate essential hypertension or toxemia of pregnancy. The pathogenic mechanism appears to involve failure of autoregulation of CBF, with forced vasodilation and hyperperfusion. Vascular necrosis and disruption of the blood-brain barrier follow, and cerebral dysfunction results. Blood pressure should be lowered at once to avoid death.

Migraine

Acute confusional migraine (ACM), i.e., migraine accompanied by delirium, occurs mostly in children and adolescents but occasionally also in adults (49–54). It has been observed in 5% of children aged 5 to 16 years suffering from migraine attacks (49). In an occasional case, ACM may be the initial manifestation of migraine and may create diagnostic problems. Headache may not be reported as part of ACM, but typical migraine headaches do develop sooner or later (49). Typically, the patient is agitated, anxious, and combative, as well as disoriented. He or she is often incoherent; unable to answer questions appropriately or obey commands, unable to recognize parents or doctors, pale, tremulous, and dizzy. Blurring of vision and visual hallucinations may occur. An attack of ACM may last for minutes or for a day or so, but its usual duration is several hours. It is usually preceded and accompanied by headache, and is followed by sleep and partial or total amnesia for the whole episode (49–54). The EEG is usually abnormal during the attack and features diffuse delta activity that tends to predominate over the left hemisphere (52). The pathophysiology of ACM is unknown. It has been suggested that a generalized, reversible dysfunction of the brain, involving the basal portion of both temporal lobes and the deep midline structures, may be responsible for the syndrome (52). It is unclear why such dysfunction should occur and be more frequent in children.

Delirious migraine, or migraine delirium, has long been recognized (55,56). Delirium may complicate an intense aura of migraine and, very rarely, may last throughout an entire attack (56). In one study, 8% of patients with severe migraine had delirium in association with an attack (55); in another study, confusion or loss of memory occurred in 6.8% of 500 migraine patients (57). Delirium tends to occur with very severe attacks and may feature visual and auditory hallucinations (55). Very rarely it may last for several days (55,56). Delirious migraine aura may resemble a nightmare (53). The relation of delirious migraine to ACM is unclear: are they the same condition, or do they represent two distinct variants of migraine? Basilar artery migraine may feature confusion. In one study, it was displayed by 32% of the patients (58). Confusion, often associated with agitation, is the most frequently encountered disturbance of consciousness in basilar artery migraine (58).

Migraine as well as cerebrovascular disease may be associated with *transient global amnesia (TGA),* which must be distinguished from delirium (59). The former is defined as rapid onset of the inability to form new memories for more than 15 minutes, but less than 48 hours, with preservation of consciousness (59). The patients are also disoriented for time and place but are said not to exhibit any other cognitive abnormalities (59). The EEG is usually normal (59). These features distinguish TGA from delirium.

Cerebral vasculitis

Vasculitis is a pathological process involving inflammation and necrosis of blood vessels (60). Most of the vasculitides are associated with immunopathogenic mechanisms. CNS dysfunction is a common feature of vasculitic and rheumatologic diseases (60–62). It is often due to damage to organs other than the brain, such as the kidney, rather than to vasculitis per se (62). In some cases, vasculitis is confined to the CNS, as in granulomatous angiitis of the nervous system (62,63). Delirium may be a feature of any vasculitic or rheumatological syndrome that affects the CNS, due either to vasculitis or to some other pathogenic mechanism. Sigal (62) classifies these syndromes into three groups: 1. primary CNS vasculitides; 2. systemic necrotizing vasculitides that often affect the CNS; and 3. rheumatological syndromes associated with CNS disease, due to vasculitis or other mechanisms. A brief review of these syndromes in relation to delirium follows. They are listed in Table 16–2.

PRIMARY CNS VASCULITIDES

Granulomatous angiitis of the nervous system is limited to the CNS. Confusion or "possible psychiatric disorder" is one of its most frequent presenting features and has been observed in 55% of the patients (62).

Cogan syndrome may cause an organic mental syndrome (62).

SYSTEMIC NECROTIZING VASCULITIDES

Cryoglobulinemia may occasionally present with encephalopathy and confusion (64).

TABLE 16–2 Vasculitides Associated With Delirium

A. Primary CNS vasculitides
   1. Granulomatous angiitis of the nervous system
   2. Cogan's syndrome
B. Systemic necrotizing vasculitides
   1. Cryoglobulinemia
   2. Giant-cell arteritis
   3. Lymphomatoid granulomatosis
   4. Polyarteritis nodosa and related conditions
   5. Wegener's granulomatosis
C. Rheumatological syndromes associated with CNS disease
   1. Behçet's syndrome
   2. Mixed connective tissue disease
   3. Progressive systemic sclerosis
   4. Rheumatoid arthritis
   5. Sjögren's syndrome
   6. Systemic lupus erythematosus
D. Miscellaneous multisystem diseases
   1. Thrombotic thrombocytopenic purpura
   2. Sarcoidosis
   3. Relapsing polychondritis
   4. Ulcerative colitis

Giant-cell arteritis comprises temporal arteritis (TA) and Takayasu's arteritis (aortic arch syndrome, pulseless disease) (61). The former is a systemic panarteritis that may affect cranial vessels, notably the temporal artery, as well as other branches of the external carotid and internal carotid arteries. It usually affects the elderly and is a common rheumatic disease in this age group (60–62,65–67). Takayasu's arteritis typically involves the aortic arch and its branches. Giant-cell arteritis is said to involve the CNS in 10% of patients (62). Headache, fatigue, malaise, fever, weight, loss, and depression are the usual nonspecific initial symptoms (60–62,65–67,68,69). Some authors claim that depression is the most common presenting feature in the prodromal phase of the disease (69). Confusion was found in 4 of 35 patients with TA in one study (60) but in only 1 of 60 patients in another (66). By contrast, some earlier writers stated that mental symptoms are common in TA, especially in patients aged 70 years and older, and may include confusion (67,69). These authors point out that such symptoms may be the main form of presentation of TA in some patients and may lead to diagnostic errors. One writer claims that confusion may dominate the clinical picture and may resolve with steroid treatment (70). Despite these discrepancies in the reported frequency of an acute confusional state in TA, there is little doubt that it does occur. Its occurrence in the presence of polymyalgia rheumatica, headache, visual disturbances (amaurosis fugax, diplopia, visual hallucinations), difficulty in swallowing, and tender temporal arteries in a patient over 50 years of age should always suggest TA. Early diagnosis is essential if treatment with prednisone is to be instituted and loss of vision prevented.

Lymphomatoid granulomatosis involves the CNS in about 20% to 30% of cases and may feature confusion (62).

Polyarteritis nodosa and related conditions (hypersensitivity or allergic angiitis, vasculitis associated with methamphetamine abuse) affect the CNS in about 20% to 40% of patients (62). Headache, seizures, blurred vision, hemiparesis, ataxia, vertigo, aphasia, and confusion are among the manifestations of CNS involvement (62–64,71,72). Mental symptoms are among the most common presenting features (61,71,72) and are caused by vasculitis. The encephalopathy usually has an insidious onset but can appear in a single day, accompanied by hypertension that can exacerbate the symptoms of cerebral ischemia (61). An organic toxic psychosis with confusion and disorientation (presumably delirium) was observed in 23% of patients in one large series, and dementia was found in about 6% of them (71). The EEG is usually abnormal, showing diffuse or focal abnormalities (71).

Wegener's granulomatosis features lesions of the respiratory tract, sinuses, arteries, and kidneys. CNS involvement is said to occur in 25% to 50% of patients (62). Either granulomatous lesions or vasculitis of the CNS may be present. Confusion may occur (61,73) but its frequency is unknown.

RHEUMATOLOGICAL SYNDROMES ASSOCIATED WITH CNS DISEASE

Behçet's syndrome (disease) involves the CNS in 10% to 30% of cases (62). "Mental disturbance" has been reported in about 60% of patients with neuro-Behçet's syndrome (74) and "clouded consciousness" in 25% (75). Psychiatric disorders can be quite prominent in this disease (76).

Mixed connective tissue disease affects the CNS in 10% to 40% of patients (62). In one study, more than one-half of 20 patients had neuropsychiatric problems, and 3 of them displayed paranoid delusions (77). These patients tend to present with aseptic meningitis and may become delirious (77).

Progressive systemic sclerosis rarely affects the CNS (62,78–80). I have found only one report of delirium apparently due to it (80). The syndrome may complicate it, however, as a consequence of renal involvement, for example.

Rheumatoid arthritis (RA), or rather rheumatoid disease, a systemic disease associated with RA, may rarely feature cerebral vasculitis with neuropsychiatric manifestations including delirium (81–85). In the handful of cases reported in the literature by 1984, "abnormal mentation" or "alterations in the level of consciousness" were the most frequent feature of RA-associated cerebral vasculitis (81). Two of the reported patients presented with typical delirium (84). Cerebral vasculitis rarely complicates juvenile RA (82). Seizures, meningismus, drowsiness, irritability, and diffusely abnormal EEG are among its features; delirium is not mentioned, but its occurence has been implied (82).

Primary Sjögren's syndrome, it was once thought, is rarely associated with CNS disease, but recent reports indicate that this is not the case (86,87). For example, a frequent extraglandular manifestation of the sicca syndrome is cutaneous vasculitis, which is associated with either peripheral or CNS disease, or both, in about two-thirds of the patients (87). Psychiatric disturbances are commonly observed, including encephalopathy and dementia, as well as what appear to be organic affective disorders (87). Almost one-half of these patients have EEG abnormalities. Moreover, aseptic meningoencephalitis can complicate Sjögren's syndrome and give rise to delirium (86).

Systemic lupus erythematosus (SLE) is often associated with neuropsychiatric complications, which occur in 25% to 75% of patients (62). Delirium is mentioned in this context in the earliest classic papers on this disease, those by Kaposi (88) and Osler (89). The former mentions nocturnal delirium in two of his patients; the latter writes that "at the height of the attack delirium may occur." One of his patients had recurrent febrile episodes accompanied by delirium and hallucinations of "all sorts of things." As Johnson and Richardson (90) put it, "If the confusional state accompanying fever and the anxiety or despondency accompanying any chronic debilitating disease are included, certainly almost all patients with SLE would be found to have disorders of mental function" (p 351).

The frequency and nature of the mental disorders developing in the course of SLE have been a subject of controversy and confusion, however. Fessel and Solomon (91) reviewed the literature up to 1960 and found 272 reported cases of psychosis with SLE over a period of 60 years. The average incidence of the psychosis among these patients was 22%; one in four cases was thought to be due to steroid therapy. Several types of psychosis are mentioned in those early publications: organic, schizoaffective, schizophrenic, and depressive. A review of 10 studies published between 1964 and 1976 reveals an average incidence of neuropsychiatric manifestations of exactly 50%; a more recent review gives their frequency as 60% (92). The nature of the reported mental diorders in SLE varies from author to author and reflects his or her diagnostic orientation. For example, O'Connor and Musher (93) studied 150 patients with SLE, 90 of whom displayed symptoms of CNS involvement and two-thirds of whom had been diagnosed as having delirium. Johnson and Richardson (90) asserted that delirium, with delusions, hallucinations and hyperactivity, is "remarkably frequent" in SLE, more so than in other systemic diseases. Heine (94) reviewed some of the relevant studies and found that four different investigators found the incidence of organic-toxic psychoses (presumably delirium) to be about 30%. A recent study found an overall prevalence of cognitive impairment of 66% in a sample of female patients with SLE (95). This impairment was demonstrated in patients with either inactive or absent neuropsychiatric symptoms, suggesting subclinical CNS involvement. Delirium has been observed in children and adolescents suffering from SLE (96).

One may conclude that while the quality and consistency of published reports on the incidence and nature of mental disorders in SLE vary greatly and leave much to be desired, at least every second patient suffering from it is likely to have one or more episodes of psychiatric illness at some stage of the disease. Delirium seems to be one of the most common mental disorders encountered in SLE, with an estimated incidence of 20% to 30%. This implies that the syndrome accounts for some 30% to 60% of diagnosable psychiatric disorders among SLE patients. Dementia appears to be much less common. The published reports make it clear that a wide range of psychiatric syndromes, both organic and functional and both psychotic and nonpsychotic, can occur in the course of SLE even in the same patient (90–98). A marked variability in clinical features, observed both cross-sectionally and longitudinally, is a hallmark of the psychopathology associated with SLE. A review of the substantial literature on this subject is outside the focus of this book.

Delirium may occur at any stage in the development of SLE but appears to come on more frequently in its early phases, usually within the first year.

The syndrome may also mark a terminal stage of the disease (94). On the whole, delirium tends to occur during acute exacerbations of SLE (99). Delirious episodes are usually relatively brief, ranging from a few hours to several days or even weeks. Delirium is often modified in its clinical appearance by affective, mostly depressive, or schizophrenia-like features (100). A wide range of neurological symptoms, such as seizures, cerebellar signs, and long tract involvement, may accompany it, but some patients fail to exhibit concomitant neurological deficits (101). Association with seizures is particularly common. Fever is often present and probably contributes to the onset of delirium. Hypertension and renal disease are found significantly more often in SLE patients with an organic mental disorder (94). Some writers assert that neuropsychiatric complications have a significantly higher association with vasculitis and thrombocytopenia (101), while others claim that the development of psychosis in an SLE patient cannot be reliably related to the involvement of another organ system or to any single laboratory finding (93).

Pathogenesis of delirium and other psychiatric manifestations in the course of SLE has been the subject of much debate and remains unclear. The following factors have been implicated:

1. Cerebral vasculitis and microvascular injury (92)
2. Antineuronal antibodies (102,103)
3. Antiribosomal P protein autoantibodies (104)
4. Humoral factors (92)

In addition, uremia, hypertension, infection, fever, and treatment with drugs, such as corticosteroids and antimalarials, can give rise to delirium.

A number of *diagnostic techniques* have been used in neuropsychiatric SLE. They include the EEG, radionuclide brain scans, computed tomography, PET, and magnetic resonance imaging (92). Some authors have found the EEG to be consistently abnormal, showing diffuse slow-wave activity and focal changes (101). Finn and Rudolf (105) report that the EEG is abnormal in all patients with psychiatric symptoms at the time of the tracing. This is valuable for assessment of the progress of SLE and helpful in distinguishing psychosis due to cerebral lupus from that caused by steroids. By contrast, Johnson and Richardson (90) assert that the EEG findings are of little diagnostic and localizing value. Bilateral diffuse slowing has been the most consistent finding in CNS SLE. This is noteworthy, since such slowing is an expected concomitant of delirium due to many different causes.

Radionuclide brain scans have given results no more consistent than those of the EEG (92). ^{15}O brain scanning has been claimed to reveal active cerebral SLE in most patients (106). In a series of 47 patients with active SLE, the scanning revealed abnormalities in 47 of 51 episodes. Ten of the patients with an abnormal ^{15}O scan had no concurrent neuropsychiatric symptoms, however. The investigators suggest that abnormalities of cerebral metabolism and blood flow revealed by the scans indicate that the brain may be involved more often in the disease process than the clinical findings suggest. CBF, using the ^{133}Xe method, has been found to be depressed during exacerbation of CNS SLE (107).

Computed tomography has been claimed to be useful in classifying clinically apparent CNS involvement and hence in establishing the prognosis (108). However, the tomogram was normal in some patients with an organic brain syndrome while showing atrophy in others (108). Other investigators have failed to find a correlation between the degree of atrophy and the presence or absence of neuropsychiatric symptoms (92). Computed tomography scanning appears to be a nonspecific means of evaluating CNS SLE (92).

PET has only begun to be used in the study of SLE. It may help to detect cerebral vaculitis even before the onset of neurological symptoms (92). Finally, magnetic resonance imaging has shown inconclusive results so far in detecting disease activity or the extent of brain involvement in CNS SLE (92). No diagnostic technique applied to date has been found to be consistently useful in the diagnosis of neuropsychiatric SLE. Moreover, no study published so far has focused specifically on delirium.

Treatment of delirium in the course of SLE involves management of the underlying condition and the symptoms. Discussion of the former is beyond the scope of this book and is reviewed elsewhere (92). Symptomatic treatment should follow the guidelines discussed in Chapter 10. Some authors warn that all the neurotropics, including haloperidol, may decrease the seizure threshold in patients with CNS SLE and are best avoided (92). They recommend the use of benzodiazepines instead, provided that the psychiatric disorder is mild. However, haloperidol has a slight tendency to lower the seizure threshold, and can be used if the patient is delirious and agitated (109).

MISCELLANEOUS MULTISYSTEM DISEASES

Several diseases that can give rise to CNS involvement and delirium should be mentioned.

Thrombotic thrombocytopenic purpura may present with delirium as the first manifestation in about one-third of the patients (110). There is probably occlusion of small vessels, as well as small infarcts and petechial hemorrhages occurring diffusely in the gray matter. About one-third of the patients presenting with an organic brain syndrome are reported to improve (110). The disease may involve the CNS in the absence of other findings, although in most cases one finds thrombocytopenia, microangiopathic hemolytic anemia, and purpura (111).

Sarcoidosis of the CNS is relatively uncommon, occurring in about 5% of cases (112). Both delirium and dementia have been reported to occur (112–119). On occasion, delirium may be a presenting manifestation (114,117,119). Both structural and metabolic changes may account for it. Space-occupying granulomas, aseptic meningitis with increased intracranial pressure, and vasculopathy are among the structural causes. Of the metabolic abnormalities, hypothalamus involvement with diabetes insipidus and other neuroendocrinological abnormalities, hypercalcemia, hepatic encephalopathy, uremia, and pulmonary insufficiency are all potential causes of delirium in this disease (114). Some writers assert that the syndrome may be secondary to diffuse parenchymal inflammation, as suggested by the computed tomography scan (116). Generalized and partial seizures can occur in neurosarcoidosis, followed by delirium. Steroids used for the treatment of pulmonary sarcoidosis have been implicated in concurrent psychiatric disorders in about 4% of treated patients (120). Treatment with steroids, however, may bring about a dramatic improvement in the mental status of patients with cerebral sarcoidosis (114).

Relapsing polychondritis, with aseptic meningitis and cerebral vasculitis, may feature delirium (121,122).

Ulcerative colitis may occasionally be associated with cerebral vasculitis and delirium (123).

Multifocal cerebral ischemia and organic mental disorders may result from several diseases of the blood.

Recurrent delirium has been reported in *mixed cryoglobulinemia* (124). Delirium may also occur in *hyperviscosity syndrome,* most often associated with macroglobulinemia and, less often, with multiple myeloma (125). *Polycythemia vera* may feature mental disorders, most often delirium, in about 40% of patients (126). *Disseminated intravascular coagulation* can rarely give rise to cerebral dysfunction and delirium (127).

Cardiovascular disorders

Cardiovascular, especially cardiac, disorders represent a major class of organic causes of delirium. They can bring it about as a result of an acute reduction of cerebral perfusion and a consequent decrease in brain oxygen

TABLE 16–3 Cardiovascular Disorders Causing Delirium

Cardiac arrhythmias
Endocarditis
Heart failure
Malignant hypertension
Myocardial infarction
Pulmonary embolism

consumption and oxidative metabolism. Impaired cognitive function and delirium can follow cerebral ischemia-hypoxia brought about by some of these disorders, notably in an older individual or one suffering from chronic brain disease or damage, or both. In some cases, thromboembolic phenomena and multifocal cerebral ischemia may be the pathogenic mechanisms leading to delirium. The more common cardiovascular disorders that may give rise to the syndrome are listed in Table 16–3, and their discussion follows.

Cardiac arrhythmias

Sudden interference with normal heart rhythm, and hence function, may result in diffuse cerebral ischemia-hypoxia and an acute confusional state (128–135). Reduced cardiac output, decreased carotid blood flow, and diminished cerebral perfusion can all be the consequences of a cardiac dysrhythmia (133). Some authors emphasize that mental confusion and related abnormal behavior are a fairly common presentation of paroxysmal cardiac arrhythmias in the elderly (128). It is essential to diagnose and treat the arrhythmia promptly in order to avoid permanent brain damage and "cardiogenic dementia" (130). Prolonged Holter monitoring has been recommended for patients who are suspected of having transient cerebral dysfunction that may be caused by a cardiac dysrhythmia (133,136). Paroxysmal tachyarrhythmias, intermittent complete heart block, bundle branch block, and severe bradycardia all seem to be capable of inducing an acute confusional state, especially in an elderly patient (128–135). Dizziness, syncope, and seizures are more common manifestations of these arrhythmias, however, than is confusion. Patients suffering from an abnormally slow heart rate due to an acquired complete heart block may show improvement in cognitive functioning after implantation of an artificial pacemaker (131,132,137).

Endocarditis

Both infective and nonbacterial thrombotic endocarditis may feature delirium. The former is discussed in Chapter 15. In one series of 99 patients with nonbacterial thrombotic endocarditis examined at autopsy, mental confusion had been the initial manifestation of the disease in 8% (138). Embolism involving the CNS was found in one-third of the patients, and malignant neoplasms were found in about 40% of the autopsies.

Heart failure

A study of the etiological factors in acute confusional states in patients aged 60 years and older admitted to a general medical unit found that heart failure was the second most common factor, accounting for about 20% of the cases (139). Over 50 years ago, Michael (140) drew attention to "psychosis with cardiac decompensation." That psychosis was actually delirium and was observed in about 1% of a large series of patients with heart failure of various etiologies. Eisenberg et al. (141) studied patients with severe congestive heart failure who showed "mental aberrations" or "mental confusion." Six of these patients had alternating states of confusion and lucidity, and thus appear to have suffered from episodes of delirium. As a group, the confused patients showed a profound reduction in cerebral perfusion and a decrease in cerebral oxygen consumption. The mean CBF was 26 ml/min/100 g, and cerebral oxygen consumption was 2.71 ml/min/100 g. The six patients with episodes of mental confusion were studied both while confused and while lucid. While confused, they showed a significant decrease in CBF, an increase in cerebral vascular resistance, and a decrease in both cerebral O_2 consumption and arterial CO_2 content. Investigators observe that the onset of mental confusion in patients with advanced congestive heart failure has grave prognostic implications, often heralding deterioration of the physical condition and death. As the prevalence of heart failure rises sharply after the age of 65 years, it is not surprising that this cardiac disorder represents a major organic cause of delirium in later life.

Malignant hypertension

This disorder and the related hypertensive encephalopathy are discussed in the first part of this chapter.

Myocardial infarction

Delirium may follow myocardial infarction (MI), especially in an elderly patient (142–147). In one large series, MI was followed by delirium in 6.6% of the patients and, predictably, it was more common among those aged 60 years and older (142). It occurred on the third or fourth day after the MI and lasted for 2 to 5 days. It is noteworthy that 37% of the delirious patients died, indicating that delirium associated with an acute MI is a grave prognostic sign. Nearly one-half of the patients in this study had abused alcohol; this may have contributed both to cardiac complications and to delirium.

The clinical presentation of MI in elderly patients has attracted much attention in recent years (143–146). One study of 777 elderly hospitalized patients with an acute MI found that 6.8% of them presented with "acute confusion" (144). The incidence of the syndrome increased with the age of the patient and was highest (about 20%) in those aged 85 years and older. The diagnosis of acute MI in the very elderly, those aged 85 years or more, can be difficult and is often delayed because of the atypical presentation (145). Chest pain and dyspnea may not be reported by the patient. By contrast, confusion is a common presenting feature, even though the very elderly may display no greater hemodynamic changes than the younger elderly (145). In a demented elderly patient, the occurrence of an MI indicates that the dementia is more likely to be due to cerebrovascular disease rather than to Alzheimer's disease (147).

Observations from coronary care units give discrepant figures on the frequency of delirium in those settings (148–150). In practical terms, however, what matters most is the fact that some delirious cardiac patients are severely agitated, and adequate sedation may be lifesaving. Haloperidol has been shown to be a safe and effective psychotropic drug in these cases. On some occasions, the drug has been given intravenously in doses of over 100 mg daily without ill effects (151). The starting dose was usually 5 mg and was rapidly increased to single boluses of 30–75 mg (151). In most cases, however, such large doses are not needed to control agitation.

Various factors have been proposed to account for delirium after MI and in coronary care units (see Chapter 6). Cerebral hypoxia in the MI patient may result from cardiac arrhythmias, congestive heart failure, or an episode of severe hypotension. Many drugs used for cardiac patients are potentially deliriogenic and should always be scrutinized if the patient develops delirium (see Chapter 11). Moderate anemia in conjunction with cerebrovascular disease predisposes elderly patients to delirium after MI even in the presence of a relatively unremarkable drop in cardiac output.

Pulmonary embolism

Pulmonary embolism (PE) may lead to a decrease in cardiac output and CBF. Delirium is a frequent feature of PE (152). It may represent the initial acute event or, more usually, may come on after recovery from coma. The patient is typically dyspneic, tachypneic, anxious, and delirious. PE should be considered in any patient who suddenly loses consciousness or becomes delirious with no obvious reason and displays tachypnea. Determination of blood gases and a lung scan are needed to establish the diagnosis. The arterial PO_2 is reduced (less than 80 mm Hg), as is the PCO_2.

References

1. Peters U. H., Gille G.: Über die körperlichen Grunde körperlich begrundbaren Psychosen. *Dtsch. Med. Wochenschr.* 1973;98:967–970.
2. Kopenen H., Hurri L., Stenback U., et al: Acute confusional states in the elderly: A radiological evaluation. *Acta Psychiatr. Scand.* 1987;76:726–731.

3. Millikan C. H., Bauer R. B., Goldschmidt J., et al: A classification and outline of cerebrovascular diseases. *Stroke* 1975;6:564–616.
4. McDowell F. H.: Transient cerebral ischemia: Diagnostic considerations. *Prog. Cardiovasc. Dis.* 1980;22:309–324.
5. Genton E., Barnett H. J. M., Fields W. S., et al: XIV. Cerebral ischemia: The role of thrombosis and of antithrombotic therapy. *Stroke* 1977;8:150–175.
6. Dunne J. W., Leedman P. J., Edis R. H.: Inobvious stroke: A cause of delirium and dementia. *Aust. N. Z. J. Med.* 1986;16:771–778.
7. De Reuck J., Sieben G., De Coster W., et al: Dementia and confusional state in patients with cerebral infarcts. *Eur. Neurol.* 1982;21:94–97.
8. Horenstein S., Chamberlin W., Conomy J.: Infarction of the fusiform and calcarine regions: Agitated delirium and hemianopia. *Trans. Am. Neurol. Assoc.* 1967;92:85–89.
9. Medina J. L., Rubino F. A., Ross E.: Agitated delirium caused by infarctions of the hippocampal formation and fusiform and lingual gyri: A case report. *Neurology* 1974;24:1181–1183.
10. Bogousslavsky J., Ferrazzini M., Regli F., et al: Manic delirium and frontal-like syndrome with paramedian infarction of the right thalamus. *J. Neurol. Neurosurg. Psychiatry* 1988;51:116–119.
11. Devinsky O., Bear D., Volpe B. T.: Confusional states following posterior cerebral artery infarction. *Arch. Neurol.* 1988;45:160–163.
12. Medina J. L., Chokroverty S., Rubino F. A.: Syndrome of agitated delirium and visual impairment: A manifestation of medial temporo-occipital infarction. *J. Neurol. Neurosurg. Psychiatry* 1977;40:861–864.
13. Prendes J. L., Rosenberg S. J.: Rip Van Winkle syndrome: Confusion and irresistible somnolence after stroke. *South. Med. J.* 1986;79:1162–1164.
14. Mori E., Yamadori A.: Acute confusional state and acute agitated delirium. *Arch. Neurol.* 1987;44:1139–1143.
15. Mullaly W., Huff K., Ronthal M., et al: Frequency of acute confusional states with lesions of the right hemisphere. *Ann. Neurol.* 1982;12:113.
16. Schmidley N. W., Messing R. O.: Agitated confusional states in patients with right hemisphere infarctions. *Stroke* 1984;15:883–885.
17. Hass W. K., Goldensohn E. S.: Clinical and electroencephalographic considerations in the diagnosis of carotid artery occlusion. *Neurology* 1959;9:575–579.
18. Hurwitz L. J., Groch S. N., Wrighter I. S., et al: Carotid artery occlusive syndrome. *Arch. Neurol.* 1959;1:491–501.
19. Shapiro S. K.: Psychosis due to bilateral carotid artery occlusion. *Minn. Med.* 1959;42:25–27.
20. Gillespie J. A. (ed.): *Extracranial Cerebrovascular Disease and Its Management.* London, Butterworths, 1969.
21. Price J., Whitlock F. A., Hall R. T.: The psychiatry of vertebrobasilar insufficiency with the report of a case. *Psychiatria Clin.* 1983;16:26–44.
22. Gaenter C. A., Braun T. E.: Fat embolism syndrome. Chest 1981;79:143–145.
23. Jacobson D. M., Terrence C. F., Reinmuth O. M.: The neurologic manifestations of fat embolism. *Neurology* 1986;36:847–851.
24. Adams H. P., Jergenson D. D., Kassell N. F., et al: Pitfalls in the recognition of subarachnoid hemorrhage. *J.A.M.A.* 1980;244:794–796.
25. Sencer W., Andiman R.: A clinical study of intracranial aneurysms. *Mt. Sinai J. Med. N Y.* 1973;40:72–81.

26. Sundt T. M., Whisnant J. P.: Subarachnoid hemorrhage from intracranial aneurysms. *N. Engl. J. Med.* 1978;299:116–122.
27. Okawara S. H.: Warning signs prior to rupture of an intracranial aneurysm. *J. Neurosurg.* 1973;38:575–580.
28. Bornstein R. A., Weir B. K. A., Petruk K. C., et al: Neuropsychological function in patients after subarachnoid hemorrhage. *Neurosurgery* 1987;21:651–654.
29. Waltimo O., Putkonen A. R.: Intellectual performance of patients with intracranial arteriovenous malformations. *Brain* 1974;97:511–520.
30. Carter L. P., Morgan M., Urrea D.: Psychological improvement following arteriovenous malformation excision. *J Neurosurg.* 1975;42:452–456.
31. Dawson D. M., Fischer E. G.: Neurologic complications of cardiac catheterization. *Neurology* 1977;27:496–497.
32. Swanson D. P., Calanchini P. R., Dyken M. L., et al: A cooperative study of hospital frequency and character of transient ischemic attacks. II. Performance of angiography among six centers. *J.A.M.A.* 1977;237:2202–2206.
33. Brust J. C. M.: Dementia and cerebrovascular disease, in Mayeux R., Rosen W. G. (eds): *The Dementias.* New York, Raven Press, 1983, pp 131–147.
34. Cummings J. L.: Multi-infarct dementia: Diagnosis and management. *Psychosomatics* 1987;28:117–126.
35. Hachinski V. C., Lassen N. A., Marshall J.: Multi-infarct dementia. A cause of mental deterioration in the elderly. *Lancet* 1974;2:207–210.
36. Editorial: "Multi-infarct" dementia: A real entity? *J. Am. Geriatr. Soc.* 1986;34:482–484.
37. Liston E. H., La Rue A.: *DSM-III* Diagnosis of multi-infarct dementia. *Compr. Psychiatry* 1986;27:54–59.
38. Erkinjuntti T.: Types of multi-infarct dementia. *Acta Neurol. Scand.* 1987;75:391–399.
39. Meyer J. S., Rogers R. L., Judd B. W., et al: Cognition and cerebral blood flow fluctuate together in multi-infarct dementia. *Stroke* 1988;19:163–169.
40. Kinkle W. R., Jacobs L., Polachini I., et al: Subcortical arteriosclerotic encephalopathy (Binswanger's disease). *Arch Neurol.* 1985;42:951–959.
41. Burger P. C., Burch J. G., Junze E.: Subcortical arteriosclerotic encephalopathy (Binswanger's disease). *Stroke* 1976;7:626–631.
42. Black D. W.: Mental changes from subdural hematoma. *Br. J. Psychiatry* 1984;142:200–203.
43. Cameron M. M.: Chronic subdural haematoma: A review of 114 cases. *J. Neurol Neurosurg. Psychiatry* 1978;41:834–839.
44. Fogelholm R., Heiskanen O., Waltimo O.: Chronic subdural hematoma in adults. *J. Neurosurg.* 1975;42:43–46.
45. Potter J. F., Fruin A. H.: Chronic subdural hematoma—the "great imitator." *Geriatrics* 1977;32:61–66.
46. Raskind R., Glover B., Weiss S. R.: Chronic subdural hematoma in the elderly: A challenge in diagnosis and treatment. *J. Am. Geriatr. Soc.* 1975;20:330–334.
47. Vicario S., Danzi D., Thomas D. M.: Emergency presentation of subdural hematoma: A review of 85 cases diagnosed by computed tomography. *Ann. Emerg. Med.* 1982;11:475–477.
48. Healton E. B., Brust J. C., Feinfold D. A., et al: Hypertensive encephalopathy and the neurologic manifestations of malignant hypertension. *Neurology* 1982;32:127–132.

49. Ehyai A., Fenichel G. M.: The natural history of acute confusional migraine. *Arch. Neurol.* 1978;35:368–369.
50. Emery E. S.: Acute confusional state in children with migraine. *Pediatrics* 1977;60:110–114.
51. Gascon G., Barlow C.: Juvenile migraine, presenting as an acute confusional state. *Pediatrics* 1970;45:628–635.
52. Pietrini V., Terzano M. G., D'Andrea G., et al: Acute confusional migraine: Clinical and electroencephalographic aspects. *Cephalalgia* 1987;7:29–37.
53. Sacquegna T., Cortelli P., Baldrati A., et al: Impairment of consciousness and memory in migraine: A review. *Headache* 1987;27:30–33.
54. Tinuper P., Cortelli P., Sacquegna T., et al: Classic migraine attack complicated by confusional state: EEG and CT study. *Cephalalgia* 1985;5:63–68.
55. Klee A.: *A Clinical Study of Migraine with Particular Reference to the Most Severe Cases.* Copenhagen, Munksgaard, 1968.
56. Sacks O. W.: *Migraine. The Evolution of a Common Disorder.* Berkeley, University of California Press, 1970.
57. Lance J. W., Anthony M.: Some clinical aspects of migraine. *Arch. Neurol.* 1966;15:356–361.
58. Sturzenegger M. H., Meienberg O.: Basilar artery migraine: A follow-up study of 82 cases. *Headache* 1985;25:408–415.
59. Miller J. W., Petersen R. C., Metter E. J., et al: Transient global amnesia: Clinical characteristics and prognosis. *Neurology* 1987;37:733–737.
60. Cohen S. B., Hurd E. R.: Neurological complications of connective tissue and other "collagen-vascular" diseases. *Semin. Arthritis Rheum.* 1981;11:190–212.
61. Moore P. M., Cupps T. R.: Neurological complications of vasculitis. *Ann. Neurol.* 1983;14:155–167.
62. Sigal L. H.: The neurologic presentation of vasculitic and rheumatologic syndromes. A review. *Medicine* 1987;66:157–180.
63. Sabharwal U. K., Keogh L. H., Weisman M. H., et al: Granulomatous angiitis of the nervous system: Case report and review of the literature. *Arthritis Rheum.* 1982;25:342–345.
64. Reik L., Korn J. H.: Cryoglobulinemia with encephalopathy: Successful treatment by plasma exchange. *Ann. Neurol.* 1981;10:488–490.
65. Allen N. B., Studenski S. A.: Polymyalgia rheumatica and temporal arteritis. *Med. Clin. North Am.* 1986;70:360–384.
66. Huston K. A., Hunder G. G.: Giant cell (cranial) arteritis: A clinical review. *Am. Heart J.* 1980;100:99–107.
67. Paulley J. W., Hughes J. P.: Giant-cell arteritis, or arteritis of the aged. *Br. Med. J.* 1960;2:1562–1567.
68. Cochran J. W., Fox J. H., Kelly M. P.: Reversible mental symptoms in temporal arteritis. *J. Nerv. Ment. Dis.* 1978;166:446–447.
69. Vereker R.: The psychiatric aspects of temporal arteritis. *J. Ment. Sci.* 1952;98:280–286.
70. Andrews J. M.: Giant-cell ("temporal") arteritis. *Neurology* 1966;16:963–971.
71. Ford R. G., Siekert R. G.: Central nervous system manifestations of periarteritis nodosa. *Neurology* 1965;15:114–122.
72. Gottwald W.: Die neurologisch-psychiatrischen und muskularen manifestationen der Vasculitis nodosa. *Fortschr. Neurol. Psychiatr.* 1977;45:475–483.
73. Delaney J. F.: Psychologic and neurologic manifestations of systemic Wegener's granulomatosis. *Psychosomatics* 1973;14:341–343.

74. Motomura S., Tabira T., Kuroiwa Y.: A clinical comparative study of multiple sclerosis and neuro-Behçet's syndrome. *J. Neurol. Neurosurgy. Psychiatry* 1980;43:210–213.
75. Shimizu T., Ehrlich G. E., Inaba G., et al: Behçet disease (Behçet syndrome). *Semin. Arthritis Rheum.* 1979;8:223–260.
76. Epstein R. S., Cummings N., Sherwood E. B., et al: Psychiatric aspects of Behçet's syndrome. *J. Psychosom. Res.* 1970;14:161–172.
77. Bennett R. M., Spargo B. H.: Neuropsychiatric problems in mixed connective tissue disease. *Am. J. Med.* 1978;65:955–962.
78. Gulledge A. D.: Scleroderma. *J. Kans. Med. Soc.* 1968;69:593–596.
79. Lee P., Bruni J., Sukenik S.: Neurological manifestations in systemic sclerosis (scleroderma). *J. Rheumatol.* 1984;11:480–483.
80. Wise T. N., Ginzler E. M.: Scleroderma cerebritis, an unusual manifestation of progressive systemic sclerosis. *Dis. Nerv. Syst.* 1975;36:60–62.
81. Gobernado J. M., Leiva C., Rabano J., et al: Recovery from rhematoid cerebral vasculitis. *J. Neurol. Neurosurg. Psychiatry* 1984;47:410–413.
82. Jan J. E., Hill R. H., Low M. D.: Cerebral complications in juvenile rheumatoid arthritis. *Can. Med. Assoc. J.* 1972;107:623–625.
83. Kim R. C.: Rheumatoid disease with encephalopathy. *Ann. Neurol.* 1980;7:86–91.
84. Siomopoulos V., Shah N.: Acute organic brain syndrome associated with rheumatoid arthritis. *J. Clin. Psychiatry* 1979;40:46–48.
85. Skowronski T., Gatter R. A.: Cerebral vasculitis associated with rheumatoid disease—a case report. *J. Rheumatol.* 1974;1:473–475.
86. Alexander E. L., Alexander G. E.: Aseptic meningoencephalitis in primary Sjögren's syndrome. *Neurology* 1983;33:593–598.
87. Alexander E., Provost T. T.: Sjögren's syndrome. *Arch. Dermatol.* 1987;12:801–810.
88. Kaposi (Moriz Kohn): Kenntniss des Lupus erythematosus. *Arch. Dermatol. Syph.* 1872;4:36–78.
89. Osler W.: On the visceral complications of erythema exudativum multiforme. *Am. J. Med. Sci.* 1895;110:629–646.
90. Johnson R. T., Richardson E. P.: The neurological manifestations of systemic lupus erythematosus. *Medicine* 1968:47:337–369.
91. Fessel W. J., Solomon G. F.: Psychosis and systemic lupus erythematosus. *Calif. Med.* 1960;92:266–270.
92. Adelman D. C., Saltiel E., Klinenberg J. R.: The neuropsychiatric manifestations of systemic lupus erythematosus; An overview. *Semin. Arthritis Rheum.* 1986;15:185–199.
93. O'Connor J. F., Musher D. M.: Central nervous system involvement in systemic lupus erythematosus. *Arch. Neurol.* 1966;14:157–164.
94. Heine B. E.: Psychiatric aspects of systemic lupus erythematosus. *Acta Psychiatr. Scand.* 1969;45:307–326.
95. Carbotte R. M., Denburg S. D., Denburg J. A.: Prevalence of cognitive impairment in systemic lupus erythematosus. *J. Nerv. Ment. Dis.* 1986;174:357–364.
96. Silber T. J., Chatoon I., White P. H.: Psychiatric manifestations of systemic lupus erythematosus in children and adolescents. *Clin. Pediatr.* 1984;23:331–335.
97. Kremer J. M., Rynes R. I., Bartholomew L. E., et al: Non-organic non-psychotic psychopathology (NONPP) in patients with systemic lupus erythematosus. *Semin. Arthritis Rheum.* 1981;11:182–189.

98. Liang M. H., Rogers M., Larson M., et al: The psychosocial impact of systemic lupus erythematosus and rheumatoid arthritis. *Arthritis Rheum.* 1984;27:13–19.
99. Bennahum D. A., Messner R. P.: Recent observations on central nervous system lupus erythematosus. *Semin. Arthritis Rheum.* 1975;4:253–266.
100. Ganz V. H., Gurland B. J., Deming W. E., et al: The study of the psychiatric symptoms of systemic lupus erythematosus. *Psychosom. Med.* 1972;34:207–220.
101. Feinglass E. J., Arnett F. C., Dorrsch C. A., et al: Neuropsychiatric manifestations of systemic lupus erythematosus: Diagnosis, clinical spectrum, and relationship to other features of the disease. *Medicine* 1976;55:323–339.
102. Denberg J. A., Carbotte R. M., Denburg S. D.: Neuronal antibodies and cognitive function in systemic lupus erythematosus. *Neurology* 1987;37:464–467.
103. How A., Dent P. B., Liao S. K., et al: Antineuronal antibodies in neuropsychiatric systemic lupus erythematosus. *Arthritis Rheum.* 1985;28:789–795.
104. Bonfa E., Golombek S. J., Kaufman L. D., et al: Association between lupus psychosis and anti-ribosomal P protein antibodies. *N. Engl. J. Med.* 1987;317:265–271.
105. Finn R., Rudolf N. de M.: The electroencephalogram in systemic lupus erythematosus. *Lancet* 1978;1:1255.
106. Pinching A. J., Travers R. L., Hughes G. R. V., et al: Oxygen-15 brain scanning for detection of cerebral involvement in systemic lupus erythematosus. *Lancet* 1978;1:898–900.
107. Kushner M. J., Chawluk J., Faze-Kas F., et al: Cerebral blood flow in systemic lupus erythematosus with or without cerebral complications. *Neurology* 1987;37:1596–1598.
108. Kaell A. T., Shetty M., Lee B. C. P., et al: Systemic lupus erythematosus. *Arch. Neurol.* 1986;43:273–276.
109. Settle E. C., Ayd F. J.: Haloperidol: A quarter century of experience. *J. Clin. Psychiatry* 1983;44:440–448.
110. Silverstein A.: Thromotic thrombocytopenic purpura. *Arch. Neurol.* 1968;18:358–362.
111. Ridolfi R. L., Bell W. R.: Thrombotic thrombocytopenic purpura. *Medicine* 1981;60:413–428.
112. Oksanen V.: Neurosarcoidosis: Clinical presentations and course in 50 patients. *Acta Neurol. Scand.* 1986;73:283–290.
113. Cahill D. W., Saleman M.: Neurosarcoidosis: A review of the rarer manifestations. *Surg. Neurol.* 1981;15:204–211.
114. Delaney P.: Neurologic manifestations in sarcoidosis. *Ann. Intern. Med.* 1977;87:336–345.
115. Jefferson M.: Sarcoidosis of the nervous system. *Brain* 1957;80:540–556.
116. Stern B. J., Krumholz A., Johns C., et al: Sarcoidosis and its neurological manifestations. *Arch. Neurol.* 1985;42:909–917.
117. Stoudemire A., Linfors E., Houpt J. L.: Central nervous system sarcoidosis. *Gen. Hosp. Psychiatry* 1983;5:129–132.
118. Waxman J. S., Sher J. H.: The spectrum of central nervous system sarcoidosis. A clinical and pathologic study. *Mt. Sinai J. Med.* 1979;46:309–317.
119. Widerholt W. C., Siekert R. G.: Neurological manifestations of sarcoidosis. *Neurology* 1965;15:1147–1154.
120. Johns C. J., Zachary J. B., Ball W. C.: A ten-year study of corticosteroid treatment of pulmonary sarcoidosis. *Johns Hopkins Med. J.* 1974;134:271–283.

121. Stewart S. S., Ashizawa T., Dudley A. W., et al: Cerebral vasculitis in relapsing polychondritis. *Neurology* 1988;38:150–152.
122. Sundaran M. B. M., Rajput A. H.: Nervous system complications of relpasing polychondritis. *Neurology* 1983;33:513–515.
123. Nelson J., Barrow M. M., Riggs J. E., et al: Cerebral vasculitis and ulcerative colitis. *Neurology* 1986;36:719–721.
124. Abramsky O., Slavin S.: Neurologic manifestations in patients with mixed cryoglobulinemia. *Neurology* 1974;24:245–249.
125. Plum F., Posner J. B.: *Diagnosis of Stupor and Coma,* ed 2. Philadelphia, FA Davis Co., 1972.
126. Calabresi P., Meyer O. O.: Polycythemia vera. Clinical and laboratory manifesations. *Ann. Intern. Med.* 1958;50:118–120.
127. Schwartzman R. J., Hill J. B.: Neurologic complications of disseminated intravascular coagulation. *Neurology* 1982;32:791–797.
128. Clark A. N. G.: Ectopic tachycardias in the elderly. *Gerontol. Clin.* 1970;12:203–212.
129. Cole S. L., Sugerman J. N.: Cerebral manifestations of acute myocardial infarction. *Am. J. Med. Sci.* 1952;223:35–40.
130. Editorial: Cardiogenic dementia. *Lancet* 1977;1:27–28.
131. Lagergren K.: Effect of exogenous changes in heart rate upon mental performance in patients treated with artificial pacemakers for complete heart block. *Br. Heart. J.* 1974;36:1126–1132.
132. Lavy S., Stern S.: Transient neurological manifestations in cardiac arrhythmias. *J. Neurol. Sci.* 1969;9:97–102.
133. Sand B. J., Rose H. B., Barker W. F.: Effect of cardiac dysrhythmia on cerebral perfusion. *Arch. Surg.* 1976;111:787–791.
134. Scheinman M., Weiss A., Kunkel F.: His bundle recordings in patients with bundle branch block and transient neurologic symptoms. *Circulation* 1973,48:322–330.
135. Van Durme J. P.: Tachyarrhythmias and transient cerebral ischemic attacks. *Am. Heart J.* 1975;89:538–540.
136. Luxon L. M., Crowther A., Harrison M. J. G., et al: Controlled study of 24-hour ambulatory electrocardiographic monitoring in patients with transient neurological symptoms. *J. Neurol. Neurosurg. Psychiatry* 1980;43:37–41.
137. Dalessio D. J., Benchimol A., Dimond E. G.: Chronic encephalopathy related to heart block. *Neurology* 1965;15:499–503.
138. Biller J., Challa V. R., Toole J. F., et al: Nonbacterial thrombotic endocarditis. *Arch. Neurol.* 1982;39:95–98.
139. Flint F. J., Richards S. M.: Organic basis of confusional states in the elderly. *Br. Med. J.* 1956;2:1537–1539.
140. Michael J. C.: Psychosis with cardiac decompensation. *Am. J. Psychiatry* 1937;93:1353–1362.
141. Eisenberg S., Madison L., Sensenbach W.: Cerebral hemodynamic and metabolic studies in patients with congestive heart failure. II. Observations in confused subjects. *Circulation* 1960;21:704–709.
142. Trubnikov G. V., Zorina Z. N.: Acute psychoses in myocardial infarction. *Kardiologia* 1973;13:76–81.
143. Applegate W. B., Graves S., Collins T., et al: Acute myocardial infarction in elderly patients. *South. Med. J.* 1984;77:1127–1129.

144. Bayer A. J., Chadha J., Farag R. R., et al: Changing presentation of myocardial infarction with increasing age. *J. Am. Geriatr. Soc.* 1986;34:263–266.
145. Day J. J., Bayer A. J., Pathy M. S. J.: Acute myocardial infarction: Diagnostic difficulties and outcome in advanced age. *Age Ageing* 1987;16:239–243.
146. Editorial: Presentation of myocardial infarction in the elderly. *Lancet* 1986;2:1077–1078.
147. Hontela S., Schwartz G.: Myocardial infarction in the differential diagnosis of dementias in the elderly. *J. Am. Geriatr. Soc.* 1979;27:104–106.
148. Cay E. L., Vetter N., Philip A. E., et al: Psychological reactions to a coronary care unit. *J. Psychosom. Res.* 1972;16:437–447.
149. Hackett T. P., Cassem N. H., Wishnie H. A.: The coronary-care unit. *N. Engl. J. Med.* 1968;279:1365–1370.
150. Parker D. L., Hodge J. R.: Delirium in a coronoary care unit. *J.A.M.A.* 1967;201:702–703.
151. Tesar G. E., Murray G. B., Cassem N. H.: Use of high-dose intravenous haloperidol in the treatment of agitated cardiac patients. *J. Clin. Psychopharmacol.* 1985;5:344–347.
152. Sharma G. V. R. K., Sasahara A. A.: Diagnosis and treatment of pulmonary embolism. *Med. Clin. North Am.* 1979;63:239–250.

17

Head Injury, Epilepsy, and Brain Tumor

This chapter deals with delirium caused by or associated with three major classes of primary disorders of the brain. Some primary intracranial diseases are discussed in other chapters to which they logically belong, for example, infectious and vascular diseases. Delirium due to primary cerebral disease does not differ in its clinical features from that caused by systemic diseases secondarily affecting the brain.

Head injury

Traumatic head injuries from all causes exceed 1 million new cases in the United States annually (1). The persons most frequently injured are males between 15 and 24 years of age, and many of the injuries are associated with alcohol (2). Closed head injury has become the most common serious neurological disorder in America (2). Severe head injuries, followed by coma lasting for 6 hours or longer, are much less common than mild ones but have a mortality rate of 50% (3). Given these statistics, one can tentatively conclude that head injury represents one of the major causes of delirium in younger adults.

Head injuries have been classified into three types: blunt, sharp, and compression (4). Blunt injuries are further subdivided into deceleration and acceleration. They are the most common types of head injury in peacetime and give rise to concussion or diffuse generalized brain injury upon which may be superimposed focal brain damage in an area distant from the site of impact. "Cerebral concussion" has been defined as the reversible or irreversible disruption of neural function by trauma occurring in a diffuse, symmetrical manner throughout the brain (4). The term comprises a graded set of clinical syndromes that follow head trauma and involve a disturbance in the level and content of consciousness of increasing severity. Such disturbance is believed to be caused by mechanically induced strains acting on the brain in a centripetal sequence. That is, in the mild cases the effects occur at the surface of the brain; with increasing severity, they extend inward to involve the diencephalic and mesencephalic areas (5). Recent studies employing magnetic resonance imaging have found cortical lesions even in patients who had not lost consciousness (6).

Confusion and disturbances of memory comprise the acute psychological effects of the milder levels of closed head injury and can occur without loss of consciousness; loss of consciousness is invariably followed by delirium and amnesia. These psychopathological manifestations occurring during the transition from coma to reorientation may persist for days or weeks (7). The lesser grades of cerebral concussion are common, and their level of severity can be assessed by the duration of the posttraumatic amnesia, whose persistence beyond 1 hour after trauma suggests a moderately severe injury (8). Another widely used indicator of the severity of head injury is the Glasgow Coma Scale (9). The scale requires evaluation of three components of consciousness, one of which is verbal responsiveness, including intelligibility of speech, orientation, and the presence of confusion. Psychological and behavioral abnormalities that fulfill the criteria for delirium or ACS may occur after brief loss of consciousness, or even when consciousness is not lost at all following head injury (7). Increased psychomotor activity, manifested as restlessness, agitation, incoherent talkativeness, and disinhibited behavior, is a common, if not an invariable, feature of posttraumatic delirium (2,7,10). Follow-up studies indicate that the nature of the psychomotor behavior after head trauma is a prognostic sign; restless patients tend to recover cognitive function better than those who displayed sluggishness and immobility (10). Acute agitation is associated with greater residual psychiatric disturbance (7,10). Disorientation for time and place, memory impairment with or without confabulation, and other cognitive-attentional abnormalities are the usual features of posttraumatic delirium. Hooper (4) speaks of the "stage of confusion" that follows coma and stupor in a patient suffering from concussion, a term he confines to those injuries in which consciousness is lost. He points out that this stage is marked by considerable symptomatic variation, as symptoms are influenced by the patient's personality, the environmental stimuli, and the severity of the diffuse brain damage. Some patients are quiet and listless, while others display psychomotor overactivity and even combativeness. Lewin (11) uses slightly different terminology and talks of the stage of delirium that passes into a state of "quiet confusion." In the latter phase, the patient tends to be cooperative and alert but is disoriented for time and place, does not know the reason for being in the hospital, and has little or no insight into his or her condition. These stages, which appear to represent symptomatic variants of delirium as here defined, follow even a very brief loss of consciousness and may last only for minutes (11). After more severe injury and a longer period of unconsciousness, the delirium may last for hours, days, or even weeks before normal levels of awareness and orientation are regained. If delirium returns after a lucid interval or becomes worse, one should immediately suspect a complication—intracranial, extracranial, or both.

The most important intracranial complications of concussion include hemorrhage, subdural hematoma, subdural effusion, cerebral edema, epileptic seizures, and infection. Each of these complications may exacerbate the delirium or cause it to return. This development calls for appropriate investigations, including EEG and a computed tomography scan. Delirium fluctuating in severity is a common feature of the chronic subdural hematoma (11).

Extracranial complications of head injury that increase the severity of delirium include respiratory acidosis or alkalosis, hypernatremia or hyponatremia, hypoxia from chest or other injuries, hypercarbia, shock, blood loss, fat embolism from long bone fracture, and malnutrition (12,13). Alcohol intoxication predisposes patients to head injury as a result of accidental falls and traffic accidents, and tends to increase the severity and duration of the posttraumatic delirium. It may induce vomiting and subsequent aspiration, as well as impair the fluid and electrolyte balance (14). An alcohol withdrawal delirium may be added to the posttraumatic one in some cases.

The pathogenesis of uncomplicated posttraumatic delirium is not well understood. A decrease in cerebral serotonergic and dopaminergic activity has been suggested (7).

Delirium after head injury may be followed by complete recovery or by dementia, amnestic syndrome, or an organic personality disorder. Other psychiatric sequelae—psychotic, neurotic, and personality—may follow and appear to reflect the personal meaning of the trauma and its consequences for the patient (15). Sleep disturbances, such as more frequent awakenings, may follow concussion (16).

Management of posttraumatic delirium should follow the general principles discussed in Chapter 10. Sedation should be used only if the patient is severly agitated or belligerent, and in danger of harming the self or another person as a result. Haloperidol may be used for this purpose.

Epilepsy

Epilepsy is an important cause of delirium in all age groups. Classification and terminology of psychiatric disorders associated with epilepsy are matters of perennial controversy and confusion. As recent reviewers of this subject point out, *DSM-III-R* does not include diagnoses of psychiatric syndromes associated with epilepsy (17). On the whole, psychopathological states in epileptic patients have been classified in regard to their temporal relationship to the ictus (i.e., periictal and interictal), a classification that is flawed, as it is often difficult to establish whether a given psychotic event was or was not causally related to a seizure (17). Bruens (18) asserts that the least controversial aspect of psychopathology associated with epilepsy is that represented by transient episodes characterized by a reduced level of consciousness, i.e., the so-called twilight states, which bear a clear relationship to a seizure. Such states may be ictal or postictal, or a combination of both. Köhler (19,20) has explored the subject of epileptic psychoses in considerable detail and has reviewed their assorted classifications. He points out that such psychoses represent a heterogeneous group of syndromes and may be classified according to psychopathological criteria, reversibility, episodic or chronic course, and other clinical features. Köhler stresses clouding of consciousness as a key characteristic of these psychoses and divides them into those with and without clouding. He classifies those with clouding, or the twilight states, into preictal, ictal, and postictal, as well as those that bear no temporal relationship to epileptic seizures. Delirious states, characterized by restlessness and mostly visual hallucinations, are included by Köhler among the twilight states. More recent writers divide brief psychotic episodes in epilepsy into confusional and nonconfusional states, which may last for hours to days (21). These states may be ictal or postictal. They show the features of delirium, as defined in this book and in *DSM-III-R* (21). They may be relatively simple or feature delusions, hallucinations, and aggressive behavior (17,21). For the sake of clarity, the following classification of epileptic delirium is proposed:

1. Ictal delirium (twilight state);
   a. Complex partial status epilepticus
   b. Generalized absence (petit mal) status
2. Postictal delirium (twilight or confusional state)
3. Interictal delirium (not temporally related to seizures)
4. Delirium due to antiepileptic drugs

Ictal delirium

This term refers to delirium occurring as a manifestation of a generalized or partial complex status epilepticus. The *generalized,* or petit mal, status was first described by Lennox (22) in 1945. It is believed to occur much more often than the partial complex status and can appear at any age, but is most commonly seen in children. In later life, it can develop in a person with no history of seizures (23,24). Its onset is usually acute. All patients show confusion and slowness of responses; some of them display a catatonic-like state, ataxic gait, repetitive movements or jerks, mutism, automatism, and rhythmic blinking (23). An altered mental state is a standard feature (24). In addition, some patients may exhibit bizarre behavior, such as suddenly singing and dancing, and may be misdiagnosed as suffering from a functional psychiatric disorder (24). Hallucinations and paranoid delusions may occur (23,24). Amnesia for the period of the attack may be total or partial (23). The usual duration of this status is between 12 hours and 4 days, but occasionally an attack may last for a month or even two (23,24). The EEG in patients with a history of absence seizures shows a 3/sec spike-wave activity, while in those without a history of such seizures it tends to show atypical spike-wave discharges (23,24). Clinical symptoms and EEG abnormalities clear transiently in response to intravenous diazepam (23,24). Precipitating factors in this form of status in later life appear to include metabolic disturbances and drug effects (24). The attacks may recur for several years despite anticonvulsant therapy (23).

The *complex partial* (psychomotor) status has been much less often reported than the preceding one, but in recent years a number of reports have been published (25). This status has been defined as either continuous or recurrent partial complex seizure activity without return to baseline function for at least 30 minutes (25). Confusion is its standard feature and may or may not be associated with clearly defined, recurrent clinical seizures (25). Decreased responsiveness or automatisms are usually present. Some patients display aphasia and motor phenomena. The EEG shows a focal seizure pattern (25).

A different form of an ictal confusional state in the elderly has been reported (26). All episodes were accompanied by periodic lateralized epileptiform discharges on the EEG. The reported patients were over 60 years of age, and most of them lacked a personal or family history of epilepsy. Each ictal episode came on abruptly. The most prominent clinical features included a fluctuating confusional state with hallucinations and incoherent thinking. The ictal manifestations were ushered in by such symptoms as anxiety, headache, nausea, vomiting, and paresthesias. Apraxia and disturbances of speech were observed in some patients during the ictal episodes. The confusional state was prolonged and recurrent. Each episode lasted for several days and was followed by partial amnesia for it. These ictal confusional states appear to represent benign form of nonconvulsive status epilepticus in the elderly (26).

Postictal delirium

Classification of postictal behavioral abnormalities is confusing. Lishman (15) speaks of "post-ictal disorders" and includes under this heading automatisms, twilight states, and "post-ictal disturbances." According to him, post-ictal automatic behavior refers to a state of clouding of consciousness that occurs immediately after a seizure, and in the course of which the patient retains control of posture and muscle tone but performs simple or complex movements and actions without being aware of what is going on (15, p 221). Such automatisms are usually brief and only occasionally last for up to an hour. The patient is confused, and may occasionally be aggressive and belligerent. Complete amnesia for the event is the rule. Postictal twilight states often last longer than automatisms, sometimes for several hours or even days (15). They feature psychomotor retardation, hallucinations, and affective disturbances. Postictal disturbances or confusional states include schizophrenia-like paranoid-hallucinatory states with clouding of consciousness.

It is not clear which of the above postictal phenomena should be viewed as examples of delirium. Niedermeyer (27), for example, speaks of "postconvulsive confusion or delirium after grand mal." Other writers claim that post-ictal confusional states show features of delirium as defined in *DSM-III* (21). It appears that such states may follow any type of seizure, generalized or complex partial, but are more common after the generalized ones. This whole issue calls for further studies.

Following a complex partial seizure, some patients display automatism, which Köhler (20) regards as a transient confusional state, or delirium. It may be difficult to tell apart from ictal automatism, is usually very brief, and seems to be uncommon (28). Prolonged EEG and video monitoring is of value in the diagnosis of both ictal and postictal automatism (29).

Interictal delirium

Some patients with temporal lobe epilepsy suffer from interictal confusional states lasting for 1 to many days (30). These episodes feature confusion with temporal disorientation, memory impairment, attentional disturbances, and subsequent partial or total amnesia for the event (30). Other features include disorganized thinking, hallucinations, and body image disturbances (30). In a series of 50 patients with temporal lobe epilepsy, 18% of them were found to have confusional states (31). The affected patients had the highest prevalence of brain damage and the most disturbed social adaptation of the whole group. Pathogenesis and incidence of interictal delirium are unknown.

Some patients reportedly developed delirium when their seizures were controlled with antiepileptic drugs (32). This phenoomenon appears to represent a manifestation of Landolt's "forced normalization" (32). An antagonistic relationship between seizures and psychosis has long been suggested. It appears that such acute psychoses after seizure control, with forced EEG normalization, are not usually delirium but rather schizophrenia-like (32). This issue remains unclear.

Delirium due to antiepileptic drugs is discussed in Chapter 11.

Brain tumor

Delirium is a common manifestation of brain tumor. Walther-Büel (33) has found evidence of mental disorder in 70% of 600 patients with a proven diagnosis of cerebral neoplasm of various pathological types and anatomical sites. Of the total group of those patients, 26% showed evidence of clouding of consciousness. This disorder, presumably delirium, was most often observed in patients with occipital, brain stem, frontal, and temporal lobe tumors. It occurred least frequently with neoplasms in the areas of the sella and cerebellum. Güvener et al. (34) found "confusion" in about 18% of 326 patients with supratentorial tumors. Disturbances of consciousness have been observed in 50% of patients with tumors of the posterior fossa, nearly all of whom showed evidence of raised intracranial pressure (35). Such disturbances have been reported in about 80% of cases of proven cerebral metastases from bronchogenic carcinoma in one series (36), but not in a single case in 70 patients with such metastases from a small cell carcinoma of the lung (37).

On the whole, the quality of published reports on psychiatric disorders in patients with brain tumor leaves much to be desired. Commonly used terms, such as "mental changes," "psychiatric disturbances," and "organic mental syndrome," do not allow any conclusion about the precise nature of the observed psychopathology. Apart from the studies quoted above, the literature gives no clear indication of the incidence of delirium associated with cerebral neoplasm. The works referred to here do, however, indicate that the syndrome occurs in at least 25% of patients with brain tumor. Delirium appears to be associated with fast-growing tumors causing raised intracranial pressure; compression of blood vessels; swelling and edema around or distant from the tumor; and epileptic seizures. Other potential contributory mechanisms include hemorrhage into the tumor, hypotension, and electrolyte imbalance (38). Transient episodes of delirium may thus occur during the development of a brain tumor as a result of these contributory factors, acting singly or in various combinations. Neuropsychological studies have found that patients with rapidly growing cerebral neoplasms are more cognitively impaired than those with slowly growing ones (39). The latter are much more likely to give rise to dementia or amnestic syndrome rather than to delirium.

It is not known whether primary cerebral neoplasms are more likely to cause delirium than the brain metastases from systemic cancer. The annual incidence of both of these types of tumor is almost equal and is estimated to be about 8 per 100,000 of the U.S. population (40). Gliomas account for about 50% of primary neoplasms, while metastatic tumors originate most often in the lungs, bronchi, and trachea in men, and in these organs and the breast in women (40). Metastatic intracranial tumors include intradural, intracerebral, and leptomeningeal ones (41). Impaired cognitive function was found in three-quarters of 162 patients with intracerebral metastases, and 31% of them presented with "behavioral and mental change" (42). It is not reported what proportion of such change constituted delirium. In one series of patients with leptomeningeal metastases, 15% initially complained of lethargy, confusion, and memory loss; after headache, such mental change was the second most common presenting complaint (43). Confusion was observed in about one-quarter of patients with central nervous system involvement by non-Hodgkin's lymphoma (44).

Glioblastoma multiforme is the single most common brain tumor of adults, and confusion is reported to be often present (45). In one series of patients with supratentorial glioma, an organic mental syndrome featuring confusion, disorientation, and forgetfulness was observed in about 45% (46). Confusion has been reported to occur in patients with primary malignant lymphoma of the CNS (47) and in astrocytoma involving the amygdaloid nucleus (48). These scattered reports give insufficient data on the incidence of delirium in primary cerebral neoplasm.

Rates of primary intracranial neoplasm increase steadily with advancing age (40). A number of published studies have focused specifically on brain tumors in *geriatric* patients (49–51). Confusion and other mental changes have been observed in about 30% of such patients with both primary and metastatic brain tumors (49–51).

Delirium associated with antineoplastic agents is discussed in Chapter 11.

Miscellaneous cerebral disorders

Multiple sclerosis may rarely feature an acute organic mental syndrome that, at least in some cases, appears to represent delirium (52).

Paget's disease may give rise to episodes of delirium. Dementia due to compression of the fourth ventricle and occult hydrocephalus is, however, the most common organic syndrome encountered in this chronic disease (53,54).

References

1. Kurtzke J.: The current neurologic burden of illness and injury in the United States. *Neurology* 1982;32:1207–1214.
2. Fisher J. M.: Cognitive and behavioral consequences of closed head injury. *Semin. Neurol.* 1985;5:197–204.

3. Jennett B., Teasdale S., Galbraith S., et al: Severe head injuries in three countries. *J. Neurol. Neurosurg. Psychiatry* 1977;40:291–298.
4. Hooper R.: *Patterns of Acute Head Injury.* Baltimore, Williams & Wilkins Co, 1969.
5. Ommaya A. K., Gannarelli T. A.: Cerebral concussion and traumatic unconsciousness. *Brain* 1974;97:633–654.
6. Jenkins H., Hadley M. D. M., Teasdale G., et al: Brain lesions detected by magnetic resonance imaging in mild and severe head injuries. *Lancet* 1986;2:445–446.
7. Levin H. S., Benton A. L., Grossman R. G.: *Neurobehavioral Consequences of Closed Head Injury.* New York, Oxford University Press, 1982.
8. Hugenholtz H., Stuss D. T., Stethem L. L., et al: How long does it take to recover from a mild concussion? *Neurosurgery* 1988;22:853–858.
9. Teasdale G., Jennett B.: Assessment of coma and impaired consciousness. A practical scale. *Lancet* 1974;2:81–84.
10. Reyes R. L., Bhattacharyya A. K., Heller D.: Traumatic head injury: Restlessness and agitation as prognosticators of physical and psychologic improvement in patients. *Arch. Phys. Med. Rehabil.* 1981;62:20–23.
11. Lewin W.: *The Management of Head Injuries.* Baltimore, Williams & Wilkins Co, 1966.
12. Clifton G. L., Robertson C. S., Grossman R. G., et al: The metabolic response to severe head injury. *J. Neurosurg.* 1984;60:687–696.
13. Kaufman H. H., Bretaudiere J. P., Rowlands B. J., et al: General metabolism in head injury. *Neurosurgery* 1987;20:254–265.
14. Steinbok P., Thompson G. B.: Metabolic disturbances after head injury: Abnormalities of sodium and water balance with special reference to the effects of alcohol intoxication. *Neurosurgery* 1978;3:9–15.
15. Lishman W. A.: *Organic Psychiatry. The Psychological Consequences of Cerebral Disorder,* ed 2. Oxford, Blackwell, 1987.
16. Parsons L. C., Ver Beek D.: Sleep-awake patterns following cerebral concussion. *Nurs. Res.* 1982;31:260–264.
17. Neppe V. M., Tucker G. J.: Modern perspectives on epilepsy in relation to psychiatry: Classification and evaluation. *Hosp. Community Psychiatry* 1988;39:263–271.
18. Bruens J. H.: Psychoses in epilepsy. *Psychiatr. Neurol. Neurochir.* 1971;74:175–182.
19. Köhler G. K.: Begriffbestimmung und Einteilung der sog. epileptischen Psychosen. *Schweiz. Arch. Neurol. Neurochir. Psych.* 1977;120:261–281.
20. Köhler G. K.: Epileptische Psychosen. *Forschr. Neurol. Psychiatr.* 1975;43:99–153.
21. McKenna P. J., Kane J. M., Parrish K.: Psychotic syndromes in epilepsy. *Am. J. Psychiatry* 1985;142:895–940.
22. Lennox W. G.: The treatment of epilepsy. *Med. Clin. North Am.* 1945,29:1114–1128.
23. Guberman A., Cantu-Reyna G., Stuss D., et al: Nonconvulsive generalized status epilepticus: Clinical features, neuropsychological testing, and long-term follow-up. *Neurology* 1986;36:1284–1291.
24. Lee S. I.: Nonconvulsive status epilepticus. Ictal confusion in later life. *Arch. Neurol.* 1985;42:778–781.
25. Ballenger C. E., King D. W., Gallagher B. B.: Partial complex status epilepticus. *Neurology* 1983;33:1545–1552.

26. Terzano M. G., Parrino L., Mazzucchi A., et al: Confusional states with periodic lateralized epileptiform discharges (PLEDs): A peculiar epileptic syndrome in the elderly. *Epilepsia* 1986;27:446–457.
27. Niedermeyer E.: Neurologic aspects of the epilepsies, in Blumer D. (ed): *Psychiatric Aspects of Epilepsy.* Washington DC, American Psychiatric Press, 1984, pp 99–142.
28. Theodore W. H., Porter R. J., Penry J. K.: Complex partial seizures: Clinical characteristics and differential diagnosis. *Neurology* 1983;33:1115–1123.
29. Willmer J. P., Brunet D. G.: The value of prolonged electroencephalographic and video monitoring in diagnosis of seizure disorders. *Can. J. Neurol. Sci.* 1986;13:327–330.
30. Glaser G. H.: The problem of psychosis in psychomotor temporal lobe epileptics. *Epilepsia* 1964;5:271–278.
31. Flor-Henry P.: Psychosis and temporal lobe epilepsy. A controlled investigation. *Epilepsia* 1969;10:363–395.
32. Pakalnis A., Drake M. E., Kuruvilla J., et al: Forced normalization. Acute psychosis after seizure control in seven patients. *Arch. Neurol.* 1987;44:289–292.
33. Walther-Büel H.: *Die Psychiatrie der Hirngesch wülste.* Vienna, Springer-Verlag, 1951.
34. Güvener A., Bagchi B. K., Calhoun H. D.: Mental and seizure manifestations in relation to brain tumors. A statistical study. *Epilepsia* 1964;5:166–176.
35. Assal G., Zander E., Hadjiantonion J.: Les troubles mentaux au cours des tumeurs de la fosse postérieure. *Arch. Swisses Neurol. Neurochir. Psychiatr.* 1975;116:17–27.
36. Schmid-Wermser I., Nagel G. A., Schmid A. H.: Zur klinischen Diagnose von Hirnmetastasen beim Bronchuskarzinom. *Schweiz Med Wochenschr* 1974;104:464–468.
37. Burgess R. E., Burgess V. F., Dibella N. J.: Brain metastases in small carcinoma of the lung. *J.A.M.A.* 1979;242:2084–2086.
38. Netsky M. G., Watson J., Mac D.: The natural history of intracranial neoplasms. *Ann. Intern. Med.* 1956;45:275–284.
39. Hom J., Reitan R. M.: Neuropsychological correlates of rapidly vs. slowly growing intrinsic cerebral neoplasms. *J. Clin. Neuropsychol.* 1984;6:309–324.
40. Walker A. E., Robins M., Weinfeld F. D.: Epidemiology of brain tumors: The national survey of intracranial neoplasms. *Neurology* 1985;35:219–226.
41. Posner J. B., Chernik N. L.: Intracranial metastases from systemic cancer. *Adv. Neurol.* 1978;19:579–592.
42. Posner J. B.: Management of central nervous system metastases. *Semin. Oncol.* 1977;4:81–91.
43. Wasserstrom W. R., Glass J. P., Posner J. B.: Diagnosis and treatment of leptomeningeal metastases. Experience with 90 patients. *Cancer* 1982;49:759–772.
44. Herman T. S., Hammond N., Jones S. E., et al: Involvement of the central nervous system by non-Hodgkin's lymphoma. *Cancer* 1979;43:390–397.
45. Salcman M.: Glioblastoma multiforme. *Am. J. Med. Sci.* 1980;279:84–94.
46. Riggs H. E., Rupp C.: A clinicoanatomic study of personality and mood disturbances associated with gliomas of the cerebrum. *J. Neuropathol. Exp. Neurol.* 1958;17:338–345.
47. Freeman C. R., Shustik C., Brisson M. L., et al: Primary malignant lymphoma of the central nervous system. *Cancer* 1986;58:1106–1111.

48. Julien J., Vital C., Vallat J. M., et al: Epilepsy and agitated delirium caused by an astrocytoma of the amygdala. *Eur. Neurol.* 1979;18:387–390.
49. Friedman H., Odom G. L.: Expanding intracranial lesions in geriatric patients. *Geriatrics* 1972;27:105–115.
50. Salcman M.: Brain tumors and the geriatric patient. *J. Am. Geriatr. Soc.* 1982;30:501–508.
51. Tomita T., Raimondi A. J.: Brain tumors in the elderly. *J.A.M.A.* 1981;246:53–55.
52. Kahana E., Leibowitz U., Alter M.: Cerebral multiple sclerosis. *Neurology* 1971;21:1179–1185.
53. Friedman P., Sklaver N., Klawans H. L.: Neurologic manifestations of Paget's disease of the skull. *Dis. Nerv. Syst.* 1971;32:809–817.
54. Kissel P., Schmitt J., Barrucand D.: Les complications neuropsychiatriques de la maladie de Paget. *Encephale* 1967;2:97–111.

Part III

Delirium in Special Patient Populations

In Part II, the diverse classes of organic causes of delirium were discussed in some detail. This part focuses on the occurrence and causes of the syndrome in patient populations that share certain distinguishing features, such as older age, exposure to surgical procedures, severe burns, or parturition. The rationale for a separate discussion of these populations is that they are liable to develop delirium as a result of usually multiple predisposing or precipitating factors, or both, related to their shared clinical characteristics.

18

Delirium in Geriatric Patients

Delirium is one of the most common and important psychiatric disorders among the elderly—those aged 65 years and older—and especially in the very old (1). As a geriatrician has stated, "Acute mental confusion as a presenting symptom holds a central position in the medicine of old age. Its importance cannot be overemphasized, for acute confusion is a far more common herald of physical illness in an older person than are, for example, fever, pain or tachycardia" (2, p 24). Delirium, or "mental confusion," as some geriatricians refer to it, has been called "the very stuff of geriatric medicine" because of its high incidence, disruptive effects, and diagnostic significance as a cerebral manifestation of many diseases and intoxication with exogenous substances, including almost all medical drugs (3). The syndrome has been referred to as equivalent in the elderly to a convulsion in an infant, namely, an acute clinical event calling for immediate diagnostic assessment (4).

Despite its acknowledged high frequency and importance in later life, delirium in geriatric patients has been little studied, and not much had been written about it until recently (1). In the past several years, however, comprehensive reviews of this subject have appeared in the literature (1,5–8). The growing interest in geriatric delirium no doubt reflects the aging of the population and the related increase in the incidence and prevalence of organic mental syndromes. In the United States, the number of elderly has more than doubled since 1950 to about 28 million in 1984, and the number of the very old (85 years and over) has more than quadrupled since 1950 to 2.6 million

(9). While in 1984 the percentage of elderly in the U.S. population was 12%, by 2020 it will be about 17% (9). The very old are currently the fastest growing-age group in the United States. The elderly population is also growing rapidly in Canada, Japan, Australia, and parts of Europe (10). These widespread demographic trends have influenced the patterns of morbidity and utilization of health care facilities (11). Alzheimer's disease and other dementing diseases have become an important cause of morbidity (12). The prevalence of severe dementia in the population older than 65 years ranges from 1.3% to 6.2%, and the prevalence of mild dementia ranges from 2.6% to 15.4% (13). Between 50% and 75% of patients suffering from dementia have Alzheimer's disease (13). The elderly occupy about 40% of the total general hospital beds and have an average stay about 30% longer than patients under age 65 (14). The frequency of moderate and severe dementia among consecutively admitted medical inpatients in a Finnish study was 12.1% for all age groups; among those aged 80 years and older, it was 20.7% (15). Moreover, of all the patients on the wards in a 1-day sample, 40% were moderately or severely demented (15). In a study by the same investigators of 2,000 consecutive patients aged 55 years and older admitted to a department of medicine, the occurrence of moderate and severe dementia was 9.1%; 41.4% of the demented patients were delirious on admission, and about 25% of all delirious patients were demented (16). This study documented the common association of delirium with dementia and the frequency of the latter in elderly medical inpatients.

These facts and figures highlight the need for a separate discussion of delirium in elderly patients because of its growing importance as a common clinical problem. Investigations of this problem are overdue. In the sections to follow, the key aspects of delirium in later life are discussed. As far as possible, repetition of information on this topic scattered in the other chapters is avoided.

Historical background

Probably the first article devoted to delirium in the elderly was that by Hood (17), published in 1870. He reported on several cases of what he called "senile delirium" and asserted that the syndrome could develop in an elderly person free of prior "mental debility." It was potentially reversible but could result in death unless its underlying cause was promptly treated. In 1904, Pickett (18) published a report on a clinical study, to my knowledge the first study in this area. He made a most important point by stressing the need to differentiate delirium and confusion, two similar and curable mental disorders of the elderly, from senile dementia. He made a distinction between delirium, a syndrome always due to an organic cause, and confusion, which may follow bereavement, for example, A seminal article by Robinson (19), published in 1939, provided a modern view of acute confusional states in later life as "reactions to general disease, just as other deliriums and confusion states are" (p 479). He hypothesized that aging processes involving the brain reduce "adjustability of cerebral functions" and thus predispose an elderly individual to delirium in response to a wide range of infectious, toxic, and metabolic insults. Robinson observed that in old age the syndrome is prolonged, lasting for weeks, and is more dangerous than in younger patients.

An important contribution to the understanding of nocturnal delirium in senile patients was an experimental study by Cameron (20), which appeared in 1941 and is described in Chapter 5. He drew attention to the hypothesized role of perceptual deprivation in the occurrence of such delirium. In the 1950s, several studies on the etiological and clinical aspects of acute confusional states in elderly patients were published (21–23). Two particularly noteworthy articles to appear in that decade are those by Litin (24) and Kennedy (25). The former author drew attention to the cognitively disorganizing impact on an elderly patient of the stress occasioned by hospitalization. He maintained that the patient's reaction to such stress may take the form of delirium. Kennedy (25) offered a thoughtful discussion of the role of psychological factors in the etiology of the syndrome in the elderly. He argued that delirium is a disorder of consciousness, one in which the individual's ability to interpret stimuli from within and without is compromised, and which bears a similarity to dreaming. Both of these mental states feature slowing of the EEG and reduced level of attention. Kennedy proposed that such factors as transfer to an unfamiliar environment and sensory deprivation contribute to delirium in an older patient, who has a reduced capacity to process information and integrate it meaningfully in the light of past experience. He stressed the importance of psychotherapy of delirium and of providing a stable sensory environment for the patient.

In the late 1950s, Kral (26,27) embarked on his pioneering studies of mental disorders in the elderly. His observations led him to conclude that lowered resistance to stress in normal old people, and even more so in patients with senile dementia, renders them susceptible to the development of acute confusional states in response to both biological and psychological acute stress. His hypothesis is discussed in more detail later on in this chapter.

This brief outline of the early studies on delirium in later life provides a historical background for a discussion of the current views on this topic. The research referred to has yielded important information on the etiology and natural history of the syndrome in the elderly. It has also generated some working hypotheses on its causation, such as those by Kral, that await empirical study to test their validity. The recent demographic changes mentioned earlier and the progressive aging of the population have brought into focus organic mental syndromes that are relatively common in the elderly. One may predict that research on delirium in this age group will grow in the coming years.

Importance of delirium in geriatrics

Delirium is important in medical practice not just because it is common. Its main clinical importance derives from the fact that in an elderly individual it is often a *presenting feature* of an acute physical illness or of exacerbation of a chronic one, or of intoxication with even therapeutic doses of commonly used (especially anticholinergic) drugs (1–8). Hence, failure to diagnose it and to identify and treat its underlying causes may have lethal consequences for the patient. Acute conditions, such as myocardial infarction or pneumonia, or an exacerbation of chronic heart failure, can initially present with an acute confusional state. In an elderly patient, notably a demented one, such a development may be mistaken for the onset of a functional psychiatric disorder or a worsening of dementia in an individual known to be afflicted with it. As a result, the patient's life-threatening physical illness may remain overlooked and untreated.

The development of delirium in an elderly patient carries the risk of serious, even deadly, *complications.* The risk of self-injury is ever-present. An agitated, confused, and fearful delirious patient may make a frantic attempt to escape from an unfamiliar environment, or from hallucinated dangers, and fall and sustain a fracture or some other serious injury. He or she may tear open sutures, pull out intravenous lines, or remove a catheter. Moreover, such an agitated patient is liable to be treated with parenteral doses of psychotropic drugs and is often physically restrained. Drugs, such as chlorpromazine hydrochloride, may induce severe orthostatic hypotension, while physical restraints carry the risk of deep vein thrombosis and pulmonary embolism (28,29). Agitation and fear, with their concomitant sympathetic nervous system hyperarousal, may be dangerous for a patient who has just suffered an MI, as a potentially lethal cardiac arrhythmia or a rise in blood pressure can result.

Medicolegal complications in the form of litigation may follow a hospitalized patient's self-injury. This problem can also arise if an elderly delirious patient was denied admission to the hospital because the underlying acute medical condition was missed and the patient died as a result. Legal and ethical complications may arise from the patient's inability to give informed consent (see Chapter 10).

Finally, the development of delirium in hospitalized patients tends to prolong their hospital stay, and hence to increase its cost. This *economic* aspect of delirium has been studied recently (30,31). Patients who became delirious after surgery for femoral neck fracture were found to have an almost four times longer hospitalization than nondelirious ones (30). Thomas et al. (31) have carried out a prospective study of the impact of delirium on the length of hospitalization and found that it was significantly prolonged for the delirious patients. They concluded that to avoid this complication, it is essential to detect delirium early and treat it appropriately.

Terminology: confusion about confusion

Terminology of mental disorders in the aged continues to be muddled. Terms such as "acute confusion," "acute organic brain syndrome," "acute brain failure," "pseudosenility," "toxic psychosis," and the like are used more or less synonymously, resulting in semantic confusion (1,8). Many writers do not bother to define these terms, and one is left to guess what they imply. This issue is discussed at length in Chapter 2 and is brought up here specifically in regard to the geriatric literature. The most often used term in this context is "confusion," a word that is ambiguous, overworked, and misused as a diagnosis. It has been applied to both the delirious and the demented elderly (32–34). This confusing term should be used either informally or when its meaning is operationally defined. For example, some investigators have developed the term "confusion rating" based on the sum of scores on orientation, communication, and memory (33). If one wants to state in a clinical situation that a patient thinks and speaks incoherently, is disoriented, and shows impairment of memory and attention, it is best to use the appropriate terms referring to these mental abnormalities. Woolly statements commonly found in the literature and the medical records, such as "the patient is confused," should be replaced by description of the patient's cognitive functioning.

Incidence and prevalence

These issues are fully discussed in Chapter 3. Given the semantic muddle discussed in the preceding section and the lack of diagnostic criteria for delirium until this decade, reported incidence and prevalence figures on acute confusional states in the elderly must be taken with a grain of salt. Epidemiological studies in this area are few and badly needed; one is in progress at Harvard University (35). Millard (36) states that "in epidemiological surveys acute confusional states are less prevalent, but in the hospital service acute confusion is all too often equated with dementia" (p 1559). Studies published to date indicate that between 10% and 40% of elderly patients are acutely confused on admission (6). However, these figures come from different clinical settings and are hardly comparable. A multicenter British study found that 35% of patients aged 65 years and older had delirium on admission or developed it during hospitalization (37). Two more recent studies found confusion in about 30% and 50% of hospitalized patients, respectively (28,29).

The patients in both of these studies were aged 70 years or older, and "confusion" is not defined by the authors. Consequently, one cannot automatically assume that these high figures reflect the actual incidence of delirium in the hospitalized elderly. A critical review of the studies published to date allows only a tentative estimate of the incidence and prevalence of delirium in elderly medical inpatients. About 15% of such patients are likely to be delirious on admission, and about 15% to 20% of those who are mentally clear when admitted will become delirious during their hospital stay. These estimates apply to patients 65 years of age and older; they are likely to be too low for those over 70 years of age. Postoperative delirium has been found in 10% to 15% of elderly patients (38), but its frequency is at least three times higher in those who have undergone an operation for a femoral neck fracture (30). Some writers claim that the incidence of postoperative delirium is likely to be underestimated and that an acute confusional state is "so common postoperatively in the elderly that it may be the norm" (39, p 42).

Course and prognosis

The natural history and prognosis of delirium in the elderly have hardly been touched by researchers. Robinson (19) claimed that the syndrome tends to last longer in such patients, but systematic data on this subject are still lacking. Delirium is, by definition, a transient disorder, but its duration is not specified in *DSM-III-R*. Some authors maintain that delirium lasting for weeks to months should be rediagnosed as dementia (40). One notes that most etiological factors said to account for so-called reversible dementia are the same as those that give rise to delirium (40,41).

In the elderly, delirium is often a prelude to death, as it is a common concomitant of terminal illnesses such as cancer. The reported mortality of delirious patients within 1 month of admission to the hospital has ranged from 17% to 33% (1,6). These high figures indicate that the development of delirium in an elderly patient should be viewed as a grave prognostic sign. In one study, 80% of the survivors recovered within a month and 5% remained confused for more than 6 months (21). The latter patients would be considered by many experts to have developed dementia. How often this chronic syndrome follows delirium in an elderly patient is unknown and should be investigated. A transition from delirium to dementia appears to be uncommon, but firm data are lacking.

Clinical features

Essential features of delirium are assumed to be the same in all age groups, including the elderly. Studies of the phenomenology of the syndrome in later life are, however, lacking, and the relevant literature is mostly anecdotal. There is suggestive evidence that some of the clinical manifestations are more or less common in the delirious elderly. For example, hallucinations and dream-like (oneiric) mentation are said to be less common among them (42). In one series, only about 40% of elderly delirious patients were believed to experience hallucinations (43). Depression is said to occur in over one-half of these patients—a higher frequency than that observed in younger patients. The fact that delirium in the aged is so often superimposed on dementia seems to influence the clinical picture. A demented patient is likely to exhibit less rich fantasy in hallucinations, for example, and to show more impaired capacity for abstract thinking during the lucid intervals, than a younger patient. Moreover, a demented individual is liable to appear relatively unimaginative, dull, and lacking in general information. A delirious patient who, when accessible, cannot tell the names of recent political leaders or the dates of World War II, for example, is likely to be demented, provided that he or she had some formal schooling. Many delirious elderly patients tend to be apathetic and hypoactive; hence, their delirium is apt to be overlooked by those who do not know them well. Physical signs often observed in such patients include slurred speech, aphasia, tremor, motor incoordination, and urinary and fecal incontinence. Such signs may, of course, be present in younger delirious patients too, but, they seem to be more common in elderly ones. Focal neurological signs are also more likely to be found in the latter group, since cerebrovascular and other brain diseases are more prevalent in later life. The EEG in elderly delirious patients, notably those suffering from Alzheimer's disease, is a less reliable indicator of delirium than in younger patient's, since slowing of the background activity may be the result of the underlying, especially degenerative, brain disease.

Pathogenesis

Pathogenesis of delirium in later life does not seem to be different from that discussed in Chapter 7. If differences do exist, they have not yet been convincingly demonstrated. However, some investigators have put forth pathogenetic hypotheses that appear to apply more specifically to delirium in the elderly. Kral (26,27), for example, hypothesized that in an older patient the syndrome represents a reaction to acute stress, mediated by abnormally high levels of circulating glucocorticoids, or by increased vulnerability of the hypothalamus to their effects, or both. He demonstrated that in response to stress, patients suffering from senile dementia show a higher and more sustained increase in plasma cortisol levels than do the nondemented elderly. He speculated that such excessive cortisol levels may bring about an acute confusional state because of their deleterious effect on the centrencephalic system.

This interesting hypothesis remains to be validated. Basal plasma cortisol concentrations have been found to be higher in patients with Alzheimer's disease than in normal control subjects and were highest in the most severely demented patients (44). Cortisol affects both cerebral and mental function and interferes with selective attention, memory, and processing of information (45). A positive correlation has been observed between urinary free cortisol excretion and the degree of cognitive impairment in depressed, especially older, patients (46). The investigators proposed that age and depression interact to produce cognitive impairment, which appears to be mediated by hypercortisolemia. Other researchers have reported high resting plasma cortisol levels in those senile patients who displayed the greatest increases in EEG slow activity (47). In another study, elderly persons under stress were found to excrete larger amounts of urinary free cortisol than did middle-aged individuals (48). Delirium has been reported in patients with Cushing's syndrome, particularly in the elderly (49). Finally, patients recovering from elective surgery who developed postoperative delirium were shown to have significant and prolonged elevation of plasma cortisol levels (50). All this admittedly circumstantial evidence indicates that hypercortisolemia could be implicated in the pathophysiology of at least some, notably stress-related, cases of delirium in later life. A study of cortisol levels in the demented and nondemented delirious elderly compared to appropriate nondelirious controls should help to clarify this issue and is worth undertaking.

A second pathogenetic hypothesis relevant to delirium in elderly patients involves *sleep pathology* (1). The diurnal sleep-wake cycle in many older adults tends to be fragmented, with a high prevalence of sleep apnea, excessive daytime somnolence, and microsleeps (51). Fragmentation of the sleep patterns has been observed in degenerative brain disease (52). Sleep apnea results in hypoxemia, which may impair the patient's cognitive functioning (51). Nocturnal delirum, common in the demented elderly, has been ascribed to awakenings from periods of REM sleep and to the occurrence of REM sleep without loss of muscle tone (1). Systematic studies of the diurnal sleep-wake cycle in delirium in later life should be given high priority to establish whether its disruption could be of pathogenetic significance in this syndrome in at least a proportion of cases.

Etiological factors

The elderly, especially the very old, are highly prone to develop delirium in response to a wide range of organic etiological factors acting singly or, more often, in combination (1–8). Thus, the etiology of the syndrome in later life is usually multifactorial. A condition such as a urinary tract infection or therapeutic doses of commonly used drugs, which would seldom induce delirium in a younger patient, may do so in an elderly one. Clearly, this vulnerability must reflect a special predisposition of the old.

Predisposing factors

A number of such factors appear to render an aged person susceptible to the development of delirium. They are listed in Table 18–1 and will be discussed presently.

Age-related *changes in the brain* are likely to play a major role in this respect (1,7). Certain parts of the brain, such as the frontal lobes, amygdala, putamen, thalamus, locus coeruleus, and central cholinergic system, show selective cell loss as a result of the aging processes (53). Atrophy of both gray and white matter occurs in relation to age (53). Senile plaques occur most often in the hippocampus, amygdala, hippocampal gyrus, and middle cerebral cortical layers. There are age-related changes in the central neurotransmitter systems (54,55). Such changes involve dopaminergic neurons, as well as the synthesis of acetylcholine (56). Some authors suggest that a subtle imbalance of several interacting neurotransmitter systems, corresponding partly to regional losses of neurons, could be reflected in the cognitive performance of the healthy elderly (53). One writer hypothesizes that compensatory mechanisms, such as regulation of the sensitivity of receptive molecules to their respective neurotransmitters, help the aging brain to function well under optimal conditions. As long as these mechanisms function adequately, the only consequence of neuronal loss will be a reduction of reserve capacity, which may become manifest under stressful conditions in the form of delirium (54).

The effect of age on CMR and CBF has been a matter of controversy (53,57–61). Some investigators conclude that normal aging may result in a global decrease in the CMR for glucose, but these changes correlate poorly with cognitive function (61). Other researchers contend that the inconsistencies in the reported studies of cerebral metabolism and blood flow in relation

TABLE 18–1 Factors Predisposing Elderly to Delirium

1. Age-related changes in the brain
2. Brain damage or disease, especially Alzheimer's disease
3. Reduced capacity for homeostatic regulation and resistance to stress
4. Changed circadian rhythms
5. Impairment of vision and hearing
6. Increased susceptibility to infection
7. High prevalence of chronic diseases and high incidence of acute diseases
8. Multiple diseases
9. Impaired mechanisms of drug distribution and metabolism
10. Malnutrition

to aging reflect differences in the health status of the subjects, and that in healthy elderly these parameters are age invariant (53). Studies in the healthy elderly have shown no relationship between cognitive performance and global CMR for glucose and oxygen or CBF (53). The significance, if any, of these findings for the vulnerability to delirium of the healthy elderly is unclear.

The issue is much clearer in the case of elderly individuals suffering from *brain damage or disease.* Reductions in CBF are greater with the appearance of cerebrovascular disease or dementia, or both, than in the healthy elderly (62). Patients with Alzheimer's disease show reduction of the CMR for glucose and oxygen in the parietal and temporal areas of the neocortex, as well as right-left asymmetry (63). The pattern of metabolic reductions is related to that of neuropsychological impairments (63). In severely demented patients, the absolute CMR tends to be significantly reduced (64). There are major neurotransmitter changes in Alzheimer's disease, notably involving a cholinergic deficit and reduction of somatostatin (64–66). Loss of indoleamines from the frontal lobe has recently been reported and its relation to behavioral changes in Alzheimer patients hypothesized (67). All these findings suggest that such patients show a number of pathological changes in the brain that could predispose them to delirium. In particular, loss of cholinergic neurons in the nucleus basalis of Meynert, located in the basal forebrain, which project to most cortical areas and are the major source of cholinergic input to the cerebral cortex, appears to be an important factor predisposing Alzheimer patients to delirium (64). The resulting cholinergic deficit renders them susceptible to any factor, such as hypoxia or the intake of anticholinergic drugs, that leads to further depletion of brain acetylcholine. An adequate supply of this neurotransmitter is necessary for normal cognitive functioning, attention, and sleep-wake cycle, and its deficiency is hypothesized to play a key pathogenetic role in the development of many, if not all, cases of delirium (56). Cell loss in the locus coeruleus and raphe nuclei has been blamed for the occurrence of nocturnal delirium in demented elderly patients (68).

After Alzheimer's disease, cerebrovascular disease is the second most common cause of dementia in the elderly (69). Also common is Binswanger's disease, an ischemic periventricular leukoencephalopathy, which represents a form of vascular dementia in later life (70). Cognitive functioning and CBF in multi-infarct dementia tend to fluctuate together (71). When vascular disease affects the brain, disturbances of CBF and CMR can be demonstrated by PET and other laboratory techniques (72). Elderly persons with even mild cerebrovascular disease show focal reduction of CBF and glucose metabolism, changes that make them highly vulnerable to hypoxia due to cardiovascular disease or any other factor. As hypoxia results in reduced acetylcholine synthesis and hence a cholinergic deficit, a patient with any degree of cerebrovascular disease may be vulnerable to delirium as a consequence of acetylcholine deficiency (56). A study of elderly patients with acute confusional states has shown a high prevalence of cerebrovascular disease in delirious compared to nondelirious subjects (73).

There is little doubt that cerebral disease, both degenerative and vascular, predisposes to delirium. There are additional factors, however, that likely contribute to this predisposition. They include reduction of the capacity for homeostatic regulation and for resistance to stress, possibly as a result of changes in hypothalamic nuclei (55,74); changed circadian rhythms involving cortisol, body temperature, and the sleep-wake cycle (75); impairment of vision and hearing (76); increased susceptibility to infections, related to suppression of the immune response involving cell-mediated immunity and possibly to interferon (77,78); a high prevalence of chronic diseases and a high incidence of acute diseases, as well as common coexistence of several of them (11); and impaired mechanisms of drug distribution and metabolism (79). Moreover, the elderly are often malnourished. This condition may have an adverse effect on their health and cognition, as well as altering their response to certain commonly used drugs (80–82).

Thus, the susceptibility of the elderly to delirium appears to reflect changes in the resistance of the aging organism to disease on the one hand, and the increased vulnerability of the aging, and especially the diseased, brain to hypoxia, electrolyte and fluid imbalance, drugs, lack of essential nutrients, and other potentially pathogenic factors on the other. Homeostatic and immune mechanisms of the older individual's body are generally less efficient, and its dynamic steady state becomes readily deranged as a result of a whole range of stressors, physical, biological, and psychosocial. Higher integrative functions of the brain may be either manifestly impaired or marginally compensated. Homeostatic disturbances brought about by any of a wide range of stressors may result in decompensation of the brain structures and mechanisms subserving cognition and attention, and become manifested clinically as delirium.

Precipitating organic factors

As stated earlier, the etiology of delirium in later life is typically *multifactorial,* meaning that several causative organic factors are concurrently implicated and have a cumulative effect on the brain (1–8). Intoxication with medical, notably anticholinergic, drugs is probably the most common single precipitating factor (1–8,76). The more common organic etiological factors are listed in Table 18–2. Several published studies indicate that the disorders and diseases most often associated with delirium in the elderly include pneumonia, congestive heart failure, urinary tract infection, cancer, uremia, mal-

TABLE 18–2 Common Organic Factors Precipitating Delirium

1. Intoxication with medical drugs: anticholinergics, sedative-hypnotics, diuretics, digitalis, antihypertensive and antiarrhythmic agents, cimetidine, lithium, hypoglycemic agents, levodopa, nonsteroidal anti-inflammatory drugs, narcotics, cancer chemotherapeutic drugs
2. Alcohol and sedative-hypnotic withdrawal
3. Metabolic disorders: fluid and electrolyte imbalance; endocrine disorders; renal, hepatic, and pulmonary failure; nutritional (including vitamin) deficiency; hypothermia and heat stroke
4. Cardiovascular disorders: myocardial infarction, congestive heart failure, cardiac arrhythmias, pulmonary embolism
5. Cerebrovascular disorders: stroke, transient ischemic attacks, subdural hematoma, multi-infarct dementia, vasculitides, orthostatic hypotension
6. Infections, notably pulmonary and of urinary tract, bacteremia, septicemia, tuberculosis, meningitis, encephalitis
7. Neoplasm; intracranial, systemic
8. Trauma: head injury, burns, surgery
9. Epilepsy

nutrition, hypokalemia, dehydration and/or sodium depletion, and cerebrovascular accidents (21–23,37,43,73,76,83,84). Systemic diseases are much more often implicated than the primary cerebral ones (76). All of these conditions are discussed in Part II, and there are frequent references to their relevance to delirium in the elderly. It would be redundant to repeat all of this material here, but some of it must be referred to again briefly to highlight its importance in the context of this chapter.

Intoxication with medical drugs

As stated earlier, this is one of the most important, if not the most common, organic causes of delirium in later life. Drug-related iatrogenesis in the elderly has been amply documented in recent years and prompted an editorial writer to ask: "Need we poison the elderly so often?" (85). That author states that increase in adverse drug reactions (ADR's) is related to the patients' age. One study has found that those over 70 were seven times more likely to have such a reaction than patients under 30. ADRs were found in 15% of 2,000 successive admissions to geriatric units, and in two-thirds of these cases the ADR contributed to the need for admission (86). Hypotensive and antiparkinsonian drugs and psychotropics carried the highest risk of ADRs, although the largest single number of them were found to be due to diuretics, which were prescribed for over 30% of the sample (86). Twenty-five percent of all prescription drugs are taken by those over 65 years of age, although this group comprises only about 12% of the total population (87). Seventy percent of persons 75 years and older receive drugs (88). ADRs are more common in the elderly than in younger persons and, if unrecognized, may prompt further prescriptions to treat the related symptoms (89). The chance of ADRs grows as the number of medications taken by the patient increases (89). ADRs often involve cognitive impairment, especially in the demented elderly (90). Such impairment commonly takes the form of delirium or dementia (1,90).

A number of factors contribute to the frequent drug-related delirium in later life (1,5–8,76,87–93). They include intrinsic susceptibility to drugs on the part of the elderly and indiscriminate prescribing for and taking of drugs by them. The following are the more important factors:

A. Altered pharmacokinetics and pharmacodynamics
   1. Hepatic detoxification, especially oxidation, is impaired. This mechanism is likely responsible for the increased susceptibility to delirium in elderly patients taking tricyclic antidepressants, benzodiazepines, anticonvulsants, and oral hypoglycemic agents.
   2. Renal excretion is reduced due to decreased glomerular filtration with age, resulting in prolonged half-life of drugs such as digoxin and gentamicin.
   3. Reduction of protein binding of drugs in plasma may enhance the effects of narcotics and certain diuretics.
   4. Target tissue sensitivity is altered. Some drugs acting on the CNS, such as sedative-hypnotics and major tranquilizers, may produce an enhanced response at a given plasma concentration.
   5. Impaired homeostasis and/or concurrent disease can increase the tendency toward drug-induced postural hypotension, hypothermia, and hyperthermia.
B. Drug-induced interactions resulting in synergism or potentiation of drug effects (88,94)
C. Drug-induced nutritional deficiencies (95)
D. Reduced thirst appreciation and thus a tendency toward hypovolemia (96)
E. Excessive prescribing and polypharmacy, partly related to multiple coexisting diseases and symptoms (97)
F. Noncompliance with and mismanagement of drug regimens by patients
G. Inadequate drug monitoring by physicians

As a result of various combinations of the above factors, drug-induced delirium is a common iatrogenic disorder in the elderly. Moreover, up to 60% of all drugs taken by them are said to be over-the-counter medications, such as antihistamine hypnotics, many of which have anticholinergic effects (87). The elderly take more drugs than the general population, and about one in four of them take four to six drugs concurrently (98). The most often prescribed drugs include diuretics, digoxin, aspirin, propranolol, methyldopa, potassium supplements, and nitroglycerin (88). In one series, diuretics, analgesics, psychotropics, sedative-hypnotics, and digitalis preparations accounted for the bulk of the prescribed drugs for the elderly (98). *Diuretics* top the list of drugs with the largest number of ADRs, followed closely by psychotropics and digitalis. Diuretics may lead to hypokalemia, hyponatremia, dehydration, hypotension, and hyperkalemia, all of which may precipitate delirium in an older patient, especially a demented one.

Psychotropic drugs deserve special mention, as they are often prescribed and abused, and are liable to induce delirium in an older patient. Widespread use of these drugs by the elderly has been well documented (99–103). For example, a study of nursing home residents found that almost one-third of them received psychotropic medications, which in 30% of cases were deemed to be inappropriate (100). According to a British study, about 10% to 15% of the elderly population take a hypnotic drug each night, and the majority of the users take hypnotics for more than 1 year (103).

Tricyclic antidepressants, neuroleptics, lithium, and benzodiazepines tend to induce an acute confusional state more readily in an elderly than in a younger patient (see Chapter 11). Mental disorders attributed to psychoactive drugs have been reported to be the main reason for admission to a psychogeriatric service in 16% of patients (104). *Benzodiazepines* are the most often prescribed psychoactive drugs in later life and are liable to cause confusion as a result of intoxication or withdrawal (87,90,105–109). Patients older than 70 years should initially receive one-half of the usual dose of a benzodiazepine drug. Drugs with a long half-life, such as flurazepam hydrochloride, should be avoided (87). If a hypnotic must be used, a low dose of an agent with a short half-life should be prescribed for a limited time. Oxazepam, a benzodiazepine with a relatively short half-life (7 hours), is generally preferable as an anxiolytic agent for an elderly patient (106).

Tricyclic antidepressants appear to induce delirium in the elderly less often than was previously reported (110). It is advisable to use a drug with low anticholinergic activity, such as desipramine or nortriptyline, to start at the lowest dose (usually 25 mg), and to not exceed a total dose of 125 mg (87,111).

Lithium is liable to induce severe adverse reactions in the elderly, in whom its half-life may reach 36 hours (108). A test dose of 50–75 mg of lithium carbonate and a gradual increase in the total daily dose to 600 mg have been recommended for the elderly (112).

Neuroleptics, like all drugs with anticholinergic effects, induce delirium more readily in the older patient. High-potency neuroleptics, such as haloperidol and fluphenazine, have relatively low anticholinergic properties compared to chlorpromazine or thioridazine but a greater tendency to induce extrapyramidal reactions. For more discussion of the deliriogenic potential of all these drugs, the reader is referred to Chapter 11.

Anticholinergic agents

The elderly are highly sensitive to the effects of these drugs (see Chapter 11). Despite this generally recognized sensitivity and the related high risk of delirium, drugs with anticholinergic properties are often prescribed for the elderly (113,114). Delirium is particularly likely to ensue if several of these drugs are used concurrently, as is often the case (113). They are probably the most common single cause of delirium in later life. Patients with dementia of the Alzheimer type are especially sensitive to the toxic effects of these agents on the CNS (115). For further discussion of this important subject, see Chapter 11.

Alcohol intoxication and withdrawal

Many elderly persons abuse alcohol (116–121). Although the prevalence of alcoholism is stated to be lower in the nonhospitalized elderly than in younger people (about 6%) surveys of hospitalized elderly patients show the prevalence of alcohol abuse to be about 18% (121). Alcoholism is often missed in elderly patients admitted to general hospitals (117). Organic mental syndromes were diagnosed in over 40% of elderly alcoholics hospitalized for alcohol abuse, and alcohol withdrawal delirium was found in about 10% of them (118). Physiological effects of alcohol in the elderly may differ due to altered absorption, hepatic metabolism, excretion, and sensitivity of the brain (121). Alcohol is toxic to the brain, and its prolonged consumption may result in cognitive impairment (119). Illness, malnutrition, or concurrent use of a hepatotoxic drug or one metabolized by the liver may result in increased sensitivity to even a relatively modest intake of alcohol by an elderly person (120). Alcohol combined with anticholinergics, including the over-the-counter antihistamine hypnotics, can produce delirium in the elderly (116). The effects of alcohol on sleep, such as reduction of both REM and non-REM sleep stages, could accentuate the changes in sleep patterns associated with aging and hence possibly increase the risk of developing delirium. Ethanol interacts with many drugs, which may potentiate its effects. This applies to the psychotropics commonly used by the elderly, such as neuroleptics, sedative-hypnotics, and tricyclic antidepressants (120,121). An elderly patient using antidiabetic drugs, such as tolbutamide, is at greater risk for hypoglycemia (121).

All of the above factors are liable to render an elderly alcoholic susceptible to delirium. Not surprisingly, in two studies of the syndrome in the elderly, alcoholism was considered a major etiological factor (43,122). A patient with a preexisting brain disease and dementia is liable to be particularly vulnerable to the deliriogenic effect of acute alcohol intake. Alcoholism is often associated with malnutrition and vitamin deficiencies, which may cause or contribute to delirium (123).

Management of alcohol withdrawal delirium in an elderly patient should include an inquiry into the patient's physical state, nutrition, and intake of drugs. Psychotropics can mask the symptoms of an alcohol withdrawal syndrome, and the patient may progress to severe delirium (117). Agitation must be controlled with chlordiazepoxide, starting with 25–50 mg and repeating that dose every 2 hours. In patients with concurrent liver disease, oxazepam or lorazepam is indicated instead. Otherwise, treatment should follow the guidelines discussed in Chapters 10 and 13.

Metabolic disorders

Metabolic encephalopathies are a common and important cause of delirium in the elderly. They are fully discussed in Chapter 13, and only selected conditions will be highlighted here.

Fluid and electrolyte imbalance are common problems in later life (124). Dehydration is their most common cause in the elderly (96). A deficit in thirst and water intake after 24 hours of water deprivation have been found in the healthy elderly men (96). Dehydration tends to occur frequently, since elderly persons often have reduced urinary concentrating power, depend heavily on adequate and consistent water intake, and become dehydrated when this is curtailed as a result of illness or confusion, for example. Consequently, a delirious elderly patient should always be checked for signs of dehydration (84). Electrolyte imbalance occurs frequently as a side effect of drugs, inadequate fluid intake, neoplasm, cerebrovascular accidents, hepatic encephalopathy, and uremia. Diuretics are among the drugs most often prescribed for the elderly and can lead to hyponatremia, hypokalemia, hypomagnesemia, and metabolic alkalosis—all of them potential causes of delirium (125). In one study, almost 30% of hyponatremic elderly patients were confused (126).

Endocrine disorders in the elderly are often associated with psychiatric disorders, including delirium (127,128). *Hyperthyroidism* and *hypothyroidism* are said to occur in 3% to 4% of elderly people (129). Some elderly thyrotoxic patients present in a state referred to as "apathetic hyperthyroidism," i.e., with lethargy, withdrawal, and apathy (127). Hypothyroidism in the elderly tends to develop unobtrusively and may remain unrecognized until late in the course (130). Both of these disorders may cause delirium. *Diabetes mellitus* accounted for nearly 15% of the etiological factors in a small sample of hospitalized, delirious elderly patients (131). Such patients can suffer from delirium as a result of hyperosmolar nonketotic hyperglycemic coma, ketoacidosis, or hypoglycemia. The elderly are highly vulnerable to hypoglycemic reactions in response to insulin, oral hypoglycemic agents, or neoplasm (132).

Typical of the older diabetic is the appearance of nonketotic hyperosmolar coma, which may present as delirium (132). Both *hypocalcemia* and *hypercalcemia* may do likewise (127). *Hepatic, renal,* and *pulmonary* failure are all relatively common causes of acute confusional states in the elderly (133). All of these conditions are discussed in Chapter 14.

Nutritional disorders are common in the elderly and include vitamin deficiency (80,134). Cognitive impairment may result from malnutrition, while reduced cognitive function may lead to reduced intake of essential nutrients (80). Malnutrition can predispose an elderly person to delirium induced by drugs, for example, while deficiency of vitamins, such as folate, may cause confusion directly (123,135). For further discussion of the role of vitamin deficiencies in delirium, see Chapter 14.

Hypothermia and heat stroke are relatively common among elderly persons and reflect impaired temperature regulation (136,137). Both of them may give rise to delirium (see Chapter 14).

Cardiovascular disorders are highly prevalent in later life and constitute one of the most important classes of etiological factors in delirium among the elderly (22,37,133,138). An acute confusional state may be a presenting feature of MI, cardiac failure, various arrhythmias, aortic stenosis, and subacute bacterial endocarditis. All of these conditions may result in cerebral ischemia-anoxia and hence delirium.

MI often occurs without pain in an elderly individual and with confusion as the chief presenting feature (139). In one large series, 6.8% of the patients presented in this manner, but of those 85 years and older, nearly 20% did so (139). Sudden development of delirium, with agitation, restlessness, and noisy behavior, may be the only initial symptom of MI in an elderly patient. Such symptoms may pass unnoticed in a demented patient, with serious consequences. Complications of MI, such as cardiac arrhythmias, pulmonary or cerebral embolism, cardiogenic shock, and congestive heart failure can result in further reduction of CBF and hence in brain hypoxia and delirium.

Orthostatic hypotension occurs more readily in the elderly than in younger persons. Its causes are many and include drug reactions. Symptoms range from lightheadedness, through varying degrees of confusion, to syncope or convulsions. Treatment of hypertension in the elderly with antihypertensive drugs may result in inadequate cerebral perfusion and delirium (140). For further discussion of cardiovascular disorders, see Chapter 16. *Cerebrovascular disorders* are also discussed in that chapter.

Infections, especially of the lungs and urinary tract, are very common in the elderly and are one of the most important causes of delirium in this group (76,141). Fever, tachycardia, leukocytosis, cough, dyspnea, and tachypnea may be absent, and delirium may be the only manifestation of bronchopneumonia in an older person (142). The elderly are highly susceptible to infection, as noted earlier in this chapter, and most infections tend to be more severe in them than in younger individuals. Various factors have been implicated in this increased susceptibility to infection, including deteriorated function of B lymphocytes and T lymphocytes, and coexisting immunosuppressive disease such as cancer, diabetes mellitus, renal insufficiency, and malnutrition (143). Cholecystitis, diverticulitis, tuberculosis, septicemia, and bacteremia may all present with delirium as the only or the most conspicuous feature. Catheterization is a common source of bladder infections, which may be followed by gram-negative bacteremia and delirium. Urinary tract infections and pneumonia are relatively common postoperative complications in the elderly and may give rise to delirium (143). For further discussion of the various infections causing the syndrome, see Chapter 15.

Neoplasm of extracerebral tissues is discussed in Chapter 14, and neoplasm of the brain is covered in Chapter 17. *Head trauma* and *epilepsy* are discussed in Chapter 17. *Postoperative delirium* is discussed in Chapter 19. It occurs in 10% to 15% of elderly patients undergoing general surgery (38) and is one of its most common complications. One type of operation—that for femoral neck fracture—deserves special mention at this point because of its growing frequency in the elderly (notably female) population, as well as the high incidence of the postoperative delirium associated with it (30,144–146). The increasing incidence of hip fractures in such patients has been called an orthopedic epidemic (147). An acute confusional state has been reported in about 50% of the elderly operated on for femoral neck fractures (30,144,146). In one study, about 40% of the patients were found to be suffering from senile dementia (145). Anticholinergic medications and a history of depression appear to be major risk factors for postoperative delirium in these cases (30). Patients with this complication had four times longer hospitalization than those without it (30). Predictors of postoperative delirium in these patients include increased age, low level of preinjury physical activity, and errors on the mental status examination performed on admission (146). The incidence of postoperative delirium after hip surgery has been reduced by the efforts of nurses to orient and educate the patients and to provide continuity of care (148). The procedures followed the guidelines for the management of delirious patients presented in Chapter 10.

Facilitating factors

The facilitating or contributory factors in delirium are discussed at length in Chapter 6, to which the reader is referred. They include psychosocial stress, sleep deprivation, sensory underload or overload, and immobilization. An etiological role of these factors in acute confusional states in later life has been postulated by a number of writers (1,5–8,24–27,68,133,149,150). Psychosocial stress occasioned by bereavement or translocation may have an adverse effect on cognitive functioning in an elderly person (151,152). Levels of sensory stimulation needed for optimal cognitive activity decline with age, rendering the elderly susceptible to sensory or information overload and its disorganizing effects on cognition (1). Sensory deprivation or underload is also hypothesized to contribute to delirium in an older person (5,20,25,133,149,150). Some writers include immobilization and social isolation among the relevant contributing factors (5). There is no conclusive evidence, however, that any of these variables can bring about an acute confusional state in the absence of an organic precipitating factor. Such a possibility exists but has not been satisfactorily demonstrated. I have proposed that the term "pseudodelirium" be adopted to designate a delirium-like transient cognitive disorder occurring in the apparent absence of an organic precipitating factor and presumably brought about by psychosocial stress or sensory deprivation alone (1). This whole issue calls for research that should involve serial EEG recordings to establish whether or not pseudodelirium is accompanied by slowing of the background activity. Sensory deprivation appears to play a contributory role in the so-called *sundown syndrome* in the institutionalized elderly patients. The relation of this syndrome to delirium remains unclear (153).

Delirium and dementia

Differential diagnosis of these two organic mental syndromes is fully discussed in Chapter 9 and need not be repeated. Delirium is one of the cardinal psychopathological manifestations of physical illness and drug toxicity in the elderly. By definition it is transient, but it may be followed by death or dementia. According to Roth (154), the transition from delirium to dementia is uncommon, but the frequency of this outcome has never been systematically investigated. However, delirium is often superimposed on dementia, which is a major predisposing factor to the syndrome (16). In one study, about 46% of 534 patients aged 60 years and older admitted to psychiatric wards of a general hospital had evidence of an acute brain syndrome (delirium), which was associated with a chronic brain syndrome (dementia) in nearly 70% of the cases (43).

In clinical practice, it is most important to distinguish delirium from dementia, whether the patient is demented or not. The fact that the two syndromes often coexist at a given time does not imply that a demented individual must be delirious or a delirious one demented. When delirium develops in a demented patient, one should assume that an organic precipitating factor—an acute physical illness or an exacerbation of a chronic one, intoxication, or withdrawal from a substance of abuse—is present and should be looked for without delay. One must never assume that a demented patient who shows signs of a superimposed delirium does so merely in response to psychosocial stress or sensory deprivation, for example. Such an assumption could result in failure to detect a potentially life-threatening illness such as MI. On the other hand, to mistake delirium for dementia could either result in such a failure or in labeling the patient "senile" and transferring him or her to a chronic facility (155). Such a misdiagnosis could thus have incalculable consequences for the patient and family.

To differentiate delirium from dementia may be difficult in some cases and calls for a clinician with good diagnostic skills. This is particularly true when the patient shows evidence of cognitive impairment on admission to the hospital and a history of the duration of such impairment is unavailable, or when the patient is known to be demented and is a resident of a nursing home. In such a case, the observation by a family member or a friend that the patient's behavior has suddenly changed, or that his or her cognition seems inexplicably worse, may be crucial in alerting the physician to the possibility of delirium. There is no evidence that a disease such as Alzheimer's disease can, by itself, cause delirium, although multi-infarct dementia appears to be capable of doing so (156, Chapter 16).

Roth (157) points out that the distinction between delirium and dementia is not sharp and the two syndromes overlap. Both of them feature global cognitive impairment. The overlap is particularly marked in the case of the so-called treatable or reversible dementias (40,158). Like delirium, they are, by definition, reversible and share many of the same etiological factors (40,158). The differential diagnosis in such cases boils down to the duration of the symptoms. It is proposed that if delirium lasts for a month or longer, the diagnosis should be changed to dementia, which may or may not prove to be fully or partially reversible or irreversible (90,159,160). Byrne (161) points out that the term "reversible dementia" is often misapplied to conditions, such as acute confusional states, which also feature globally impaired cognitive function. There is an obvious need for clearer diagnostic criteria for such conditions, as well as for prospective studies of the patients displaying their features.

Whenever doubt exists about whether delirium or dementia is present, it is preferable to assume tentatively that the patient suffers from delirium and to plan investigations accordingly. What really matters is that the underlying etiological factor, or factors, be searched for and treated. An elderly delirious patient tends to be lethargic rather than agitated, or shifts from psychomotor underactivity and reduced alertness to agitation and restlessness. Such a patient may be overlooked or else may attract attention because of his or her noisiness, combativeness, tendency to wander away, paranoid delusions, visual hallucinations, and nocturnal exacerbation of symptoms. This last feature is of particular diagnostic importance, as it is so typical of delirium. When such behavior appears suddenly in a previously cognitively intact elderly person, or one known to be demented, delirium should be presumptively diagnosed; viewed as a possible manifestation of physical illness or drug toxicity, or both; and immediately investigated.

Prevention

Whenever possible, one should try to prevent delirium in order to avoid the related risks and prolonged hospitalization (31,162). Modest success in prevention has been reported (148). Drug intake by the elderly patient needs to be closely monitored, unnecessary polypharmacy avoided, and concurrent use of anticholinergic drugs resisted. Patients at high risk for the development of delirium should be identified and closely observed (146). They include the very old, the demented, the depressed, and those with impaired vision and hearing (162). One should pay particular attention to the appearance of prodromal or early symptoms of delirium, such as anxiety during the day and insomnia and disturbing dreams at night. The staff should be familiar with the features of delirium; otherwise, they may overlook or misdiagnose it (31). As the syndrome often becomes manifest first during a sleepless night, observations by the night nursing staff are particularly important for early detection. Continuity of nursing care should be maintained (148). Patients at particular risk for the development of delirium must be provided with an environment that avoids both extremes of sensory stimulation (see Chapter 10).

Mangement

Treatment of delirium in an elderly patient does not differ basically from that discussed in Chapter 10. Most essential is to search for and treat or remove organic etiological factors. Prevention of injury to the patient or other people as a result of agitation, restlessness, fear, and combativeness is necessary. Mechanical restraints are best avoided because of the associated risk of serious complications (28,163). Nursing care is crucially important (146,148,150 Chapter 10).

If the patient is agitated and restless, sedation is called for and may be lifesaving. No ideal sedative exists for an agitated, elderly delirious patient. However, high-potency neuroleptics, such as haloperidol, have been most consistently recommended because of their relatively low anticholinergic, sedating, and hypotensive potential (1,164,165, Chapter 10). Haloperidol is the drug of choice for acute agitation. It is effective, has a wide margin of safety, and is relatively free from cardiovascular, hepatotoxic, and deliriogenic effects. It does have extrapyramidal side effects, to which the elderly are prone (164). In Europe, chlormethiazole is popular for the treatment of delirium (166). Haloperidol can be used as liquid, tablets, or parenterally. A low dose, such as 0.5 mg given orally or intramuscularly twice a day, may be sufficient, but if the patient is severly agitated, higher doses may be required (Chapter 10). The goal is to produce light sedation, as an oversedated patient is at risk of falls, dehydration, deep vein thrombosis, and pressure sores. It is important for the patient to be alert during the day and asleep at night. As haloperidol is not a hypnotic, night sleep may be ensured with hydroxyzine hydrochloride, a safe antihistamine drug, in doses of 10–50 mg at bedtime. It is best to avoid benzodiazepines unless the patient has alcohol withdrawal delirium or hepatic encephalopathy, or both.

References

1. Lipowski Z. J.: Transient cognitive disorders (delirium, acute confusional states) in the elderly. *Am. J. Psychiatry* 1983;140:1426–1436.
2. Hodkinson H. M.: *Common Symptoms of Disease in the Elderly.* Oxford, Blackwell Scientific, 1976, p 24.
3. Brocklehurst J. C., Hanley T.: *Geriatric Medicine for Students.* Edinburgh, Churchill Livingstone, 1976.
4. Anderson W. F.: The inter-relationship between physical and mental disease in the elderly, in Kay D. W. K., Walk A. (eds): *Recent Developments in Psychogeriatrics.* Asford, Kent, Headley Brothers, 1971, pp 19—24.
5. Beresin E. V.: Delirium in the elderly. *J. Geriatr. Psychiatry Neurol.* 1988;1:127–143.
6. Levkoff S. E., Besdine R. W., Wetle T.: Acute confusional states (delirium) in the hospitalized elderly. *Annu. Rev. Gerontol. Geriatr.* 1986;6:1–26.
7. Lipowski Z. J.: Acute confusional states (delirium) in the elderly, in Albert M. L. (ed): *Clinical Neurology of Old Age.* New York, Oxford University Press, 1984, pp 277–297.
8. Liston E. H.: Delirium in the aged. *Psychiatr. Clin. North Am.* 1982;5:49–66.
9. Siegel J. S., Taeuber C. M.: Demographic perspectives on the long-lived society. *Daedalus* 1986;115:77–117.
10. Grundy E.: Demography and old age. *J. Am. Geriatr. Soc.* 1983;31:325–332.
11. Rowe J. W.: Health care of the elderly. *N. Engl. J. Med.* 1985;312:827–835.
12. Schoenberg B. S., Kokmen E., Okazaki H.: Alzheimer's disease and other dementing illnesses in a defined United States population: Incidence rates and clinical features. *Ann. Neurol.* 1987;22:724–729.
13. Council on Scientific Affairs: Dementia. *J.A.M.A.* 1986;256:2234–2238.
14. US Department of Health and Human Services: *Utilization of Short-Stay Hospitals: Annual Summary for the United States, 1980.* Series 13, No 64. Washington, DC, National Center for Health Statistics, 1982.
15. Erkinjuntti T., Autio L., Wikström J.: Dementia in medical wards. *J. Clin. Epidemiol.* 1988;41:123–126.
16. Erkinjuntti T., Wikström J., Palo J., et al: Dementia among medical inpatients. Evaluation of 2000 consecutive admissions. *Arch. Intern. Med.* 1986;146:1923–1926.

17. Hood P.: On senile delirium. *The Practitioner* 1870;5:279–289.
18. Pickett W.: Senile dementia: A clinical study of two hundred cases with particular regard to types of the disease. *J. Nerv. Ment. Dis.* 1904;31:81–88.
19. Robinson G. W.: Acute confusional states of old age. *South. Med. J.* 1939;32:479–485.
20. Cameron D. E.: Studies in senile delirium. *Psychiatr. Q.* 1941;15:47–53.
21. Bedford P. D.: General medical aspects of confusional states in elderly people. *Br. Med. J.* 1959;2:185–188.
22. Flint F. J., Richards S. M.: Organic basis of confusional states in the elderly. *Br. Med. J.* 1956;2:1537–1539.
23. Roth M.: Some diagnostic and aetiological aspects of confusional states in the elderly. *Gerontol. Clin.* 1959;1:83–95.
24. Litin E. M.: Mental reaction to trauma and hospitalization in the aged. *J.A.M.A.* 1956;162:1522–1524.
25. Kennedy A.: Psychological factors in confusional states in the elderly. *Gerontol. Clin.* 1959;1:71–82.
26. Kral V. A.: Confusional states: Description and management, in Howells J. G. (ed): *Modern Perspectives in the Psychiatry of Old Age.* New York, Brunner/Mazel, 1975, pp 356–362.
27. Kral V. A.: Stress and mental disorders of the senium. *Med. Serv. J. Canada* 1962;18:363–370.
28. Gillick M. R., Serrell N. A., Gillick L. S.: Adverse consequences of hospitalization in the elderly. *Soc. Sci. Med.* 1982;16:1033–1038.
29. Warshaw G. A., Moore J. T., Friedman S. W., et al: Functional disability in the hospitalized elderly. *J.A.M.A.* 1982;248:847–850.
30. Berggren D., Gustafson Y., Eriksson B., et al: Postoperative confusion after anesthesia in elderly patients with femoral neck fractures. *Anesth. Analg.* 1987;66:497–504.
31. Thomas R. I., Cameron D. J., Fahs M. C.: A prospective study of delirium and prolonged hospital stay. *Arch. Gen. Psychiatry* 1988;45:937–940.
32. Simpson C. J.: Doctors and nurses use of the word confused. *Br. J. Psychiatry* 1984;142:441–443.
33. Vardon V. M., Blessed G.: Confusion ratings and abbreviated mental test performance: A comparison. *Age Ageing* 1986;15:139–144.
34. Williams M. A., Ward S. E., Campbell E. B.: Confusion: Testing versus observation. *J. Gerontol. Nurs.* 1988;14:25–30.
35. Levkoff S. E.: Personal communication.
36. Millard P. H.: Editorial: Last scene of all. *Br. Med. J.* 1981;283:1559–1560.
37. Hodkinson H. M.: Mental impairment in the elderly. *J. R. Coll. Physicians Lond.* 1973;7:305–317.
38. Seymour G.: *Medical Assessment of the Elderly Surgical Patient.* London, Croom Helm, 1986.
39. Seibert C. P.: Recognition, management, and prevention of neuropsychological dysfunctions after operation, in Hindman B. J. (ed): *Neurological and Psychological Complications of Surgery and Anesthesia.* Boston, Little, Brown, 1986, pp 39–58.
40. Mahler M. E., Cummings J. L., Benson D. F.: Treatable dementias. *West. J. Med.* 1987;146:705–712.
41. Barry P. P., Moskowitz M. A.: The diagnosis of reversible dementia in the elderly. *Arch. Intern. Med.* 1988;148:1914–1918.

42. Robinson G. W.: The toxic delirious reactions of old age, in Kaplan O. J. (ed): *Mental Disorders in Later Life.* Stanford, Stanford University Press, 1956, pp 227–255.
43. Simon A., Cahan R. B.: The acute brain syndrome in geriatric patients. *Psychiatr. Res. Rep.* 1963;16:8–21.
44. Davis K. L., Davis B. M., Greenwald B. S., et al: Cortisol and Alzheimer's disease, 1: Basal studies. *Am. J. Psychiatry* 1986;143:300–305.
45. Carpenter W. T., Gruen P. H.: Cortisol effects on human mental functioning. *J. Clin. Psychopharmacol.* 1982;2:91–101.
46. Rubinow D. R., Post R. M., Savard R., et al: Cortisol hypersecretion and cognitive impairment in depression. *Arch. Gen. Psychiatry* 1984;41:279–283.
47. Muller H. F., Grad B.: Clinical-psychological, electroencephalographic, and adrenocortical relationships in elderly psychiatric patients. *J. Gerontol.* 1974;29:28–38.
48. Jacobs S., Mason J., Kosten T., et al: Urinary free cortisol excretion in relation to age in acutely stressed persons with depressive symptoms. *Psychosom. Med.* 1984;46:213–221.
49. Regestein Q. R., Rose L. I., Williams G. H.: Psychopathology in Cushing's syndrome. *Arch. Intern. Med.* 1972;130:114–117.
50. McIntosh T. K., Bush H. L., Yeston N. S., et al: Beta-endorphin, cortisol and postoperative delirium: A preliminary report. *Psychoneuroendocrinology* 1985;10:303–313.
51. Dement W. C., Miles L. E., Carskadon M. A.: "White Paper" on sleep and aging. *J. Am. Geriatr. Soc.* 1982;30:25–50.
52. Loewenstein R. J., Weingartner H., Gillin J. C., et al: Disturbances of sleep and cognitive functioning in patients with dementia. *Neurobiol. Aging* 1982;3:371–377.
53. Creasey H., Rapoport S. I.: The aging human brain. *Ann. Neurol.* 1985; 17:2–10.
54. Carlsson A.: Neurotransmitter changes in the aging brain. *Dan. Med. Bull.* 1985;32 (Suppl 1): 40–43.
55. Simpkins J. W., Millard W. J.: Influence of age on neurotransmitter function. *Endocrinol. Metab. Clin.* 1987;16:893–917.
56. Blass J. P., Plum F.: Metabolic encephalopathies in older adults, in Katzman R., Terry R. D. (eds): *The Neurology of Aging.* Philadelphia, FA Davis Co, 1983, pp 189–220.
57. Gur R. C., Gur R. E., Obrist W. D., et al: Age and regional cerebral blood flow at rest and during cognitive activity. *Arch. Gen. Psychiatry* 1987;44:617–621.
58. Horwitz B., Duara R., Rapoport S. I.: Age differences in intercorrelations between regional cerebral metabolic rates for glucose. *Ann. Neurol.* 1986;19:60–67.
59. Pantano P., Baron J. C., Lebrun-Grandie P., et al: Regional cerebral blood flow and oxygen consumption in human aging. *Stroke* 1984;15:635–641.
60. Takeda S., Matsuzawa T., Matsui H.: Age-related changes in regional cerebral blood flow and brain volume in healthy subjects. *J. Am. Geriatr. Soc.* 1988;36:293–297.
61. Stoessl A. J., Tuokko H., Martin W. R. W., et al: Cerebral glucose metabolism in normal aging. *Neurology* 1986;36 (Suppl 1):104.
62. Shaw T. G., Mortel K. F., Meyer J. S., et al: Cerebral blood flow changes in benign aging and cerebrovascular disease. *Neurology* 1984;34:855–862.

63. Friedland R. P. (moderator): Alzheimer disease: Clinical and biological heterogeneity. *Ann. Intern. Med.* 1988;109:298–311.
64. Cummings J. L., Benson D. F.: The role of the nucleus basalis of Meynert in dementia: Review and reconsideration. *Alzheimer Dis. Associated Disorders* 1987;1:128–145.
65. Katzman R.: Alzheimer's disease. *N. Engl. J. Med.* 1986;314:964–973.
66. Whitehouse P. J.: Neurotransmitter receptor alterations in Alzheimer disease: A review. *Alzheimer Dis. Associated Disorders* 1987;1:9–18.
67. Palmer A. M., Stratmann G. C., Procter A. W., et al: Possible neurotransmitter basis of behavioral changes in Alzheimer's disease. *Ann. Neurol.* 1988;23:616–620.
68. Hishikawa Y., Lijima J., Shimizu T., et al: A dissociated sleep state "stage 1-REM" and its relation to delirium, in Baldy-Moulinier M. (ed): *Actualités en Médecine Expérimentale.* Montpellier, Editions EUROMED, 1981.
69. Fields W. S.: Multi-infarct dementia. *Neurol. Clin.* 1986;4:405–413.
70. Roman G. C.: Senile dementia of the Binswanger type. A vascular form of dementia in the elderly. *J.A.M.A.* 1987;258:1782–1788.
71. Meyer J. S., Rogers R. L., Judd B. W., et al: Cognition and cerebral blood flow fluctuate together in multi-infarct dementia. *Stroke* 1988;19:163–169.
72. Heiss W. D., Böcher-Schwarz H. G., Pawlik G., et al: PET, CT, and MR imaging in cerebrovascular disease. *J. Comput. Assist. Tomogr.* 1986;10:903–911.
73. Koponen H., Hurri L., Stenbäck U., et al: Acute confusional states in the elderly. A radiological evaluation. *Acta Psychiatr. Scand.* 1987;76:726–731.
74. Samorajski T., Hartford J.: Brain physiology of aging, in Busse E. W., Blazer D. G. (eds): *Handbook of Geriatric Psychiatry.* New York, Van Nostrand Reinhold, 1980.
75. Sherman B., Wysham C., Pfohl B.: Age-related changes in the circadian rhythm of plasma cortisol in man. *J. Clin. Endocrinol. Metab.* 1985;61:439–443.
76. Organic mental impairment in the elderly. *J. R. Coll. Physicians Lond.* 1981;15:141–167.
77. Phair J. P.: Aging and infection: A review *J. Chronic Dis.* 1979; 32:535–540.
78. Rytel M. W.: Effect of age on viral infections: Possible role of interferon. *J. Am. Geriatr. Soc.* 1987;35:1092–1099.
79. Schmucker D. L.: Aging and drug disposition: An update. *Pharamcol. Rev.* 1985;37:133–148.
80. Goodwin J. S., Goodwin J. M., Garry P. J.: Association between nurtritional status and cognitive functioning in a healthy elderly population. *J.A.M.A.* 1983;249:2917–2921.
81. Gupta K. L., Dworkin B., Gambert S. R.: Common nutritional disorders in the elderly: Atypical manifestations. *Geriatrics* 1988;43:87–97.
82. Lamy P. P.: The elderly, undernutrition, and pharmacokinetics. *J. Am. Geriatr. Soc.* 1983;31:560–562.
83. Kay D. W. K., Roth M.: Physical accompaniments of mental disorder in old age. *Lancet* 1955;2:740–745.
84. Seymour D. G., Henschke P. J., Cape R. D. T., et al: Acute confusional states and dementia in the elderly: The role of dehydration/volume depletion, physical illness and age. *Age Ageing* 1980;9:137–146.
85. Editorial: Need we poison the elderly so often? *Lancet* 1988;2:20–22.
86. Williamson J., Chopin J. M.: Adverse reactions to prescribed drugs in the elderly: A mutlicentre investigation. *Age Ageing* 1980;9:73–80.

87. Everitt D. E., Avorn J.: Drug prescribing for the elderly. *Arch. Intern Med.* 1986;146:2393–2396.
88. Lamy P. P.: The elderly and drug interactions. *J. Am. Geriatr. Soc.* 1986;34:586–592.
89. Ostrom J. R., Hammarlund E. R., Christensen D. B., et al: Medication usage in elderly population. *Med. Care* 1985;23:157–164.
90. Larson E. B., Kukull W. A., Buchner D., et al: Adverse drug reactions associated with global cognitive impairment in elderly persons. *Ann. Intern. Med.* 1987;107:169–173.
91. Cutler N. R., Narang P. K. (eds): *Drug Studies in the Elderly.* New York, Plenum Medical, 1986.
92. Medication for the elderly. *J. R. Coll. Physicians Lond.* 1984;18:7–17.
93. Vestal R. E.: Drug use in the elderly: A review of problems and special considerations. *Drugs* 1978;16:358–382.
94. Gosney M., Tallis R.: Prescription of contraindicated and interacting drugs in elderly patients admitted to hospital. *Lancet* 1984;2:564–567.
95. Roe D. A.: Drug effects on nutrient absorption, transport, and metabolism. *Drug-Nutrient Interact.* 1985;4:117–135.
96. Phillips P. A., Rolls B. J., Ledingham J. G. G., et al: Reduced thirst after water deprivation in healthy elderly men. *N. Engl. J. Med.* 1984;311:753–759.
97. Kroenke K.: Polypharmacy. Causes, consequences, and cure. *Am. J. Med.* 1985;79:149–152.
98. Williamson J.: Prescribing problems in the elderly. *The Practitioner* 1978;220:749–755.
99. Buck J. A.: Psychotropic drugs practice in nursing homes. *J. Am. Geriatr. Soc.* 1988;36:409–418.
100. Burns B. J., Kamerow D. B.: Psychotropic drug prescriptions for nursing home residents. *J. Fam. Pract.* 1988;26:155–160.
101. Helling D. K., Lemke J. H., Semla T. P., et al: Medications use characteristics in the elderly: The Iowa 65+ rural health study. *J. Am. Geriatr. Soc.* 1987;35:4–12.
102. James D. S.: Survey of hypnotic drug use in nursing homes. *J. Am. Geriatr. Soc.* 1985;33:436–439.
103. Morgan K., Dallosso H., Ebrahim S., et al: Prevalence, frequency, and duration of hypnotic drug use among the elderly living at home. *Br. Med. J.* 1988;296:601–602.
104. Kayne R. C.: Acute brain symdrome in an elderly patient. *Drug Intell. Clin. Pharm.* 1974;8:476–482.
105. Foy A., Drinkwater V., March S., et al: Confusion after admission to hospital in elderly patients using benzodizepines. *Br. Med. J.* 1986;293:1072.
106. Meyer B. R.: Benzodiazepines in the elderly. *Med. Clin. North Am.* 1982;66:1017–1035.
107. Morgan K.: Sedative-hypnotic drug use and ageing. *Arch. Gerontol. Geriatr.* 1983;2:181–199.
108. Thompson R. L., Moran M. G., Nies A. S.: Psychotropic drug use in the elderly. *N. Engl. J. Med* 1983;308:134–138.
109. Whitcup S. M., Miller F.: Unrecognized drug dependence in psychiatrically hospitalized elderly patients. *J. Am. Geriatr. Soc.* 1987;35:297–301.
110. Meyers B. S., Mei-Tal V.: Psychiatric reactions during tricyclic treatment of the elderly reconsidered. *J. Clin. Psychopharmacol.* 1983;3:2–6.

111. Salzman C.: Geriatric psychopharmacology. *Ann. Rev. Med.* 1985;36:217–228.
112. Foster J. R., Gershell W. J., Goldfarb A. I.: Lithium treatment in the elderly. 1. Clinical usage. *J. Gerontol.* 1977;32:299–302.
113. Blazer D. G., Federspiel C. F., Ray W. A., et al: The risk of anticholinergic toxicity in the elderly: A study of prescribing practices in two populations. *J. Gerontol.* 1983;38:31–35.
114. Seifert R., Jamieson J., Gardner R.: Use of anticholinergics in the nursing home: An empirical study and review. Drug Intell. Clin. Pharm. 1983;17:470–473.
115. Sunderland T., Tariot P. N., Cohen R. M., et al: Anticholinergic sensitivity in patients with dementia of the Alzheimer type and age-matched controls. *Arch. Gen. Psychiatry* 1987;44:418–426.
116. Atkinson J. H., Schuckit M. A.: Geriatric alcohol and drug misuse and abuse. *Adv. Substance Abuse* 1983;3:195–237.
117. Beresford T. P., Blow F. C., Brower K. J. et al: Alcoholism and aging in the general hospital. *Psychosomatics* 1988;29:61–72.
118. Finlayson R. E., Hurt R. D., Davis L. J., et al: Alcoholism in elderly persons: A study of psychiatric and psychosocial features of 216 inpatients. *Mayo Clin. Proc.* 1988;63:761–768.
119. Freund G.: The interaction of chronic alcohol consumption and aging on brain structure and function. *Alcoholism* 1982;6:13–21.
120. Hartford J. T., Samorajski T.: Alcoholism in the geriatric population. *J. Am. Geriatr. Soc.* 1982;30:18–24.
121. Scott R. B., Mitchell M. C.: Aging, alcohol, and the liver. *J. Am. Geriatr. Soc.* 1988;36:255–265.
122. Gaitz C. M., Baer P. E.: Characteristics of elderly patients with alcoholism. *Arch. Gen. Psychiatry* 1981;24:372–378.
123. Mitra M. L.: Confusional states in relation to vitamin deficiencies in the elderly. *J. Am. Geriatr. Soc.* 1971;19:536–545.
124. Exton-Smith A. N., Caird F. I. (eds): *Metabolic and Nutritional Disorders in the Elderly.* Chicago, Year Book Medical Publishers, 1985.
125. Hyams D. E.: The elderly patient. A special case for diuretic therapy. *Drugs* 1986;31(Suppl 4):138–153.
126. Sunderam S. G., Mankikar G. D.: Hyponatremia in the elderly. *Age Ageing* 1983;12:77–80.
127. Gambert S. R., Benson D., Grosenick D. J., et al: Psychiatric manifestations of common endocrine disorders in the elderly. *Psychiatr. Med.* 1984;1:407–427.
128. Meites J. (ed): *Neuroendocrinology of Aging.* New York, Plenum Press, 1983.
129. Morrow L. B.: How thyroid disease presents in the elderly. *Geriatrics* 1978;31:42–45.
130. Rosenthal M. J., Hunt W. C., Garry P. J., et al: Thyroid failure in the elderly. *J.A.M.A.* 1987;258:209–213.
131. Freedman D. K., Troll L., Mills A. B., et al: *Acute Organic Disorder Accompanied by Mental Symptoms.* Sacramento, Calif, Dept of Mental Hygiene, 1965.
132. Podolsky S.: Hyperosmolar nonketotic coma in the elderly diabetic. *Med. Clin. North Am.* 1978;62:815–828.
133. Rockwood K.: Acute confusion in elderly medical patients. *J. Am. Geriatr. Soc.* 1989;37:150–154.
134. Gupta K. L., Dworkin B., Gambert S. R.: Common nutritional disorders in the elderly: Atypical manifestations. *Geriatrics* 1988;43:87–97.

135. Marcus D. L., Freedman M. L.: Folic acid deficiency in the elderly. *J. Am. Geriatr. Soc.* 1985;33:552–558.
136. Celestino F. S., Van Noord G. R., Miraglia C. P.: Accidental hypothermia in the elderly. *J. Fam. Pract.* 1988;26:259–267.
137. Levine J. A.: Heat stroke in the aged. *Am. J. Med.* 1969;47:251–258.
138. Coodley E. L. (ed): *Geriatric Heart Disease.* Littleton, Mass, PSG Publishing Company, 1985.
139. Bayer A. J., Chadha J., Farag R. R., et al: Changing presentation of myocardial infarction with increasing age. *J. Am. Geriatr. Soc.* 1986;34:263–266.
140. Jones J. V., Graham D. I.: Hypertension and cerebral circulation—its relevance to the elderly. *Am Heart J.* 1978;96:270–271.
141. Levkoff S. E., Safran C., Cleary P. D., et al: Identification of factors associated with the diagnosis of delirium in elderly hospitalized patients. *J. Am. Geriatr. Soc.* 1988;36:1099–1104.
142. Murphy E.: The confused elderly patient. *J. Ir. Med. Assoc.* 1978;61:99–103.
143. Polly S. M., Sanders W. E.: Surgical infections in the elderly: Prevention, diagnosis, and treatment. *Geriatrics* 1977;32:88–97.
144. Campion E. W., Jette A. M., Cleary P. D., et al: Hip fracture: A prospective study of hospital course, complications, and costs. *J. Gen. Intern. Med.* 1987;2:78–82.
145. Haljamäe H., Stefansson T., Wickström I.: Preanesthetic evaluation of the female geriatric patient with hip fracture. *Acta Anaesth. Scand.* 1982;26:393–402.
146. Williams M. A., Campbell E. B., Raynor W. J., et al: Predictors of acute confusional states in hospitalized elderly patients. *Res. Nurs. Health* 1985;8:31–40.
147. Wallace W. A.: The increasing incidence of fractures of the proximal femur: An orthopaedic epidemic. *Lancet* 1983;2:1413–1414.
148. Williams M. A., Campbell E. B., Raynor W. J., et al: Reducing acute confusional states in elderly patients with hip fractures. *Res. Nurs. Health* 1985;8:329–337.
149. Oster C.: Sensory deprivation in geriatric patients. *J. Am. Geriatr. Soc.* 1976;24:461–464.
150. Wolanin M. O., Phillips L. R. F.: *Confusion. Prevention and Care.* St Louis, CV Mosby Co, 1981.
151. Avorn J.: Biomedical and social determinants of cognitive impairment in the elderly. *J. Am. Geriatr. Soc.* 1983;31:137–143.
152. Schulz R., Brenner G.: Relocation of the aged: A review and theoretical analysis. *J. Gerontol.* 1977;32:323–332.
153. Evans L. K.: Sundown syndrome in institutionalized elderly. *J. Am. Geriatr. Soc.* 1987;35:101–108.
154. Roth M.: The psychiatric disorders of later life. *Psychiatr. Ann.* 1976;6:417–445.
155. Glassman M.: Misdiagnosis of senile dementia: Denial of care to the elderly. *Social Work* 1980;25:288–292.
156. Balter R. A., Fricchione G., Sterman A. B.: Clinical presentation of multi-infarct delirium. *Psychosomatics* 1986;27:461–462.
157. Roth M.: Some problems of geriatrics common to medicine and psychiatry, in Agate J. N. (ed): *Medicine in Old Age.* Philadelphia, J. B. Lippincott Co, 1965, pp 99–112.
158. Barry P. Moskowitz M. A.: The diagnosis of reversible dementia in the elderly. A critical review. *Arch. Intern. Med.* 1988;148:1914–1918.
159. Larson E. B., Reifler B. V., Featherstone H. J. et al: Dementia in elderly outpatients: A prospective study. *Ann. Intern. Med.* 1984;100:417–423.

160. Larson E. B., Reifler B. V., Sumi S. M., et al: Diagnostic evaluation of 200 elderly outpatients with suspected dementia. *J. Gerontol.* 1985;40:536–543.
161. Byrne E. J.: Reversible dementia. *Intern. J. Geriatr. Psychiatry* 1987;2:73–81.
162. Lipowski Z. J.: Delirium in the elderly patient. *N. Engl. J. Med.* 1989;320:578–582.
163. Evans L. K., Strumpf N. E.: Tying down the elderly. *J. Am. Geriatr. Soc.* 1989;37:65–74.
164. Salzman C.: Treatment of the elderly agitated patient. *J. Clin. Psychiatry* 1987;48 (Suppl 5):19–22.
165. Steinhart M. J.: The use of haloperidol in geriatric patients with organic mental disorder. *Curr. Ther. Res.* 1983;33:132–143.
166. Haar H. W. ter: A comparison of chlormethiazole and haloperidol in the treatment of elderly patients with confusion of organic and psychogenic origin: A double-blind crossover study. *Pharmocotherapeutica (Berl.)* 1977;1:563–569.

19

Delirium after Surgery, Burns, and Childbirth

Postoperative delirium

Historical introduction

Delirium following surgery has been known for centuries. The famous French surgeon Paré (1), who was active in the sixteenth century, discussed at some length delirium complicating surgical conditions and procedures. He referred to it as a transient disorder featuring "raving, talking idly, or doting" and occurring in association with fever and pain due to wounds, after loss of blood during an operation, and as a complication of gangrene. Dupuytren (2), another eminent French surgeon, gave an excellent description of what he referred to as "traumatic" or "nervous" delirium:

> The delirium manifests itself by a singular confusion of things, places, and persons; the patient is deprived of sleep, and is possessed by some predominant idea, which is generally connected with his profession, habits, age, or sex. The limbs are constantly tossed about; the upper part of the body is covered with abundant sweat; the eyes are bright and injected; the face is animated and flushed; individuals affected with this species of delirium are often so extremely insensible, that patients with commuted fracture of the lower extremity, have dragged off all the dressing, and walked about on the broken limb, without exhibiting any sign of pain; others, whose ribs were broken, tossed themselves about, and sung without seeming to suffer; finally, it has happened that a patient who had been operated on for hernia, introduced his fingers into the wound, and amused himself by unrolling his intestines as if he were acting on a dead body (p. 922).

Dupuytren observed that delirium is particularly likely to occur in persons injured as a result of a suicide attempt, lasts no longer than 6 days but can be rapidly fatal, and can be treated successfully with enemas of laudanum.

Graves (3) hypothesized that traumatic delirium resulted from an injury acting on the nerves leading to loss of sleep and excitement. In 1870, Croft (4) wrote an article devoted to delirium tremens in surgical patients and reported on 31 patients, 4 of whom had died. Savage (5), another nineteenth-century writer, drew attention to the role of anesthetics in producing "insanity" and asserted that some patients exposed to them during surgery might develop not only a transient but also a permanent mental illness, such as progressive dementia. In his view, hereditary factors appeared to predispose a patient to such an outcome. Haward (6) claimed that, apart from withdrawal from alcohol, lack of food or loss of sleep and the presence of fatigue or anxiety were needed for delirium tremens to develop in a surgical patient. He observed that old people might develop a different form of delirium after surgery, marked by "subdued but constant talkativeness," and referred to it as "senile delirium." Unless a patient displaying it was taken out of bed and mobilized, he might die. Delirium, according to this writer, was frequently seen with severe burns.

At the beginning of this century, several authors addressed the problem of what had been labeled "postoperative psychosis" or "insanity." Da Costa (7), a professor of surgery in Philadelphia, wrote one of the best accounts of that syndrome. He asserted that various forms of mental disorder could follow surgery, including delirium, hysterical excitement, obsessions, confusion, hypochondria, and melancholy. No mental disorder was characteristic of the postoperative period. Acute confusional insanity was the most common such disorder encountered in surgical practice; it featured confusion of thought, inchoherent speech, illusions, hallucinations, and delusions. Fear and worry were the most important causes of this disorder, which could become manifest immediately after an operation and was probably caused by anesthesia, but usually came on 3 to 4 days after surgery. Da Costa stated at one point that postoperative delirium could be mistaken for insanity, but elsewhere in his paper wrote that the "analysis of the mental state of a delirious patient shows us that delirium is identical with confusional insanity" (p 581); evidently, Da Costa himself was a bit confused about the nature of this condition. His whole description of it, however, suggests that he was speaking of delirium as this term is currently applied. He observed that this syndrome was most often encountered in children and the elderly, usually appeared initially in the period between sleep and full wakefulness, and might clear up as the patient became fully awake, only to return with the onset of drowsiness. Interestingly, Da Costa contended that delirium postoperatively might be caused by morphine: "In every unexplained case of delirium think of the possibility of morphinism and search for the drug" (p 582). He urged that in every case of postoperative mental disorder, a careful history should be obtained, a thorough physical examination made, and a neurologist be asked to see the patient. This enlightened advice reflected Da Costa's opinion that the patient's disturbed mental state after an operation should be taken seriously. He made this clear when he concluded that the "entire subject of postoperative psychoses is extremely interesting and highly important. There remains much to learn about it" (p 584). Had this view been shared by more surgeons and psychiatrists, our ignorance in this area today would have been less conspicuous.

Da Costa's pioneering paper appeared in 1910. A year earlier, Kelly (8) reported on 40 patients with postoperative psychoses, over one-third of whom had "acute hallucinatory confusional insanities." Thus, despite a terminological muddle, a reasonably coherent picture of delirium as the most common postoperative psychosis had emerged. As Abeles (9) summed it up, most observers agree that the majority of postoperative psychoses fall into "the same syndrome as the toxic-exhaustive and infective states. There is a combination of confusion, delusions, hallucinations, and disturbances in motility" (p 1189). He himself found confusion, manifested by disorientation, memory impairment, bewilderment and hallucinations, in 17 of 23 patients with postoperative psychosis, and stressed its multifactorial etiology. The latter involves various combinations of metabolic disturbances, general anesthesia, infection, vascular disease, vitamin deficiency, use of sedatives, and psychodynamic factors. Doyle (10) reported on 28 consecutive cases of postoperative psychosis observed at the Mayo Clinic and concluded that "clinically postoperative psychosis is best classified with delirium" (p 199).

This brief historical review shows that, different terminology notwithstanding, the early writers on the subject of postoperative psychosis recognized delirium as its most common type. They also acknowledged that the etiology of this syndrome involves an interplay of multiple factors, both organic and psychological. Those writers noticed that postoperative delirium typically occurred after 2 to 5 days, an observation that remains valid and unexplained to this day. On the other hand, Savage (5) noted that some patients who became delirious after surgery showed from the beginning "unusual depression, heaviness, drowsiness, or irritability," suggesting that they may have been delirious from the time of regaining consciousness, but that their delirium became recognized only when they began to show agitation and other more conspicuous manifestations of a disordered mental state. These assorted features of postoperative delirium have been largely reaffirmed by more recent investigators. On the whole, however, the syndrome has been relatively neglected by researchers, except for its occurrence after cardiac and cataract surgery. Many questions about the causes and outcome of postoperative delirium remain unanswered and clamor for more clinical research.

Incidence

The true incidence of postoperative delirium is virtually unknown. There is a dearth of epidemiological studies in this important area. What reports can be found have come mostly from anesthetists and usually refer to what they call "emergence delirium or excitement." Bastron and Moyers (11) stated that its incidence ranges from 3% to 20%. Eckenhoff et al. (12) reviewed the records of 14,436 patients admitted to the surgical recovery room at the Hospital of the University of Pennsylvania over a 4-year period and noted references to emergence delirium in 5.3% of them. The highest incidence of the syndrome was found in children and in patients given barbiturates for premedication or anesthetized with cyclopropane or ether, or both. Tonsillectomy, thyroidectomy, circumcision, and hysterectomy were most often associated with postoperative delirium. Emotional factors, according to these authors, were responsible for a high incidence of the syndrome after breast and thyroid operations. Pain seemed to facilitate its occurrence. Coppolino (13) came up with an incidence figure very close to that of Eckenhoff et al. Kuhn and Savage (14) found delirium in about 20% of patients premedicated with scopolamine hydrobromide. A similar incidence was reported by Greene (15), who observed emergence delirium in 10.2% and 8.1% of two groups of patients. He concluded that drug-induced CNS depression, usually aggravated by pain, was responsible for the delirium in his cases. Scopolamine, used as a premedicant, appeared to be a major etiological factor, a hypothesis supported by the finding that in 19 of 21 patients who had received physostigmine intravenously, delirium was relieved in less than 5 minutes. Titchener et al. (16) diagnosed delirium in 7.8% of 200 surgical patients; the syndrome accounted for about 30% of postoperative psychoses. Knox (17) estimated the incidence of "postoperative psychosis" to be about 1 per 1,600 surgical procedures, a figure that seems improbably low. By contrast, Hammes (18) estimated this psychosis as 1 in 400 operations.

The above quotations reflect the wide discrepancy in the reported incidence of postoperative delirium. It is hardly surprising that Seibert (19) concludes, in a recent review of this subject, that "so many widely divergent estimates have been made regarding the incidences of postoperative delirium that the figures are virtually useless except to note that the problem is extremely common" (p 42). The incidence is liable to vary according to such factors as the age of the patients, the type of surgery, the drugs used for premedication and general anesthesia, and the use of narcotics for pain. One may tentatively conclude that postoperative delirium occurs in about 5% to 10% of patients undergoing general surgery and in 10% to 15% of the elderly ones (20). Delirium was diagnosed in 20.7% of 150 postoperative patients referred for psychiatric consultation (21). Its reported incidence in surgical intensive care units ranges from 2% to 40% (22–24). The highest figure comes from a study of patients confined to a windowless intensive care unit (24). However, the author does not provide any information on the type of surgery performed or on his method of case identification; his reported incidence figure seems unusually high.

Because many authors use the diagnostically nondescript term "postoperative psychosis," few reported incidence figures provide any meaningful information about the forms of mental disorders occurring postoperatively. Future epidemiological studies will have to apply explicit diagnostic criteria for such disorders, including delirium. Moreover, for research purposes, they should distinguish between *emergence* delirium, occuring during the first 24 hours after an operation and lasting for up to 1 day, and *interval* delirium, appearing 24 hours to 1 week after surgery (10,25). These two subtypes are liable to differ in etiology and clinical significance.

Etiology and pathogenesis

Postoperative delirium appears to be the outcome of multiple factors acting synergistically to bring about widespread cerebral dysfunction. While one or another of these factors may play a predominant etiological role in a given case, it is important to consider the possibility that other factors may have contributed and should be eliminated or corrected. The following review of the more important and common causes of delirium after surgery should help the clinician to search for them and treat the patient accordingly. Moreover, it is most important to try to prevent delirium whenever feasible.

The etiological factors most often resulting in postoperative delirium are listed in Table 19–1. A number of recent authors have addressed the etiology of the syndrome, and their views are worth summarizing (12,15,18–20,25–29). Hammes (18) has classified postoperative phychoses into four categories: withdrawal psychoses, toxic psychoses, psychoses of circulatory and respiratory origin, and functional psychoses. The first three of these catagories are, in most cases, nothing but delirium. The fourth category comprises brief reactive, paranoid, affective, and atypical psychotic disorders, which, by definition, are not due to cerebral dysfunction caused by organic etiological factors. Withdrawal psychosis or delirium is caused by withdrawal of alcohol or a sedative-hypnotic drug, or both, from a person addicted to one or more of these substances. "Toxic psychosis" is an imprecise and obsolete term that may refer to delirium or some other transient organic mental syndrome, such as an organic hallucinosis, caused by an exogenous toxic substance. Finally, "psychoses of circulatory and respiratory origin" are almost invariably delirium due to hypoxemia, hypo- or hypercarbia, acidosis or alkalosis, and other metabolic encephalopathies induced by dysfunction of the circulatory or respiratory system, or both (30). This classification leaves out some relevant eti-

TABLE 19–1 Etiological Factors in Postoperative Delirium

A. Predisposing factors
   1. Age of 60 years and over
   2. Cerebral disease
   3. Chronic renal, cardiac, hepatic, or pulmonary disease
   4. Addiction to alcohol and/or sedative-hypnotics
   5. Personal history of delirium or functional psychosis
   6. Family history of psychosis (?)
   7. Paranoid personality (?)
   8. Depression (?)

B. Contributory (facilitating) factors
   1. Sensory environment of the intensive care unit (sensory deprivation, overload)
   2. Sleep deprivation
   3. Immobilization
   4. Psychological stress

C. Precipitating organic factors
   1. Intoxication with drugs, including agents for premedication (anticholinergics), anesthesia, and analgesia (notably morphine)
   2. Metabolic disturbances: hypoxemia, hypercarbia, hypocarbia, dehydration, electrolyte imbalance, acid-base imbalance, hepatic or renal failure
   3. Hemodynamic disturbances: hypotension, hypovolemia, cardiac failure
   4. Respiratory disorder: hypopnea or apnea, pulmonary embolism
   5. Infection: pneumonia, septicemia, bacteremia
   6. Acute cerebral disorder: trauma, edema, stroke, fat embolism, metastases
   7. Alcohol and/or sedative-hypnotic withdrawal syndrome
   8. Malnutrition, vitamin deficiency
   9. Cerebral seizures
   10. Porphyria

ological factors but has the merit of drawing attention to the most important ones.

Kaufer (26) reviewed the causes of postoperative "consciousness disturbances," or delirium, based on a study of 100 patients. He observed that in many cases it was impossible to establish the etiology of the delirium. Kaufer found the following groups of factors to be most often implicated: cerebral-organic, respiratory, hemodynamic, infectious-toxic, and metabolic. Cerebral-organic factors included trauma, vascular occlusion, neoplasm, and fat embolism, and accounted for about 30% of the identifiable causes. The next most important group of etiological factors involved postoperative infections, such as wound infections, peritonitis, or septicemia, as well as intoxications. Withdrawal delirium occurred in 7% of the patients. Metabolic factors ranked third in frequency and constituted the main etiology in 15% of the delirious patients. They included hepatic encephalopathy, electrolyte and acid-base disturbances, renal failure, and hydration disorders. Kaufer stressed that in one-third to one-half of all the patients, more than one causal factor was involved. He emphasized that every disturbance in a postoperative patient's state of consciousness is a grave prognostic sign; 39% of his delirious surgical patients died.

One of the best studies of the etiology of postoperative delirium published to date is that by Morse and Litin (27–29). They studied 60 patients aged 30 years and older who developed the syndrome, as well as a matched control group who were not delirious. Factors that were found to distinguish the delirious patients from the controls included the following variables:

1. Age 60 years and over; 2. greater proportion of abnormal laboratory findings; 3. duration of the operation of more than 4 hours; 4. emergency surgery; 5. the presence of other postoperative complications; 6. intake of more than five drugs in the postoperative period; 7. fear of death before surgery; 8. alcoholism; 9. current or previous depression; 10. family history of psychosis; 11. personal history of delirium in the past; 12. preoperative insomnia; 13. paranoid personality disorder; 14. current or previous functional psychosis; 15. personal history of postoperative psychosis of any type; and 16. problems related to retirement. Once again, the *multifactorial* etiology of postoperative delirium has been highlighted by this study. Metabolic disturbances, high surgical stress, infection, intoxication with drugs, age of 60 years and over, and preexisting brain disease were all positively correlated with the syndrome. Sensory and sleep deprivation also appeared to play a role. Organic factors were essential, but those related to the patient's psychological features and psychosocial stress also seemed to play an etiological role in at least some cases (27).

More recent studies have tended to focus on single etiological or pathogenetic factors. Tune et al. (31) carried out a prospective study of the relation between serum levels of *anticholinergic drugs* and the occurrence of delirium following cardiac surgery. They found that most patients who developed the syndrome postoperatively had higher serum levels of these drugs than those who did not develop it. Other investigators have focused on the putative etiological role of *morphine* (32,33). They found that it produced a profound disruption of nocturnal sleep, i.e., reduction in both REM and slow-wave sleep stages, as well as an increase in awakenings. Standard analgesic doses of this narcotic were more disruptive of sleep than 3 hours of isoflurane anesthesia. The researchers postulated that administration of morphine during the first 24 hours after surgery suppresses REM sleep, which rebounds as the narcotic is withdrawn on subsequent days. Such rebound enhances the morphine-induced ventilatory depression and the resulting hypoxemia, which, in turn, precipitates delirium. The arterial oxygen saturation has been found to be reduced during both wakefulness and sleep in the first week after abdominal surgery, notably during REM sleep on night 4 (34). Rebound of REM activity was associated with frequent episodes of hypopnea or apnea, with a consequent increase in the incidence and severity of periods of oxygen desaturation (35). These interesting findings and hypotheses suggest that in many cases postoperative delirium could be prevented by avoiding administration of relatively large doses of narcotics after surgery.

Disturbances of sleep after surgical procedures have also been documented by other investigators (36–39). Sleep stages 3 and 4, as well as REM, have been found to be severely or completely suppressed on the first 2 to 4 postoperative nights (36,38,39). Elderly patients appear to be particularly affected (39). Several possible factors have been postulated to cause the postoperative sleep disturbances, including the use of opiates, changes in CBF, metabolic disturbances, pain, fear, and conditions in the intensive care unit (32,39). Some authors have proposed that a direct effect on the brain by the general anesthetic or the systemic reaction to surgical trauma may bring about a disorder of the sleep-wake cycle regulating mechanism (36). Anesthetics, such as halothane, as well as opiates, seem to play a major role in this disorder (32,33,36,39,40). The hypothesis, referred to earlier—that morphine-induced disturbances of both sleep and breathing may result in hypoxemia, and consequent cerebral dysfunction and delirium—is plausible and calls for further research. Elderly patients are especially vulnerable to the deliriogenic effects of hypoxemia, and hence are at risk. Rebound of REM sleep following morphine administration may increase that risk (35).

Anxiety or fear is mentioned by some authors as a contributory factor in postoperative delirium (7,27), but a recent study found no relationship between preoperative anxiety and the development of the syndrome (41). On the contrary, high preoperative anxiety tended to be associated with less rather than more impairment in cognitive performance postoperatively. However, none of the patients in this study developed unequivocal delirium; hence, the contributory role of anxiety in at least some cases remains a possibility.

The deliriogenic potential of the various *anesthetic agents,* both general and local, is discussed in Chapter 11. Ketamine is of particular interest in this regard (42). Administration of lorazepam or midazolam is reported to reduce the incidence of delirium associated with ketamine anesthesia (42). A major toxic effect of both general and local anesthetics on the CNS is irritability, which may result in *seizures* and postictal delirium (43).

An interesting contribution to the study of pathogenetic mechanisms in postoperative delirium concerns the role of *beta-endorphin* and *cortisol* (44). The investigators studied seven male patients, 42 to 65 years old, who underwent elective surgery. They found that delirium was associated with a significant and unusually prolonged postoperative increase in circulating levels of both beta-endorphin and cortisol. The researchers postulated that an alternation of the hypothalamic-pituitary-adrenal axis, reflected in a disruption of the normal circadian rhythms of these two substances, may contribute to the development of postoperative delirium. Psychological stress occasioned by the operation and the environment of the intensive care unit might be responsible for the disruption of the normal circadian rhythms of plasma beta-endorphin and cortisol, and hence may contribute to delirium in some patients. This hypothesis deserves further study.

In summary, the etiology of postoperative delirium appears to be multifactorial, and to involve a combination of various organic factors, as well as psychological and environmental facilitating or contributory factors. There is little doubt that the role of the organic factors is essential. Hypoxemia and anticholinergic drug-induced acetylcholine deficiency are likely to be the main pathogenetic factors. A disruption of circadian rhythms of the endogenous opiate system and the hypothalamic-pituitary-adrenal axis has also been suggested as a putative pathogenetic mechanism, but its role remains uncertain.

Postoperative delirium in the elderly

Delirium is one of the most common postoperative complications in elderly patients, especially those older than 75 years. This subject is discussed briefly in Chapter 18, with special emphasis on delirium that often follows surgery for a broken hip. Because of the high susceptibility of the elderly patient to delirium due to any potentially pathogenic factor, its importance in surgical practice deserves a separate discussion.

As mentioned earlier, the reported incidence of postoperative delirium in elderly surgical patients ranges from 10% to 15% (20). However, writers on this subject offer widely divergent estimates of the incidence of this complication. While one writer states that "an acute confusional state is so common in the elderly that it may be the norm" (19), other authors claim that "most normal elderly patients will experience no ill effects from general anesthesia. Recovery of presurgical mental status is generally rapid" (45, p 40). While more epidemiological studies are clearly needed to resolve this issue, there is little doubt that postoperative delirium in an elderly patient is clinically important, as it often interfers with postoperative care; alerts the surgeon to previously unsuspected physical disease or drug intoxication or withdrawal; may lead to serious complications as a result of the treatment of agitation or lack of proper investigations to identify its cause; and is a grave prognostic sign (20). Moreover, in an unknown proportion of cases, delirium in an elderly patient may herald irreversible dementia (25,46,47). Such a patient, especially one with preexisting cerebral disease, is highly vulnerable to cerebral hypoxia of any origin, including that associated with general anesthesia, surgical trauma, and intraoperative and postoperative complications, all of which may result in hypoxemia manifested by delirium. The appearance of the latter should draw attention to the possibility that brain damage may occur as a consequence of reduced cerebral perfusion, and the patient may either develop or suffer an exacerbation of the already present dementia (25,46,47). A century ago, Savage (5) warned that a "progressive dementia" may follow in the wake of surgery.

More recently, Bedford (46,47) has also drawn attention to this possible outcome. He found 120 patients, aged 65 years and older, whose relatives had reported that they had never been the same since an operation. This comment seemed to reflect the development of various cognitive deficits and personality changes dating back to the postoperative period. Bedford studied 18 elderly patients with severe dementia with postoperative onset. He tested them both before and after surgery and found that they displayed confusion (presumably delirium) postoperatively, a state followed by irreversible dementia. Such an outcome is rare, according to this investigator, but the fact that it does occur warrants taking precautionary measures. The appearance of delirium after surgery in an older patient, argues Bedford, must be viewed as a warning sign that cerebral hypoxia or some other pathogenic factor is present, and calls for immediate diagnosis and treatment if permanent brain damage and dementia are to be prevented. He contends that potent hypnotics and analgesics should not be used either before or immediately after surgery in an elderly patient (46,47).

Interval delirium, occurring after a lucid interval of one or more days after an operation, is the most frequent form of postoperative delirium in an elderly patient (12,20). By contrast, *emergence* or postanesthetic delirium, which comes on within minutes of regaining consciousness to 24 hours, is most often found in otherwise healthy children (12). In the majority of cases the delirium resolves in a few days.

The *etiology* of postoperative delirium in an elderly patient involves the same factors as those listed in Table 19-1. Some factors, however, are more important and call for a brief discussion.

Preoperative risk factors in elderly general surgical patients are reported to include an age of 75 years and over, male sex, preoperative medical problems, and preexisting brain damage or disease (20,25,48–50). Postoperative precipitating factors involve physical complications of surgery, use of narcotics, intravenous infusion, infection, blood loss, fluid and electrolyte imbalance, alcohol and/or drug withdrawal, and pulmonary embolism (20,25,48–50). The importance of *anticholinergic drugs* has already been mentioned. The elderly patient, especially one with Alzheimer's disease, is highly sensitive to the effects of these drugs, as well as those of sedative-hypnotics. Preoperative intake of tricyclic antidepressants for depression or insomnia could predispose to delirium (51), and anesthetic agents with anticholinergic properties could precipitate it (52).

Spinal *anesthesia* for an elderly patient is followed by delirium less often than general anesthesia (51). *Shock* may result from heart failure, hypovolemia, decreased vasomotor tone, or markedly increased resistance to blood flow (53). Effective management of this perioperative complication is especially important in the elderly, who are so vulnerable to *hypoxemia* and reduced cerebral perfusion.

Hypoxemia and cerebral hypoxia may also result from impaired pulmonary function and inadequate ventilation. The elderly are highly prone to develop postoperative *infections* (53). Poor nutritional state, diminished resistance to stress, and impaired immune mechanisms all appear to contribute to this susceptibility (Chapter 18). Catheterization may lead to urinary tract infection and delirium. Bacteremia and other postoperative infections may initially present with the syndrome (53, Chapter 15). *Fluid* and *electrolyte imbalance* often follow surgery with general anesthesia and may precipitate an acute confusional state (46).

Postoperative alcohol withdrawal delirium

The subject of alcohol withdrawal delirium is fully discussed in Chapter 13, to which the reader is referred. The occurrence of the syndrome as a serious postoperative complication has been recognized for over a century (4,6). Da Costa (7) offers a vivid account of it and states that an alcoholic typically experiences a sleepless night after an injury or operation, or may have brief periods of sleep filled with terrifying dreams. The next day he is likely to be tremulous, restless, and apprehensive. Bouts of hallucinations appear and the withdrawal syndrome may then end, but in some cases a full-blown delirium follows and usually lasts for 2 to 4 days.

The importance and pitfalls of postoperative alcohol withdrawal delirium have been fully recognized by recent writers (54–58). Bruce (54), in particular, has written an informative review of alcoholism and its complications in relation to surgery and anesthesia. Any patient with a history of drinking at least one pint of whisky or its equivalent for at least 10 out of 14 days immediately prior to admission is at risk for developing withdrawal delirium after surgery (55). Patients operated on for cancer of the oral cavity and laryngopharynx are often alcohlics; hence, delirium is a frequent complication in head and neck surgery (57). Cirrhosis or enlargement of the liver, a history of alcohol withdrawal delirium, and the presence of early withdrawal symptoms are associated with an increased probability of postoperative delirium tremens (55). Some writers claim that an alcoholic who has abstained from alcohol for months may still develop withdrawal delirium after an accident or operation (27), but in my opinion, this seems improbable. It is more likely that, in such cases, one is dealing with cirrhosis of the liver or with brain damage due to previous alcohol abuse, which render the patient more susceptible to delirium of any origin.

Alcohol withdrawal delirium is liable to become manifest on the second to fourth postoperative day (57). Within the next 24 hours the delirium is likely to grow in severity, and delirium tremens follows. In some cases, the withdrawal syndrome may present initially with a general convulsion (56). An occasional patient, notably one who is also abusing benzodiazepines, may develop the delirium as long as a week after surgery. The symptoms are described in Chapter 13. When they occur postoperatively, they carry the risk of complications related to removal of or interference with sutures, dressings, intravenous catheters, skin flaps, and tracheostomy or drainage tubes (57). Other complications are discussed by Bruce (54). Postoperative delirium tremens is claimed to have the same mortality as that arising in other settings (55).

Prevention and *management* of alcohol withdrawal delirium in surgery are important and challenging tasks (54,56). Preoperative evaluation by an anesthetist willing to spend the time to obtain an adequate history of the patient's drinking patterns, the duration of alcohol abuse, the concurrent use of other drugs, the previous episodes of withdrawal symptoms, and the dietary habits is crucial (54). The anesthetic management of an alcholoic patient calls for special consideration in choosing the anesthetic agent and its dose, careful medical evaluation preoperatively, and cardiorespiratory monitoring and support postoperatively (54). While it is not essential to delay emergency surgery because withdrawal delirium is thought to be highly probable, postponement of an operation whenever reasonable is advised (55). Prophylactic use of a benzodiazepine drug is recommended in such a case (see Chapter 13). It is also advisable to administer a high-potency vitamin B complex preparation parenterally, both before and after surgery, to avoid the confounding effects of vitamin deficiency common among chronic alcoholics. Attention to concurrent liver disease, if any, is essential if hepatic encephalopathy is to be avoided (55). Subdural hematoma should always be ruled out in an alcoholic patient, especially if there is a history of recent head injury. Finally, an alcoholic may be concurrently abusing sedative-hypnotics and withdrawal from them could precipitate seizures and exacerbate delirium due to alcohol withdrawal. Such drugs should be continued during the perioperative period. If symptoms of withdrawal appear or frank delirium develops postoperatively, the treatment should follow the guidelines discussed in Chapter 13. The use of high doses of midazolam given by a constant infusion to control agitation in a surgical patient with delirium tremens has recently been reported (59).

Prevention, management, and prognosis of postoperative delirium

Treatment of delirium is discussed in detail in Chapter 10. Pharmacotherapy of the syndrome in the intensive care unit is the subject of a recent review (60). An essential aspect of prevention is to identify patients at high risk for the development of postoperative delirium, including the elderly, the demented, the alcoholic, and the sedative-hypnotic addict. Other identifying features are mentioned earlier in this chapter and are listed in Table 19-1. Bedside testing of cognitive function, including spatiotemporal orientation, memory, and attention, should be performed prior to surgery to identify patients already cognitively impaired and hence at risk of becoming delirious. Such testing should also be carried out postoperatively in order to detect changes in cognitive functioning early. Narcotic analgesics and anticholinergics should be avoided as much as possible in patients considered to be at risk for delirium.

Intraoperative monitoring of the EEG can help assess brain integrity and depth of anesthesia (61–63). Potentially hazardous cerebral dysfunction can be detected early and treated appropriately. The cerebral function analyzing monitor has been developed to monitor EEG and evoked potentials (61). This technique allows visual and quantitative assessment of the depth of anesthesia. The potentials recorded in the EEG reflect the level of CBF and oxygen metabolism (63). A recently reported technique involves phase space plotting of EEG data in a patient undergoing general anesthesia (62). Its potential advantage is the possibility of differentiating deep anesthesia from hypoxemia (62). Thus, abnormal cerebral activity may be detected as soon as it develops, allowing timely therapeutic intervention before delirium becomes manifest or permanent brain damage occurs, or both.

A most important aspect of the management of postoperative delirium is its *early detection.* Severe delirum seldom arises without prodromal symptoms of restlessness, insomnia, nightmares, and anxiety or lethargy. Such symptoms are typically accentuated at night and should be observed and reported by the nurses. A nurse's observations, however, will make little difference unless the surgeon takes note of them. All too often in my experience, the surgeon requests a psychiatric consultation at a point when the patient is obviously delirious, disturbed, combative, and generally difficult to manage. Almost invariably, such a patient had shown prodromal or early signs of delirium for at least a day, but they were ignored by the surgical staff even though nurses' notes in the patient's chart contained a clear description of them. It follows that early identification and proper management of the syndrome necessitate a high level of awareness of its prodromal symptoms on the part of both the nursing and the surgical staff.

Little information on the *prognosis* of postoperative delirium can be found in the literature. It appears, however, that the outcome is usually benign, even in elderly patients (20,50). In an unknown proportion of cases, especially in the elderly, delirium may be followed by death, dementia, or some other chronic organic mental syndrome (16,29,46).

One may conclude that even though postoperative delirium appears to result in full recovery of cognitive functioning in the majority of patients, it must never be taken lightly, notably in an elderly patient. It is a sign of brain disorder that, in a proportion of cases, may be followed by cerebral damage and dementia or organic personality disorder, with disastrous consequences for the patient and the family. Moreover, litigation against the surgeon or the anesthetist, or both, may result from such a mishap. It follows that prevention as well as timely recognition and adequate treatment of postoperative delirium are always important.

Postoperative delirium in special conditions

HEART SURGERY

This type of surgery has generated more studies and publications on postoperative delirium than any other. A recent review of the reports on this complication after open-heart surgery indicates that during the past 25 years the incidence of postcardiotomy delirium has remained fairly steady despite claims to the contrary (64).

The first report of psychiatric disturbances following *mitral commissurotomy* appeared in 1954 and stated an incidence of about 20% (65). Subsequent studies confirmed this finding and documented the clinical features of the postoperative syndromes involved. The latter were stated to be most often delirium and a schizophreniform psychosis. Some authors speculated that the symbolic meaning of the heart as the organ of life was a key variable in bringing about the psychiatric complications, while others emphasized the importance of organic etiological factors such as chronic heart disease, cerebral hypoxia, and preexisting brain disease due to rheumatic fever (66). As surgical techniques improved, the incidence of postoperative psychoses was claimed to decline (67).

The earlier reports on neuropsychiatric complications of *open-heart surgery* began to appear in the mid-1960s (68,69). Some 21 studies on this subject appeared between 1964 and 1979 and reported on a total of about 1,820 cases of cardiotomy, with the incidence of postoperative psychiatric disturbances ranging widely from 13% to 100%. Fifteen of the 21 studies found this incidence to be between 30% and 60%; only 4 studies gave an incidence figure of less than 30%. One study reported an incidence as low as 13%, but the definition of delirium applied by the investigators was skewed: they included only those patients who displayed hallucinations or severe disorientation; those with "mild confusion" were excluded (70). A Canadian study reported that the incidence of delirium after open-heart surgery was cut to about 5% by administering diazepam, 2.5–5 mg intravenously six times a day, after the operation (71). Some authors claim that between 1965 and 1969 the frequency of delirium dropped from 38% to 24% as a result of decreased time on cardiopulmonary bypass (72).

Smith and Dimsdale (64) reviewed 44 studies of psychiatric complications following open-heart surgery published between 1963 and 1987. According to their review, the total incidence of postcardiotomy delirium during the years 1963–1974 and 1975–1987 was 32.41% and 32.95%, respectively. Thus the reported total incidence of this complication has not changed over 25 years. The more recent reports contain fewer cases of delirium that feature hallucinations, paranoid delusions, or agitation, and more cases of delirium with spatiotemporal disorientation. No single risk factor has been consistently identified in the reviewed studies, despite claims by some authors that such factors as the duration of bypass time and sleep deprivation and immobilization in the intensive care unit are related to the incidence of postcardiotomy delirium. A slight correlation has been found between age and the occurrence of the syndrome; children, however, are reportedly less prone to delirium after open-heart surgery. Six of seven studies on the effect of the severity of illness found a small correlation between this variable and delirium. The presence of brain damage or abnormal neurological signs before surgery was found to correlate with the incidence of the syndrome. Postoperative EEG abnormality correlated with it, as did serum levels of anticholinergic drugs (31). The authors of this valuable review conclude that the etiology of delirium following open-heart surgery is not yet known. There is evidence that the syndrome develops in one-third of these patients—a high incidence.

Some studies have reported an incidence of postcardiotomy delirium far lower than 30% (71,73–75). For example, a retrospective study of open-heart surgery performed at the Montreal Heart Institute over 4 years found an incidence of delirium of only 3% (74). In one study of such surgery in 100 consecutive patients 80 years of age or older, the incidence was 12% (73). The reasons for such a wide discrepancy in the reported incidence are unknown; an understanding of them could offer valuable clues regarding prevention of delirium in this setting. For example, three studies found that preoperative psychiatric intervention was associated with the lower incidence of the syndrome (64).

Delirium after open-heart surgery appears to be of two types in terms of time of onset: (1) with an onset on the first postoperative day and (2) with onset after a lucid interval of at least 2 days after the operation (75). According to some writers, in less than 10% of the cases the onset occurs on the first day. The majority of the reports, however, do not mention the onset times, and this issue remains unresolved (64). About one-half of the patients are delirious for 1 or 2 days, about one in four for 3 to 4 days, and only about 12% remain delirious for 10 or more days. Hallucinations and delusions, if any, tend to arise on the third postoperative day. In one series, the mean day of onset was 4.2 and the mean day of recovery was 5.9 (75). An early onset appears to be more common in elderly patients.

Etiology. The etiology of postcardiotomy delirium remains unknown (64). A wide range of preoperative, intraoperative, and postoperative factors have been postulated to play an etiological role, but few of them have been firmly established (64). A causative factor proposed by one group of investigators is often discounted by others (64). It is likely that the etiology of the syndrome is multifactorial (72). Table 19–2 lists the postulated etiological variables found in the literature.

In summary, no single etiological factor is generally recognized as being both necessary and sufficient to cause postcardiotomy delirium. Its etiology is most likely multidetermined (79). Which of the factors carries the greatest risk for this complication is still a matter of controversy, as exemplified by opposing views on the importance of cardiopulmonary bypass time and hypotension during or after it (80). Similarly, while sleep disturbances are

TABLE 19–2 Etiological Factors in Postcardiotomy Delirium

A. Preoperative factors
   1. Age over 50 years; very low incidence in children (72)
   2. Evidence of cerebral disease before surgery (64)
   3. Severe cardiac functional incapacity (64)
   4. Abnormal neurological signs (64)
   5. Marked anxiety before surgery (72)
   6. Use of psychotropic drugs (64)
   7. Language barrier (76)

B. Intraoperative factors
   1. Long cardiopulmonary bypass time (not accepted by all authors) (64,72)
   2. Hypotension (64)
   3. Surgical complications (64)
   4. Multiple-valve and aortic-replacement procedures (72)

C. Postoperative factors
   1. Low cardiac output (77)
   2. High serum level of anticholinergic drugs (31)
   3. Tracheostomy (64)
   4. Hypoxemia (64)
   5. Hypokalemia (64)
   6. Pneumonitis (64)
   7. Sleep deprivation (78)
   8. Altered sensory environment: sensory deprivation, noise, monotony (69,75)

common after open-heart surgery, patients who display them need not be delirious (81). It has been suggested that rather than being a cause of delirium, sleep loss appears to be its consequence (82). There is little doubt that organic factors play a key etiological role in the syndrome, while that of psychological and environmental factors is at best contributory (64).

Pathophysiology. This aspect of delirium after open-heart surgery has been the subject of much speculation. Extracorporeal circulation during the operation has attracted particular attention as a suspected major source of pathophysiological variables responsible for delirium (80,83–88). Two major pathogenetic factors related to bypass have emerged: particulate and air *microemboli* and *cerebral hypoperfusion* (80,84–88). EEG studies, as well as those of CBF and CMR during cardiopulmonary bypass have provided evidence of cerebral damage and dysfunction related temporally to this technique (85,89–92). Lee et al. (93) found that patient subjected to various cardiac operative procedures without the use of extracorporeal circulation showed neither neurological deficits nor psychiatric complications postoperatively. By contrast, patients who underwent cardiac surgery with such circulation exhibited neurological deficits or psychiatric complications, or both, in the postoperative period. These investigators hypothesize that a microvascular perfusion defect is the basic pathophysiological condition responsible for the neuropsychiatric complications. Microemboli consisisting of platelets, blood cells, or air are believed to result in defective microvascular perfusion and ischemic brain damage (83–93). Factors such as hypotension, hypoxemia, low cardiac output, and hypocapnia may contribute to cerebral dysfunction. Some researchers, however, failed to find a relationship between low perfusion pressure and neurophychiatric complications (87). Thus, the role of microemboli appears to be more firmly established than that of any other putative pathogenetic factor (80,84,87,88,90,91). Some writers speak of "microembolic encephalopathy" (94). Cardiopulmonary bypass causes significant depression of CBF and CMR. Continuous EEG monitoring during open-heart surgery has provided evidence of abnormal brain function and correlates with the development of neuropsychiatric abnormalities (83,89,91,92). Monitoring of CNS function during open-heart surgery is crucial (83).

The hazards to the integrity of the brain have been reduced by improvements in operative technique, and a measure of protection against brain damage has been achieved (85–87). Despite these refinements, however, delirium continues to follow open-heart surgery as often as before their introduction (64). Some writers assert that diffuse brain damage, reversible or not, follows most cardiac operations (85). *Cerebral hypoxia* and *ischemia* appear to be the best-documented and most important pathophysiological factors in postcardiotomy delirium and in other manifestations of cerebral dysfunction and damage.

Some investigaors propose that additional factors contribute to the delirium. Metabolic acidosis, fluid and electroloyte imbalance, accumulation of cerebrotoxic metabolites, and intracerebral hemorrhages have been suggested as potential pathphysiological mechanisms (95).

Prognosis. The prognosis of delirium after open-heart surgery appears to be favorable. Heller et al. (96) found that its occurrence bore no relation to the psychological outcome 1 year after the operation. Kaplan et al. (97) studied children who underwent open-heart surgery for the correction of various congenital abnormalities. Five of them became delirious, and all of them recovered without demonstrable deficits. Tufo et al. (98) carried out a prospective study of 100 open-heart surgery patients and found confusion, disorientation, and/or delirium in about 42% of the survivors. At discharge, about 20% of the delirious subjects still exhibited nocturnal confusion and decreased intellectual performance. Branthwaite (99) found "confusion" in 22 patients, all of whom recovered without any gross impairment of cognitive functioning. Such impairment does occur following open-heart operations, but its relationship to postoperative delirium is unclear.

In terms of neuropsychological assessment, the long-term outcome after open-heart surgery has shown evidence of permanent neurological and cognitive abnormalities in a proportion of patients (85,100–103). Henriksen (85) contends that transient neuropsychiatric disturbances following extracorporeal circulation should be regarded as a potentially harmful development. He found slightly reduced CBF in 11 patients studied 1 year after surgery, and believes that the diffuse decrease in CBF indicates that open-heart surgery may cause generalized neuronal cell damage or cell loss. Sotaniemi et al. (102) carried out a prospective, 5-year neuropsychological, neurological, and EEG study in 44 patients who had undergone open-heart surgery for valve replacement. There was a correlation between the immediate postoperative clinical outcome and long-term neuropsychological performance. Harmful effects of long extracorporeal circulation were reflected in reduced performance on neuropsychological tests on follow-up. Savageau et al. (100) studied 245 patients before and 6 months after coronary bypass and cardiac valve operations. They concluded that sustained neuropsychological dysfunction 6 months after cardiac operations is rare but does occur. Taylor (88) asserts that while disturbances of consciousness after operation are usually transient, persistent cerebral dysfunction may follow, resulting in minor degrees of intellectual and memory impairment and personality changes. These sequelae can cause considerable handicap and suffering for the patients and their families. Their incidence remains unclear, but they do occur in a proportion of patients and call for preventive measures.

Prevention and management. Prevention of postcardiotomy delirium involves more than improvements in surgical technique and decreases in bypass and anesthesia times (104). There is evidence that psychological preparation of the patient prior to surgery helps to reduce the incidence of delirium (64). Psychiatric consultation pre- and postoperatively is advisable for patients who have a history of mental disorder or display marked anxiety, or both (104). Patients need to be warned that perceptual and other disturbances of mental function may be experienced after the operation and should be reported to the staff without delay. Sleep should be monitored during the first few postoperative nights and ensured as far as possible (104). Open-heart surgery is a stressful procedure, as indicated by markedly elevated levels of serum cortisol, beta-endorphin, and noradrenaline (105). It follows that mea-measures aimed at reducing such stress are worthwile and may help to reduce the incidence of postoperative delirium (106). After surgery, provision of a stable environment that avoids extremes of sensory stimulation is important (79,107). Frequent reorientation should be part of the intensive care nursing routine and may help to reduce the severity and duration of delirium (79,108).

Essentially, management of postcardiotomy delirium is no different from that recommended for delirium generally (Chapter 10). Haloperidol is the drug of choice; its intravenous use has been advocated to control postoperative agitation (60,109).

CORONARY ARTERY BYPASS SURGERY

A number of studies have focused on neuropsychiatric complications after coronary artery bypass surgery (110–114). The reported incidence of delirium after such surgery varies widely: from 0% (111) to 28% (113). The most recent reports give the lowest incidence figures (111,112). Calabrese et al. (111) state that none of their 59 patients exhibited delirium on the sixth postoperative day, but 6.8% of them showed "transient signs of confusion" on postoperative day 1. These authors suggest that refinement of surgical technique coupled with improved monitoring of intra- and perioperative hemodynamic function may account for the low overall incidence of delirium in their series of patients. Nevertheless, they observed significant, if subtle, cognitive deficits on the sixth postoperative day. Carella et al. (112) found delirium in 3.4% of their patients but noted that 48% of the total series showed neurological signs 8 days postoperatively and 5.7% had either permanent or severe neurological deficits. Pump time appeared to be the main predictor of such deficits. Breuer et al. (110) reported that 11.6% of their 421 patients were "encephalopathic" (presumably delirious) on postoperative day 4, and in 20% of them, mental status abnormalities were still evident at the time of discharge. Hypoxia, medications, and fever/sepsis appeared to be the main etiological factors. No statistically significant pre- or intraoperative factors were found to account for the encephalopathy, which appeared to be of multifactorial etiology, Kornfeld et al. (113) studied 100 consecutive patients undergoing coronary artery bypass surgery, 28% of whom developed postoperative delirium. A history of MI and the severity of the illness in the recovery room were two variables that correlated significantly with the incidence of the syndrome. Age, severity of cardiac disease, and cardiopulmonary bypass time did not show a significant association with such incidence. Nor did any psychological variable reach the .05 level of significance. The researchers postulate that the presence of a lucid interval between the operation and the onset of delirium indicates that variables such as sensory monotony, sleep deprivation, and anxiety could have played an etiological role.

A report on over 5,000 patients 65 years of age and older who underwent coronary bypass surgery at the Cleveland Clinic mentions neither delirium nor cognitive functioning postoperatively (115). Other investigators maintain that age is not a crucial factor in determining the prognosis in such patients (110,116). Bass (117) notes, however, that age was the only demographic variable associated with an adverse psychological outcome in his study. More long-term studies of cognitive functioning in all (especially elderly) patients undergoing coronary artery bypass surgery are needed.

CARDIAC TRANSPLANTATION

This form of heart surgery is reported to be followed by delirium (118–124). Hotson and Pedley (120) reviewed 83 patients who had received cardiac transplants at Stanford University Medical Center. An "acute psychosis" developed in 12% of these patients, a further 12% suffered from metabolic encephalopathy, and 34% had a CNS infection. As far as one can discern from this report, about one-half of the patients experienced delirium of some severity. The authors state that "behavioral changes" or intellectual impairment were the most frequent neuropsychiatric manifestations in their patients, and that CNS infection was the most common, and sometimes unrecognized, etiological factor in postoperative delirium. This infection was mostly fungal or viral and could cause the syndrome weeks or even a few months after transplantation.

More recent studies indicate that delirium does occur after this type of surgery, but its incidence is not very high, i.e., about 20% to 25% (119,124). One group of investigators states that while virtually all of their patients displayed confusion for 1 to a few days after surgery, this was detectable without a detailed examination of the mental status in only 25.9% of the cases (122). Preoperative psychopathological symptoms did not predict postoperative neuropsychiatric complications. Hallucinations and delusions were not observed in the delirious patients. In another study, postoperative delirium appeared to be related to administration of steroids and to metabolic disturbances (119). After organ transplantation, patients are immunosuppressed and hence more susceptible to infections, which may lead to delirium (125).

The famous case of Dr. Clark, the world's first recipient of a mechanical heart (he was ineligible for heart transplantation), is worth noting. He suffered a prolonged confusional state after surgery (126).

Liver and *kidney* transplantation are discussed in Chapter 14, and their neuropsychiatric complications have recently been reviewed (125). Delirium has been reported in 70% of *lung* transplantation patients (127). Cyclosporine A plasma levels were significantly correlated with its occurrence.

Delirium has been observed in 77% of patients undergoing pulmonary thromboendartectomy (128). It was significantly associated with deep hypothermia and total circulatory arrest times.

EYE SURGERY

Delirium has been a recognized complication of eye surgery for over a century. One of the early reports on it appeared in 1863 (129). It followed cataract surgery and was thought to be due to occlusion of the eyelids. Some patients appeared to suffer from delirium tremens. None of them were younger than 60 years. The duration of the delirium was brief. Sichel, the author of the report, recommended "moral treatment" for the delirious patient, i.e., telling him where he is and why, and letting him open his eyes and look around so that he may orient himself for place and space.

Several other observers reported similar cases at about the same time, but the condition attracted little attention until Schmidt-Rimpler (130) devoted an article to it in 1879. His paper focused on delirium after closure of the eyes and in dark rooms. The author claimed that every eye surgeon must have encountered delirium after cataract extraction. He observed that the syndrome could also occur, without eye surgery, in eye patients kept in dark rooms, and argued that sudden exclusion of visual cues through patching and placement in a dark room induced it in some individuals. Thus, the author of this early report anticipated future theories of the putative deliriogenic effect of sensory deprivation.

The above two pioneering papers introduced a sizable literature on the nature, incidence, and etiology of mental disturbances after eye, notably cataract, surgery. Both of them drew attention to two variables that are still considered important in the etiology of delirium in eye surgery today: old age and patching of the eyes. In 1887, Chisolm (131) published an article, "The Revolution in the After-Treatment of Cataract Operations," in which he challenged traditional methods of such treatment and advocated a drastic departure from them. He announced optimistically that "hereafter there will be no more bandaging, dark rooms, bed operations, bed restraints, diet lists, isolation or smoked glasses needed," i.e., methods that "cruelty kept up for days in the name of progressive surgery" (p 156). Chisolm claimed that allowing patients to move about immediately after surgery and not patching the good eye resulted in better operative results and shorter convalescence. Unfortunately, his "revolution" spread slowly, and delirium after cataract surgery continued to be reported.

Posey (132) reported on 24 cases of delirium after such surgery. All of his patients had both eyes bandaged. The delirium featured restlessness, hallucinations, and delusions of persecution. The author believed that the patients' preoccupation with the eyes was a decisive factor in precipitating the syndrome. Kipp (133) found 12 cases of delirium in patients who had had eye sugery or were suffering from eye injury. The majority of his patients had been treated in a well-lighted room and had one or both eyes unpatched. Most of them had been hospitalized for more than a week when the delirium developed, and they remained delirious until discharge. Kipp postulated that his patients suffered this complication as a result of a change in their environment and of nostalgia. Bruns (134) noted that not one of a group of over 200 patients who had undergone cataract extraction and been treated on an ambulatory basis developed delirium. By contrast, several patients hospitalized for such surgery became delirious, and three of them committed suicide. Bruns believed that the delirium was due to old age and the dread of the unknown. He wrote that "the stranger, the darker, the stiller, the lonelier the after-treatment, the more likely is the mental disturbance to occur" (p 720). The ambulatory patients avoided become delirious, since they had the advantage of returning at once to familiar surroundings.

A thorough review of psychiatric complications of eye surgery prior to 1920 is provided by Fisher (135). He credited Dupuytren with being the first author to report, in 1819, delirium after cataract surgery, and refers to 29 other publications on this subject. He quoted Fromaget, who claimed that occlusion of the eyes put the patient into a hypnotic state and induced sleep, dreams, and delirium. Fisher listed the putative etiological factors he was able to find in the papers under review. They included bandaging of the eyes, loneliness, nervousness, exhaustion, disturbances of CBF, fear of blindness, withdrawal of alcohol, administration of atropine, and homesickness.

The next major paper on delirium after cataract surgery was by Greenwood (136), who gave its incidence as being 2.5% to 3%. Old age and blindfolding are the main etiological factors, according to this author. Anxiety over the outcome of the anticipated operation also seems to play a significant role. Greenwod observed wisely that "the establishment of a mutual feeling of confidence between the physician and the patient is of major importance" (p 1713). If delirium does develop, removal of the bandage from the unoperated eye should speed up recovery.

Several papers published between 1950 and 1970 are worth mentioning (137–143). Bartlett (138) compared visual hallucinations in elderly patients with bilateral cataracts to the phantom limb phenomenon and argued that deprivation of normal visual stimuli facilitated their occurrence. Linn et al

(141) studied 21 patients operated on for bilateral senile cataracts and observed "some alteration of behavior" (a meaningless term) in the course of index hospitalization in 95% of the cases. Only four patients exhibited some disorientation for time, while eight of them displayed spatial disorientation. Only 3 patients experienced visual hallucinations, while 11 of them had abnormal EEG, a finding suggestive of the presence of brain damage or dysfunction. It is impossible to conclude from this inadequate report what proportion of these patients were delirious. In a later publication, the chief investigator in the above study stated that as a result of advances in postoperative care of cataract patients, notably leaving the unoperated eye uncovered and lifting restrictions on mobility, the incidence of major psychiatric complications had dropped to "well below 1 percent" (140). This low incidence had already been reported over 50 years earlier (145). Jackson (139) studied 78 patients undergoing eye surgery, 60 of them for cataract extraction. He focused on the role of sensory deprivation as a possible factor in the development of postoperative psychiatric complicatons and concluded that the evidence for it was inconclusive. This study stands out for its sound methodology, but it lacks acceptable precision in the use of diagnostic terms for the psychiatric disturbances. Ziskind (144) carried out a well-designed study of such disturbances following surgery for cataract and for repair of detached retina. He observed a higher incidence of these problems in patients undergoing retinal surgery. A history of alcoholism, double eye patching, and a language barrier were the variables associated with psychiatric symptoms. Ziskind, like Jackson, stated that the cognitive disturbances observed in his patients could best be accounted for by sensory deprivation, but, unlike Jackson, he concluded that his hypothesis was valid. He proposed that such disturbances could be viewed as "aberrations of half-sleep, half-wakefulness" and constituted a "hypnoid syndrome." Reduced sensory input enhances and prolongs this state of reduced awareness, one necessary for the development of hallucinations, confusion, anxiety, restlessness, and noncompliant behavior observed in some patients after eye surgery. This interesting hypothesis calls for studies involving EEG and sleep monitoring in order to test its validity. Other investigators argued that such variables as dehydration (137) and the use of sedatives and analgesics (146) were the main etiological factors in delirium after cataract surgery.

One other study published prior to 1970 deserves mention, as it offers practical guidelines for the management of the eye surgery patient. Weisman and Hackett (143) treated six patients who were delirious after such surgery. They assumed that the delirium had been precipitated by deprivation of visual cues, with resulting impairment of reality testing. Consequently, they applied a therapeutic approach that tried to compensate for this deprivation. They substituted auditory, tactile, gustatory, and olfactory perceptual cues for the missing visual ones. This approach improved the patients' reality testing and counteracted the delirium. Weisman and Hackett emphasized the importance of a good doctor–patient relationship. Even though the premises on which these authors based their therapeutic approach are open to criticism, the value of offering the patients reassurance, orienting cues, and information, which they advocate, is undeniable.

The etiological role of sensory deprivation in delirium after eye surgery remains controversial. For example, Stonecypher (142) argued that clinical examples show that such deprivation does not really occur. The unoperated eye is usually left unpatched and the patched one has lost so much of its function that it required surgery in the first place. Stonecypher proposes instead that the "black-patch psychosis," as he calls it, is due to psychological stress and concomitant fear. The patient prone to develop it tends to be one with a history of marginal social adjustment, long-standing disability, and a previous episode of psychosis while hospitalized. Management of a delirious patient should involve orientation and emotional support, the approach so persuasively advocated by Weisman and Hackett (143).

A number of reports on delirium following cataract extraction have appeared in the past decade (148–153). A carefully designed Finnish study involving 1,505 patients who had undergone cataract surgery found the incidence of postoperative psychiatric complications to be 3.3% (149). The authors concluded that increased age, markedly deteriorated vision, and anticholinergic eye drops appeared to be the significant etiological factors. They followed their patients for 5 years and noted increased mortality among those who had been delirious postoperatively (150). They suggested that the patients likely to develop the delirium were demented at the time of surgery. Finally, Summers and Reich (153) asserted that postcataract-surgery delirium may be an acute anticholinergic syndrome.

In summary, delirium after cataract surgery occurs in about 1% to 3% of patients. A number of etiological factors have been proposed to account for its development and are summarized in Table 19–3. A constellation of these factors is most likely to be involved: one or another of them may predominate in a given patient. Cataract surgery is usually performed on elderly patients, who, due to many factors, are generally more susceptible to delirium than younger individuals (Chapter 18). Unfamiliarity of the environment, reduction of visual cues, and fear are likely to facilitate the onset of delirium in the aged. Preexisting dementia is a predisposing factor in delirium. Sensory deprivation alone is unlikely to cause delirium in the absence of organic etiological factors. Mobilizing the patient early, leaving one eye unpatched, testing cognitive function pre- and postoperatively, and good nursing care are the factors credited with the decline of delirium after cataract surgery. If it does occur, the therapeutic measures discussed in Chapter 10 should be applied.

TABLE 19–3 Etiological Factors in Postcataract-Surgery Delirium

A. Predisposing factors
   1. Age of 65 years and over
   2. Preexisting dementia
   3. Severe bilateral loss of vision
   4. Alcoholism
B. Precipitating factors
   1. Anticholinergic drugs, including eye drops
   2. Dehydration
C. Facilitating factors
   1. Eye patching
   2. Unfamiliar environment (?)
   3. Fear (?)

It appears that the therapeutic "revolution" launched by Chisolm (131) a century ago has prevailed, with the consequent reduction of postcatarectomy delirium.

Delirium after burns

Delirium is the main early psychiatric complication of severe burns. Its incidence in this context has been reported to range from 5% to 57% (154–158). The lowest incidence was found in children, and the authors assert that more attention to fluid balance and avoidance of topical agents with neurotoxic properties, such as hexachlorophene and tannic acid, has resulted in reduced frequency of neuropsychiatric complications in recent years (157). The term "burn encephalopathy" that some authors use (155,157) has been criticized for being nondescript, as it designates neither a specifc type of structural cerebral change nor a specific syndrome (159). I agree that this term is indeed vague. Three of the published studies refer specifically to delirium and report its incidence as being 30% to 57% (154,156,158).

Delirium is more likely to occur in the older and more severely burned patient (154,158). It typically develops in the first month after burn injury and in patients with burns covering more than 40% of the body surface area. The syndrome occurs only rarely after grafting has been completed. Its incidence in patients isolated in a bed-sized plenum laminar air flow ventilation unit has been reported to be 40% (156). It is claimed that treatment in this environment results in a greater risk of developing delirium than the standard management of burn patients in open cubicles, where orientation is easier to maintain (156).

A number of etiological factors, both organic and psychologic-environmental, have been proposed to account for the frequent occurrence of delirium following burns (155–158,160). In the earliest stages, hypoxia and hypovolemic shock are the most important, and potentially fatal, causes of delirium. The patient is usually frightened and in pain, yet may appear calm and lucid. Many patients, however, are agitated and restless, and suffer from insomnia and nightmares (154). Delirium may appear at any time. It usually follows a benign course but, depending on its etiology, may be followed by coma and death. After the first week, infection becomes the most important cause of the syndrome, which tends to develop gradually over a period of several days and most often after 2 to 3 weeks following burn injury. Prompt improvement usually follows the application of skin homografts. Acidosis, hyponatremia, hypocalcemia, and seizures may also contribute to the development of the syndrome. Cerebral edema has been blamed for its occurrence in some cases (161). It has been ascribed to hyponatremia with water intoxication, hypoxia, prolonged hypotension, a toxin produced by the burned tissue, and hexachlorophene treatment of burns.

In addition to the above organic factors, psychological and environmental ones have been postulated to contribute to delirium in burn patients (156). The burn injury itself is often the result of an accident involving negligence, child abuse, or intoxication with alcohol or drugs. The patient tends to experience terror and pain, followed by prolonged immobilization, painful procedures, total dependence on the hospital staff, and uncertainty about the extent of future disfigurement and its social consequences (154,158,162). Patients are often preoccupied with these issues (162). Depression or posttraumatic stress disorder, or both, tend to develop in patients hospitalized for more than a month (154,158). Immobilization, sensory deprivation, and boredom add to the overall psychological stress and possibly increase the risk of delirium. Insomnia is very common; it precedes, accompanies, and follows the syndrome (163). All these factors must be taken into account in the management of the burned patient.

The EEG changes in burn patients have been observed by several groups of investigators (160,164,165). Petersen et al. (160) studied 58 patients with burns of moderate severity. In 31% of them the EEG changes involved diffuse or focal abnormalities, or both; the degree of abnormality correlated with the extent of the burns. Eight patients were delirious, and all of them showed EEG abnormalities. Similar findings have been reported by other investigators (164,165). Some patients show epileptiform activity on the EEG and may develop seizures (161,165). All of these abnormal tracings tend to occur 3 to 11 days after the burn.

Management of delirium after burns should follow the guidelines discussed in Chapter 10. Psychological managment is crucial, as it may influence the long-term outcome (162). Both severe burns and the delirium that may follow them are highly stressful experiences that may profoundly affect the patient long after the initial stage has passed (162). The role of the consulting psychiatrist on a burn unit is important; this person may provide crisis intervention and psychotherapy for the patients and advice on their management for the staff (162,166).

Haloperidol has been reported to induce extrapyramidal side effects in burn patients more readily than in those who are delirious in other settings (167). Consequently, the use of chlorpromazine has been recommended instead.

In summary, delirium occurs in about 15% to 40% of patients who sustain severe burns. Its onset has two peaks: the first within the first week after the burn, the second 2 to 3 weeks after it. The main etiological factors in the early stages involve various metabolic disturbances, while in the later stages infection is the chief cause. Etiology of the delirium is multifactorial, involving both organic and psychological factors (Table 19–4).

Postpartum delirium

Delirium in the postpartum period is rare today. Recent reports on psychiatric illness associated with childbirth either do not mention it at all or give its incidence at 1% to 2% of puerperal psychoses (168,169). On the other hand, Hamilton (170) maintains that delirium is one of the main variants of such psychosis. These contradictory reports appear to reflect problems with terminology, as well as certain atypical clinical characteristics of the puerperal psychoses, notably "confusion" (171–175). This vague term is usually applied to disorientation and other cognitive deficits and abnormalities (175). In one series, "confusion" was observed in about one-third of the patients with post-

TABLE 19–4 Etiological Factors in Delirium after Burns

A. Organic precipitating factors
    1. Hypoxia due to inhalation of CO and other toxic gases
    2. Hypovolemia related to initial shock and dehydration, resulting in cerebral hypoxia
    3. Hyponatremia due to loss of sodium from the surface of extensive burns
    4. Infection of burned areas leading to septicemia, bacterial meningitis, septic cerebral embolism, etc.
    5. Acidosis
    6. Hypocalcemia
    7. Seizures
    8. Hypertensive encephalopathy
    9. Direct brain damage in severe burns of the head
    10. Administration of analgesics and hypnotics

B. Psychological and environmental factors
    1. Pain
    2. Fear
    3. Sleep loss
    4. Immobilization
    5. Isolation in a plenum laminar air flow ventilation unit

partum psychosis and was distributed more or less evenly across the diagnostic spectrum (172). Some writers use the term "cofusional-oneiroid syndrome" in this regard and claim that it is particularly common in patients with manic symptoms (175). Dean and Kendell (171) noted disorientation, visual hallucinations, or organic impairment in about 25% of patients with puerperal illness, most of whom showed no evidence of an organic cause of such symptoms.

The first known description of a psychiatric disorder during the puerperium was given by Hippocrates and appeared to be delirium (166). Subsequently, many writers over the centuries described "puerperal insanity," a syndrome bearing striking similarity to delirium, if not actually identical with it. Marcé (177), in his classical treatise on puerperal psychosis, speaks of acute delirium *(Délire aigu)* as a potentially lethal complication of the puerperium. Silbermann et al. (176) assert that postpartum delirium is a typical puerperal psychosis, featuring a fluctuating level of consciousness, perplexity, extreme anxiety, delusions, and psychomotor hyperactivity. These authors suggest that this syndrome resembles the "toxic delirium" of the English-language literature. Arentsen (178) diagnosed delirium in about 20% of women who became psychotic in the first 6 months after childbirth. In about 60% of the patients, the cause of the delirium could not be established.

As pointed out earlier, many reports are at variance with those just quoted. Foundeur et al. (179) failed to find any delirium in 100 women with postpartum mental illness treated betwen 1944 and 1952. Other investigators point out that the frequency of postpartum delirium had dropped sharply by the 1950s as a result of improved obstetric technique, introduction of antibiotics, and changed diagnostic criteria (180–182). With the development of modern obstetric practice and the consequent prevention of puerperal sepsis, delirium has become rare.

A study by Melges (183) is worth mentioning in the present context. He found no cases of delirium among 100 women suffering from postpartum mental illness and concluded that it was erroneous to claim that this syndrome is a common form of puerperal psychosis. None of his 15 patients who had had an EEG showed any abnormal changes suggestive of delirium. Moreover, even though 18% of his patients displayed confusion and disorientation, their performance on the serial 7s and the digit-span tests was no different from that of patients who had been hospitalized more than 2 weeks after childbirth. This study provides some support for the contention that the "confusion" displayed by many women with puerperal psychosis is not really delirium but could be regarded as pseudodelirium. This issue could be finally resolved if the women exhibiting delirium-like symptoms underwent EEG, a study that Melges did not carry out.

Postpartum psychoses that do not meet the criteria for an organic mental disorder or any other specific psychotic disorder are classified in *DSM-III-R* as "atypical psychoses" (184). This classification does not, of course, settle the issue of whether the puerperal psychoses featuring "confusion" should or should not be viewed as organic mental syndromes. The majority of puerperal psychoses are currently diagnosed as being either depressive, manic, or schizoaffective; schizophrenic disorders are less often diagnosed (168,171,172,174,175). A recent large epidemiolgical study found that 73% of psychiatric admissions in the puerperium were for affective disorders (185). There is no doubt that delirium due to infection in the postpartum period has almost disappeared. Terms such as "puerperal psychosis" and "postpartum delirium," as used in the literature, are no longer acceptable, as they are vague and misleading. There is no evidence so far that an organic factor unique to the postpartum period gives rise to the delirium-like psychoses. Ergotism has recently been suggested (186). Meanwhile, one is struck by the similarity between such psychoses and those due to the administration of corticosteroids (Chapter 11) or arising in the course of SLE (Chapter 16). The same mixture of affective, schizophrenia-like, and delirium-like features often characterizes all of these conditions. It is unknown whether this phenomenological similarity signifies common pathophysiological mechanisms, but the possibility has not been ruled out.

In summary, the incidence of delirium in the puerperium is low. However, a substantial proportion of women suffering from a psychotic illness after childbirth display features, usually referred to as "confusion," that strongly resemble delirium. There is a need for a prospective study of such postpartum psychoses, employing serial EEG recordings, laboratory tests, and a battery of neuropsychological tests, in order to establish whether these psychoses do or do not represent delirium as this syndrome is currently defined.

References

1. *The Works of That Famous Chirurgion Ambrose Parey.* Trans T. Johnson. London, Cotes and Young, 1634.
2. Dupuytren, Baron: On nervous delirium (traumatic delirium).—Successful employment of laudanum lavements. *Lancet* 1834;2:919–923.
3. Graves R. J.: *A System of Clinical Medicine.* 3rd American ed. Philadelphia, Barrington and Haswell, 1848, p 389.
4. Croft J.: Delirium tremens in surgical cases. *St. Thomas Hosp. Rep.* 1870;1:451–463.
5. Savage G. H.: Insanity following the use of anesthetics. *Br. Med. J.* 1887;2:1199–1200.
6. Haward W.: Delirium tremens and other forms of surgical delirium. *Intern. Clin.* 1893;4:119–127.
7. Da Costa J. C.: The diagnosis of postoperative insanity. *Surg. Gynecol. Obstet.* 1910;11:577–584.

8. Kelly H. A.: Postoperative psychoses. *Am. J. Obstet.* 1909;59:1035–1039.
9. Abeles M. M.: Post-operative psychoses. *Am. J. Psychiatry* 1938;94:1187–1203.
10. Doyle J. B.: Postoperative psychosis. *Mayo Clin. Proc.* 1928;3:198–199.
11. Bastron R. D., Moyers J.: Emergency delirium. *J.A.M.A.* 1967;200:179.
12. Eckenhoff J. E., Kneale D. H., Dripps R. D.: The incidence of etiology of post-anesthetic excitement. *Anesthesiology* 1961;22:667–673.
13. Coppolino G. A.: Incidence of post-anesthetic delirium in a community hospital: A statistical study. *Milit. Med.* 1963;128:238–241.
14. Kuhn J. A., Savage G. H.: Belladonna alkaloid psychosis. *Del. Med. J.* 1974;46:239–242.
15. Greene L. T.: Physostigmine treatment of anticholinergic-drug depression in postoperative patients. *Anesth. Analg.* 1971;50:222–226.
16. Titchener J. L., Zwerling I., Gottschalk L., et al: Psychosis in surgical patients. *Surg. Gynecol. Obstet.* 1956;102:59–65.
17. Knox S. J.: Severe psychiatric disturbances in the postoperative period: A five-year survey of Belfast hospitals. *J. Ment. Sci.* 1961;107:1078–1083.
18. Hammes E. M.: Postoperative psychoses. *Lancet* 1957;77:55–60.
19. Seibert C. P.: Recognition, management, and prevention of neuro-psychological dysfunction after operation, in Hindman B. J. (ed): *Neurological and Psychological Complications of Surgery and Anesthesia.* Boston, Little, Brown, 1986, pp 39–58.
20. Seymour G.: *Medical Assessment of the Elderly Surgical Patient.* London, Croom Helm, 1986.
21. Golinger R. C.: Delirium in surgical patients seen at psychiatric consultation. *Surg. Gynecol. Obstet.* 1986;163:104–106.
22. Hale M., Koss N., Kerstein M., et al: Psychiatric complications in a surgical ICU. *Crit. Care Med.* 1977;5:199–203.
23. Katz N. M., Agle D. P., De Palma R. G., et al: Delirium in surgical patients under intensive care. *Arch. Surg.* 1972;104:310–313.
24. Wilson L. M.: Intensive care delirium. *Arch. Intern. Med.* 1972;130:225–226.
25. Scott J.: Postoperative psychosis in the aged. *Am. J. Surg.* 1960;100:38–42.
26. Kaufer C.: Etiology of consciousness disturbances in surgery. *Minn. Med.* 1968;51:1509–1515.
27. Morse R. M.: Postoperative delirium: A syndrome of multiple causation. *Psychosomatics* 1970;11:164–168.
28. Morse R. M., Litin E. M.: Postoperative delirium: A study of etiologic factors. *Am. J. Psychiatry* 1969;126:388–395.
29. Morse R. M., Litin E. M.: The anatomy of a delirium. *Am. J. Psychiatry* 1971;128:111–116.
30. Salem M. R.: Hypercapnia, hypocapnia, and hypoxemia. *Semin. Anesth.* 1987;6:202–215.
31. Tune L. E., Holland A., Folstein M. F., et al: Association of post-operative delirium with raised serum levels of anticholinergic drugs. *Lancet* 1981;2:651–654.
32. Knill R. L., Moote C. A., Skinner M. I., et al: Morphine-induced ventilatory depression is potentiated by non-REM sleep. *Can. J. Anaesth.* 1987;34:S101.
33. Moote C. A., Knill R. L., Skinner M. I., et al: Morphine produces a profound disruption of nocturnal sleep in humans. *Can. J. Anaesth.* 1987;34:S100.
34. Knill R. L., Rose E. A., Skinner M. I., et al: Episodic hypoxaemia during REM sleep after anaesthesia and gastroplasty. *Acta Anaesth. Scand.* 1987;31(Suppl 86):102.

35. Knill R. L., Moote C. A., Rose E. A., et al: Marked hypoxemia after gastroplasty due to disorders of breathing in REM sleep. *Anesthesiology* 1987;67:A552.
36. Aurell J., Elmqvist D.: Sleep in surgical intensive care unit: Continuous polygraphic recording of sleep in nine patients receiving postoperative care. *Br. Med. J.* 1985;290:1029–1032.
37. Helton M. C., Gordon S. H., Nunery S. L.: The correlation between sleep deprivation and the intensive care unit syndrome. *Heart Lung* 1980;9:464–468.
38. Kavey N. B., Altshuler K. Z.: Sleep in herniorrhaphy patients. *Am. J. Surg.* 1979;138:682–687.
39. Lehmkuhl P., Prass D., Pichlmayr I.: General anesthesia and post-narcotic sleep disorders. *Neuropsychobiology* 1987;18:37–42.
40. Kay D. C., Eisenstein R. B., Jasinski D. R.: Morphine effects on human REM state, waking state and NREM sleep. *Psychopharmacologia (Berl).* 1969;14:404–416.
41. Simpson C. J., Kellett J. M.: The relationship between pre-operative anxiety and post-operative delirium. *J. Psychosom. Res.* 1987;31:491–491.
42. White P. F.: Ketamine update: Its clinical uses in anesthesia. *Semin. Anesth.* 1988;7:113–126.
43. Steen P. A., Michenfelder J. D.: Neurotoxicity of anesthetics. *Anesthesiology* 1979;50:437–453.
44. McIntosh T. K., Bush H. L., Yeston N. S., et al: Beta-endorphin, cortisol and postoperative delirium: A preliminary report. *Psychoneuroendocrinology* 1985;10:303–313.
45. LaRue A., Schaeffer J.,: Psychologic reactions of elderly patients to illness and surgery. *Semin. Anesth.* 1986;5:36–43.
46. Bedford P. D.: Adverse cerebral effects of anaesthesia on old people. *Lancet* 1955;2:259–263.
47. Bedford P. D.: Cerebral damage from shock due to disease in old people. *Lancet* 1957;2:505–509.
48. Millar H. R.: Surgery and anaesthesia, in Kay D. W. K., Burrows G.: *Handbook of Studies on Psychiatry and Old Age.* New York, Elsevier, 1984, pp 217–234.
49. Millar H. R.: Psychiatric morbidity in elderly surgical patients. *Br. J. Psychiatry* 1981;138:17–20.
50. Seymour D. G., Pringle R.: Post-operative complications in the elderly surgical patient. *Gerontology* 1983;29:262–270.
51. Chung F., Meier R., Lautenschlager E., et al: General or spinal anesthesia: Which is better in the elderly? *Anesthesiology* 1987;67:422–427.
52. Ries D. I., Gaines G. Y.: Anesthetic considerations for patients with Alzheimer's disease. *Tex. Med.* 1985;81:45–48.
53. Polly S. M., Sanders W. E.: Surgical infections in the elderly: Prevention, diagnosis, and treatment. *Geriatrics* 1977;32:88–97.
54. Bruce D.: Alcoholism and anesthesia. *Anesth. Analg.* 1983;62:84–96.
55. Glickman L., Herbsman H.: Delirium tremens in surgical patients. *Surgery* 1968;64:882–890.
56. Gower W. E., Kersten H.: Prevention of alcohol withdrawal symptoms in surgical patients. *Surg. Gynecol. Obstet.* 1980;151:382–384.
57. Helmus C., Spahn J. G.: Delirium tremens in head and neck surgery. *Laryngoscope* 1974;84:1479–1488.
58. Mays E. T., Ransdell H. T., de Weese B. M.: Metabolic changes in surgical delirium tremens. *Surgery* 1970;67:780–788.

59. Lineaweaver W. C., Anderson K., Hing D. N.: Massive doses of midazolam infusion for delirium tremens without respiratory depression. *Crit. Care Med.* 1988;16:294–295.
60. Figge H., Huang V., Kaul A. F., et al: The pharmacotherapy of the behavioral manifestations of the ICU syndrome. *J. Crit. Care* 1987;2:199–205.
61. Frank M., Prior P. F.: The cerebral function analysing monitor: Principles and potential use, in Rosen M., Lunn J. N. (eds): *Consciousness, Awareness and Pain in General Anaesthesia.* London, Butterworths, 1987, pp 61–71.
62. Watt R. C., Hameroff S. R.: Phase space eletroencephalography (EEG): A new mode of intraoperative EEG analysis. *Int. J. Clin. Monitoring Comput.* 1988;5:3–13.
63. Prior, P. F., Maynard D. E.: *Monitoring Cerebral Function,* ed 2. Amsterdam, Elsevier, 1986.
64. Smith L. W., Dimsdale J. E.: Postcardiotomy delirium: Conclusions after 25 years: *Am. J. Psychiatry* 1989;146:452–458.
65. Fox H. M., Rizzo N. D., Gifford S., et al: Psychological observations of patients undergoing mitral surgery. *Psychosom. Med.* 1954;16:186–208.
66. Abram H. S.: Psychological reactions to cardiac operations: Historical perspective. *Psychiatr. Med.* 1970; 1:277–294.
67. Knox S. J.: Psychiatric aspects of mitral valvulotomy. *Br. J. Psychiatry* 1963;109:656–668.
68. Blachly P. H., Starr A.: Post-cardiotomy delirium. *Am. J. Psychiatry* 1964;121:371–375.
69. Egerton N., Kay J. H.: Psychological disturbances associated with open-heart surgery.*Br. J. Psychiatry* 1964;110:433–439.
70. Gilberstadt H., Sako Y.: Intellectual and personality changes following open-heart surgery. *Arch. Gen. Psychiatry* 1967;16:210–214.
71. McClish A., Andrew D., Tetreault L.: Intravenous diazepam for psychiatric reactions following open-heart surgery. *Can. Anaesth. Soc. J.* 1968;15:63–79.
72. Heller S. S., Frank K. A., Malm J. R., et al: Psychiatric complications of open-heart surgery. *N. Engl. J. Med.*1979;283:1015–1020.
73. Edmunds H. H., Stephenson L. W., Edie R. N., et al: Open-heart surgery in octogenarians. *N. Engl. J. Med.* 1988;319:131–136.
74. Morin P., Coupal P.: Delirium post-chirurgie cardiaque avec circulation extracorporelle: Aspects cliniques et observations dans un centre spécialisé. *Can. J. Psychiatry* 1982;27:31–39.
75. Kornfeld D. S., Zimberg S., Malm J. R.: Psychiatric complications of open-heart surgery. *N. Engl. J. Med.* 1965;273:287–292.
76. Danilowicz D. A., Gabriel H. P.: Postoperative reactions in children: "Normal" and abnormal responses after cardiac surgery. *Am. J. Psychiatry* 1971;128:185–188.
77. Heller S. S., Kornfeld D. S., Frank K. A., et al: Postcardiotomy delirium and cardiac output. *Am. J. Psychiatry* 1979;136:337–339.
78. Johns M. W., Large A. A., Masterton J. P., et al: Sleep and delirium after open-heart surgery. *Br. J. Surg.* 1974;61:377–381.
79. Sadler P. D.: Incidence, degree, and duration of postcardiotomy delirium. *Heart Lung* 1981;10:1084–1092.
80. Slogoff S., Girgis K. Z., Keats A. S.: Etiologic factors in neurospychiatric complications associated with cardiopulmonary bypass. *Anesth. Analg.* 1982;61:903–911.

81. Orr W. C., Stahl M. L.: Sleep disturbances after open-heart surgery. *Am. J. Cardiol.* 1977;39:196–201.
82. Harrell R. G., Othmer E.: Postcardiotomy confusion and sleep loss. *J. Clin. Psychiatry* 1987;48:445–446.
83. Barash P. G.: Cardiopulmonary bypass and postoperative neurologic dysfunction. *Am. Heart J.* 1980;99:675–677.
84. Blauth C. I., Arnold J. V., Schulenberg W. E., et al: Cerebral embolism during cardiopulmonary bypass. *J. Thorac. Cardiovasc Surg.* 1988;95:668–676.
85. Henriksen L.: Evidence suggestive of diffuse brain damage following cardiac operations. *Lancet* 1984;1:816–820.
86. Nevin M., Adams S., Colchester A. C. F., et al: Evidence for involvement of hypocapnia and hypoperfusion in aetiology of neurological deficit after cardiopulmonary bypass. *Lancet* 1987;2:1493–1495.
87. Nussmeier N. A., Arlund C., Slogoff S.: Neuropsychiatric complications after cardiopulmonary bypass: Cerebral protection by a barbiturate. *Anesthesiology* 1986;64:165–170.
88. Taylor K. M.: Brain damage during open-heart surgery. *Thorax* 1982;37:873–876.
89. Barash P. G., Katz J. D., Kopriva C. J., et al: Assessment of cerebral function during cardiopulmonary bypass. *Heart Lung* 1979;8:280–287.
90. Henriksen L., Hjelms E., Lindenburgh T.: Brain hyperperfusion during cardiac operations. *J. Thorac. Cardiovasc. Surg.* 1983;86:202–208.
91. Malone M., Prior P., Scholtz C. L.: Brain damage after cardiopulmonary by-pass: Correlations between neurophysiological and neuropathological findings. *J. Neurol. Neurosurg. Psychiatry* 1981;44:924–931.
92. Salerno T. A., Lince D. P., White D. N., et al: Monitoring of electroencephalogram during open-heart surgery. *J. Thorac. Cardiovas. Surg.* 1978;76:97–100.
93. Lee W. H., Brady M. P., Rowe J. M., Miller W. C.: Effects of extracorporeal circulation upon behavior, personality and brain function. 11. Hemodynamic, metabolic and psychometric correlations. *Ann. Surg.* 1971;173:1013–1023.
94. Brennan R. W., Patterson R. H., Kessler J.: Cerebral blood flow and metabolism during cardiopulmonary bypass: Evidence of microembolic encephalopathy. *Neurology* 1971;21:655–672.
95. Speidel H., Dahme B., Flemming B., et al: Psychische Störungen nach offenen Herzoperationen. *Nervenarzt* 1979;50:85–91.
96. Heller S. S., Frank K. A., Kornfeld D. S., et al: Psychological outcome following open-heart surgery. *Arch. Intern. Med.* 1974;134:908–914.
97. Kaplan S., Achtel R. A., Callison C. B.: Psychiatric complications following open-heart surgery. *Heart Lung* 1974;3:423–428.
98. Tufo H. M., Ostfeld A. M., Shekelle R.: Central nervous system dysfunction following open-heart surgery. *J.A.M.A.* 1970;212:1333–1340.
99. Branthwaite M. A.: Neurological damage related to open-heart surgery. *Thorax* 1972;27:748–753.
100. Savageau J. A., Stanton B. A., Jenkins C. D.:Neuropsychological dysfunction following elective cardiac operation. II. A six-month reassessment. *J. Thorac. Cardiovasc. Surg.* 1982;84:595–600.
101. Sotaniemi K. A.: Five-year neurological and EEG outcome after open-heart surgery. *J. Neurol. Neurosurg. Psychiatry* 1985;48:569–575.
102. Sotaniemi K. A., Mononen H., Hokkanen T. E.: Long-term cerebral outcome after open-heart surgery. A five-year neuropsychological follow-up study. *Stroke* 1986;17:410–416.

103. Willner A. E., Rabiner C. J.: Psychopathology and cognitive dysfunction five years after open-heart surgery. *Compr. Psychiatry* 1979;20:409–418.
104. Sveinsson I. S.: Postoperative psychosis after heart surgery. *J. Thorac. Cardiovasc. Surg.* 1975;70:717–726.
105. Naber D., Bullinger M.: Neuroendocrine and psychological variables relating to post-operative psychosis after open-heart surgery. *Psychoneuroendocrinology* 1985;10:315–324.
106. Kornfeld, D. S., Heller S. S., Frank K. A., et al: Personality and psychological factors in postcardiotomy delirium. *Arch. Gen. Psychiatry* 1974;31:249–253.
107. Peuhkurinen K. J., Korhonen U.: Diagnosis and management of early postoperative complications in open heart-surgery. *Ann. Clin. Res.* 1987;19:365–373.
108. Budd S., Brown W.: Effect of reorientation technique on postcardiotomy delirium. *Nurs. Res.* 1974;23:341–348.
109. Sos J., Cassem N. H.: Managing postoperative agitation. *Drug Ther.* 1980;10:103–106.
110. Breuer A. C., Furlan A. J., Hanson M. R., et al: Central nervous system complications of coronary artery bypass graft surgery: Prospective analysis of 421 patients. *Stroke* 1983;14:681–687.
111. Calabrese J. R., Skwerer R. G., Gulledge A. D., et al: Incidence of postoperative delirium following myocardial revascularization. A prospective study. *Cleve. Clin. J. Med.* 1987;54:29–32.
112. Carella F., Travaini G., Gontri P., et al: Cerebral complications of coronary bypass surgery. A prospective study. *Acta Neurol. Scand.* 1988;77:158–163.
113. Kornfeld D. S., Heller S. S., Frank K. A., et al: Delirium after coronary artery bypass surgery. *J. Thorac. Cardiovasc. Surg.* 1978;76:93–96.
114. Kornfeld D. S., Heller S. S., Frank K. A., et al: Psychological and behavioral responses after coronary artery bypass surgery. *Circulation* 1982;66(Suppl 111):24–28.
115. Loop F. D., Lytle B. W., Cosgrove D. M., et al: Coronary artery bypass graft surgery in the elderly. *Cleve. Clin. Med. J.* 1988; 55:23–34.
116. Folks D. G., Franceschini J., Sokol R. S., et al: Coronary artery bypass surgery in older patients: Psychiatric morbidity. *South. Med. J.* 1986; 79:303–306.
117. Bass C.: Psychosocial outcome after coronary artery bypass surgery. *Br. J. Psychiatry* 1984;145:526–532.
118. Brennan A. F., Davis M. H., Buchholz D. J., et al: Predictors of quality of life following cardiac transplantation.*Psychosomatics* 1987;28:566–571.
119. Freeman A. M., Folks D. G., Sokol R. A., et al: Cardiac transplantation: Clinical correlates of psychiatric outcome. *Psychosomatics* 1988;29:47–54.
120. Hotson J. R., Pedley T. A.: The neurological complications of cardiac transplantation. *Brain* 1976;99:673–694.
121. Kraft I.: Psychiatric complications of cardiac transplantation. *Semin. Psychiatry* 1971;3:58–69.
122. Kuhn W. F., Myers B., Brennan A. F., et al: Psychopathology in heart transplant candidates. *J. Heart Transplant* 1988;7:223–226.
123. Lunde D. T.: Psychiatric complications of heart transplants. *Am. J. Psychiatry* 1969;126:369–372.
124. Mai F. M., McKenzie F., Kostuk W. J.: Psychiatric aspects of heart transplantation: Preoperative evaluation and postoperative sequelae. *Br. Med. J.* 1986;292:311–313.

125. House R. M., Thompson T. L.: Psychiatric aspects of organ transplantation. *J.A.M.A.* 1988;260:535–539.
126. Berenson C. K., Grosser B. I.: Total artificial heart implantation. *Arch. Gen. Psychiatry* 1984;41:910–916.
127. Craven J. L.: Post-operative organic mental syndromes in lung transplant recipients. *Am. J. Psychiatry,* in press.
128. Wragg R. E., Dimsdale J. E., Moser K. M., et al: Operative predictors of delirium following pulmonary thromboendarterectomy: A model for postcardiotomy delirium? *J. Thorac. Cardiovasc. Surg.* 1988;96:524–529.
129. Sichel: Sur une espéce particuliére de délire senile, qui survient quelquefois aprés l'extraction de la cataracte. *Union Med.* 1863;17:149–150.
130. Schmidt-Rimpler H.: Delirien nach Verschluss der Augen und in Dunkel-Zimmern. *Arch. Psychiatr.* 1879;9:233–243.
131. Chisolm J. J.: The revolution in the after-treatment of cataract operations. *Am. J. Ophthalmol.* 1887;4:153–156.
132. Posey W. C.: Mental disturbances after operations upon the eye. *Ophthalmol. Rev.* 1900;19:235–237.
133. Kipp C. J.: The mental derangement which is occasionally developed in patients in eye hospitals. *Arch. Ophthalmol.* 1903;32:375–387.
134. Bruns H. D.: On the ambulant after-treatment of cataract extraction, with a note on postoperative delirium and on striped keratitis. *Ann. Ophthalmol.* 1916;25:718–723.
135. Fisher W. A.: Delirium following cataract and other eye operations. *Am J. Ophthalmol.* 1920;3:741–747.
136. Greenwood A.: Mental disturbances following operations for cataract. *J.A.M.A.* 1928;91:1713–1716.
137. Abrahamson I. A., Abrahamson I. A.: Dehydration—a cause of psychosis following cataract extraction. *Eye Ear Nose Throat Monthly* 1968;47:144–146.
138. Bartlett J. E. A.: A case of organized visual hallucinations in an old man with cataract, and their relations to the phenomena of the phantom limb. *Brain* 1951;74:363–373.
139. Jackson C. W.: Clinical sensory deprivation: A review of hospitalized eye-surgery patients, in Zubek J. P. (ed): *Sensory Deprivation: Fifteen Years of Research.* New York, Appleton-Century-Crofts, 1969, pp 332–373.
140. Linn L.: Psychiatric reactions complicating cataract surgery. *Int. Ophthalmol. Clin.* 1965;5:143–154.
141. Linn L., Kahn R. L., Coles R., et al: Patterns of behavior disturbance following cataract extraction. *Am. J. Psychiatry* 1953; 100:281–289.
142. Stonecypher D. D.: The cause and prevention of postoperative psychoses in the elderly. *Am. J. Ophthalmol.* 1963;55:605–610.
143. Weisman A. D., Hackett T. P.: Psychosis after eye surgery. *N. Engl. J. Med.* 1958;258:1284–1289.
144. Ziskind E.: An explanation of mental symptoms found in acute sensory deprivation: Researchers 1958–1963. *Am. J. Psychiatry* 1965;121:939–946.
145. Parker W. R.: Postcataract extraction delirium. *J.A.M.A.* 1913;61:1174–1177.
146. Fasanella R. M. (ed): *Complications in Eye Surgery,* ed 2. Philadelphia, WB Saunders, 1965.
147. Stonecypher D. D.: The cause and prevention of postoperative psychoses in the elderly. *Am. J. Ophthalmol.* 1963;55:605–610.

148. Burrows J., Briggs R. S., Elkington A. R.: Cataract extraction and confusion in elderly patients. *J. Clin. Exp. Gerontol.* 1985;7:51–70.
149. Karhunen U., Orko R.: Psychiatric reactions complicating cataract surgery: A prospective study. *Ophthalmic Surg.* 1982;13:1008–1012.
150. Karhunen U., Raitta C.: Psychiatric reactions complicating intracapsular cataract surgery. A 5 year follow-up. *Acta Ophthalmol.* 1985;63:45–49.
151. Lavelle P. A., Chung F., McDonald S.: Cataract operation—inpatient or outpatient? *Anesth. Analg.* 1987;66(Suppl 1):101.
152. Lavelle P. A., Chung F., McDonald, N. J., et al: Mental function after neuroleptic anaesthesia for cataract surgery. *Can. J. Anaesth.* 1987;34(Suppl):103.
153. Summers W. K., Reich T. C.: Delirium after cataract surgery: Review and two cases. *Am. J. Psychiatry* 1979;136:386–391.
154. Andreasen N. J. C., Noyes R., Hartford C. E., et al: Management of emotional reactions in seriously burned adults. *N. Engl. J. Med.* 1972;286:65–69.
155. Antoon A. Y., Volpe J. J., Crawford J. D.: Burn encephalopathy in children. *Pediatrics* 1972;50:609–616.
156. May S. R., Ehleben C. M., De Clemente F. A.: Delirium in burn patients isolated in a plenum laminar air flow ventilation unit. *Burns* 1984;10:331–338.
157. Mohnot D., Snead O. C., Benton J. W.: Burn encephalopathy in children. *Ann. Neurol.* 1982;12:42–47.
158. Steiner H., Clark, W. R.: Psychiatric complications of burned adults: A classification. *J. Trauma* 1977;17:134–143.
159. Mettler F. A.: Burn encephalopathy as a "diagnosis." *J. Med. Soc. N.J.* 1974;71:817–823.
160. Petersen I., Sörbye R., Johanson B.: Electroencephalographic and psychiatric study of burn cases. *Acta Chir. Scand.* 1965;129:359–366.
161. Hughes J. R., Cayaffa J. J.: Seizures following burns of the skin. *Dis. Nerv. Syst.* 1973;34:203–211.
162. Blank K., Perry S.: Relationship of psychological processes during delirium to outcome. *Am. J. Psychiatry* 1984;141:843–847.
163. Miller W. C., Gardner N., Mlott S. R.: Psychosocial support in the treatment of severely burned patients. *J. Trauma* 1976;15:722–725.
164. Andreasen N. J. C., Hartford C. E., Knott J. R., et al: EEG changes associated with burn delirium. *Dis. Nerv. Syst.* 1977;38:27–31.
165. Hughes J. R., Cayaffa J. J., Boswick J. A.: Seizures following burns of the skin. III. Electroencephalographic recordings. *Dis. Nerv. Syst.* 1975;36:443–447.
166. Billowitz A., Friedson W., Schubert D. S. P.: Liaison psychiatry on a burn unit. *Gen. Hosp. Psychiatry* 1980;2:300–305.
167. Huang V., Figge H., Demling R.: Haloperidol complications in burn patients. *J. Burn Care* 1987;8:269–273.
168. Davidson J., Robertson E.: A follow-up study of postpartum illness, 1946–1978. *Acta Psychiatr. Scand.* 1985;71:451–457.
169. Protheroe C.: Psychiatric illness associated with childbirth. *The Practitioner* 1981;225:1245–1251.
170. Hamilton J. A.: Puerperal psychoses. *Gynecol. Obstet.* 1977;2:1–8.
171. Dean C., Kendell R. E.: The symptomatology of puerperal illnesses. *Br. J. Psychiatry* 1981;139:128–133.
172. McNeil T. F.: A prospective study of postpartum psychoses in a high-risk group. 1. Clinical characteristics of the current postpartum episodes. *Acta Psychiatr. Scand.* 1986;74:205–216.

173. Munoz R. A.: Postpartum psychosis as a discrete entity. *J. Clin. Psychiatry* 1985;46:182–184.
174. O'Hara M. W.: Post-partum 'blues', depression, and psychosis: A review. *J. Psychosom. Obstet. Gynecol.* 1987;7:205–227.
175. Schöph J., Bryois C., Jonquiére M., et al: On the nosology of severe psychiatric post-partum disorders. *Eur. Arch. Psychiatr. Neurol. Sci.* 1984;234:54–73.
176. Silbermann R. M., Beenen F., de Jong H.: Clincial treatment of postpartum delirium with perphenazine and lithium carbonate. *Psychiatr. Clin.* 1975;8:314–326.
177. Marcé L. V.: *Traité de la Folie des Femmes Enceintes.* Paris, JB Bailliere, 1858.
178. Arentsen K.: Postpartum psychoses. *Dan. Med. Bull.* 1968;15:97–100.
179. Foundeur M., Fixsen C., Triebel W. A., et al: Postpartum mental illness. *Arch. Neurol. Psychiatry* 1957;77:503–512.
180. Stevens B. C.: Psychoses associated with childbirth: A demographic survey since the development of community care. *Soc. Sci. Med.* 1971;5:527–543.
181. Thomas C. L., Gordon J. E.: Psychosis after childbirth: Ecological aspects of a single impact stress. *Am. J. Med. Sci.* 1959;238:363–388.
182. Wilson J. E., Barglow P., Shipman W.: The prognosis of postpartum mental illness. *Compr. Psychiatry* 1972;13:305–316.
183. Melges F. T.: Postpartum psychiatric syndromes. *Psychosom. Med.* 1968;30:95–108.
184. *Diagnositc and Statistical Manual of Mental Disorders,* ed 3 revised. Washington, DC, American Psychiatric Association, 1987.
185. Kendell R. E., Chalmers J. C., Platz C.: Epidemiology of puerperal psychoses. *Br. J. Psychiatry* 1987;150:662–673.
186. Iffy L., Lindenthal J. J., McArdle J. J., et al: Ergotism: A possible etiology for puerperal psychoses. *Obstet. Gynecol.* 1989;73:475–477.

Author Index

Subject Index

The italic letter *t* after a page number indicates a table reference.